Pharmaceutical Practice

9/11/92

Pharmaceutical Practice

Edited by

Diana M. Collett BPharm Phd MRPharmS
Principal Lecturer in Pharmacy Practice and Clinical Studies, Leicester Polytechnic, Leicester, UK

Michael E. Aulton BPharm PhD MRPharmS
Reader in Pharmacy and Principal Lecturer in Pharmaceutics, Leicester Polytechnic, Leicester, UK

CHURCHILL LIVINGSTONE
EDINBURGH LONDON MELBOURNE AND NEW YORK 1990

CHURCHILL LIVINGSTONE
Medical Division of Longman Group UK Limited

Distributed in the United States of America by Churchill
Livingstone Inc., 1560 Broadway, New York, N.Y. 10036, and
by associated companies, branches and representatives
throughout the world.

First published 1990

ISBN 0-443-03644-6

British Library Cataloguing in Publication Data
Pharmaceutical practice.
  1. Great Britain. Pharmaceutical products.
  Manufacture
  I. Collett, D. M.   II. Aulton, Michael E.
  615′.191′0941

Library of Congress Cataloging in Publication Data
Pharmaceutical practice/edited by Diana M. Collett, Michael
  E. Aulton.
       p.   cm.
    Replaces: Cooper and Gunn's Dispensing for
  pharmaceutical students. 12th ed. 1975.
    Companion v. to Pharmaceutics/edited by Michael
  E. Aulton. 1988
    Includes index.
    ISBN 0-443-03644-6
    I. Collett, Diana M.   II. Aulton, Michael E.
  III. Cooper, John W. (John William), 1896–
  Dispensing for pharmaceutical students.
  12th ed.   IV. Pharmaceutics.
    [DNLM: 1. Dosage Forms.   2. Drug Compounding.
   3. Pharmacy.   QV
  778 95355]
  RS91.P44   1990
  615′.4 — dc20
  DNLM/DLC
  for Library of Congress   89-17268
                                                  CIP

Produced by Longman Singapore Publishers (Pte) Ltd.
Printed in Singapore

Preface

This first edition of *Pharmaceutical practice* replaces the 12th edition of *Cooper and Gunn's Dispensing for pharmaceutical students* published in 1975 by Pitman Medical. There has been a change in the editorship, a change in the title and a completely redesigned and updated content. The text has been written by a number of authors, each of whom has experience and expertise in a particular field of pharmacy education and practice.

The changes in the subject matter of the book reflect the changes that have taken place in the role of the practising pharmacist and that have been described in the report of the Nuffield Inquiry into pharmacy. (*'Pharmacy' The Report of a Committee of Inquiry appointed by the Nuffield Foundation 1986.*) Whilst becoming increasingly patient orientated the pharmacist continues to maintain the traditional product-orientated expertise in the formulation, compounding, packaging, storing and dispensing of medicines.

The overall philosophy of the book is unchanged; that is to provide a sound base for all aspects of good pharmaceutical practice.

The reader of this book is referred to the companion volume *Pharmaceutics: the science of dosage form design*, (Aulton 1988, Churchill Livingstone) for an account of the scientific principles which underlie the formulation of drug delivery systems, for the principles of pharmaceutical microbiology and for the techniques used in large-scale manufacture of pharmaceutical products. Specific cross-references to Aulton (1988) are given throughout this book.

1989

D.M.C.
M.E.A.

Acknowledgements

The editors wish to take this opportunity to thank the following who have assisted with the preparation of the text:

Mr Sidney Carter, who edited this book under its previous title of *Cooper and Gunn's Dispensing for pharmaceutical students* for passing on to us the opportunity to edit this new edition.

The many pharmacists from all spheres of practice who have helped during the planning and writing of this edition to ensure that it corresponds as closely as possible with current pharmaceutical practice.

The contributing authors for the time and effort that they have given to the task of preparing text, often under pressure from numerous other commitments and from us. The many unnamed typists and artists who assisted the authors.

Our families for patience and help in many ways which enabled us to spend time on this book.

The Royal Pharmaceutical Society of Great Britain and the National Pharmaceutical Association for prompt responses to requests for information and advice.

Those publishing companies who have given their permission to reproduce material here. Specific acknowledgements are made throughout the text but a general acknowledgement is made here to the Controller of Her Majesty's Stationery Office for permission to reproduce material from the British Pharmacopoeia, and to the Pharmaceutical Press for permission to reproduce material from the British Pharmaceutical Codex (1973), Pharmaceutical Codex and the British National Formulary.

D.M.C.
M.E.A.

Contributors

Malcolm G. Aiken BPharm MRPharmS
Principal Lecturer in Pharmacy Practice, Pharmacy
Department, Brighton Polytechnic, Brighton, UK

Andrew Auld MSc MRPharmS MCPP
Information Pharmacist, Queen Elizabeth Medical
Centre, Birmingham, UK

Alan Broad BSc (Hons) MRPharmS
Principal Pharmacist, Sterile Fluids Manufacturing
Unit, Queen Elizabeth Medical Centre, Birmingham,
UK

Carol E. Bude BPharm (Hons) MRPharmS
Compounding Manager, Baxter Healthcare Ltd,
Thetford, Norfolk, UK

Christine Hirsch BPharm MSc MRPharmS
Clinical Pharmacist, Queen Elizabeth Medical Centre,
Birmingham, UK

Diana M. Collett BPharm PhD MRPharmS
Principal Lecturer in Pharmacy Practice and Clinical
Pharmacy, Department of Pharmacy, Leicester
Polytechnic, Leicester, UK

Clive Edwards BPharm PhD MRPharmS
Senior Lecturer in Clinical Pharmacy, Wolfson Unit
of Clinical Pharmacology, University of Newcastle
upon Tyne, UK

Stuart R. Hesselwood BPharm PhD MRPharmS
Regional Radiopharmacist, Department of Physics
and Nuclear Medicine, Dudley Road Hospital,
Birmingham, UK

Steven A. Hudson BPharm MPharm MRPharmS
Principal Pharmacist Lothian Health Board, Western
General Hospital, Edinburgh; Lecturer in Clinical
Pharmacy, University of Strathclyde, Glaslow, UK

Micheal H. Jepson MRPharmS
Lecturer in Pharmaceutics, Pharmacy Practice
Research Group, Department of Pharmaceutical
Science, Aston University, Birmingham, UK

Robert Lund BSc (Hons) MSc MRPharmS
District Quality Controller, Central Birmingham
Health Authority, Pharmacy Department, Queen
Elizabeth Medical Centre, Birmingham, UK

Alan L. G. Pugh BPharm PhD MIBiol CBiol MRPharmS
Senior Lecturer in Pharmacy Practice, Department of
Pharmacy, Brighton Polytechnic, Brighton, UK

Judith A. Rees MRPharmS
Lecturer in Pharmaceutics, Department of Pharmacy,
University of Manchester, Manchester, UK

R. M. E. Richards BPharm PhD DSc FRPharmS Phc
(Thai) Phc (Zimb)
Head of School of Pharmacy, Robert Gordon's
Institute of Technology, Aberdeen, UK

Linda Titcomb BSc MRPharmS MCPP
Principal Pharmacist, Birmingham and Midland Eye
Hospital, Birmingham, UK

Roger W. Walker BPharm PhD MRPharmS
Principal Lecturer and Director of Pharmacy Practice
Unit, School of Pharmaceutical Sciences, Sunderland
Polytechnic, Sunderland, UK

About this book

Current pharmaceutical practice embraces the techniques of preparation and presentation of medicines, a knowledge of the biological fate of drugs and medicines, the symptomatic treatment of minor ailments and the abilities to relate to and communicate with the patient, the prescriber and other members of the health-care team.

This book provides a practical guide to those aspects of pharmaceutical practice encountered in a hospital department concerned with the provision of pharmaceutical services and in a pharmacy serving a local community.

Part 1 describes the basic principles of compounding, i.e. the manufacture of medicines on a small scale. The reader is introduced to the types of dosage form currently prescribed and to the weights and measures and units used in pharmaceutical preparations.

Numeracy in the pharmaceutical context is a vital skill and a chapter on pharmaceutical calculations provides practical examples of commonly encountered procedures.

The operations fundamental to compounding — weighing, measurement of liquids, dissolution, filtration, mixing, size reduction and size separation are described in Chapter 4. This is followed by a summary of the codes of good pharmaceutical practice.

The practical aspects of formulation of dosage forms are described together with the principles of appropriate storage and packaging to minimize deterioration of the products.

Dispensing may be defined as the supply of a medicine to an individual patient in accordance with the prescription of a practitioner. Chapters 9 and 10 deal with the response by the pharmacist to different types of prescription and the labels to be attached to the dispensed product.

In Part 2, different types of dispensed product are considered in detail in terms of their formulation, compounding, packaging and labelling, together with appropriate examples. The types of dispensed product are grouped according to the physical nature of the product which has a major influence on the method of preparation.

High standards of cleanliness and hygiene are required for the preparation of all pharmaceutical products. However, some preparations, notably those for parenteral and ophthalmic use must be totally free from microbial and particulate contamination. Part 3 of the book introduces the reader to the basic principles of sterilization and to the preparation of medicines in an aseptic environment.

The methods for testing to ensure the absence of contaminating micro-organisms are also explained.

Pharmaceutical products containing a radionuclide pose additional handling and storage problems. The techniques involved and some commonly used radiopharmaceutical preparations are described in Part 4.

The role of the pharmacist includes the supply of surgical dressings, elastic hosiery, stoma appliances and medical gases. These products are introduced in Part 5.

The preparation and supply of medicinal products comprises part of the overall practice of pharmacy. Of increasing importance is the relationship of the pharmacist with the patient and with the prescriber and other health-care professionals.

The extent to which patients take or use the prescribed medication in accordance with the advice of the prescriber is described as 'patient compliance'. Counselling of the patient by the pharmacist on the appropriate use of medicines helps to improve compliance and is an important activity of the pharmacist both in the hospital and in the community. Communication and counselling skills are discussed in Part 6. In the community, patient medication records form a valuable database for counselling patients on the use of both prescribed and purchased medicines and these are discussed in Chapter 38.

The giving of advice and treatment for the symptomatic relief of minor ailments has long been a part of the traditional role of the pharmacist. Part 6 therefore also includes guidance in responding to symptoms for which advice may be sought from the community pharmacist.

Diagnostic tests, such as pregnancy tests and blood pressure measurements, which may be carried out by pharmacists in the community are also described in Part 6.

More recent additions to the role of the pharmacist, particularly in the hospital, include providing the prescriber with information and advice on pharmaceutical and therapeutic aspects of drugs. Whilst it is beyond the scope of this book to deal with the science of therapeutics, the principles involved in the choice of a drug regimen are discussed and the contribution of the pharmacist to the selection of appropriate therapy emphasized.

The effects produced by drugs in the body, whether pharmacological or toxicological, are generally related to the concentration of the drug at different sites within the body. Pharmacokinetics is concerned with the study of the absorption, distribution, metabolism and excretion of drugs. The mathematical description of drug handling in the body is a powerful tool in the design of dosage schedules to provide for maximum therapeutic benefit with minimum adverse effects.

The measurement of the concentration of drugs in body fluids provides a guide to their safe and effective use and the pharmacist has an important contribution to make in the field of therapeutic drug monitoring. A practical guide to pharmacokinetic principles and therapeutic drug monitoring is provided in Part 7.

A number of patients unfortunately suffer from unwanted effects of drug therapy. Many of these adverse effects are an extension of known pharmacological actions of the drugs and are thus predictable. Other adverse effects are unpredictable. The pharmacist may help to reduce the incidence of adverse reactions if predictions and/or early recognition of unwanted symptoms are made.

Since the early 1970s the provision by the pharmacist of drug information has become an important speciality. The role of the pharmacist as a source of up-to-date and evaluated information on drugs and medicines is also discussed in Part 7.

Many aspects of pharmaceutical practice are the subject of legislative control. The Pharmaceutical legislation in force at the time of publication of this book is summarized in Appendix 1 which also refers the reader to more detailed sources of relevant information. Appendix 2 provides a brief guide to NHS pharmaceutical services.

Undergraduate students and preregistration graduates are often confused by the terminology of clinical medicine, particularly in abbreviated form. Appendix 3 provides a list of commonly encountered abbreviations for medical terms. Prescribers in the UK are strongly advised that titles of drugs and preparations should be written in full and that directions should be stated in English without abbreviation. Nevertheless the use of some Latin abbreviations persists. In Appendix 4 the reader is provided with a list of Latin terms and abbreviations which may be encountered in practice; and commonly encountered abbreviations for the qualifications of practitioners are listed in Appendix 5.

The metric system has been used for dispensing in the UK since 1969. Appendix 6 contains information on imperial weights and measures for the benefit of readers in countries still using the imperial system.

The current public interest in homeopathy is reflected by the inclusion of Appendix 7 on homeopathic preparations.

Finally, a description of the more important sources of information for compounding and dispensing is provided in Appendix 8, particularly for the student new to the practice of pharmacy.

This book is intended as a practical guide for undergraduate students of pharmacy and trainee technicians; and also as a reference text for qualified and preregistration pharmacists and technicians in all branches of the profession of pharmacy.

This book is a companion volume to 'Pharmaceutics: the science of dosage form design', edited by M. E. Aulton and published by Churchill Livingstone (1988). The reader is referred to this book for details of the background science of dosage form design and aspects of the physicochemistry of pharmaceutical materials, bioavailability, design and formulation of drug delivery systems, pharmaceutical microbiology and large-scale manufacture. Whilst the books are intended to 'stand alone', there are frequent cross-references throughout the text, when the term 'Companion Volume' is used.

D.M.C.
M.E.A.

General notices

Throughout this book frequent reference is made to substances and preparations of the *British Pharmacopoeia*. The use of capital letters, e.g. White Soft Paraffin, Magnesium Trisilicate Mixture, etc. indicates that a substance or preparation is of pharmacopoeial standard.

The following standard abbreviations are used:

BP	*British Pharmacopoeia*
BPC	*British Pharmaceutical Codex*
BNF	*British National Formulary*
DPF	*Dental Practitioners Formulary*
EP	*European Pharmacopoeia*
PC	*Pharmaceutical Codex*
USP	*United States Pharmacopeia*

The term 'official' is used in this book to indicate a formula published in the BP, BPC, or other publication 'specified' under the Medicines Act. Pharmacopoeial formulae are quoted in this book simply in order to illustrate pharmaceutical principles and should be considered as such. The reader should always use the appropriate (and current) official publication as a formulary source.

The editions current at the time of writing are BP 1988, BNF 16th edition (1988). The BPC was last published in 1973. Readers should always refer to the most recent addendum of the most recent edition.

The information included in Appendix 1 ('Current UK pharmaceutical legislation') and Appendix 2 ('NHS dispensing') was current at the time of writing (1989). Readers should always consult the most recent source of information available.

D.M.C
M.E.A

Contents

Preface   v
Acknowledgements   vii
Contributors   ix
About this book   x
General notices   xii

PART 1
Basic principles of compounding and dispensing

1. Types of dosage form   3
   D. M. Collett

2. Weights, measures and units   11
   D. M. Collett

3. Calculations for compounding and dispensing   13
   D. M. Collett

4. Fundamental operations in compounding   21
   D. M. Collett

5. Good pharmaceutical practice in compounding and dispensing   29
   D. M. Collett

6. Formulation of dispensed products   35
   J. A. Rees

7. Storage and stability of dispensed products   45
   J. A. Rees

8. Containers and closures for dispensed products   53
   J. A. Rees

9. Responding to the prescription   61
   M. G. Aiken, A. L. G. Pugh

10. Labelling of dispensed medicines   73
    M. G. Aiken, A. L. G. Pugh

PART 2
Pharmaceutical preparations

11. Solutions   87
    D. M. Collett

12. Suspensions   99
    D. M. Collett

13. Emulsions and creams   109
    D. M. Collett

14. Ointments, pastes and gels   125
    D. M. Collett

15. Suppositories and pessaries   135
    D. M. Collett

16. Powders and granules   145
    D. M. Collett

17. Oral unit dosage forms   151
    D. M. Collett

18. Therapeutic aerosols   157
    D. M. Collett

PART 3
Sterile pharmaceutical preparations

19. Principles of sterilization   165
    R. M. E. Richards

20. Heat sterilization   171
    R. M. E. Richards

21. Non-heat methods of sterilization   181
    R. M. E. Richards

22. Aseptic technique   189
    R. M. E. Richards

23. Design and operation of clean rooms   193
    A. Broad

24. Parenteral products   209
    A. Broad

25. Intravenous additives   227
    A. Auld

26. Dispensing of cytotoxic agents   233
    C. Hirsch

27. Total parenteral nutrition 241
C. E. Bude

28. Ophthalmic products 257
L. Titcomb

29. Principles of quality assurance 273
R. Lund

30. Sterility testing 285
R. M. E. Richards

PART 4
Radiopharmacy

31. Techniques in radiopharmacy 301
S. R. Hesselwood

32. Clinical applications of radiopharmaceuticals 309
S. R. Hesselwood

PART 5
Additional pharmaceutical products

33. Wound management products and surgical
dressings 315
D. M. Collett

34. Elastic hosiery 321
D. M. Collett

35. Stoma care and incontinence appliances 325
D. M. Collett

36. Medical gases 333
D. M. Collett

PART 6
Relating to the patient

37. Patient compliance and counselling 339
M. H. Jepson

38. Patient medication records 351
J. A. Rees

39. Responding to symptoms 357
C. Edwards

40. Diagnostic tests 373
D. M. Collett

PART 7
Relating to the prescriber

41. Therapeutics in practice 379
S. A. Hudson, R. W. Walker

42. Practical pharmacokinetics 385
S. A. Hudson, R. W. Walker

43. Therapeutic drug monitoring 403
S. A. Hudson, R. W. Walker

44. Adverse drug reactions 413
S. A. Hudson, R. W. Walker

45. Drug information and pharmaceutical advice 421
S. A. Hudson, R. W. Walker

PART 8
Appendices

A1. Current UK pharmaceutical legislation 435
M. G. Aiken, A. L. G. Pugh

A2. NHS dispensing 443
M. G. Aiken, A. L. G. Pugh

A3. Medical abbreviations 451
D. M. Collett

A4. Latin terms and abbreviations 455
D. M. Collett

A5. Qualifications of practitioners 457
D. M. Collett

A6. The imperial system of weights and measures 459
D. M. Collett

A7. Homeopathic preparations 461
D. M. Collett

A8. Sources of information for compounding and
dispensing 463
D. M. Collett

Index 467

PART 1

Basic principles of compounding and dispensing

INTRODUCTION

This part of the book is an introduction to the disciplines of good pharmaceutical practice. The student, new to pharmacy, will find a brief description of the forms in which medicines can be administered to patients and a detailed account of the manipulative skills necessary to prepare medicines on a bench scale. The basic principles underlying the selection of ingredients, choice of storage conditions, packaging and labelling of medicines are described in this part of the book together with the competencies that are required for good dispensing practice.

1. Types of dosage form

D. M. Collett

Introduction

Dosage forms are the means by which drug molecules are delivered to sites of action within the body. The pharmacological effects of a drug are generally related to the concentration of the drug at its sites of action and include both the undesirable (toxic) effects and the desirable (therapeutic effects). The aim of successful drug therapy is to deliver the appropriate concentration of drug molecules to the appropriate sites in order to achieve maximum therapeutic benefit with minimum toxicity. Some dosage forms are designed to produce only a local effect of the drug on the skin or on mucous membranes, including those of the eye, nose, stomach, rectum, vagina or respiratory tract. Although systemic absorption from such formulations should be minimal, some drug inevitably enters the blood stream with potentially undesirable effects.

Many dosage forms are designed to produce significant absorption of the drug into the blood stream from the gastrointestinal tract, through the skin or from mucous membranes at various sites in the body.

Parenteral dosage forms are designed for administration by injection to various depths beneath the skin surface.

The absorption and distribution of drugs in the body is largely influenced by the release of the drug from the dosage form and the ability of the drug to cross biological membranes.

A discussion of the factors affecting the bioavailability of drugs from different dosage forms can be found in the companion volume (Aulton 1988).

Routes of administration for systemic effects

Oral route

The most commonly used route of administration is the oral route. It is convenient for self administration and effective for most drugs except for those that are rapidly inactivated by gastric or intestinal secretions or by passage via the hepatic portal circulation through the liver.

The oral route is unsuitable for surgical patients immediately pre- and post-operatively, for patients who are unconscious or vomiting and for those with malabsorption states.

Buccal route

The buccal route is useful for self-administered drugs and may be used to overcome some of the problems of the oral route. Blood flow through the buccal mucosa is high and drugs are absorbed into the systemic rather than the hepatic portal circulation, thus avoiding immediate inactivation by the liver. This route may also be used in the unconscious patient.

Rectal route

Drugs administered into the rectum are absorbed mainly into the systemic circulation although some entry into the hepatic portal circulation may occur. Absorption from the rectal mucosa is less predictable than from the small intestine following oral administration. However, the rectal route is useful for the systemic administration of drugs known to cause gastrointestinal irritation or to a patient who is unconscious or vomiting.

Inhalational route

The high blood flow through the lungs and the large surface area of the alveolar membrane provide a route for rapid absorption of drugs into the general circulation. Anaesthetic gases, volatile liquids and drugs that can be dispersed in an aerosol form may be administered by inhalation in order to produce a systemic effect. The nasal mucosa may also be used as route of systemic administration.

Transdermal route

Drugs applied to the skin surface may be absorbed slowly into the systemic circulation. This route is useful

3

for drugs with a short duration of action after oral administration, particularly those rapidly metabolized by the liver, and may provide a sustained concentration of the drug in the circulation.

Parenteral routes

Drugs may be administered directly into the circulation by the intravenous route. Distribution of the drug throughout the circulatory system is rapid and this route bypasses many biological membranes which may delay absorption into the circulation. The dose volume of an intravenous injection may vary from a fraction of a millilitre given as a bolus injection to 500 ml or more given as a slow infusion.

Intra-arterial injections are used mainly for diagnostic purposes and rarely for the administration of drugs except in neonates.

Fairly rapid absorption of drugs in aqueous solution follows administration by the intramuscular route while slower absorption usually follows the administration of small volume injections into the subcutaneous tissues. Other parenteral routes include intra-articular (into a joint), intra-ocular (into the eye), intracardiac (into the heart muscle) and intracisternal (into the cerebrospinal fluid).

Routes of administration for local effects

Oral route

Dosage forms of adsorbents, antimicrobial compounds and antacids may be designed to exert a local effect within the gastrointestinal tract after oral administration.

Topical route

Application of a dosage form to the epithelium covering one of the body surfaces may be used to exert a local effect at the site of application. Examples include preparations applied to the skin, the cornea of the eye, the nasal, rectal, vaginal or urethral mucosa.

Types of dosage form

The different forms in which drugs may be supplied to a patient are described briefly in this section. All dosage forms should be free from gross microbial contamination and standards of cleanliness in preparation must be high. For some dosage forms, sterility, that is a total absence of micro-organisms, is essential. Sterile pharmaceutical preparations are discussed in detail in Part 3 of this book.

Some of the dosage forms described below may be prepared extemporaneously for an individual patient, other dosage forms may be prepared by the pharmacist as stock products. Many of the dosage forms supplied routinely to patients on prescription are manufactured and packaged by the pharmaceutical industry.

Aerosol inhalations (see below 'Pressurized inhalations')

Aerosol sprays (see below 'Pressurized dispensers')

Applications

Applications are fluid or semi-fluid preparations intended for application to the skin. Usually they are suspensions or emulsions.

Cachets

The shells of cachets are moulded from rice paper and are used to enclose quantities of medium-density dry powder up to 2 g in weight. Cachets are now rarely dispensed in the UK but in the past were used to administer unpleasantly tasting powdered drugs in a tasteless form. Because of the large size, cachets should be immersed in water for a few seconds before swallowing with a draught of water.

Capsules

The shells of capsules are made from gelatin and, like cachets, may be used as oral dosage forms to mask the unpleasant taste of their contents. There are two main types of capsule:

Hard gelatin capsules are generally used for solid medicaments. They consist of a cylindrical body and cap which fit together after filling. Most of the capsules prescribed in the UK are manufactured by the pharmaceutical industry but the pharmacist may occasionally be required to fill hard capsules extemporaneously, particularly in a hospital pharmacy.

Soft gelatin capsules are one-piece capsules and are formed, filled and sealed in one manufacturing operation. The contents of soft capsules are usually solutions or dispersions of drugs in non-aqueous liquids.

Capsules should be swallowed whole with a draught of water.

Collodions

These are fluid preparations for application to the skin. Pyroxylin is dissolved in a volatile vehicle (usually ether and ethanol) and forms a protective film on the skin after evaporation of the solvent. Collodions may also be used to provide prolonged contact between the skin and a dissolved medicament like salicylic acid.

Creams

These are semi-solid emulsions for external use. There are two kinds, aqueous and oily creams, in which the emulsions are oil-in-water and water-in-oil respectively. Aqueous creams are relatively non-greasy. Creams may be used to exert emollient or moisturizing effects on the skin or to deliver drugs for percutaneous absorption. Creams intended for application to large open wounds should be sterile.

Draughts

These are now rarely used liquid oral preparations with a dose volume of the order of 50 ml. Each dose was supplied in a separate container.

Dusting powders

These are free-flowing very fine powders for external use but not for use on open wounds unless the powders are sterilized.

Ear drops

Ear drops are solutions, suspensions or emulsions of drugs that are instilled into the ear with a dropper.

Elixirs

Elixirs are pleasantly flavoured clear liquid oral preparations of potent or nauseous drugs. The vehicle may contain a high proportion of ethanol or sucrose together with antimicrobial preservatives which confer stability to the preparation.

Elixirs containing drugs which are unstable in solution, such as some antibiotics, may be prepared by dissolving dry granules in water immediately before issue to the patient.

Emulsions (see below 'Oral emulsions')

Enemas

Enemas are solutions, suspensions or emulsions for rectal administration.

Eye drops

These are sterile solutions or suspensions of one or more medicaments intended for instillation into the con-

junctival sac. They may be packed in single dosage forms or in multiple application containers.

Eye lotions

Eye lotions are sterile aqueous solutions used usually undiluted for bathing the eye. Sterile solutions containing no bactericide may be used for first aid and should be discarded within 24 hours of opening the container.

Eye ointments

These are sterile semi-solid preparations intended for application to the conjunctiva or eyelid margin. They contain one or more medicaments dissolved or dispersed in a suitable non-irritant base.

Gargles

Gargles are aqueous solutions used in the prevention or treatment of throat infections. Usually they are prepared and dispensed in a concentrated solution with directions for the patient to dilute with warm water before use.

Gels

Gels are translucent or transparent non-greasy semi-solid preparations mainly used externally. The gelling agent may be gelatin or a carbohydrate such as starch, tragacanth, sodium alginate or a cellulose derivative. Gels intended for application to large open wounds should be sterile.

The term 'gel' is also applied to colloidal suspensions of aluminium or magnesium hydroxides used as antacids.

Granules

Granules for oral administration are small irregular particles from 0.5 to 2 mm in diameter often supplied in single-dose sachets. Some granules are placed on the tongue and swallowed with a draught of water, others are intended to be dissolved in water before taking. Effervescent granules evolve carbon dioxide when added to water.

Inhalations

These are liquid preparations consisting of, or containing, volatile substances. They are used to relieve congestion and inflammation of the respiratory tract. Some are volatile at room temperature and may be inhaled from a handkerchief or other fabric. Proprietary products may be enclosed in soft gelatin capsules from which the liquid is expressed before inhaling. Other types of inhalation are added to hot, but not boiling, water (about 65°C is suitable) and the vapour inhaled for about 10 minutes. This second type of inhalation includes simple solutions of medicaments, dissolved in either alcohol or an alcoholic preparation, and aqueous dispersions containing light magnesium carbonate to adsorb and distribute the volatile ingredients.

Injectable preparations (see below 'Parenteral preparations')

Implants

These are sterile disks or cylinders introduced surgically into body tissues and designed to release one or more medicaments over an extended period of time.

Insufflations

These are medicated powders designed to be blown into the ear, nose, throat or body cavities by means of a device known as an *insufflator*. Bulk insufflation has largely disappeared and has been replaced by individual doses of powdered drugs supplied in hard capsules and inhaled from a device which breaks the capsule and allows the patient to inhale the powder. This type of insufflation is used mainly for drug delivery into the respiratory tract by inhalation.

Irrigation solutions

These are sterile, pyrogen-free solutions usually intended for irrigation of body cavities, operation cavities, wounds or the urogenital system.

Linctuses

Linctuses are viscous, liquid oral preparations that are usually prescribed for the relief of cough. They usually contain a high proportion of syrup and glycerol which have a demulcent effect on the membranes of the throat. The dose volume is small (5 ml) and, to prolong the demulcent action, they should be taken undiluted.

Liniments

Liniments are fluid, semi-fluid or, occasionally, semi-solid preparations intended for application to the skin. They may be alcoholic or oily solutions or emulsions. Most are massaged into the skin (counter-irritant or stimulating types) but some are applied on a warm dressing or with a brush (analgesic and soothing types). Liniments should not be applied to broken skin.

Lotions

These are fluid preparations for external application without friction. They are either dabbed on the skin or applied on a suitable dressing and covered with a waterproof dressing to reduce evaporation.

Lozenges

Lozenges are solid preparations consisting mainly of sugar and gum, the latter giving strength and cohesiveness to the lozenge and facilitating slow release of the medicament. They are used to medicate the mouth and throat and for the slow administration of indigestion or cough remedies.

Mixtures

Mixtures are liquid oral preparations consisting of one or more medicaments dissolved or suspended in an aqueous vehicle. Official mixtures are not usually formulated for a long shelf-life.

Mouthwashes

These are similar to gargles but are used for oral hygiene and to treat infections of the mouth.

Nasal drops and sprays

Drugs in solution may be instilled into the nose from a dropper or from a plastic squeeze bottle. The drug may have a local effect, e.g. antihistamine, vasoconstrictor, decongestant. Alternatively the drug may be absorbed through the nasal mucosa to exert a systemic effect, e.g. the peptide hormones oxytocin and vasopressin.

The use of oily nasal drops should be avoided because of possible damage to the cilia of the nasal mucosa. Prolonged use of nasal vasoconstrictors may result in rebound vasodilatation and further nasal congestion.

Ointments

Ointments are semi-solid, greasy preparations for application to the skin, rectum or nasal mucosa. The base is usually anhydrous and immiscible with skin secretions. Ointments may be used as emollients or to apply suspended or dissolved medicaments to the skin. Ointments intended for application to large open wounds should be sterile.

Oral emulsions

The term 'oral emulsion' as an oral dosage form may be defined as 'a fine dispersion of droplets of an oily liquid in an aqueous liquid which forms the continuous phase'. Drugs may be dissolved in either of the phases or suspended in the emulsion.

Oral liquids

Oral liquids are homogeneous preparations containing one or more active ingredients dissolved or suspended in a suitable vehicle. Elixirs, linctuses, mixtures, oral drops, oral emulsions, oral solutions and oral suspensions are included in the general category of oral liquids.

Paints

Paints are liquids for application to the skin or mucous membranes. Skin paints often have a volatile solvent that evaporates quickly to leave a dry resinous film of medicament. Throat paints are more viscous due to a high content of glycerol, designed to prolong contact of the medicament with the affected site.

Parenteral preparations (injectable preparations)

These are sterile dosage forms containing one or more medicaments and designed for parenteral administration.

Injections are sterile solutions, suspensions or emulsions in a suitable aqueous or non-aqueous vehicle and are usually classified according to their route of administration.

Powders for injections are sterile solid substances to be dissolved or suspended by adding a prescribed volume of the appropriate sterile fluid. The solution or suspension is usually prepared immediately prior to use to avoid deterioration of the product on storage.

Intravenous infusions are sterile aqueous solutions or emulsions, free from pyrogens and usually made isotonic with blood. They do not contain added antimicrobial preservatives or buffering agents and are designed for intravenous administration in volumes usually greater than 10–15 ml.

Pastes

Pastes are semi-solid preparations for external application that differ from similar ointments and gels in that they contain a high proportion of finely powdered medicaments. The base may be anhydrous (liquid or soft paraffin) or water soluble (glycerol or a mucilage). Their stiffness makes them useful protective coatings. Pastes intended for application to large open wounds should be sterile.

Pastilles

Pastilles are solid medicated preparations designed to dissolve slowly in the mouth. They are softer than lozenges and their basis is either glycerol and gelatin, or acacia and sugar.

Pessaries

Pessaries are solid medicated preparations designed for insertion into the vagina where they melt or dissolve. The medicaments may then exert a local action or in some cases may be absorbed from the vaginal mucosa. There are three types. *Moulded pessaries* are cone shaped and prepared in a similar way to moulded suppositories. *Compressed pessaries*, or *vaginal tablets*, are made in a variety of shapes and are prepared by compression in a similar manner to oral tablets. *Vaginal capsules* are similar to soft gelatin oral capsules differing only in size and shape.

Pills

Pills are oral dosage forms which consist of spherical masses prepared from one or more medicaments incorporated with inert excipients. Pills are now rarely used. The term 'pill' is used colloquially (yet incorrectly) as a synonym for oral contraceptive tablets which are actually prepared by compression.

Poultices

Poultices are paste-like preparations used externally to reduce pain and inflammation because they retain heat well. After heating, the preparation is spread thickly on a dressing and applied as hot as the patient can bear, to the affected area.

Powders (oral)

There are two kinds of powder intended for internal use.

Bulk powders usually contain non-potent medicaments such as antacids since the patient measures a dose by volume using a 5 ml medicine spoon. The powder is then usually dispersed in water or, in the case of effervescent powders, dissolved before taking.

Divided powders are packaged individually — each dose is separately wrapped in paper or sealed into a sachet.

Powders for mixtures

These are powders mixed in the proportions of standard suspension type mixtures, e.g. Magnesium Trisilicate Mixture BP. The mixed powders may be conveniently stored in the dry form and the mixture prepared by the pharmacist when required for dispensing, by suspension of the powders in the appropriate vehicle with the addition of any liquid ingredients.

Pressurized dispensers (aerosol sprays)

Several different types of pharmaceutical product may be packaged in pressurized dispensers, popularly known as 'aerosols'. Surface sprays producing droplets of 100 μm diameter or greater may be used as surface disinfectants, as wound or burn dressings, to relieve the irritation of bites and stings or as counter-irritants in the relief of muscular aches.

Spray-on dusting powders are also available from pressurized containers.

Foam dispensers are used for some spermicidal preparations and rectal foams are packed in metered dose dispensers. Metered dose aerosols are available for the delivery of glyceryl trinitrate in droplet form to the buccal mucosa for rapid absorption.

Pharmacists should be aware that the abuse of aerosol propellants, as with abuse of other solvents, may cause hallucinations, severe toxicity and possible death.

Pressurized inhalations (aerosol inhalations)

Aerosol inhalations are solutions, suspensions or emulsions of drugs in a mixture of inert propellants held under pressure in an aerosol dispenser. Release of a dose of the medicament in the form of droplets of 50μm diameter or less from the container is achieved by means of a spring-loaded valve incorporating a metering device. The patient then inhales the released drug through a mouthpiece. In some types of product the valve is actuated by finger pressure, in other types the valve is actuated by the patient breathing in through the mouthpiece.

Solutions

Solutions are liquid preparations containing one or more dissolved ingredient. They may be used for a variety of purposes as both internal or external dosage forms.

Solution tablets

These are compressed tablets that are dissolved in water to produce solutions for application to the skin or mucous membranes. They are usually uncoated biconvex discs but those containing poisons may be distinctive in shape or colour. They are formulated to dissolve quickly.

Sprays

Sprays are preparations of drugs in aqueous, alcoholic or glycerol-containing media. They are applied to the mucous membranes of the nose or throat with a suitable atomizer or nebulizer.

Suppositories

Suppositories are solid medicated preparations designed for insertion into the rectum where they melt, dissolve or disperse and exert a local or, less often, a systemic effect.

Syrups

These are concentrated aqueous solutions of a sugar, usually sucrose. Flavoured syrups are a convenient form of masking disagreeable tastes, although the prolonged use of sugar-based medicines is inadvisable because they encourage dental decay. Sorbitol syrups are advantageous in this latter respect.

Tablets

Tablets are prepared by compression of medicaments with a variety of excipients into a solid dosage form. Each tablet contains a single dose of the drug(s). Tablets for oral administration are usually swallowed with water but it may be recommended that they be chewed before swallowing or dissolved in water before taking. Oral tablets are designed to release the medicament within the gastrointestinal tract for absorption into the circulation or, more rarely for a local effect. (See also 'Solution tablets' and 'Pessaries'.)

Vitrellae

Vitrellae are thin-walled glass capsules containing a volatile ingredient and are protected by absorbent cotton wool and an outer silk bag. The wrapped capsule is crushed in order to release the vapour for inhalation. This dosage form was used for the administration of volatile nitrites in the treatment of angina pectoris and has been superseded by newer dosage forms.

Intermediate products used in compounding

The products described below may be prepared extemporaneously by the pharmacist as stock products or purchased from pharmaceutical manufacturers and used in the preparation of compounded medicines.

Extracts

These are concentrated preparations containing the active principles of vegetable or animal drugs which have been extracted with suitable solvents and concentrated to form liquid, soft or dry extracts.

Glycerins

These are solutions of medicaments in glycerol with or without the addition of water.

Infusions

Infusions are dilute solutions containing the readily soluble constituents of crude drugs and prepared by diluting 1 part of concentrated infusion to 10 parts with water. Concentrated infusions are prepared by cold extraction of crude drugs with 25% ethanol.

Oxymels

These are preparations in which the vehicle is a mixture of acetic acid and honey.

Spirits

Spirits are alcoholic or aqueous alcoholic solutions of volatile substances used as flavouring agents.

Tinctures

These are alcoholic preparations containing the active principles of vegetable drugs. They are relatively weak compared with extracts.

Waters (aromatic waters)

These are aqueous solutions, usually saturated, of volatile oils or other volatile substances, e.g. chloroform, that are used mainly as flavouring agents. Aromatic waters are prepared by diluting the concentrated water with 39 times its volume of freshly boiled and cooled purified water.

REFERENCE

Aulton M E (ed) 1988 Pharmaceutics: the science of dosage form design. Churchill Livingstone, Edinburgh

2. Weights, measures and units

D. M. Collett

The International System of Units (SI) is generally accepted for use in pharmacy.

Units of mass (weights)

The base unit for mass is the kilogram (kg).

1 kilogram is the mass of the International Prototype Kilogram

The units of mass commonly encountered in pharmacy are:

Name	Abbreviation	Equivalent
1 kilogram	kg	1000 g
1 gram	g	1000 mg
1 milligram	mg	1000 μg (mcg)
1 microgram	μg (mcg)	1000 ng
1 nanogram	ng	1000 pg
1 picogram	pg	1/1000 ng

In order to avoid confusion between the abbreviations for milligram, microgram and nanogram it is recommended that, in pharmacy, the latter terms be written in full where possible.

Quantities should be written as whole numbers, e.g. 50 mg not 0.05 g, 100 micrograms not 0.1 mg. When decimals are unavoidable the decimal point should always be preceded by a zero, e.g. 0.5 g not .5 g.

Units of amount of substance

The base unit for amount of substance is the mole (mol).

1 mole is the amount of substance of a system containing as many formula units (atoms, molecules, ions, electrons, quanta or other entities) as there are in 12 g of the pure nuclide carbon-12.

The units of amount of substance encountered in pharmacy are:

Name	Abbreviation	Equivalent
1 mole	mol	1000 mmol
1 millimole	mmol	1000 μmol
1 micromole	μmol	1/1000 mmol

Units of capacity (volumes)

Although the litre (l) is not part of SI its use as the unit of volume is likely to continue. The use of litre and millilitre are virtually universal in pharmacy practice.

1 litre is defined in the UK as 1 cubic decimetre.

The units of capacity commonly encountered in pharmacy are:

Name	Abbreviation	Equivalent
1 litre	l	1000 ml
1 millilitre	ml	1000 μl
1 microlitre	μl	1/1000 ml

Units of concentration

In the SI system concentration may be expressed in two ways:

Mass concentration: expressed as g per l (g per dm^3).

Amount of substance concentration: expressed as mol per l.

In pharmacy the concentrations of drugs in solution are conventionally expressed as mass concentration (g per l). The concentrations of electrolyte solutions for parenteral use are conventionally expressed as amount of substance concentration (mol per l). The concentrations of substances normally present in the blood, electrolytes, creatinine, glucose, urea, etc. are also expressed in terms of mol per l. An exception is the amount of haemoglobin which is usually expressed as g per dl (g per 100 ml).

Units of length

The metre (m) is the base unit. Other units include:

Name	Abbreviation	Equivalent
1 centimetre	cm	1000 mm
1 millimetre	mm	1000 μm
1 micrometre	μm	1000 nm
1 nanometre	nm	1/1000 μm

Units of radiation

Activity of a radioactive source

The SI unit of activity is the becquerel (Bq) equal to 1 disintegration or nuclear transformation per second.

The curie is the traditional unit of activity.

Name	Abbreviation	Equivalent
1 curie	Ci	3.7×10^{10} Bq
1 millicurie	mCi	3.7×10^7 Bq
1 microcurie	μCi	3.7×10^4 Bq
1 nanocurie	nCi	3.7×10 Bq

Absorbed dose of ionizing radiation

The SI unit is the gray (Gy), equal to 1 joule per kilogram (J kg^{-1}).

The rad (radiation absorbed dose) is the traditional unit.

Name	Abbreviation	Equivalent
1 rad	rad	10^{-2} Gy
1 megarad	Mrad	10^4 Gy
1 gray	Gy	100 rads

Dose equivalent The SI unit is the sievert (Sv), equal to 1 joule per kilogram (J kg^{-1}).

The rem (rad-equivalent-man) is the traditional unit.

Name	Abbreviation	Equivalent
1 rem	rem	10^{-2} sievert
1 millirem	mrem	10^{-5} sievert
1 sievert	Sv	100 rem

Energy of radiation The traditional unit of measurement of the energy of ionizing radiation is the electron volt (eV). 1 eV is the kinetic energy acquired by an electron when it is accelerated through a potential difference of 1 volt. The SI replacement is the attojoule (aJ $= 10^{-18}$J).

Name	Abbreviation	Equivalent
1 electron volt	eV	1.60×10^{-19} joule
		$= 0.16$ aJ
1 joule	J	6.24×10^{18} eV

3. Calculations for compounding and dispensing

D. M. Collett

Most of the calculations required for compounding and dispensing involve relatively simple arithmetic. The welfare of patients depends on the accuracy of pharmaceutical calculations.

Careless calculations cost lives

Errors are less likely to occur if a disciplined approach to calculations is adopted. It is recommended that the following sequence is followed:

1. *Set out the calculation clearly.* This assists accurate calculation and facilitates checking.
2. *Work methodically through the calculation.* A series of small steps is less likely to lead to an error than a 'short cut' and is also easier to re-check.
3. *Simplify the calculation as far as possible.* The avoidance of awkward figures by making a slight excess of a product assists accuracy. Making ten-fold steps in dilutions to eliminate odd factors also helps to avoid arithmetic mistakes.
4. *Write clear figures and avoid alterations.* Cross out an incorrect figure rather than change it by superimposing the correct one. A zero should always precede a decimal point.
5. *Check the completed calculation.* If possible check the result by using a different method of calculation. For calculations involving very potent substances a second check by a colleague is a wise precaution.

TYPES OF CALCULATION

Working from a master formula

In order to prepare a pharmaceutical product it is necessary to make a list of the quantities of the ingredients. The 'master' or source formula may list the ingredients for a total quantity greater than or less than the amount required to be prepared. The formula must therefore be scaled down or scaled up as appropriate.

Examples 3.1–3.5 show a range of types of these calculations.

Example 3.1

Calculate the amounts of the ingredients for 150 ml Opiate Squill Linctus BP 1988

Ingredients	Master formula (from BP)	Scaled quantities
Squill Oxymel	300 ml	50 ml
Camphorated Opium Tincture	300 ml	50 ml
Tolu Syrup	300 ml	50 ml
Check		
Total volume	900 ml	150 ml

The sum of the scaled quantities is the correct fraction of the sum of the master quantities.

Example 3.2

Calculate the amounts of the ingredients for 200 ml Chloral Mixture BP 1988

Ingredients	Master formula (from BNF*)	Scaled quantities
Chloral Hydrate	1 g	20 g
Syrup	2 ml	40 ml
Water	to 10 ml	to 200 ml

Check by comparing the figures —
2 is 1/5 of 10: is 40 1/5 of 200?
1 is half of 2: is 20 half of 40?

* BNF 1988 16th. Edition

Example 3.3

Calculate the amounts of the ingredients for 30 g Paraffin Ointment BP 1988

Ingredients	Master formula (from BP)	Scaled quantities
White Beeswax	20 g	0.6 g
Hard Paraffin	30 g	0.9 g
Cetostearyl Alcohol	50 g	1.5 g
White Soft Paraffin	900 g	27.0 g
Check		
Total weight	1000 g	30.0 g

Example 3.4

Calculate the amounts of the ingredients to prepare 25 g of a paste to the following prescribed formula

Ingredients	Master formula (from prescriber)	Scaled quantities
Coal Tar	6 g	1.5 g
Starch	20 g	5.0 g
Zinc Oxide	20 g	5.0 g
Yellow Soft Paraffin	54 g	13.5 g
Check		
Totals	100 g	25.0 g

Compare the figures —
6 is 1/9 of 54: is 1.5 1/9 of 13.5?
20 is 1/5 of 100: is 5.0 1/5 of 25.0?

Example 3.5

Calculate the amounts of the ingredients for 100 ml Turpentine Liniment BP 1988

Ingredients	Master formula (from BP)	Scaled quantities
Soft Soap	75 g	9 g
Camphor	50 g	6 g
Turpentine Oil	650 ml	78 ml
Purified Water freshly boiled and cooled	225 ml	27 ml
Check		
Sum of units	1000 units	120 units

Note that the quantities in this formula are expressed in mixed units of weights and volumes. Although the figures add up to 1000 units, they will not produce 1000 ml of liniment. A convenient excess in order to produce 100 ml of liniment is 20% (120 units).

Dealing with percentage concentrations

Many pharmaceutical preparations consist of solutions of solids in liquids, solutions of liquids in liquids, admixtures of liquids in solids or mixtures of solids with solids. The proportions of the different components of these systems are often expressed as 'percentages'. The term 'percentage' in pharmaceutical calculations should be qualified to indicate whether the solution is weight in volume (w/v), weight in weight (w/w) or volume in volume (v/v).

Percentage weight in volume (% w/v)

Definition: percentage w/v indicates the number of grams of ingredient in 100 millilitres of product.

Note that unless otherwise specified the strength of a pharmaceutical solution of a solid in a liquid is expressed as % w/v (Example 3.6).

Example 3.6

Prepare 100 ml Sodium Chloride Solution BP 1988

Ingredients	% w/v	for 100 ml
Sodium Chloride	0.9%	900.0 mg
Purified Water freshly boiled and cooled	to 100.0%	to 100.0 ml

To prepare the solution 900 mg sodium chloride is dissolved in part of the solvent and the volume adjusted to 100 ml at room temperature (20°C).

Note that *adding* 900 mg to 100 ml would result in a volume slightly greater than 100 ml and is therefore incorrect.

Percentage weight in weight (% w/w)

Definition: percentage w/w indicates the number of grams of ingredient in 100 grams of product.

Note that unless otherwise specified the strength of a pharmaceutical solution of a gas in a liquid is expressed as % w/w (e.g. Strong Ammonia Solution BP contains 27.0–30.0% w/w ammonia (calculated as NH_3)).

The strength of some solutions of solids in liquid is expressed as a % w/w (Example 3.7).

Example 3.7

Prepare 100 g Syrup BP 1988

Ingredients	% w/w	for 100 g
Sucrose	66.7%	66.7 g
Purified Water freshly boiled	to 100.0%	to 100.0 g

To prepare the solution 66.7 g sucrose is dissolved in part of the heated solvent and the weight adjusted to 100 g with hot solvent.

Note that the temperature at which the adjustment is made is not specified when adjusting to weight. Note also that the volume of the final product will be less than 100 ml because the weight per ml of the product is greater than unity.

The strength of solutions or admixtures of liquid in solid is usually expressed as a % w/w (e.g. Liquefied Phenol BP which is a solution of phenol in water containing 80% w/w phenol. Many semi-solid preparations include liquid ingredients included as % w/w (Example 3.8).

Example 3.8

Calculate the amounts of the ingredients for 25 g Coal Tar Ointment (prescriber's formula)

Ingredients	% w/w	for 25 g
Coal Tar Solution	12%	3 g
Hydrous Wool Fat	12%	3 g
Yellow Soft Paraffin	to 100%	19 g
Check		Total 25 g

Note that for ointments the base is not added 'to' 100% because it is inconvenient to adjust the weight during preparation; it is more convenient to calculate the amount of base required. See Chapter 14 for methods of preparation of semi-solid dosage forms. Note also that in order to 'send' 25 g a small excess (5 g) would be prepared to allow for manipulative losses.

The strength of mixtures of solid in solid is also expressed as % w/w (Example 3.9).

Example 3.9

Calculate the amounts of the ingredients for 1000 g Chlorhexidine Dusting Powder BP 1988

Ingredients	% w/w	for 1000 g
Chlorhexidine Hydrochloride	0.5%	5 g
Sterilizable Maize Starch	to 100.0%	995 g
		(to 1000 g)

Percentage volume in volume (% v/v)

Definition: percentage v/v indicates the number of millilitres of ingredient in 100 millilitres of product.

Note that unless otherwise specified the strength of a pharmaceutical solution of a liquid in a liquid is expressed as % v/v (Examples 3.10, 3.11).

Example 3.10

Calculate the amounts of the ingredients for 300 ml Wintergreen Liniment (patient's recipe)

Ingredients	% v/v	for 300 ml
Methyl Salicylate	25%	75 ml
Eucalyptus Oil	10%	30 ml
Arachis Oil	to 100%	to 300 ml

Example 3.11

Calculate the amounts of the ingredients to prepare 100 ml Formaldehyde Lotion (from BNF 1988 16th edn)

Ingredients	% v/v	for 100 ml
Formaldehyde Solution	3%	3 ml
Water for preparations	to 100%	to 100 ml

Note that Formaldehyde Solution BP is a 34–38% w/w (mean 36% w/w) aqueous solution of formaldehyde gas. (See also Examples 3.18 and 3.19.)

Concentrations expressed as parts

The strengths of some pharmaceutical solutions are expressed as 'parts' of dissolved substance in 'parts' of solution (e.g. 1 in 1000). For solutions of solid in liquid this is understood to mean parts by weight (grams) in parts by volume (millilitres) of the *final* solution. For solutions of liquid in liquid it is understood to mean parts by volume (millilitres) of the dissolved liquid in parts by volume (millilitres) of the final solution. In order to prepare solutions of a particular concentration it is useful to convert 'parts' into 'percentages'.

For example:

1 in 100 = 1.0%
1 in 200 = 0.5%
1 in 500 = 0.2%
1 in 800 = 0.125%
1 in 1000 = 0.1%, etc.

Preparing dilutions

It is often necessary to prepare a dosage form by dilution of a more concentrated product. Potential errors arise in the choice of diluent, in the calculation of the dilution factor and in the expression of the concentration of the diluted product on the label. Guidance on the choice of appropriate diluents for different types of pharmaceutical preparations may be found in Part 2 of this book.

Antiseptic solutions prepared from concentrates

Concentrated solutions of antiseptics and disinfectants are generally more stable than dilute solutions of the same substances and require less storage space. It is often necessary to prepare an antiseptic solution for dispensing from a commercially available concentrate (Examples 3.12, 3.13).

Example 3.12

Calculate the amount of Benzalkonium Chloride Solution BP 1988 required to prepare 150 ml of a solution of benzalkonium chloride 10% w/v

Benzalkonium chloride is available only as Benzalkonium Chloride Solution BP 1988 which contains 50% w/v.

Method 1
Calculation of dilution factor:

$$\frac{\text{Strength of concentrate}}{\text{Strength of dilute solution}} = \text{dilution factor}$$

e.g. $\dfrac{50\%}{10\%} = 5$ times

The dilute solution is obtained by diluting 150/5 = 30 ml of concentrate to 150 ml.

Method 2
Using the product of volume and concentration:
$V_c \times C_c = V_d \times C_d$
Where:

V_c = Volume of concentrate	?
C_c = Concentration of concentrate	50% w/v
V_d = Volume of dilute solution	150 ml
C_d = Concentration of dilute solution	10% w/v

$V_c \times 50 = 150 \times 10$
$V_c = 30$ ml

Formula for preparation

Benzalkonium Chloride Solution BP	30.0 ml
Water	to 150.0 ml

Note that a 10% w/v solution of benzalkonium chloride is equivalent to a 1 in 5 (or 20% v/v) solution of Benzalkonium Chloride Solution BP 1988.

Example 3.13

Calculate the amount of Strong Cetrimide Solution BP 1988 required to prepare 200 ml of Cetrimide Solution BP

Strong Cetrimide Solution BP (1988) contains 40% w/v cetrimide. Cetrimide Solution BP 1988 is a 1% w/v solution

Method 1
Calculation of dilution factor

$$\frac{\text{Strength of concentrate}}{\text{Strength of dilute solution}} = \text{dilution factor}$$

$$\frac{40\%}{1\%} = 40 \text{ times}$$

The dilute solution is obtained by diluting $200/40 = 5$ ml of concentrate to 200 ml.

Method 2
Using the products of volume and concentration
$V_c \times C_c = V_d \times C_d$
(see Example 3.12)
$V_c \times 40 = 200 \times 1$
$V_c \quad\quad = 5$ ml

Formula for preparation

Strong Cetrimide Solution BP (40% w/v)	5.0 ml
Purified Water freshly boiled and cooled	to 200.0 ml

Antiseptic solutions for dilution by the patient

Solutions of some antiseptics and disinfectants may be dispensed as concentrates with instructions to the patient or nurse for making the appropriate dilution immediately before use. The user should be reminded to discard any unused diluted solution immediately after use (Examples 3.14 and 3.15).

Example 3.14

1. Calculate the quantity of potassium permanganate required to prepare 200 ml of a 0.25% w/v solution and give dilution directions for 100 ml quantities of a 0.0125% solution of potassium permanganate

Formula for concentrated solution

Ingredients	% w/v	for 200 ml
Potassium permanganate	0.25%	0.5 g
Water	to 100.00%	to 200.0 ml

Calculation of dilution factor

$$\frac{\text{Strength of concentrate}}{\text{Strength of dilute solution}} = \text{dilution factor}$$

$$\frac{0.25\%}{0.0125\%} = 20 \text{ times}$$

The dilute solution is obtained by diluting $100/20 = 5$ ml of concentrate to 100 ml.

Label
The label should include the following information:

Potassium Permanganate
Solution 0.25% w/v
5 ml diluted to 100 ml with water
(or 5 ml diluted with 95 ml water) before use
gives a 0.0125% w/v solution

Note that if the solution is for issue to a patient some explanation of the dilution is necessary.

2. Give dilution directions for 500 ml quantities of a 1 in 5000 solution of potassium permanganate from the 0.25% solution above

Conversion to % w/v
1 in 100 = 1%
1 in 1000 = 0.1%
1 in 5000 = 0.02%

Calculation of dilution factor

$$\frac{\text{Strength of concentrate}}{\text{Strength of dilute solution}} = \text{dilution factor}$$

$$\frac{0.25\%}{0.02\%} = 12.5 \text{ times}$$

The dilute solution is obtained by diluting $500/12.5 = 40$ ml of concentrate to 500 ml.

Label
The label should include the following information:

Potassium Permanganate
Solution 0.25% w/v
40 ml diluted to 500 ml with water
gives a 1 in 5000 solution.

Example 3.15

Calculate the quantity of proflavine hemisulphate required to prepare 300 ml of a 1 in 1000 solution and give dilution directions for preparing 200 ml quantities of a 1 in 4000 solution.

Conversion to % w/v
1 in 100 = 1%
1 in 1000 = 0.1%
1 in 4000 = 0.025%

Formula for concentrated solution

Ingredients	% w/v	for 300 ml
Proflavine Hemisulphate	0.1%	0.3 g
		(300 mg)
Water	to 100.0%	to 300.0 ml

Calculation of dilution factor

$$\frac{\text{Strength of concentrate}}{\text{Strength of dilute solution}} = \text{dilution factor}$$

$$\frac{0.10\%}{0.025\%} = 4$$

The dilute solution is obtained by diluting 200/4 = 50 ml of concentrate to 200 ml

Label
The label should include the following information:

> Proflavine Hemisulphate
> Solution 1 in 1000
> 50 ml diluted to 200 ml
> (or 50 ml diluted with 150 ml)
> gives a 1 in 4000 solution

Concentrated stock solutions

Concentrated solutions containing ingredients required regularly for dispensing may be used providing that the storage conditions and shelf-life have been fully researched. Examples of 'official' concentrates include Concentrated Waters (used for flavouring). Chloroform Water, Double Strength BP (1988) (used as flavouring and preservative), and Amaranth Solution BP (1988) (used for colouring) (Example 3.16).

Example 3.16

Calculate the amount of Concentrated Cinnamon Water BP 1988 required to prepare 300 ml of Cinnamon Water BP 1988

Cinnamon Water is prepared by diluting:
1 part by volume of Concentrated Cinnamon Water 'with' 39 parts by volume of water, or 1 part by volume 'to' a total of 40 parts by volume.

General formula	*Parts by volume*	
Concentrated Cinnamon Water	1	1
Water	39	to 40

Formula for 300 ml Cinnamon Water BP 1988		
Concentrated Cinnamon Water	7.5 ml	7.5 ml
Water	292.5 ml	to 300.0 ml

Ethanol dilutions

Ethanol 96 per cent BP is a solution of ethanol in water containing 96–96.6% v/v (average 96.3%) ethanol. The volumes of Ethanol (96 per cent) BP required to produce 1 litre quantities of the 'official' dilute ethanols are listed in the BP. For other dilutions, the following formula may be used:

$$\frac{\text{Volume required} \times \text{percentage required}}{\text{Percentage ethanol used}}$$

= volume of stronger ethanol to be used

(See Example 3.17).

On mixing ethanol with water a contraction in volume and a rise in temperature occur. It is therefore necessary to cool the solution to 20°C (room temperature) before the final adjustment of volume is made.

The turbidity that is often produced at first is due to air bubbles released from the ethanol on dilution because air is less soluble in water than in ethanol.

Example 3.17

Calculate the amount of Ethanol (96 per cent) BP 1988 required to prepare 250 ml of Ethanol 60 per cent BP 1988 (Ethanol (96 per cent) BP contains 96.0–96.6% v/v mean 96.3% v/v) ethanol.

$$\frac{\text{Volume required} \times \text{\% required}}{\text{\% of stronger ethanol}} = \begin{array}{l}\text{volume of stronger}\\\text{ethanol to be used}\end{array}$$

$$= \frac{250 \text{ ml} \times 60\%}{96.3\%} = 155.8 \text{ ml}$$

Formula		
Ethanol (96 per cent)		155.8 ml
Water	to	250.0 ml

Dilutions of formaldehyde solution

When formaldehyde solutions are ordered it is essential to distinguish solutions containing a particular percentage w/w of formaldehyde gas from solutions containing a particular percentage by volume of the 'official' *solution* (Examples 3.18, 3.19).

Example 3.18

Calculate the amount of Formaldehyde Solution BP 1988 required to prepare 250 ml of a 4% solution of formaldehyde

This is a w/w solution of formaldehyde gas and may be prepared from Formaldehyde Solution BP 1988 which contains 34–38% w/w (average 36%) formaldehyde gas.

To calculate the amount to prepare:
The weight per ml of Formaldehyde Solution BP is about 1.08, therefore 250 ml will weigh about 270 g. In order to produce 250 ml, 270 g must be prepared.

For dilutions of w/w solutions, the following formula may be used:

$$\frac{\text{Weight required} \times \text{\% required}}{\text{\% of stronger solution}} = \begin{array}{l}\text{Weight of stronger}\\\text{solution to be used}\end{array}$$

$$= \frac{270 \text{ g} \times 4\%}{36\%} = 30 \text{ g}$$

Formula	
Formaldehyde Solution BP	30 g
Water	240 g
Check (by adding)	270 g
Supply 250 ml	

Label
This would be labelled:

```
Formaldehyde solution
4% w/w
```

Example 3.19
Calculate the amount of Formaldehyde Solution BP 1988 to prepare 250 ml of a solution containing 4% formalin

The requirement is not for a solution containing 4% formaldehyde. Formalin is a synonym for Formaldehyde Solution BP. Therefore 4% v/v of the 'official' solution must be supplied.

Formula

Formaldehyde Solution BP	10 ml
Water	to 250 ml

Label
This would be labelled:

```
Formalin solution
4% v/v
```

Dilutions of creams and ointments

Sometimes dilutions of proprietary creams or ointments are prescribed. The strength of the preparation should normally be expressed on the label in terms of the percentage w/w of active ingredient(s) in the final product rather than by the degree of dilution (Example 3.20).

Example 3.20
Calculate the quantities of the ingredients required to prepare 20 g diflucortolone valerate ointment 0.025%

Ointment containing diflucortolone valerate 0.1% w/w is available. The recommended diluent for this product is white soft paraffin (see BNF).

Calculation

$$\frac{\text{weight required} \times \% \text{ required}}{\% \text{ of concentrated}} = \frac{\text{weight of concentrated}}{\text{ointment to be used}}$$

$$= \frac{20 \text{ g} \times 0.025\%}{0.1\%} = 5 \text{ g}$$

Formula

Diflucortolone valerate 0.1% ointment	5 g
White Soft Paraffin	15 g
Check total	20 g

Label
This would be labelled

```
Diflucortolone ointment
containing diflucortolone
valerate
0.025% w/w
```

In order to fulfil a prescription for 20 g it would be advisable to make a small excess, e.g. 5 g.

Dilutions of liquid oral dosage forms

If a dose less than, or not a multiple of, 5 ml is prescribed a liquid dosage form may be diluted so that the patient can measure the dose in 5 ml spoonfuls. For 'official' products containing more than one active ingredient the degree of dilution may be used on the label to indicate the strength. For products containing a single active ingredient the label should state the amount of active ingredient in a 5 ml dose volume (Examples 3.21, 3.22).

Example 3.21
Chloral Elixir Paediatric BP 1988 is a stock preparation in your pharmacy. How would you respond to a prescription for 25 ml Chloral Elixir Paediatric to be labelled: 2.5 ml to be given at night?

The preparation should be diluted to a 5 ml dose volume. The recommended diluent is Syrup BP (see BNF).

Calculation
The number of doses ordered is 25/2.5 = 10 doses.
10 × 5 ml doses of the *diluted* preparation must be supplied

Formula

Chloral Elixir, Paediatric	25 ml
Syrup	to 50 ml

Label
The label should include the following information:

```
Chloral Elixir Paediatric BP
50% v/v
containing 100 mg Chloral
Hydrate
in each 5 ml spoonful
```

Example 3.22
Calculate the amounts of the ingredients required to prepare 100 ml of salbutamol syrup containing 1.5 mg in each 5 ml dose

Syrup containing salbutamol 2 mg in 5 ml is available. The recommended diluent is Purified Water, freshly boiled and cooled (see BNF).

Calculation
The number of doses ordered is 100/5 = 20 doses
  Each dose of the diluted syrup is to contain 1.5 mg. 20 doses will contain 20 × 1.5 = 30 mg.
  Each 5 ml of the concentrated syrup contains 2 mg. 30 mg will be contained in 30/2 × 5 ml of the concentrated syrup = 75 ml.

Formula

| Salbutamol syrup (2 mg/5 ml) | 75 ml = 30 mg salbutamol |
| Purified Water freshly boiled and cooled | to 100 ml |

Label
A suitable label would be

> Salbutamol syrup
> each 5 ml spoonful
> contains 1.5 mg salbutamol

Triturations

The term 'trituration' is applied to the dilution of an active substance by an inert diluent, usually in order to obtain smaller quantities of the active substance than could be otherwise weighed or measured. (See Chapter 5 for minimum measurable quantities.)

Small quantities in powders

In order to obtain an amount of an active substance too small to be weighed, the minimum weighable quantity of the substance is mixed with an inert substance such as lactose in order to produce a 1 in 10 or a 1 in 100 dilution (Example 3.23). Great care must be taken to ensure effective mixing (see Chapter 4).

Example 3.23

Calculate the amounts of the ingredients required to prepare 4 powders each containing 500 micrograms diazepam

It is usual to prepare enough material for one extra powder in order to allow for manipulative losses. An inert diluent (lactose) is used to produce the recommended minimum weight (120 mg) for a divided powder.

Formula	*for 5 powders*
Diazepam	2.5 mg*
Lactose	597.5 mg
Total	600.0 mg

* Since this quantity is too small to measure directly (see Chapter 4), it must be incorporated as a triturate.

Trituration 1

Diazepam	100 mg
Lactose	900 mg
Total	1000 mg (each 100 mg contains 10 mg diazepam)

Trituration 2

Triturate 1	100 mg
Lactose	900 mg
Total	1000 mg (each 100 mg contains 1 mg diazepam)

Trituration 3

Triturate 2	250 mg (= 2.5 mg diazepam)
Lactose	350 mg
Total	600 mg

Each 120 mg aliquot of Triturate 3 contains 0.5 mg (500 micrograms) diazepam.
(See Ch. 16 for method of preparation of divided powders.)

Small quantities in solution (w/v)

These may be obtained by making suitable solutions and taking appropriate aliquot portions. 1 in 1000 (100 mg in 100 ml) or 1 in 100 (100 mg in 10 ml) solutions are usually convenient (Example 3.24). It is necessary to take into account the solubility of the substance and also the final volume of the product being prepared.

Example 3.24

Calculate the amounts of the ingredients required to prepare 50 ml of an elixir to the following formula

Ingredients	Master formula from prescriber	Scaled quantities
Diamorphine Hydrochloride	4 mg	40 mg*
Ethanol 90%	0.5 ml	5 ml
Syrup	1.0 ml	10 ml
Chloroform Water	to 5.0 ml	to 50 ml

*Again, this quantity is too small to be weighed accurately and must be incorporated as a triturate, as follows.

The trituration is performed in the diluent i.e. Chloroform Water. Diamorphine hydrochloride is freely soluble in water (1 in 1.6). Since the total volume of the elixir is 50 ml, a 1 in 100 dilution is appropriate.

Formula for Trituration

| Diamorphine Hydrochloride | 100 mg |
| Chloroform Water | to 10 ml (4 ml contains 40 mg) |

  Difficulties may arise if the vehicle of the product is unsuitable for making a trituration. Potent substances included in linctuses are usually dissolved in a small quantity of water before making to volume with a viscous vehicle such as syrup or glycerol (Example 3.25).

Example 3.25

Calculate the amounts of the ingredients required to prepare 50 ml of a linctus to the following formula

Ingredients	Master formula from prescriber	Scaled quantities
Diamorphine Hydrochloride	4 mg	40 mg*
Water	0.05 ml	0.5 ml
Oxymel	1.5 ml	15.0 ml
Syrup	to 5.0 ml	to 50.0 ml

* Unweighable and thus requires a trituration.

The viscous vehicle syrup is unsuitable for preparing a trituration. The preferred method would be to make an excess of the preparation and to discard the excess. An alternative method would be to make a trituration by weight using the small quantity of water.

Calculation
Require 40 mg diamorphine hydrochloride plus 0.5 ml (500 mg) water:
i.e. 40 mg diamorphine hyd. in 540 mg 'solution'
i.e. 1 mg diamorphine hyd. in 13.5 mg 'solution'
or 100 mg diamorphine hyd. in 1350 mg (13.5 g) 'solution'.
It would be incorrect to prepare a triturate containing 40 mg diamorphine hydrochloride in 0.5 ml of 'solution' since this would contain slightly less than the required 0.5 ml of water.

Formula for trituration
Diamorphine hydrochloride	100	mg
Water		1.25 g
Total		1.35 g

(540 mg at trituration contains 40 mg diamorphine together with 0.5 g (0.5 ml) water)

REFERENCES

British National Formulary 1988 16th edn. British Medical Association and Royal Pharmaceutical Society of Great Britain, London (updated twice yearly)

Small quantities in solution (w/w)

For solutions of the w/w type the triturate must be dissolved in a suitable weight of solution and an aliquot portion by weight taken (Example 3.26).

Example 3.26

Calculate the amounts of the ingredients required to prepare 30 g Cetomacrogol Cream BP (Formula A)

Ingredients	Master formula	Scaled quantities
Cetomacrogol Emulsifying Ointment	300 g	9.0 g
Chlorocresol	1 g	30 mg*
Purified Water freshly boiled and cooled	699 g	20.97 g*
Check	1000 g	30.00 g

* The 30 mg or chlorocresol is too small to measure accurately. The trituration can be approached as follows.

Require 30 mg chlorocresol plus 20.97 g water:
i.e. 30 mg chlorocresol in 21 g 'solution'
i.e. 1 mg chlorocresol in 700 mg 'solution'
or 100 mg chlorocresol in 70 g 'solution'
i.e. a 1 in 700 w/w solution of chlorocresol in water is required.
It would be incorrect to prepare a triturate containing 30 mg chlorocresol in 21 ml 'solution' since this would contain an unknown weight of water.

Trituration
Chlorocresol	100	mg
Purified Water freshly boiled and cooled	69.9	g
	(to 70.0	g)

21 g of this trituration contains 30 mg chlorocresol together with 20.97 g water, i.e. exactly as required, see * in formula.
(see Ch. 4 for method of dissolving chlorocresol and Ch. 13 for method of preparing creams.)

British Pharmacopoeia 1980 HMSO, London (and addenda 1982, 1983 and 1986)
British Pharmacopoeia 1988 HMSO, London

4. Fundamental operations in compounding

D. M. Collett

Compounding is concerned with the preparation of medicines from basic ingredients on a small scale. The formulation and production of medicines on a large scale is discussed in the companion volume. The accurate and elegant compounding of medicines requires expertise in several fundamental operations; namely weighing, measurement of liquids, dissolution, filtration, mixing, size reduction and size separation. The basic principles underlying each of these operations are the same for large- or small-scale manufacture. However, the techniques vary according to the batch size and the equipment available.

This chapter introduces the beginner to the equipment and techniques used in the dispensing laboratory, in the hospital pharmacy department and in the community pharmacy where compounding is carried out on a small scale.

WEIGHING

Balances

Weighing instruments used in a trade, e.g. retail transactions, must comply with the current Weights and Measures Regulations. For a description of the Statutes affecting Pharmacy see Dale & Appelbe (1983). Balances which comply with the prescribed limits of error for beam scales are defined as 'Class B' and dispensing balances are usually of this class. The weights used must also comply with regulations covering shape, composition and limits of error.

The traditional dispensing balance (shown in Fig. 4.1) consists of a simple, light but rigid, equal-armed horizontal beam with central and terminal knife edges. The beam turns about the central fulcrum under the influence of loads placed on pans suspended from the terminal knife edges. The oscillations of the beam are dampened to allow readings to be made quickly and easily and deflection of the beam is indicated by movement of a pointer fixer below the centre of the beam. Although the pointer moves over a calibrated scale, this

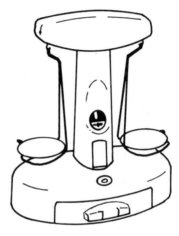

Fig. 4.1 Dispensing balance

should be used for guidance only. Appropriate weights and the central zero on the scale should be used for accurate weighing.

Electronic balances are replacing mechanical balances for many weighing purposes. A wide range of electronic balances are available with differing degrees of sensitivity to serve differing functions.

It is important to note the characteristics of any balance to be used, in particular the maximum capacity of the balance and the smallest weight to which the balance will respond when loaded to capacity. 'Class B' dispensing balances generally have a maximum capacity of 50 g and a sensitivity of 20 mg under load. The capacity and sensitivity of electronic balances vary with manufacturer and model and should be checked prior to use. It is essential to use a balance with characteristics appropriate for the particular task in hand.

Minimum weighable amounts

The recommended minimum weighable quantity of any substance to be used in compounding is 50 mg provided

21

that a 'Class A' sensitive balance is available. For quantities less than 50 mg losses in transferance of the weighed material become excessive. The recommended minimum weighable quantity for a 'Class B' balance is 100 mg, although for highly potent substances a higher limit may be preferred.

Approximations

Approximations should be avoided if possible. If approximations are unavoidable the figure should be rounded to two places of decimal places of grammes and the rounded figure shown in brackets beside the original weight, e.g. 17.784 g (17.78 g)

Weighing technique for the dispensing balance

(The instructions given below are for right-handed personnel.) The balance should always be sited on a convenient level surface away from the influence of draughts.

1. Clean the balance and pans if necessary. A clean sheet of white demy paper placed under the pans helps to contain spillage and protect the balance.

2. Select a suitable weighing vessel or paper. Balance pans are usually made of glass or stainless steel and are resistant to contact direct with most medicaments with a few exceptions. For soluble solids in a liquid preparation the most accurate method of transfer is by rinsing from the balance pan with the solvent. The pan should never be tapped on the side of the container. Weighing papers are convenient for bulky powders and may facilitate transfer from the balance. For greasy or waxy constituents greaseproof paper should be used since white demy partly absorbs greasy substances and transfer from the paper is difficult. Small, lightweight, disposable weighing boats are a useful alternative to weighing papers since they may also be used for viscous substances such as coal tar or ichthammol and for non-viscous liquids such as coal tar solutions which are usually weighed. If containers such as glass beakers or porcelain evaporating dishes are used as weighing vessels care should be taken to avoid exceeding the total (50 g) capacity of the balance.

3. Check that the pointer is at the null point but is able to move freely. Counterbalance the weighing vessel if necessary.

4. Place the required weights on the left-hand pan. Use forceps to avoid contamination of the weights with consequent alteration in mass (especially small weights).

5. Close the balance drawer. This prevents spills from contaminating the weights.

6. Collect the medicament from the shelf. Check the label word for word with the formula — there are many similarly named substances. Record the batch number.

7. Hold the bottle in the left hand. Keep the label uppermost so that it is visible during weighing.

8. Remove the lid or stopper. If possible hold the stopper between the little finger and the palm of the right hand. The thumb and remaining fingers of the right hand remain free to use a spatula. If it is not possible to hold the lid it should be placed top uppermost on a clean tile to protect against atmospheric contamination.

9. Use a spatula to transfer medicament to the right-hand pan until the pointer returns to the null point. Powders should not be shaken onto the pan.

10. Close the stock container.

11. Recheck the weights and the medicament against the formula.

12. A check by a second person may be made before the stock bottle is returned to the shelf. It may be departmental policy in some pharmacies for all procedures to be double checked. For students in training it is usual for a member of staff to check weighings of substances subject to the more stringent legal controls.

13. Return the stock container tidily to the shelf.

14. Return the weights to the drawer and carefully clean the balance.

Variations in weighing technique for the electronic balance

Step 2. Materials are not weighed directly onto the pans of electronic balances, a weighing vessel or paper is always used.

Step 3. Check that the balance is set at zero. Many electronic balances have a 'built-in counterbalance' — the scale may be reset to zero with the weighing vessel in place.

For high grade 'analytical' balances it may first be necessary to record the weight of the weighing vessel. This weight is then added to the required weight of medicament in order to calculate the final balance reading (These figures should be included in the record.)

Steps 4 and *5* are unnecessary.

Step 9. Medicament is transferred to the pan until the required weight is read on the scale.

Step 14. Reset the balance reading to true zero and carefully clean the balance.

Taring the weighing vessels

Some procedures in compounding (e.g. adjustment of a product to weight) require a knowledge of the weight of the vessel containing the preparation. With an electronic balance the weight of the empty vessel may be easily recorded. Alternatively, the balance may be reset to zero and the tare automatically retained provided that no one alters the adjustment before the preparation is completed.

For mechanical beam balances it is usually inconvenient to obtain the weight of the vessel and the following procedure may be used.

Two small containers with lids are required, one containing a quantity of small lead shot. The vessel to be tared is placed on one balance pan and the empty container on the other, and shot is poured into the container until balance is obtained. This container is then retained and used as a tare for the vessel when required.

Weighing by difference

When very viscous substances are weighed it is difficult to transfer them completely from the weighing vessel. The alternative is to weigh by difference — that is to weigh a slight excess of the substance which remains in the weighing vessel after the correct amount has been transferred. For the dispensing balance the following procedure may be used:

1. Place a weighing vessel on the right-hand (RH) pan of the balance and counterbalance with a similar weighing vessel and, if necessary a little lead shot.

2. Put weights for the required amount of substance on the left-hand (LH) pan.

3. Add the substance to the RH vessel until balance is obtained and then add an excess.

4. Place more lead shot on the LH pan to restore the balance.

5. Remove the weights from the LH pan and carefully transfer the substance from the RH pan until the balance is again restored, when the appropriate weight of substance will have been removed. Discard the excess.

MEASUREMENT OF LIQUIDS

The traditional dispensing measures are conical (shown in Fig. 4.2) or, for large volumes, beaker shaped. Although less accurate than the cylindrical measures used in laboratories the use of conical measures has persisted in compounding because they offer a number of advantages.
Conical measures are:

a. Easier to fill without spilling liquid on the sides above the required level.

b. Easier to drain out the preparation.

c. Easier to rinse out the residue left after draining viscous liquids into the preparation.

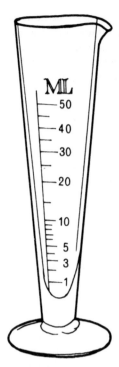

Fig. 4.2 Conical dispensing measure

d. Easier to clean after use.

e. Harder to read the meniscus accurately — the error increases with height because of the slope of the side.

f. Harder to estimate volumes between graduations.

Like balances, measures used in trade must comply with the current Weights and Measures Regulations and should be so stamped.

Minimum measurable amounts

The recommended minimum measurable quantity for a small (10 ml) conical measure is 1 ml. For highly potent substances or viscous liquids a higher limit may be preferred. A graduated pipette may be used to deliver volumes of 0.1 ml. For smaller volumes a trituration should be made (see Ch. 3).

Measuring technique for conical measures

(The instructions given below are for right-handed personnel.) The measure should always be clean and dry.

1. Choose the smallest measure that will hold the required volume. If possible do not split the volume between two measurements because this will increase the error.

2. Collect the medicament from the shelf. Check the label word for word with the formula — there are many similarly named substances. Record the batch number.

3. Hold the bottle in the right hand. Keep the label uppermost so that it is visible during measuring and so that any trickles after use do not obscure the label.

4. Remove the lid or stopper. If possible hold the stopper between the little finger and the palm of the left hand. The thumb and remaining fingers of the left hand remain free to hold the measure. If it is not possible to hold the lid it should be placed top uppermost on a clean tile to protect against atmospheric contamination.

5. Straighten the measure by aligning the appropriate guide-line on the rear of the measure with the graduation on the front.

6. Carefully pour the liquid into the centre of the measure; any that falls on the sides should be allowed to drain down before the volume is finally adjusted; this means that measurement takes longer, especially for viscous liquids.

7. Hold the measure at eye level and re-align the guide-line corresponding to the required volume with the appropriate graduation. This prevents parallax errors. For volumes for which no guide-line is provided the nearest line and corresponding graduation are used. Measurement errors are lower if the measure is steadied by resting on the bench or a shelf.

8. Align the top of the graduation line with the lowest part of the liquid surface, i.e. the true meniscus. If a finger is held horizontally just below the graduation line, then the true meniscus is seen as a pink line. For very dark liquids the true meniscus is often invisible and it is recommended that such liquids should be *measured by difference* (see below).

9. Close the stock container.

10. Recheck the volume and the medicament against the formula.

11. A check by a second person may be made before the stock bottle is returned to the shelf. It may be departmental policy in some pharmacies for all procedures to be double checked. For students in training it is usual for a member of staff to check measurements of substances subject to the more stringent legal controls.

12. Return the stock container tidily to the shelf.

13. Pour the liquid into the vessel in which the preparation is being made and thoroughly rinse the measure into the same vessel. With coloured preparations it is easy to see when rinsing is complete. Before transferring viscous liquids, add a small volume of vehicle and mix with a glass rod. When rinsing, use the rod again and finally rinse into the preparation any liquid adhering to the rod. If it is very hard to rinse out a measure containing a viscous liquid, e.g. where the vehicle itself is viscous, the volume should be measured by difference.

Variations in measuring technique for pipettes.

Graduated pipettes of the drain-out type may be used to measure volumes under 1 ml or to measure dark-coloured liquids by difference.

Step 3. Place the bottle on the bench with the label facing you so that it is visible during measuring.

Steps 5–8: use of a pipette teat

a. Place a teat of appropriate size over the mouth of the pipette. Do not push down too far onto the pipette or it will be difficult to remove.

b. Squeeze the teat gently with the right hand and immerse only a small length of the pipette in the medicament because liquid on the outside may cause inaccuracy in the volume delivered.

c. Control the teat with the right hand and suck up liquid to well above the relevant graduation (but not up into the teat!).

d. Flick off the teat with the thumb of the right hand and, before the liquid has fallen to the required mark, place the forefinger over the mouth of the pipette.

e. Control the outflow precisely to the required level

Step 13. Drain the liquid into the vessel in which the preparation is being made.

Use of tared containers

Whenever possible liquid preparations are adjusted to final volume in a measure. For preparations such as suspensions and emulsions sedimentation of the disperse phase may make transfer to the final container difficult. Viscous preparations may also present transfer problems. For such preparations the final container may be calibrated and the volume adjusted finally in the container. The appropriate volume of water, accurately measured, is introduced carefully into the bottle and the meniscus marked with the upper edge of a small adhesive (tare) label. The bottle is then emptied and inverted on a tile to allow the water to drain out completely. Calibration of containers introduces an additional potential source of error and should therefore be reserved for those preparations where transfer from a measure would be likely to introduce a greater error.

Measurement by difference

For dark-coloured liquids a small excess of the amount required is taken into a cylindrical measure or pipette. The required amount of liquid is delivered into the preparation and the remainder discarded. Although the true meniscus cannot be seen, both readings will be of the same 'false meniscus' and the difference will be an accurate measure. Viscous liquids may also be measured by difference in a measure to avoid an excessive time for drainage.

DISSOLUTION

Many dosage forms consist of a solution of a solid in a liquid, most commonly water. The extent to which different substances dissolve in water or other solvents may be found in the pharmacopoeias and is usually quoted as 'the number of parts by volume of solvent required to dissolve one part by weight of the solid'. It is useful to check the solubility of any ingredient before attempting dissolution. The factors affecting the solubility and the dissolution rates of solids in liquids are discussed in detail in the companion volume. Briefly, the rate of solution of a solid in a liquid is increased by:

1. Finely powdering the solid to increase the surface area from which molecules can diffuse into the liquid.
2. Agitation, which produces eddies that quickly disperse the solute through the bulk of the solution once it has diffused the boundary layer.
3. Raising the temperature, which reduces the thickness of the boundary layer by decreasing viscosity and increasing the diffusion coefficient. In addition the solubility of most substances is increased at elevated temperature.

Dissolution technique

1. Select a vessel in which to prepare the solution. A conical flask that will hold the final volume of the preparation is the preferred vessel. The advantages of conical flasks over other vessels are:
   a. contents can be agitated by shaking with little risk of spillage;
   b. contents can be readily heated if required;
   c. contents can be rapidly cooled under running water with little risk of contamination.
2. Powder the medicament (except for substances already in fine powder and freely soluble substances). A porcelain mortar is generally preferred for size reduction (see below), although glass mortars should be used for substances that taint or stain.
3. Weigh the medicament. Note that powdering should precede weighing because of the difficulty in removing all the dry powder from the mortar. In order to avoid powdering a large excess of the medicament which would then be wasted, an approximate weight plus a little excess may be weighed and transferred to the mortar. For readily soluble substances to be dissolved in the mortar, powdering may follow weighing, e.g. menthol in eucalyptus oil.

4. Agitate the solution. Shaking the flask or stirring with a glass rod will aid solution. For slowly soluble substances a mechanical stirrer is to be preferred. A simple stainless steel propeller that will pass through the neck of a flask is most useful. The propeller may be driven by a variable-speed electric motor.

5. Heat the solution (only if necessary and if it does not damage the medicament). Heating is appropriate for substances that are:
   a. more soluble at high temperature, e.g. proflavine hemisulphate;
   b. non-heat labile;
   c. non-volatile (unless special precautions are taken see below).

6. Check that solution is complete. Examine the solution critically for traces of undissolved solid on the neck of the flask, in the bottom of the flask or in suspension in the solvent.

7. Restore the solution to room temperature (if necessary).

8. Transfer to a measure and adjust to final volume (see above 'Measuring technique for conical measures').

Some solutions require filtration which is discussed below.

Special techniques for volatile substances

Volatile solvents

Some solvents contain volatile ingredients (e.g. Chloroform Water BP and Peppermint Water BP) and should not be heated if this can be avoided. Since most of these waters are prepared at the time of use by diluting a concentrated solution with water, it may be practicable to make a solution of the medicament in hot water and add the concentrate after cooling.

Volatile solutes

A number of very volatile substances, of which chlorbutol and chlorocresol are commonly used examples, present special difficulty. They dissolve very slowly in the cold even with size reduction and mechanical stirring. When solutions must be made quickly, heat is required. A suitable small-scale method is as follows:

   a. Measure as much water as the formula allows and transfer to a conical flask suitable for stoppering.
   b. Heat the water to approximately 60°C. *The flask must not be heated with the stopper in place.*

c. Add to the hot water the substance to be dissolved.

d. Quickly insert the stopper and shake vigorously until solution is complete.

FILTRATION

Unwanted particulate matter may be removed from solutions by the process of filtration. Mechanisms of filtration and factors affecting the rate of filtration are discussed in detail in the companion volume. Briefly, the rate of filtration can be increased by:

1. Increasing the pressure differences across the filter. In an ordinary open filter the pressure difference is produced by the head of liquid above the filtration medium. It can be increased by applying a vacuum below the medium (e.g. by using a Buchner flask and a vacuum pump) or by applying pressure to the surface of the liquid (e.g. with air from a compressor).

2. Reducing the viscosity of the liquid. Heating lowers viscosity and therefore decreases the resistance to flow.

3. Increasing the surface area of the filter. A pleated filter paper increases the filter area.

4. Using a filtration medium of high porosity. Filter papers, sintered glass filters and membrane filters are obtainable in a range of porosities. The filtration rate may be inconveniently slow if unnecessarily fine medium is used.

Straining (coarse filtration)

This is used to remove large foreign particles from:

a. Preparations in which traces of fine particulate matter are tolerable (e.g. solutions for use on intact skin or solutions of disinfectants and antiseptics not intended for use on or in the body).

b. Heterogeneous systems (e.g. emulsions and suspensions).

c. Viscous preparations.

The materials commonly used for this purpose are:

1. A plug of absorbent cotton wool or cotton gauze placed in a conical funnel, well rinsed to remove loose fibres (useful for category a above).

2. Well-rinsed muslin held taut across a special strainer (useful for categories b and c above).

Fine filtration

For oral solutions and solutions for application to mucous membranes or broken skin a higher degree of clarification is necessary. This is achieved with filter papers or sintered glass filters. (Special requirements for sterile products are discussed in Part 3 of this book.)

Table 4.1 The characteristics of Whatman series filter papers

No.	Relative filtration time (rate)	Size of particle removed	Average pore size (μm)
54	1 (fast)	Coarse	3.4–5.0
1	4 (medium fast)	Medium	2.1–2.8
50	23 (slow)	Fine	0.4–1.1

Filter papers

Many grades are available. In the Whatman series three of the most useful are numbers 1 (suitable for general filtration purposes), 50 (better if a particularly clean filtrate is required) and 54 (suitable for acid and alkaline solutions). The characteristics of these papers are shown in Table 4.1.

Sintered glass filters

The most suitable grades are numbers 3 (for filtration of small volumes by gravity) and 4 (for large or small volumes by vacuum or pressure).

These filters are expensive and require special cleaning and therefore are not universally available in practice. They are particularly useful for substances that attack filter paper, e.g. potassium permanganate (oxidizes) and zinc chloride (dissolves).

Adjustment to volume after filtration

It is preferable to adjust solutions to volume through the filter. A suitable procedure is as follows:

a. Wash through the filter with a little of the vehicle and discard.

b. Make the solution almost to volume and pass through the filter into a measure.

c. Rinse through the filter with sufficient vehicle to make to final volume.

It may be convenient to make up to volume through a sintered filter incorporated in a vacuum line. A slight loss in volume of solutions adjusted to volume before filtration is to be expected during transfer through the filter and from the collecting vessel. This must not be re-adjusted with solvent.

MIXING

Many pharmaceutical products consist of homogeneous mixtures of two or more components. These may be mixtures of solids, semi-solids or liquids. The theory of mixing is discussed in detail in the companion volume (Chapter 32, Aulton 1988). There are four main classes of mixture, as below.

Mixtures of liquids

Homogeneous mixtures (solutions)

The mixing of liquids is easy if they are miscible and mobile because the operation merely accelerates a process that would eventually occur by diffusion. All that is necessary is to encourage flow of the liquids by shaking or stirring. It is quicker and easier to use an electric stirrer if the liquids are not readily miscible or have very different viscosities or densities.

Heterogeneous mixtures (emulsions)

For the production of a stable emulsion from two immiscible liquids the mixing must be very efficient because the components tend to separate unless work is continually expended on them. Two requirements must be fulfilled:

1. Localized mixing, in which shear is applied to the globules of liquid.
2. A general movement to take all of the material through the shearing zone and thus ensure a uniform product.

On a small scale a pestle and mortar is suitable for preparing an emulsion; shear forces are produced between the flat head of the pestle and the flat bottom of the mortar, while a general movement is created by wider movements of the pestle and by frequent use of a spatula to return liquid from the sides of the mortar to the end of the pestle or the bottom of the mortar.

Mechanical mixer-emulsifiers are also available for medium-scale production.

Mixtures of liquids and solids

Homogeneous mixtures (solutions)

In this case the aim of mixing is to produce a physical change, i.e. the solution of a soluble solid. Like the mixing of miscible liquids this will occur eventually by diffusion and therefore agitation will usually effect solution (see above 'Dissolution')

Heterogeneous mixtures (suspensions)

The components of suspensions, like those of emulsions, tend to separate and the same requirements must be fulfilled to obtain a good mixture. On a small scale suspensions are usually made with a pestle and mortar.

Mixtures of solids

It can be very difficult to ensure the effective mixing of powders because they do not mix spontaneously. The problem is greatest if the proportion of one ingredient is very small.

As with emulsions and suspensions, localized shear is necessary to move the particles relative to one another while a general circulation is required to bring the bulk of the material into the region of shear.

For small quantities a pestle and mortar may be used. A porcelain mortar is generally preferred except for materials that taint or stain. However, it is important to use a sufficiently large mortar since the powder bed will dilate during mixing and space for adequate circulation of the mix should be allowed. Mortars should be perfectly dry before mixing dry powders. The following procedure is suitable:

1. Add to the mortar the ingredient present in the lowest bulk.
2. Add a quantity of the second ingredient that approximately doubles the bulk already in the mortar.
3. Mix lightly since undue pressure may cause caking.
4. Occasionally loosen the powder from the bottom of the mortar and scrape it from the sides using a large flexible spatula.
5. At each addition, add a quantity that approximately doubles the bulk already in the mortar.

Mixtures containing semi-solids

This type of mixture involves incorporating a solid and/or a liquid into a base consisting of one or more semi-solids. Examples are found in ointments, pastes and suppositories.

A suitable procedure is as follows:

1. Prepare the base (if necessary).

The bases of ointments and pastes may contain liquids (e.g. liquid paraffin), semi-solids (e.g. wool fat and soft paraffin) and solids (e.g. cetostearyl alcohol and hard paraffin). To ensure homogeneity, the ingredients are melted together in a dish over a water-bath and stirred well taking care to avoid overheating any labile substances. To avoid separation of the constituents with higher melting points, the mixture must be stirred until cold.

2. Incorporate any solid medicaments

Solids are first rubbed down with a little of the base which may need prior warming or melting depending on its consistency. The rest of the base is added gradually and mixing continued until the preparation has cooled enough to hold the medicament in suspension and prevent separation of the ingredients of the base.

3. Incorporate any liquid medicaments

To prevent separation, liquids are not incorporated until the base is fairly cool. Volatile liquids (e.g. methyl salicylate) and labile liquids (e.g. coal tar preparations) should not be added until the temperature of the base is below 40°C.

The incorporation of solid or liquid ingredients may be achieved on a large warm tile using a large flexible spatula or alternatively in a warm mortar using a pestle.

SIZE REDUCTION OF SOLIDS

It is an advantage to use fine powders in pharmaceutical preparations because:

1. They mix more uniformly and suspend more easily.
2. If soluble, they dissolve more quickly.
3. They are absorbed more readily from the gastrointestinal tract.
4. They yield preparations that are relatively free from grittiness; consequently oral powders and suspensions are more pleasant to take and external powders are less irritating to apply.

A detailed discussion of particle size reduction is to be found in the companion volume (Chapter 34, Aulton 1988). On a small scale there are two main methods of size reduction, dry grinding and wet grinding.

Dry grinding

The material is broken down in a mortar and pestle. The mechanisms are 'compression', between the flat head of the pestle and the bottom of the mortar, and 'attrition', by the shearing action of the pestle.

Wet grinding (levigation)

For aqueous suspensions the material is made into a paste with the vehicle and ground in a mortar. Effort put in while the paste is thick, before the addition of more vehicle, produces most effect.

For semi-solid preparations the medicament is rubbed down with the warm base on a warm tile or in a warm mortar.

SIZE SEPARATION

The methods available for the separation of particles on a large scale are discussed in the companion volume (Chapter 35, Aulton 1988). On a small scale the separation of particles of the required size from a medicament is achieved by sifting. Generally wire mesh sieves are used, the most suitable grades being those with mesh diameter 180 μm (for dusting powders and for ingredients required to be in the form of a 'fine' powder) and 250 μm (for external preparations when no particular grade of powder is required and for oral powders).

Wire mesh sieves are made from a variety of materials, particularly brass and stainless steel. Stainless steel is best because it is attacked by very few of the powders commonly used in compounding. (Note that salicylic acid and resorcinol both corrode brass sieves.)

Powders must not be forced through sieves as this distorts the apertures. Particles of the correct size pass through easily if the sieve is tapped or gently stroked with a bristle brush.

Since some material is retained by the sieve, powders should always be sifted before weighing and a fresh sieve used for each ingredient.

Sifting tends to separate powders of different densities, and after mixtures such as dusting powders have been sifted they are remixed in a mortar, or if the quantity is small, with a large spatula on paper.

Sometimes, sifting aids mixing by splitting up aggregates of fine powder that have resisted breakdown in a mortar. The distribution of colouring matter in powders is often better after sifting and remixing.

REFERENCES

Aulton M E 1988 Pharmaceutics: the science of dosage form design. Churchill Livingstone, Edinburgh
Dale J R, Appelbe G E 1989 Pharmacy law and ethics, 4th edn. Pharmaceutical Press, London

5. Good pharmaceutical practice in compounding and dispensing

D. M. Collett

In dispensing, a medicine is supplied to an individual patient usually in response to a prescription written by a practitioner. In a community pharmacy some medicines may also be sold to patients on the recommendation of the pharmacist (counterprescribed) or on the request of the patient at the discretion of the pharmacist (a sale). The medicines supplied to an individual patient may be:

1. Compounded extemporaneously on receipt of the prescription or request.

2. Weighed or measured from stock which has been previously compounded from basic ingredients on a small scale in the pharmacy.

3. Weighed, measured or counted from stock purchased from a manufacturer.

4. Supplied in a manufacturer's original pack.

RESOURCES

The resources that are required for good compounding and dispensing practice include:

A. Suitable, well-maintained premises.
B. An adequate supply of equipment.
C. Well-trained personnel.
D. Strict control procedures to assure quality of the products.
E. Readily accessible information sources.

A. The premises

The premises from which a pharmaceutical service is provided should inspire confidence in the users of the service. They should be clean and hygienic, well organized, tidy, accessible and secure. The premises should provide suitable environmental conditions for both personnel and products.

Table 5.1 Equipment for compounding and dispensing

Working surface of adequate size with impervious surface
Sink with hot and cold water
Supply of mains (potable) water
Heating ring (means of boiling water)
Hot water-bath
Storage units for raw materials and manufactured products
Refrigerator
Typewriter or labeller
Electric stirrer
Accurate 'Class B' dispensing balance and weights
Other appropriate balances, e.g. 'Class A', top pan, etc.
A range of glass and earthenware mortars and pestles
A range of glass beakers and conical flasks
A range of accurate, graduated conical measures
A range of graduated pipettes
Large and small glass or ceramic tiles
A range of spatulas and glass rods
Thermometers
A range of containers for each type of dosage form
A suitable range of labels
A means of counting tablets and capsules
Appropriate information sources
A telephone

B. The equipment

The equipment in the pharmacy should be suitable and adequate for the work to be undertaken. A basic range of equipment is listed in Table 5.1. A pharmacy in which compounding is carried out extensively will require more equipment than a pharmacy largely concerned with the supply of pre-packed medicines. All equipment must be maintained in accurate working order and checked for cleanliness prior to each use.

C. The personnel

There should be an adequate number of trained personnel, i.e. pharmacists and technicians together with appropriate support staff. Standards of personal hygiene should be high and appropriate protective clothing worn. Eating, drinking and smoking should not be permitted in any area where medicines are prepared or supplied.

D. Control procedures

In order to assure the quality of all medicines prepared and/or supplied, stringent control procedures are necessary.

Quality of materials

All materials purchased for use in compounding and dispensing should be of suitable quality and obtained from a licensed source. Where facilities exist, an 'in house' check of quality may be made on starting materials. The materials should be fully identifiable at all times and carry a clear batch identification and expiry date. Appropriate storage conditions should be maintained and out-of-date stock safely disposed.

Supervision

The compounding and dispensing of medicines should be carried out by a pharmacist or by other suitable personnel (trained or in training) under the personal supervision of a pharmacist.

Documentation

All compounding procedures should be fully documented and the record should include the following details:

1. The name of the product.
2. A written master formula (it may be useful to record the source of the formula, e.g. BP, BNF, prescriber, etc.).
3. The working formula of the batch being prepared.
4. The method of preparation.

The detail recorded should be sufficient to allow consistency in the method used for different batches of the same product.

5. The names, quantities and identification of each starting material (supplier, batch number and date received).
6. The date of manufacture.
7. An identification allocated to the batch of product being made.
8. The appropriate container and closure.
9. The required storage conditions.
10. A copy of the label.

The records of dispensing procedures that need to be made are described in Chapter 9 and Appendix 1. All records of compounding and dispensing procedures should be retained for 2 years.

Packaging and labelling

The containers used should comply with any current legal standards for containers and with current professional opinion. Containers and closures used presently for medicines are discussed in Chapter 8.

Containers should be labelled immediately after filling.

Labelling for stock

The labelling requirements for dispensed medicines are discussed in detail in Chapter 10. Medicines that are sufficiently stable may be prepared for dispensary stock. The following labelling requirements apply to 'in-house' stock:

1. The quantity in the container.
2. The name of the medicine.
3. The strength of the medicine.
4. Batch identification.
5. Date of preparation.
6. Storage conditions.
7. Expiry date.
8. Shake the bottle (if appropriate).
9. An indication if the product is for external use.
10. Name and address of the pharmacy.

Storage conditions

Storage conditions for medicines should be selected to prevent contamination and to minimize the inevitable deterioration of the product and allow for the maximum possible shelf-life. The factors affecting the stability of dosage forms are discussed fully in Chapter 7. Appropriate storage conditions for products compounded to an 'official' formula are usually given in the monograph. For 'unofficial' products the storage conditions for the individual ingredients should be noted.

Expiry date

The shelf-life of a product compounded in the pharmacy may be predicted from stability tests under storage conditions or by accelerated stability testing under extreme conditions. The data may be obtained from the literature or may be determined empirically. It may be necessary to state an expiry date for unopened packs, together with a statement further limiting the shelf-life after opening.

Table 5.2 Suggested maximum shelf-life for preparations extemporaneously prepared or diluted

Type of formulation	Additional information	Suggested shelf-life	
		As pharmacy stock	After issue to patient
'Official' full formula	No comment	Total shelf-life 12 mth, reduce to 3 mth if opened	4 weeks
'Official' full formula	To be recently prepared	Total shelf-life 1 mth, therefore 2 weeks as stock	2 weeks
'Official' full formula	To be freshly prepared	Prepared not more than 24 h before issue	2 weeks
Diluted 'official'	See official book	Usually prepared not more than 24 h before issue	2 weeks
'Unofficial' unresearched	None	Prepared not more than 24 h before issue	2 weeks
'Unofficial' researched	See data	Refer to stability data	
Particularly unstable	See data	Prepared just before issue	Refer to data
Aqueous antiseptic solution	Non-sterile	Prepared just before issue	1 week
Oral liquid prepared from granules or powder just before issue	See product literature	Prepared just before issue	1 week or 2 weeks see literature
Diluted proprietary product	See product literature	Usually prepared not more than 24 h before issue	Usually 2 weeks

Most hospital pharmacy departments have guide-lines for expiry dates based on their own stability data and experience. Students may find the maximum storage times recommended in Table 5.2 a useful guide.

E. Information sources

The effective use of information sources is an essential part of dispensing. A list of basic sources of information for compounding and dispensing is provided in Table 5.3. Further sources of information are described in Appendix 8. Additional information may be obtained from specialist information services in local and regional drug information centres.

Table 5.3 Basic information sources for compounding and dispensing*

Alder Hey Book of Children's Doses (ABCD)
ABPI Data Sheet Compendium
British National Formulary (BNF)
British Pharmacopoeia (BP)
Drug Tariff
Guide to Good Dispensing Practice
Martindale: The Extra Pharmacopoeia
Medicines, Ethics and Practice — A Guide for Pharmacists
Medicines and Poisons Guide
Monthly Index of Medical Specialities (MIMS)
Paediatric Vade Mecum
Pharmaceutical Codex (PC)
Pharmaceutical Handbook

* For more detailed lists, see Appendix 8.

GUIDELINES FOR STUDENTS

It is essential to develop a high standard of professional practice during training. Arrive for your class well prepared and try to work independently. Confidence in your own ability will grow with self reliance. Remember that teaching staff are usually a more reliable source of help than fellow students. Mistakes are an inevitable and useful part of the learning process so long as they are recognized and corrected.

The premises and equipment are provided in the dispensing laboratory of your School to simulate the situation in practice.

Personal standards

1. *Wear a freshly laundered coat overall:* This is to protect the medicines from contamination as well as to protect your clothes. For the same reason long hair should be tied back and preferably covered. Hands should be clean and any open lesions covered.

2. *Provide personal equipment:* An adequate supply of pens, pencils and a ruler will be required. An electronic calculator and a pair of scissors are also essential. A clean glass cloth should be used to polish bottles and a duster is useful for wiping dry spills. Borrowing from other students is an inconvenience to all concerned.

3. *Work in a clean and tidy manner:* The working space should be kept clear of books and papers whilst compounding and used equipment should be cleared away at once. One ingredient should be collected at a time and the stock container returned to the correct shelf immediately after use.

4. *Avoid contamination of all materials:*

— Do ensure all equipment is clean before use.
— Do keep the bench clear of all unnecessary items.
— Do not leave stoppers off containers.
— Do not return material to stock containers.
— Do not leave weighed or measured ingredients uncovered and unlabelled on the bench.
— Do not allow raw materials or dispensed products to come into direct contact with the hands (if necessary wear disposable gloves).

5. *Accuracy is essential:* Take care to select the correct ingredient or medicine — many have similar-looking names. Weigh and measure carefully, and avoid approximations where possible.

Documentation

It is important to develop a systematic approach to documentation in order to:

— Provide a data base for future class work.
— Prepare for a practice environment.

The record sheet for products compounded in the dispensing class should contain all the information listed under 'D. Control procedures: Documentation' above. In addition, it is useful to record details of equipment on the first occasion of use, e.g. filter media, sieves, suppository moulds, etc. for future reference.

A systematic approach to compounding

a. Copy out the formula onto your record sheet.
b. Check the legal categories and doses of ingredients.
c. Confirm that there are no pharmaceutical or pharmacological incompatibilities in the preparation.
d. Look up the appropriate storage conditions for the preparation.
e. Select the appropriate container and closure.
f. Prepare the label.
g. Check the calculations.
h. Select the correct method of preparation.
i. Make the preparation.
j. Check the preparation, the records and the label.
k. Pack the preparation, affix the label and polish the bottle (if appropriate).

A similar systematic approach to the dispensing of prescriptions is described in Chapter 9.

Learning to use information sources

It is important that you develop the ability to find relevant information quickly since this is an essential attribute of the practising pharmacist.

— Become familiar with all the information sources in Table 5.3.
— Compare information from several reference sources.
— Make a note on your record of the source(s) used.
— Always use current editions of texts (unless a previous edition is specified).

Competencies

The competencies that are required for good dispensing practice include:

1. Establishing the validity of the prescription.
2. Interpreting the wishes of the prescriber.
3. Checking the suitability of the prescription.
4. Exercizing the skills of formulation and compounding.
5. Predicting the shelf-life and storage requirements.
6. Selecting a suitable container and closure.
7. Assuring the quality of all medicines supplied.
8. Preparing appropriate labels.
9. Providing an information service for patients and for prescribers.
10. Maintaining necessary records.

Details of each of these competencies are to be found in various parts of this book.

BIBLIOGRAPHY

Alder Hey Book of Children's Doses 1982 4th edition Liverpool Health Authority, Liverpool
ABPI Data Sheet Compendium, current edition Datapharm

Publications, London (updated annually)
British National Formulary 1988 16th edn. British Medical Association and Royal Pharmaceutical Society of Great

Britain, London (updated twice yearly)

British Pharmacopoeia 1980 HMSO, London (and addenda 1982, 1983 and 1986)

British Pharmacopoeia 1988 HMSO, London

Department of Health and Social Security 1983 Guide to good pharmaceutical manufacturing practice HMSO, London

Drug Tariff current edition HMSO, London (updated monthly)

Dunn W R, Hamilton D D 1986 Identification of competencies required by a pharmacist practising in community pharmacy. Appendix to determining the continuing education priorities for pharmacists. Pharmaceutical Journal 237: 225–228

Insley J, Wood B (eds) 1986 Paediatric vade mecum, 11th edn. Lloyd-Luke, London

Kalman S H, Schlegel J F 1979 Standards of Practice for the Profession of Pharmacy. American Pharmacy NS19: 133–147

Martindale, see Reynolds J E F

Medicines, ethics and practice — a guide for pharmacists 1989 No. 3. Royal Pharmaceutical Society of Great Britain, London (updated twice yearly)

Monthly Index of Medical Specialities (MIMS). Medical Publications Ltd, London

Pearce M E (ed) 1984 Medicines and poisons guide, 4th edn. Pharmaceutical Press, London (with cumulative amendments in the *Pharmaceutical Journal*)

Pharmaceutical Codex 1979 11th edn, incorporating the British Pharmaceutical Codex. Pharmaceutical Press, London

Pharmaceutical Society 1979 Guide to good dispensing practice. Pharmaceutical Journal 233: 157–158

Pharmaceutical Society 1971 Guide to good small-scale pharmaceutical manufacturing practice for pharmacists in retail pharmacy business. Pharmaceutical Journal 207: 195–196

Pharmaceutical Society 1981 Self-assessment of professional practice Pharmaceutical Journal 227: 250–254

Pharmacy 1986 The Report of a Committee of Inquiry appointed by the Nuffield Foundation. Nuffield Foundation, London

Reynolds J E F (ed) 1989 Martindale, the Extra pharmacopoeia, 29th edn. Pharmaceutical Press, London

United States Pharmacopeia Dispensing Information 1986 United States Pharmacopeial Convention, Rockville, MD

Wade A (ed) 1980 Pharmaceutical Handbook, 19th edn. Pharmaceutical Press, London

6. Formulation of dispensed products

J. A. Rees

Formulation is the process whereby a drug or drugs are combined with other substances (adjuvants or excipients) to produce a dosage form (or formulation) suitable for administration to or by a patient.

A modern formulation should be an elegant, stable preparation, which is acceptable to the patient but at the same time is designed to provide the correct dose of drug in a therapeutically active and bioavailable form. The reader is referred to the companion volume (Aulton 1988) for a more detailed discussion of many aspects of the formulation of dosage forms.

Patient acceptability

In order to be acceptable to the patient, the formulated product must comply with certain criteria. Most importantly, the formulation should not offend the patient's senses of sight, feel, taste and smell; on first appearance the formulation should look, feel, taste and smell good. Obviously, all four senses will not always be used to assess all products, for example, patients are not normally expected to taste ointments and lotions. However, an 'ideal' formulated product should have an acceptable uniform colour and consistency as well as having no unpleasant odour, taste or feel. For example, formulated products for oral use should have both an acceptable and preferably pleasant taste and odour. Unpleasant aftertaste should be avoided if at all possible. Oral liquids should be easy to pour, easy to resuspend (if necessary), pleasant to taste, easy to swallow and ideally non-cariogenic (that is, does not cause dental caries). Capsules and tablets should not appear to be a formidable size to patients. External products, such as ointments and creams, should be ideally non-irritant, non-allergenic, non-staining, easy to apply and cause a pleasant feeling to the skin.

If a formulated product is to be acceptable to the patient then it is equally important that the product is seen to be suitable for the purpose or role for which it is prescribed. For example, ointments should spread and soften on the skin, products for insertion into body cavities should be of a suitable shape and size, lotions should be easy to apply, etc. However, problems may arise when a product does not appear to the patient to be suitable for treating his or her condition. For example, suppositories may be prescribed for the relief of asthma or rheumatoid arthritis, and some systemically active drugs are delivered by the transdermal route. In such cases the pharmacist must inform and reassure the patient that the prescribed product is suitable for the relief of their condition.

Finally, all formulated products ideally should be non-toxic, non-harmful, incapable of supporting the growth of micro-organisms and as free as possible from side-effects.

Routes of administration

There are various routes of administration for drugs and each route will present the formulator with the choice of several different types of formulations. Table 6.1

Table 6.1 Some of the routes of administration of drugs and some possible formulations

Route of administration	Possible formulations
Oral	Liquid medicines, e.g. mixtures, suspensions, syrups, elixirs Solid medicines, e.g. tablets, capsules, powders
Parenteral	Aqueous and oily injections Emulsions Intravenous fluids
Rectal	Suppositories Creams and ointments Aerosols
Topical	Creams and ointments Gels Lotions Liniments Transdermal delivery devices

shows some of the routes of administration as well as some of the possible formulations for each route. It can be seen, for example, that the oral route presents numerous different types of formulations. The different formulations lend themselves to different drugs for different conditions, as well as for different patients. For example, formulations for young children are invariably in a liquid form for ease of administration, whereas the same drug formulated for adults would probably be in a solid oral dosage form. Drugs that are difficult to tablet may well be presented in capsule form. Oils can be formulated as emulsions or encapsulated in a soft gelatin shell. For more detail on routes of administration, see the companion volume (Aulton 1988).

Formulation

Before formulating a drug into a dosage form it is essential to know the physicochemical characteristics of the drug as well as its therapeutic action. A consideration of these factors will enable the formulator to decide which types of formulation and routes of administration are feasible. For example, a drug which rapidly hydrolyses to inactive or toxic product(s) should not be formulated as an aqueous solution, whilst drugs which are inactivated in the stomach should not be formulated into an oral dosage form unless enteric coated.

All formulations consist of the drug plus at least one other substance (adjuvant or excipient). The main adjuvant is usually termed the vehicle, and the vehicle determines the physical form of the final formulation. The physical form of the formulation along with the vehicle and types of formulations can be seen in Table 6.2.

Besides the vehicle, most formulations will contain a number of other substances or excipients. Which excipients are included in the formulation will depend on the physicochemical nature of the final dosage form and the method of preparation. Excipients can be broadly categorized as:

1. Those providing an essential part of the dosage form.
2. Those preventing the degradation of the formulation.

The former category of excipients includes such substances as emulsifiers, suspending agents, gelling agents, binders, mould and die-wall lubricants. Without these substances the production of the formulation would be an impossible task. Excipients included in the formulation to prevent degradation include antioxidants, antibacterial and fungicidal preservatives and u.v. absorbers. It could be that without due care the excipients used to prepare the formulation may be more likely to degrade than the drug itself. Again the physicochemical nature of the formulation will dictate which excipients are required, for example, oils are susceptible to oxidation, so antioxidants are included in their formulation, while aqueous solutions support the growth of microorganisms and will need water-soluble preservatives. More examples will be found in the chapter on stability and storage (Ch. 7).

At all stages during the formulation of a pharmaceutical product it is important to consider whether the final product will be stable for a sufficient period of time to enable the product to be marketed and distributed to the final consumer. Therefore, it is essential that methods are devised to assess the stability of the product. What is required is a stability-indicating assay and accelerated stability tests.

Table 6.2   Final physical form of formulation, main vehicle and types of formulations

Final physical form	Main vehicle	Types of formulations
Liquid	Aqueous or oily liquid	Solutions, suspensions or emulsions
Solid	Powder	Powders, capsules, tablets
Semi-solid	Waxes and oils or emulsions	Ointments, creams
Aerosol	Organic solvents	Aerosols

Table 6.3   Examples of constraints in formulation reproduced with permission from the author and Elsevier/North Holland Biomedical Press (Jones 1977).

Scientific	— Instability of drug in biological fluids
Technical	— Poor suspendability/compressibility of drug
	— Absence of theoretical knowledge on pharmaceutical processes
Patient	— Age, disease, intelligence, diet Acceptance and compliance
Therapeutic	— Site and duration of activity
Drug	— Potency v. size of dose
Market	— Bulk/unit packs
	Environmental conditions of transport and storage
Economic	— Degree of sophistication of technology
	— Ingredient and process costs
	— Capital expenditure
Legal	— Variations in registration acceptability, e.g. excipients
	— Patents
Time	— Integration in overall R & D activity

It can be seen that the formulation of a drug into a suitable dosage form is a complex process. Table 6.3 shows some of the overall constraints in the formulation process. This list is not comprehensive nor in an order of priority, but serves to illustrate the complexity of the formulation process. The reader is referred to the companion volume (Aulton 1988) for detailed information.

Certain general aspects of formulation not considered in great detail elsewhere in this book, will be described in the following pages.

COLOUR

Pharmaceutical preparations are coloured for the following reasons:

1. *To mask an unpleasant appearance.* As stated previously pharmaceuticals should look good in order to inspire confidence in them and aid patient compliance. Therefore, an unpleasant appearance, such as a pale, insipid-looking mixture or mottled tablets, can be improved by the addition of colour.

2. *To increase their acceptability to patients.* It is generally believed that brightly coloured liquids and flesh-tinted ointments are more likely to be used because they are attractive.

3. *To prepare products of a consistent colour.* For example, natural calamine is not constant in colour and has been replaced by an artificially prepared material tinted with a form of ferric oxide.

4. *To aid identification.* Colours may be used to distinguish between two or more different strengths of a tablet or capsule. However, the use of colour to identify drugs has its objectors. Some objectors believe that coloured oral dosage forms increase the danger of children mistaking them for sweets. Also, the general reliance on colour as a means of identification may lead to the dangerous assumption that a particular colour is always associated with a particular drug. On the other hand, in the case of accidental poisoning by drugs, then colours can often expedite recognition of a product and allow more effective treatment of poisoning to commence sooner.

5. *To give warning.* Colours may be used to indicate preparations that should not be taken internally. A violet dye in mineralized methylated spirits is used to distinguish it from surgical spirit. Antiseptic solutions may also be coloured for hospital use.

Desirable properties of a colouring agent

1. It should be harmless to health and should have no pharmacological activity.

2. It should be a definite chemical compound because then its colouring power will be reliable, its assay practicable, and it will be easier to ensure freedom from harmful impurities.

3. Ready solubility in water is desirable in most cases but some oil-soluble and spirit-soluble colours are necessary.

4. Its tinctorial (colouring) power should be high so that only small quantities are required.

5. It should be unaffected by light, tropical temperatures, hydrolysis and micro-organisms and thus be stable on storage.

6. It should not be affected by oxidizing or reducing agents or by pH changes.

7. It should be compatible with medicaments and not interfere with the tests and assays to which the preparations containing it are subject.

8. It should not be appreciably adsorbed on to suspended matter.

9. It must be free from objectionable taste and odour.

10. It must be readily available and inexpensive.

Selection of the appropriate colouring agent

It is usual to employ a colour appropriate to the flavour of the medicine and vice versa, e.g. red with cherry, strawberry, or raspberry flavour, yellow with citrus fruits and banana, and green with mint flavours. The colouring dyes selected must be permitted for use in the country concerned. In the UK, most dyes permitted for use in foods may also be used in medicines. In approving a permitted list, account is taken of the European Economic Council Directive on food colours. The Ministry of Agriculture, Fisheries and Food prepares a list of permitted food additives. Most of these permitted items are allocated a serial number. The serial numbers are used to facilitate specific declaration and make identification more certain on labels. Below is a list of some permitted colours.

Number	Colour range	Example
100–110	yellows	E102 Tartrazine
120–128	reds	E123 Amaranth
131–133	blues	E131 Patent blue V
140–142	greens	E140 Chlorophyll
150–155	black and browns	E150 Caramel
170–175	metallic	E172 Iron oxides

Tartrazine

Tartrazine is a colouring agent which is known to give rise to hypersensitivity in certain individuals, especially those sensitive to aspirin. Tartrazine was included in a number of official and commercial preparations but is gradually being replaced. (If older BPC formulations which contain tartrazine are ordered for sensitive patients, the products can be prepared specially omitting the dye.

FLAVOURING AGENTS

One of the aims of formulation is to produce a palatable and hopefully pleasant-tasting medicine. An objectionable taste may lead to nausea and vomiting and refusal to take the preparation regularly or at all. On the other hand, a pleasant flavour may well encourage the continuation of the treatment and patient compliance. For these reasons it is usual to use flavouring agents to mask unpleasant tastes and make medicines more acceptable to the patient.

Identification of flavours

Complex mechanisms are involved in the appreciation of flavour. The taste buds of the tongue are sensitive to a number of basic tastes, i.e. sweet, sour, bitter, salt and, possibly, metallic and alkaline, but their response is modified by additional factors such as the temperature, physical nature and special characteristics (e.g. astringency and pungency) of the flavoured material. Also, since many flavours are odorous, the brain receives additional impulses from the olfactory receptors in the nose which it coordinates with the gustatory stimuli to produce the mingled sensation that is recognized as the flavour of a substance.

Problems of flavouring

The acceptance of a flavour is influenced by age. In general, children like fruit-flavoured syrups, adults prefer a more acid taste, while many old people find mint or wine flavours more agreeable. The threshold values at which individuals detect and like or dislike flavours differ, and blindness to certain tastes is known. Response may not be the same in health and disease, while a flavour that is acceptable for a short time may become objectionable if treatment is prolonged.

The selected flavour must be non-toxic, soluble (if for a clear product like an elixir) and stable in and compatible with the preparation.

Sweetening agents that raise blood sugar or increase calorie intake cannot be included in formulations for diabetics or patients on restricted diets.

Principles of flavouring

The creation of an acceptable flavour is more of an art than a science and the most useful background is practical experience, but, even with a wealth of this, much trial and error may be unavoidable.

Ideally, an unpleasant taste should be masked completely but this may be impossible or attainable only by creating a flavour that is no more acceptable than the original; in these circumstances the flavourist has to be satisfied with making the preparation palatable.

Often, the flavour is built upon a sweetened base, which is usually a syrup but may be a mucilage prepared from a cellulose ester or an alginate and containing a synthetic sweetener. Apart from sweetness, these viscous materials give the product a better 'feel' in the mouth.

An important means of selecting flavouring agents for addition to the base is to taste the objectionable medicament and attempt to recognize undertones reminiscent of pleasant flavours. Use of such flavours may significantly improve the taste of the drug. Blending of tastes in this way is generally more effective than adding a large excess of a powerful but unrelated flavour. Examples of satisfactory blending are citrus and mint flavours with bitter drugs, butterscotch and caramel flavours with salty drugs and fruit flavours with acid drugs.

Bitterness is the hardest basic taste to cover. Some bitter medicaments leave a persistent and unpleasant after-taste which occasionally can be overcome by a lingering flavour such as chocolate or apricot, or by including adjuncts, such as glycine and monosodium glutamate, that have been found to reduce this effect.

Other additives include menthol and peppermint oil, which appear to have a mild local anaesthetic action on the taste buds, sodium chloride and sodium citrate, which help to reduce bitterness, and citric acid, which obscures some types of bitter taste and sometimes improves the ability of citrus flavours to cover acid tastes.

Tests should be performed on the complete preparation because other ingredients, such as antimicrobial preservatives, may modify the taste.

There are a number of rather specialized methods of obscuring an unpleasant taste:

1. Formulation of the medicament as a sweet; amethocaine, used to anaesthetize the throat before bronchoscopy, has been dispensed in lollipops.

2. Use of a virtually insoluble and, therefore, comparatively tasteless derivative of a drug; e.g. chloramphenicol cinnamate or palmitate instead of the very bitter parent antibiotic.

3. Use of effervescent powders, granules or tablets. These contain the medicament, a sweetener, sodium or

potassium bicarbonate and citric or tartaric acid. When the preparation is added to water the carbonated, sweetener solution obscures the taste of salines such as potassium citrate.

Types of flavouring

Sweetening agents

Sucrose Sucrose is used in lozenges and tablet coatings and, as Syrup BP (sometimes refered to as simple syrup), as the base flavour in linctuses and some elixirs.

Invert syrup This is made from the mixture of fructose and glucose obtained by acid hydrolysis of sucrose. It is sweeter than simple syrup because fructose is sweeter than sucrose. The relative sweetness of four important sugars is — sucrose 100, fructose 173, dextrose 74 and lactose 16. Sometimes, on standing, sucrose crystals separate from preparations containing simple syrup; this can be reduced by replacing part of the simple syrup by invert syrup. Fructose is relatively thermolabile and the syrup darkens if not kept cool.

Sorbitol This hexahydric alcohol is used as a 70% w/w solution which is about half as sweet as simple syrup. Its compatibility and stability are good and it does not separate in preparations, such as elixirs, containing up to 40% of ethyl alcohol. When taken orally there is no rise in blood sugar and thus it can be used to replace simple syrup in formulations for diabetics. Like invert syrup, it can be mixed with simple syrup to prevent crystallization on storage.

Saccharin Saccharin and saccharin sodium are both used and are between 300 and 500 times as sweet as sucrose. The former is less palatable and leaves an unpleasant after-taste. A convenient method of adding saccharin sodium is in the form of a 10% w/v solution. 1% v/v of this concentrate is suitable for most liquids. Hydrolysis takes place in water and the decomposition product is bitter; breakdown is very slow in the cold (less than 1% after 6 months) but more serious if the solution is heated, particularly if acids and fruit juices are present. It is non-toxic and is excreted unchanged within 24 hours.

Saccharin sodium is also used to sweeten tablets, since it is less likely than carbohydrates to cause dental caries; it is used in toothpastes and other preparations for oral hygiene. Products for patients on diabetic or slimming diets can be sweetened with it and if a viscous preparation is desired, a mucilage made from an alginate (e.g. 2.5% sodium alginate), a cellulose ester (e.g. 1.5% sodium carboxymethylcellulose) or tragacanth (1.5%) is suitable.

Flavoured syrups

Fruit-flavoured syrups These are made from fruit juices (e.g. blackcurrant, raspberry and cherry) or indirectly, from the peel of citrus fruits (e.g. lemon and orange). Fruit juice syrups are acceptable to children, and all syrups, particularly the citrus types, are useful for disguising acid or sour flavours. Lemon Syrup BP contains citric acid which gives it a pleasant tart flavour that blends well with acid drugs. Blackcurrant, citrus and raspberry syrups are suitable for cough mixtures, salines and bitter drugs (e.g. sulphonamides), respectively.

Syrups with weak therapeutic activity A number of flavouring agents are made from vegetable extracts with weak therapeutic activity. For example, the pleasantly aromatic odour and pungent taste of ginger syrup makes it a satisfactory flavour for laxative mixtures containing rhubarb, while its carminative action (ability to relieve flatulence) is helpful in such a preparation.

Liquorice liquid extract has a mild expectorant action that is useful in cough mixtures in which its powerful, lingering, sweet flavour is excellent for covering salty tastes. Unfortunately, its flavour is not widely liked.

Cocoa syrup This is popular in America for disguising bitter drugs in paediatric preparations.

Aromatic oils

Volatile oils, such as anise (aniseed), caraway, cinnamon, clove, dill, ginger, lemon, orange and peppermint, are used as flavouring agents in a variety of forms. The vehicles of mixtures are often aromatic waters while alcoholic or hydroalcoholic solutions of oils (tinctures or, more often, spirits) provide convenient concentrated preparations for flavouring purposes (lemon, peppermint and compound orange spirits, and strong ginger tincture are examples).

Certain oils have become associated with particular types of preparation; for example, anise (cough mixtures and lozenges), peppermint (indigestion mixtures), dill (gripe waters), clove (dentifrices) and volatile bitter almond oil (emulsions).

Flavours containing aromatic oils (except lemon and orange) are more suitable than fruit syrups for neutral preparations.

Lemon and orange oils keep badly and develop an unpleasant turpentine-like taste. By removing most of the terpenes, terpeneless oils are produced which, compared with the natural oils, are about 20 times stronger in flavour and odour, are more readily soluble and have better stability.

Synthetic flavours

In addition to synthetic sweeteners other synthetic chemicals are used in flavouring. There are often preferred to natural materials because of their more constant composition, more ready availability, lower cost, greater stability and more predictable incompatibilities.

Chloroform has an agreeable, warm, sweet taste and Chloroform Water BP is widely used as a vehicle for mixtures. The spirit and emulsion of chloroform are alternative, more concentrated preparations.

For emulsified products, soft flavours like benzaldehyde and vanillin are most suitable. Benzaldehyde has the odour of bitter almonds and is a substitute for wild cherry syrup and volatile bitter almond oil. Vanillin is useful when, as with liquid paraffin emulsions, the medicament has a bland taste. Fractionated coconut oil, a non-aqueous vehicle for oral preparations, is difficult to flavour because of its oily nature; imitation ground-almond and olive oil flavours are suitable.

A variety of organic compounds, such as alcohols, aldehydes, esters, fatty acids, ketones and lactones, are used, alone or combined with essential oils, in the formulation of imitation flavours.

Flavour assessment

Understandable aversion to tasting drugs makes volunteers hard to find. Luckily flavourists often eliminate their less successful efforts by tests on themselves. It is wise to subject new volunteers to a preliminary test in which each tastes three samples, two of which are the same while the other is only slightly different; an acceptable volunteer must detect the odd one. Only a few samples should be examined at each session because repeated tasting numbs the taste buds and so raises the taste threshold. The full dose of the preparation must be taken and the experiment should be designed to minimize the effects of personal variation and other factors such as temperature, age, environment and time of day.

Stability of flavours

When a satisfactory flavour has been created it is necessary to confirm that it is stable in the preparation and unaffected by the container. Deterioration of flavours may be accelerated by alkaline pH (e.g. cinnamon oil), hydrolysis (e.g. esters) and oxidation (e.g. citrus oils), while loss may occur through volatilization from an imperfectly fitting closure or by adsorption into certain plastics. The preparation should be subjected to an accelerated storage test to show that none of these problems exists.

INCOMPATIBILITY

Incompatibility occurs when the components of a medicine interact in such a way that the properties of that medicine are adversely affected. Incompatibility may be detected by changes in the physical, chemical and therapeutic qualities of the medicine. Such changes may affect the safety, efficacy and appearance of the medicine.

Today's pharmacist is unlikely to see many incompatibilities because he/she mainly dispenses proprietary preparations or prepares medicines from official formulae. However, the possibility of incompatibility occurs when proprietary medicines are diluted or mixed together or placed in an unsuitable container or package. If the doctor prescribes a special formula containing a list of names and quantities of ingredients then the pharmacist should be on the look out for possible incompatibilities. Obviously any pharmacist employed as a formulator in the pharmaceutical industry should be aware of possible incompatibilities in new or proposed formulations.

Incompatibility may be pharmaceutical or therapeutic.

Therapeutic incompatibility arises when a medicine contains two or more antagonistic substances, the effect of which counteract or enhance each other, or when the action of one component in the body affects the action of another component. For example, a medicine containing an expectorant and a cough suppressant drug would be considered to be a therapeutic incompatibility.

Pharmaceutical incompatibility arises when the components of the medicine interact either physically or chemically to give an unsuitable product. Examples of pharmaceutical incompatibility are given below.

Physical incompatibility

Physical incompatibility is usually demonstrated in pharmaceutical formulations as immiscibility or insolubility. Such incompatibility can cause unsightly, non-uniform products from which it is difficult to remove the correct dose.

Immiscibility

1. Oils are immiscible with water, a problem that may be overcome by emulsification or solubilization.

2. Care is necessary when concentrated hydro-alcoholic solutions of volatile oils, such as spirits and concentrated waters, are used as adjuncts (e.g. flavouring agents) in aqueous preparations. To prevent the oil separating in relatively large globules, the hydroalcoholic solution should either be gradually diluted with the vehicle before admixture with the remaining ingredients or poured slowly into the vehicle with constant stirring.

3. Addition of high concentrations of electrolytes to mixtures in which the vehicle is a saturated aqueous solution of a volatile oil causes the oil to separate and collect as an unsightly surface layer. This happens with Potassium Citrate Mixture BPC in which the large quantity of soluble solids salts out the lemon oil and, to disperse this evenly, quillaia tincture is added as a suspending and emulsifying agent.

Insolubility

1. In liquid preparations, containing indiffusible solids such as chalk and sulphadimidine (in mixtures) and calamine and zinc oxide (in lotions), a thickening agent is necessary to obtain an elegant product from which uniform doses can be removed.

2. Some insoluble powders such as sulphur and certain corticosteroids and antibiotics are difficult to wet with water. Wetting agents (e.g. saponins, for sulphur-containing lotions, and polysorbates, for parenteral suspensions of corticosteroids and antibiotics) are used to distribute the powder and prevent formation of a slowly dispersing, solid-stabilized foam on shaking.

3. The deflocculating action of excess surface-active agent may cause claying. This may be controlled by reducing the surfactant concentration.

4. When a preparation contains a *potent* insoluble medicament, failure to shake thoroughly or delay in removing the dose before significant sedimentation has re-occurred, may lead to dangerously high concentrations of the drug in the last few doses. Sometimes it is possible to substitute a chemically equivalent amount of a soluble derivative of the drug, e.g. an alkaloidal salt for an alkaloid.

5. Dispersions of hydrophilic colloids such as polysaccharide mucilages are precipitated by high concentrations of alcohol or salts but significant amounts are tolerated if well diluted and added in small amounts with vigorous stirring.

6. High concentrations of electrolytes cause cracking of soap emulsions by salting out the emulgent.

7. Sometimes, vehicles consisting of, or containing, one or more organic liquids (usually termed cosolvent solutions) are used to dissolve medicaments of low solubility. Water-soluble adjuncts, particularly inorganic salts, may be precipitated in such vehicles. The reader is referred to the companion volume for more information on physical incompatibilities (Aulton 1988).

Chemical incompatibility

This section will also include incompatibilities which may be described as physicochemical processes.

pH effects

Medicaments are often salts of weak acids and bases. These salts are usually soluble in water while most of the unionized acids and bases are practically insoluble. Consequently, if a solution of a salt of a weakly basic drug is made alkaline, the free base may be precipitated, while precipitation of free acid may occur if a solution of a weakly acidic drug is acidified. Whether precipitation occurs or not depends on:

1. The solubility of the unionized acid or base.
2. The pH of the solution.
3. The dissociation constant (pK_a) of the acid or base.

pH and disperse systems

Emulsions made with soaps, or emulgents, like self-emulsifying monostearin which contain soap, are incompatible with mineral acids which destroy the emulgent by precipitating the fatty acid.

Outside an optimum pH range, dispersions of natural polysaccharides, carbomer or sodium carboxycellulose lose viscosity — very rapidly in some instances. Below pH 3, alginic acid is precipitated from dispersions of sodium alginate and strong acids precipitate carboxymethylcellulose from mucilages of the sodium derivative. The gelling property of bentonite is greatly reduced in acid media but improved by adding alkaline substances.

When a disperse system, e.g. a cream, is mixed with another of different pH, precipitation and/or degradation of active ingredients may occur. Diluents for disperse systems must be chosen with care.

Soap emulsions and polyvalent cations

Emulsions prepared with alkali-metal, ammonium and triethanolamine soaps are incompatible with salts producing polyvalent cations. Double decomposition yields a polyvalent soap which inverts the emulsion.

Any incompatibility that causes phase inversion in an emulsified product may lead to poor release of any dissolved medicament.

Complexation

Many macromolecular adjuncts used in formulation form complexes in which medicaments and preservatives are bound to the macromolecules or trapped within micelles. This behaviour is most common with non-ionic macromolecules. Because these complexes are too large to penetrate cell membranes, the activity of the medicament or preservative may be greatly reduced. Further details on the process of complexation can be found in the companion volume (Aulton 1988).

Complex formation may be reversible and when unbound drug in the preparation has been utilized, it is replaced from the complex. When this situation permits an adequate level of medication, complexation may be used as a method of depot therapy. The complex provides a reservoir of drug from which a safe but sufficient concentration is available to the tissues over a prolonged period. A 10–15 per cent aqueous solution of povidone (polyvinyl-pyrrolidone) has been found suitable for this purpose.

Complex formation may also reduce the irritancy and improve the stability of a drug, as in the iodophores, which are complexes of iodine in which the halogen is bound to a water-soluble polymer (e.g. povidone) or solubilized in the micelles of surfactants (e.g. certain macrogol ethers).

On the other hand, therapeutic activity or adjunct efficiency may be seriously impaired by complex formation, particularly as many suspending agents (e.g. polysaccharides), emulgents (e.g. macrogol esters and ethers) and solubilizers, (e.g. polysorbates) exhibit the phenomenon. Instances of the complexation of preservatives are common.

Cationic and anionic compounds of high molecular weight

The valuable pharmaceutical and pharmacological properties of many organic compounds are associated with a large cation or a large anion. Interaction of ions of opposing types yields salts of very high molecular weight which, usually, are almost or entirely insoluble in water and lack the useful properties of the ions.

The salt may precipitate from solution, as in the following instances:

1. When an aqueous solution of chlorpromazine hydrochloride is mixed with certain anionic drugs such as phenobarbitone sodium, pentobarbitone sodium and benzylpenicillin potassium (May & Baker 1970, Riley 1970). Such mixtures must not be made prior to injection.

2. When anionic or cationic dyes are mixed together or with drugs or adjuncts of opposite ionic type. For example:

a. The soluble, edible coal tar dyes used for colouring internal medicines (e.g. amaranth and tartrazine) are sodium salts of organic acids (i.e. anionic compounds) and should not be dispensed with cationic dyes such as the derivatives of thiazine (e.g. methylene blue) and triphenylmethane (e.g. crystal violet). The precipitation, which may be slow and detectable only after long storage, results in loss of colour. With medicinally active dyes, such as brilliant green, crystal violet and the acridines, the interaction may, additionally, cause loss of therapeutic effect.

b. Anionic dyes may react with cationic drugs, such as phenothiazine derivatives (e.g. chlorpromazine salts) and antihistamines.

c. Cationic dyes may be precipitated by soaps and clays.

Precipitation is not always apparent because the salt may dissolve in excess of one of the reactants or in other constituents of the preparation. The incompatibility is detected by other changes, of which the following is an example:

Creams made with an anionic emulgent, e.g. a soap of Emulsifying Wax BP, may:

a. cream or crack if mixed with a cream in which a cationic emulgent, e.g. Cetrimide Emulsifying Wax BPC 1973, has been used,

b. hinder release of cationic medicaments to the tissues, or

c. lower the antimicrobial activity of a cationic medicament or preservative.

Many important antimicrobial agents are cationic organic compounds, e.g. the quaternary ammonium compounds (cetrimide, cetylpyridinium chloride, benzalkonium salts and domiphen bromide), chlorhexidine salts, dequalinium salts, acridines, triphenylmethane dyes and neomycin sulphate. Any incompatibility may reduce therapeutic activity, when the substance is present as a medicament, or lead to growth of contaminants, when it is added as a preservative.

The interaction of anionic compounds with cationic antibacterial agents is important in another context. Several cationic bactericides are used as skin disinfectants and, before they are applied, the skin should be thoroughly rinsed to remove traces of soap that might otherwise cause inactivation.

Care must be taken to avoid cationic-anionic incompatibilities when choosing a vehicle for a formulation. For example, the activity of cationic medicaments and preservatives may be impaired in suspensions made with anionic suspending agents such as clays, carbomer and sodium alginate. Coagulation and sedimentation of the suspension may also occur, due to neutralization of the charges of the dispersed particles.

Cation–anion incompatibilities are prevented by carefully examining the chemical structure of the medicaments and adjuncts in a proposed formulation so that the combined use of cationic and anionic ingredients can be avoided. For emulsified systems containing an ionic medicament or preservative it is often advantageous to use a non-ionic emulgent.

Reducing agents

Reducing agents often cause fading of dyes. Anionic dyes are most stable at acid pHs. For example, in experiments with solutions containing sodium metabisulphite, the pH above which fading began was 5 for amaranth and 4 for tartrazine (Pharmaceutical Society Laboratory Report 1856a,b). Some basic dyes (e.g. methylene blue, crystal violet and indigo carmine) are converted to a colourless (leuco) form.

Detection of incompatibility

It is the pharmacist's responsibility to consider whether an incompatibility is likely to occur. In some cases, the occurrence of an incompatibility will be obvious, e.g. a cracked cream. However, some incompatibilities will only be detected by sophisticated analytical techniques, e.g. hydrolysis may not be visible to the naked eye, but detectable by u.v. or h.p.l.c. analysis. It must always be borne in mind that some interactions may not occur instantly but over a time period resulting in delayed discoloration, precipitation, etc.

Incompatibility with containers

When formulating a dosage form it is important to remember that the dosage form will require some form of final container or package before presentation to the patient. Incompatibility can occur between the formulation and the packaging materials. A classic example is the softening of plastic containers by methyl salicylate ointment. More examples of unsuitable packaging will be found in Chapter 8 on 'Containers and closures for dispensed products'.

IMPROVIZATION

On occasions a pharmacist may have to improvize in order to satisfy the prescriber's requirements. The types of prescription which usually require improvization are:

1. For a product of a different strength from that normally marketed by a manufacturer.
2. For a mixture (usually paediatric) when the drug is unavailable in pure powder form, but is available as a tablet or capsule.

In order to obtain a product of a different strength, the pharmacist will dilute a stronger product. Examples where the product may be diluted are mixtures, linctuses, lotions, creams and ointments. The diluent is usually the vehicle used in the preparation of the product, or that specified under the relevant entries in the BNF or Pharmaceutical Codex. When a formulated product is diluted, there is the possibility that the stability of the final product will be reduced.

When a drug is available only as a tablet or capsule, but is required in a liquid form, then the quantity of drug required in the mixture may be obtained by using the relevant number of capsules or tablets. A suspending agent is added to the capsule contents or ground-up tablets and a suspension prepared extemporaneously. Chloroform water may be added as the preservative while simple colouring and flavouring agents may be added if necessary to improve the appearance of the final product. Unless stability data is available, the product should not be used later than 7 days after dispensing. Chapter 12 gives more details: see 'Suspensions as emergency formulations'.

BIBLIOGRAPHY

Aulton M E (ed) 1988 Pharmaceutics: the science of dosage form design. Churchill Livingstone, Edinburgh
British National Formulary 1988, No. 16. British Medical Association and Pharmaceutical Society of Great Britain, London
Brookes L G 1965 Use of synthetic sweetening agents in pharmaceutical preparations and foods. Chemist and Druggist 183: 421–423
Department of Health and Social Security 1983 Guide to good pharmaceutical manufacturing practice. HMSO, London
Food additives: identification by serial numbers. 1985 MAFF, HMSO, London
Jones T M 1977 In: Polderman J (ed) Formulation and preparation of dosage forms. Amsterdam, Elsevier/North Holland Biomedical Press

May and Baker 1970 Largactil in general medicine and anaesthesia. May and Baker, Dagenham
Pharmaceutical Society laboratory report 1956a Pharmaceutical Journal 176: 345
Pharmaceutical Society laboratory report 1956b Pharmaceutical Journal 177: 383–384
Pharmaceutical Society 1979 Guide to good dispensing practice. Pharmaceutical Journal 223: 157–158
Pharmaceutical Society 1981 Self-assessment of professional practice. Pharmaceutical Journal 227: 250–254
Pharmaceutical Society 1971 Small scale manufacturing in retail pharmacy. Pharmaceutical Journal 207: 195
Riley B B 1970 Incompatibilities in intravenous solutions. Journal of Hospital Pharmacy 28: 228–240

7. Storage and stability of dispensed products

J. A. Rees

It is true to say that no pharmaceutical product is stable indefinitely and certainly the majority of products are stable only for a limited time.

The instability of pharmaceutical products may be demonstrated as drug or excipient degradation. All instability is thermodynamic in nature, but this inherent instability may be exacerbated by poor formulation, poor packaging and poor storage conditions.

Rhodes (1984) has reported six possible results of pharmaceutical product instability. This list is not meant to be fully comprehensive or exhaustive.

1. Loss of active drug (e.g. aspirin hydrolysis, oxidation of adrenaline).

2. Loss of vehicle (e.g. evaporation of alcohol from alcoholic mixtures, evaporation of water from oil-in-water creams).

3. Loss of content uniformity (e.g. impaction of suspensions, creaming of emulsions).

4. Reduction in bioavailability (e.g. ageing of tablets resulting in a change in dissolution profile).

5. Loss of pharmaceutical elegance (e.g. fading of coloured solutions and tablets).

6. Production of potentially toxic materials (e.g. breakdown products from drug degradation).

It is usual to classify the degradation of pharmaceutical products as being due to chemical, physical and biological mechanisms. In some cases the degradation may be due to one or more of these mechanisms or what appears to be the result of one mechanism may be the result of another mechanism. For example, a cracked emulsion (a physical effect) may be the result of microbial degradation of the emulsifier.

CHEMICAL DEGRADATION

Solvolysis

Solvolysis involves the degradation of the drug or excipients through reaction with the solvents present in the formulations. In most pharmaceutical products the solvent is water so that the degradation will be hydrolysis. However, in some pharmaceutical products the solvent may include such cosolvents as ethyl alcohol, propylene glycol and glycerol together with water.

Most of the solvolysis reactions involved in the degradation of drugs and excipients involve 'labile' carbonyl compounds, such as esters, amides, lactones and lactams. Examples include esters such as aspirin and the local anaesthetics, amides such as sulphonamides and chloramphenicol, lactones such as spironolactone and pilocarpine, and lactams such as the penicillins and cephalosporins.

Oxidation

Oxidation is an extremely common cause of drug and excipient degradation. This method of degradation occurs in both water- and oil-soluble drugs, as well as fixed and volatile oils.

A substance is said to be oxidized if it gains electronegative atoms or radicals or loses electropositive atoms or radicals. Oxidation often involves the addition of oxygen or removal of hydrogen. There are two types of oxidation processes which affect pharmaceutical products:

1. Those involving atmospheric oxygen.
2. Those involving the reversible loss of electrons.

The latter process can proceed under anaerobic conditions and is independent of atmospheric oxygen. Examples of drugs undergoing such an oxidation process are riboflavine, ascorbic acid, adrenaline and ferrous salts. Oxidation is usually demonstrated in the latter stages by a change in colour, e.g. adrenaline solution changes from a clear to a red-coloured solution.

Oxidation processes involving atmospheric oxygen, at ambient temperatures, are usually referred to as autoxidation. Autoxidation is usually a chain reaction involving the formation of free radicals in the initiation stage. In the propagation stage, the formation of peroxy radicals from oxygen and the free radicals produced in the initiation stage react with intact drug to produce hydroperoxides and more free radicals. These free radicals then combine with more molecular oxygen to form peroxy radicals and so on. Therefore in the propagation stage the products of the oxidation process are used to induce more oxidation, and so once the process has started it becomes self propagating until all the free drug has been used up and the termination stage reached. At this point the peroxy radicals and hydroperoxides combine to form inactive products.

Photolysis

Degradation of drugs or excipient molecules can be brought about by light, either room light or sunlight. Such reactions are termed photolysis and light-sensitive drugs are known as photolabile.

The shorter the wavelength of the light then the more potentially damaging is the light. Thus, u.v. light is more harmful than red/orange light. However, in order to cause a photolytic reaction the energy from the light radiation must be absorbed by the molecules. If the energy absorbed is sufficient to achieve the activation energy, then degradation of the molecule is possible. In some cases, the molecules absorbing the light do not themselves take place in the reaction, but pass on their increased energy to other molecules, which then degrade. In such cases, the light energy absorbing drug or molecule is said to be a photosensitizer.

Although the energy obtained from light may be the initiator of a reaction, the reaction itself may be an oxidation process, polymerization or ring rearrangement, etc. Also, since light energy may be converted to heat, photolysis may be accompanied by a thermal reaction. Alternatively, a photolytic reaction may produce a catalyst, which catalyses a thermal reaction. Once a thermal reaction is started it may proceed when the light source is removed.

Photolytic reactions include the decomposition of chlorpromazine hydrochloride, and other phenothiazines, the darkening of morphine and codeine, the fading of tartrazine dye and the initiation of many autoxidation processes.

Polymerization

Polymerization involves the combination of two or more identical molecules to form a much larger and complex molecule. Degradation of pharmaceutical products by polymerization is not very common and such reactions may occur after the initial degradation of the drug. Such an example of polymerization is the production of a straw-coloured solution after the autoclaving of dextrose injection. The coloured solution is attributed to the polymerization of the initial major degradation product, 5-hydroxymethyl furfural.

Optical isomerization

A change in the optical activity of a drug may result in a change in its biological activity. Racemization is the main type of optical isomerization which affects drug molecules and it occurs when the optically active form of the drug is converted into its enantiomorph. Racemization continues until 50% of the original drug has been converted to its enantiomorph. In most cases the enantiomorph has less therapeutic effect than the original drug. An example of racemization is the conversion of (−)-hyoscyamine into the racemic mixture of (+)- and (−)-hyoscyamine. Other examples include adrenaline, tetracycline and pilocarpine (Nunes & Brochmann-Haussen 1974).

Other methods of chemical degradation include hydration, dehydration, decarboxylation, dimerization, acylation and transesterification.

PHYSICAL DEGRADATION

Polymorphism

Polymorphs are different crystal forms of the same compound. Polymorphs differ from one another in their crystal energies, the more energetic ones converting to the least energetic (or most stable) one. Different polymorphs of the same drug may exhibit different solubilities and melting points. These physicochemical properties have significant implications for pharmaceutical dosage forms. For example, theobroma oil used in the preparation of suppositories has two polymorphs. The β form has a melting point at 37°C, whilst the α form has a melting point at 30°C. Conversion by excessive heating of the β form to the α form makes the theobroma oil unsuitable as a suppository base. Another well-documented example is the conversion of cortisone acetate to a less soluble form when the drug is formulated in aqueous suspension. The less soluble polymorph forms an insoluble cake in the aqueous suspension (Macek 1954).

This type of phenomena also occurs in ointments and creams when the presence of a less soluble drug gives a gritty feel to the product and poor release characteristics.

Vaporization

Many drugs and excipients may be lost from pharmaceutical products at ambient temperatures through vaporization. These drugs and excipients possess a sufficiently high vapour pressure that they are volatile at room temperatures. Examples of such drugs are glyceryl trinitrate, alcohols, camphor, menthol, chloroform and volatile oils. These drugs may be lost from the product because of a loose-fitting closure.

Water loss

Evaporation of water from liquid preparations will cause concentration of the drug with the possibility of crystallization occurring if the solubility of the drug in the solvent is exceeded. Water loss from oil-in-water creams may result in a decrease in volume and a surface rubbery feel. Further evaporation of the water will cause the emulsion to crack. Some drugs are efflorescent, which means that they will lose water to the atmosphere resulting in a concentration of the drug and overall weight loss. Water loss to the atmosphere can be prevented by storing the pharmaceutical product in a well-closed container.

Absorption of water

Water will be absorbed from the atmosphere by some drugs and pharmaceutical products. For example, some drugs are deliquescent (calcium chloride and potassium citrate), whereas others are hygroscopic (glycerol and dry plant extracts). Effervescent powders and tablets will deteriorate if stored in a moist atmosphere.

Particle sedimentation

This is mainly seen as creaming of emulsions when the disperse phase contains large globules as a result of coalescence and aggregation of smaller globules.

FACTORS INFLUENCING DEGRADATION

Temperature

An increase in temperature generally increases the rate of reactions and thus the degradation of pharmaceutical products is generally increased with an increase in temperature. The Arrhenius equation quantitatively describes the relationship between reaction (or degradation) rate (k) to temperature (T).

$$k = Ae^{\frac{-E_a}{RT}} \tag{7.1}$$

where A is the frequency factor, R is the gas constant, E_a is the activation energy and T is the temperature in degrees absolute.

Because an increase in temperature results in an increased rate of degradation, then one method of preventing or reducing degradation is to store the pharmaceutical product at low temperatures. For example, Insulin injections are normally required to be stored between 2°C and 8°C.

However, storage at low temperatures of some pharmaceutical products may not decrease the degradation rate as much as would be expected from the Arrhenius equation. For example, although the rate of oxidation is decreased at low temperatures, the solubility of oxygen in solution is increased. This increase in solubility may promote the oxidation process, so that the overall result is usually a decrease in oxidation but not as much as would have been predicted. An example of non-Arrhenius behaviour has been reported by Savello & Shangraw (1971) who showed an increased degradation rate of ampicillin solution on freezing.

A change of temperature, besides influencing chemical reaction rates, may also affect physical degradation rates. For example, an increase in temperature can cause creams and emulsions to become unfit for use and separate into two phases. Alternatively, freezing creams and emulsions will usually damage the emulsion structure due to the crystallization of water at 0°C. On reheating to ambient temperature the emulsion does not reform.

A decrease in temperature may cause a drug to exceed its solubility and crystallize · out from the solution. Sodium Lactate Infusion Compound BP (1988) (Hartman's solution) frequently exhibits crystallization at temperatures just below ambient.

An increase in temperature may result in an increased loss of volatile material or increased loss of water from pharmaceutical products. Such products should be stored in a cool place.

Solvent

Drugs may be placed in a variety of solvents in order to produce a suitable dosage form. However, the different solvents used may influence the degradation of the drug. Solvents alter the activity coefficients of the reactant molecules, but the change in solvent can also cause a change in pK_a, surface tension or viscosity, thus affecting the reaction rate (Fung 1979).

The most commonly used solvent is water and unfortunately many drugs hydrolyse in water. The hydrolysis rate can be catalysed by the presence of acids or alkalis which supply hydrogen ions or hydroxyl ions to the solution. The rate of hydrolysis may vary depending on the pH of the solution and a plot of log of the degradation rate against pH usually shows a pH at which the hydrolysis rate is at a minimum. Thus, one method of reducing drug degradation due to hydrolysis is to prepare the solution at the pH at which hydrolysis is minimized (if this pH is physiologically suitable). Buffer salts may be used to obtain the optimum pH. However, buffer salts may give rise to increased hydrolytic degradation due to general acid-base catalysis. General acid-base catalysis arises in the presence of some buffer salts but not with others. For example, the rate of degradation of hydrocortisone in aqueous solution is enhanced in the presence of phosphate and borate buffers (Hansen & Bundgaard 1979).

Oxidation of drugs in aqueous solution can be reduced by lowering the pH to between 3 and 4. The susceptibility of a drug to oxidation is related to its oxidation-reduction potential. This value is influenced by the pH of the solution. As the hydrogen ion concentration is increased, so the oxidation-reduction potential of the drug is increased resulting in the system becoming less oxidizing.

The addition of buffer salts and other ionic compounds to aqueous solutions may influence the degradation of a drug according to Equation 7.2.

$$\log k = \log k_o + 1.02\, Z_A Z_B \sqrt{\mu} \qquad (7.2)$$

where μ is ionic strength, k is the rate constant of degradation, k_o is the rate constant at infinite dilution and $Z_A Z_B$ are the charges carried by the reacting species. A plot of log k against μ should be a straight line if the degradation rate is influenced by the ionic strength of the solution. If the charges on the ions are the same then an increase in $\sqrt{\mu}$ will increase the degradation rate. If the charges on the ions are opposite then an increase in $\sqrt{\mu}$ will decrease the degradation rate. A summary of this effect is shown in Table 7.1.

Since many drugs are poorly water soluble, the addition of a non-aqueous solvent, such as alcohol, glycerol

and propylene glycol to an aqueous solution will improve the solubility characteristics of the drug. Also, non-aqueous solvents have been used to replace some or all of the water in a solution in order to reduce the hydrolysis of a drug. However, changing the solvent will alter the activity coefficients of the drug and other excipient molecules and the activation product which may lead to a change in degradation rates.

The relationship between the degradation rate and the relative solubilities of the drug and decomposition product in the solvent is given by Equation 7.3.

$$\log k = \log k_o + \frac{V}{2.30RT}(\triangle \delta_A + \triangle \delta_B - \triangle \delta^\star) \quad (7.3)$$

where k is the degradation rate constant, k_o is the rate constant at infinite dilution, V is the molar volumes of A,B and the activation product, R is the gas constant, T is the temperature in degrees absolute, $\Delta \delta_A$, $\Delta \delta_B$, $\Delta \delta^\star$ represent the differences between the solubility parameters of the reactants A and B and the activation complex* and those of the solvent. From Equation 7.3 it can be shown that if the degradation products have similar relative solubilities to the solvent, and the drug has dissimilar relative solubilities to the solvent, then the degradation will be favoured in that solvent and the degradation rate will be increased. In other words if the degradation product is more soluble than the original drug in the solvent then the degradation rate will be increased. Conversely, if the drug is more soluble than the degradation product in the solvent, then the degradation will be minimized (see Table 7.1).

The addition of a non-aqueous solvent, besides altering the relative solubilities, will cause a change in dielectric constant. The influence of the dielectric constant of the solvent will depend on the presence or absence of an electrical charge on the drug molecule. A generalized equation relates the rate constant (ln k) in the solvent system to the dielectric constant (D).

$$\ln k = \ln k_{D=\infty} - f \cdot \frac{1}{D} \qquad (7.4)$$

where ln $k_{D=\infty}$ is the rate constant in a solvent of infinite dielectric constant, f, is a variable depending on the reacting species present in the solvent.

If other ions such as OH^- or H^+ are present, then f becomes:

$$\frac{N\, Z_A\, Z_B\, e^2}{RTr^\star} \qquad (7.5)$$

where Z_A and Z_B are charges on the two ionic species, e is the charge on the electron, N is Avogadro's number and $r^\star$ is the distance between the ions in the activated complex.

Table 7.1 Effects of increasing dielectric constant and ionic strength on the rate of different reaction types

Reaction type	Effect on reaction rate of increasing:	
	Dielectric constant	Ionic strength
Two dipoles	Increase	No effect
Two ions		
Same signs	Increase	Increase
Opposite signs	Decrease	Decrease
Ion and dipole	Decrease	Increase

If a dipole and an ion are present in the solvent, then f becomes:

$$\frac{-N Z_A^2 e^2}{2RT}\left(\frac{1}{ra} - \frac{1}{r^\star}\right) \qquad (7.6)$$

where Z_A is the charge on the ionic species, ra is the radius of the ionic species and $r^\star$ is the radius of the activated complex.

Plotting $\ln k$ against $1/D$ should give a straight line relationship. If Z_A and Z_B have the same signs then the slope will be negative. In such cases, decreasing the dielectric constant by replacing water by some water-miscible solvent will decrease the degradation rate. Conversely if Z_A and Z_B have opposite signs, then the slope will be positive and replacing water by another solvent of lower dielectric constant will increase the degradation rate. If one of the reacting species is a dipole, then decreasing the dielectric constant of the solvent will increase the degradation rate. Table 7.1 summarizes the effects of both dielectric constant and ionic strength on degradation rates.

Moisture (atmospheric)

Moisture or humidity can adversely affect the stability of dry drug formulations, such as tablets and capsules. For example, gelatin capsules become soft and swell in the presence of moisture and the drug content of tablets may undergo surface hydrolysis (Cartensen & Pothisiri 1975). The presence of moisture may encourage the growth of micro-organisms.

Additives

Buffer salts

These may be used to adjust and maintain the pH of a formulation. However, they may cause general acid-base catalysis and ionic effects (see companion volume, Aulton 1988).

Surfactants

Surfactants may be added to formulations as solubilizers or emulsifiers. However, the presence of a surfactant may increase, decrease or leave unchanged the degradation of a drug or the excipients. Acceleration of degradation in the presence of surfactants acting as micellar catalysts is well documented (Fendler & Fendler 1975). Other references demonstrate the ability of surfactants to decrease the hydrolysis of poorly water-soluble drugs (Reigelman 1960). The presence of surfactants in aqueous solution have been shown to protect some drugs from oxidation (Amin & Bryan 1973). Some surfactants will trap

microbial preservatives within the micelles and so reduce the preservative content of the aqueous phase, resulting in the possibility of microbial degradation of the product.

Complexing agents

Some drugs have been mixed with other substances to produce a complex which is more stable than the uncomplexed drug. Examples of complexation include benzocaine and procaine complexed with caffeine to reduce hydrolysis (Higuchi & Lachman, 1955). More recently, Uekema et al (1983) have improved the thermal and photochemical stability of benzaldehyde in water by complexing the drug with α, β and γ cyclodextrins.

Antioxidants

Antioxidants are added to drug formulations to prevent or reduce oxidation. They can be conveniently classified according to the mechanism of action into:

1. Antioxygens
2. Reducing agents
3. Chelating agents

Antioxygens act by providing the necessary electrons and easily available hydrogen ions which are accepted by the free radicals and this stops the chain reaction in auto-oxidation. Antioxygens act as chain breakers. Examples of antioxygens are the gallates, α tocopherols and butylated hydroxyanisoles/hydroxytoluenes.

Reducing agents are substances which are preferentially oxidized and offer protection to the drug until they themselves are used up or until all the oxygen in the container has been removed. Sodium metabisulphite is the most commonly used reducing agent. Other reducing agents include hypophosphorous acid, dextrose, sulphurous acid and ascorbic acid.

Chelating agents act by complexing or chelating heavy metals present in solution which may be responsible for acting as catalysts in the oxidation process. Examples of chelating agents are sodium edetate and 2,3-dimercapto-propane sodium in vitamin C injection.

The reader is referred to the companion volume (Chapter 7, Aulton 1988) for further details on reaction kinetics, stability and stability testing.

STORAGE

In order to maintain the stability of a drug formulation, it should be suitably packed and stored. Storage conditions are laid down in the various compendial monographs and, in the case of manufactured goods, the manufacturer will define the appropriate storage conditions for the product. It is important that these storage conditions are adhered to and thus all pharmaceutical products should be labelled indicating the required storage conditions which will maintain the stability of the product for a known time. Because, even 'good' storage conditions will not maintain the stability of a product for ever, all pharmaceutical products should be labelled with an expiry date or a 'not to be used later than . . . . . .' date.

Storage in practice — stock control

Drug formulations are goods of a special type and although they should follow basic stock control principles they do have special considerations.

1. Drugs have a limited shelf-life and cannot be stored for ever.
2. Incorrect handling and storage may contribute to their degradation and hence shorten their shelf-life.
3. Drugs are prescribed to prevent diseases which may be of a seasonal or epidemic nature. Therefore the demand for drugs is difficult to predict.
4. Where alternative drug therapies exist, drugs may be prescribed at the whim of the prescriber, thus complicating demand predictions.

Whatever accommodation is chosen for storing pharmaceuticals, it is important that the following points are considered:

1. The accommodation has the correct combination of storage facilities.
2. Selection of drugs can be carried out with the minimum of effort.
3. Handling of drugs should be minimized.
4. The space should be used effectively.

Thus, in planning and choosing accommodation for storing drug formulations it is important that a dry, adequately ventilated, shady and cool room is chosen. Within the store room special facilities will be situated such as fridges, deep freezers and security cabinets. Inflammable goods should be stored in a special building equipped with fire-extinguishing facilities.

Pharmaceutical products should be stored according to some system, such as alphabetically, so that they are easily found. The only products not stored in such a system are those requiring special storage facilities. If drug formulations are stored alphabetically then the assembly of a collection of drugs for an order is a relatively simple task, even for new or unskilled staff. However, such a system may entail the collector covering a considerable floor area for the collection of just a few items. Where drugs are demanded very frequently then it may be possible to place them close to the dispensing area for ease of use. This would cut down the time required to assemble a collection. However, the staff would need to know and remember the location of the drugs and problems would arise with inexperienced or new staff. Even with this disadvantage many stores combine a popularity system with an alphabetical system.

A suitable stock control system and storage area should ensure adequate turnover of stock without excessive stock handling. Turnover is the ratio of annual purchases to average stock levels. Thus for the same yearly purchases, an item with a low turnover is indicated by a high average stock level, whereas an item with a high turnover is indicated by a low average stock level. Generally a low stock turnover implies that too much money is tied up in stock, on the other hand a very high stock turnover may result in high order preparation costs, since goods will be frequently ordered. Thus, a compromise must be sought between excessively low and excessively high turnovers. However, it must always be remembered that some drugs, by virtue of their special nature, may be prescribed only rarely, thus giving a low turnover. In such cases, the possibility of ordering when required, rather than keeping a stock, should be considered.

It is essential that drugs are stored so that packs received first are also the first to be issued. One method of ensuring the first-in, first-out rule is that stock is always taken from the front of the shelf and replenishment stock refilled onto shelves from the back.

Since drug formulations have a limited shelf-life, then it is essential that expiry dates on the packages are noted and recorded. Some system must be devised to enable the storekeeper to quickly identify drug formulations that are nearing their expiry date, so that action can be taken.

The store area itself should be designed to make the maximum use of the space available, whilst allowing ease of access and use to the staff employed. It should be well lit and free of obstructions.

REFERENCES

Amin M I, Bryan J T 1973 Kinetic factors affecting stability of methylprednisolone in aqueous formulation. Journal of Pharmaceutical Sciences 62(11): 1768–71

Aulton M E (ed) 1988 Pharmaceutics: the science of dosage form design. Churchill Livingstone, Edinburgh

Cartensen J T, Pothisiri P 1975 Decomposition of p-aminosalicylic acid in the solid state. Journal of Pharmaceutical Sciences 64: 37–44

Fendler J H, Fendler E J 1975 Catalysis in micellar and macromolecular systems. Academic, New York

Fung H L 1979 In: Barrier G S, Rhodes D T (eds) Modern pharmaceutics. Marcel Dekker, New York

Hansen J, Bundgaard H 1979 Studies on the stability of corticosteroids. I. Kinetics of degradation of hydrocortisone in aqueous solution. Archiv. for Pharmaci og Chemi, Scientific Edition 7: 135

Higuchi T, Lachman L 1955 Inhibition of hydrolysis of esters in solution by formation of complexes. I. Stabilization of benzocaine with caffeine. Journal of the American Pharmaceutical Association (Scientific Edition) 44: 521–526

Macek T J 1954 US Patent 2, 671, 750 (9 March 1954)

Nunes M A, Brochmann-Haussen E 1974 Hydrolysis and epimerization kinetics of pilocarpine in aqueous solution. Journal of Pharmaceutical Sciences 63: 716–721

Rhodes C T 1984 An overview of kinetics for the evaluation of the stability of pharmaceutical systems. Drug Development and Industrial Pharmacy 10: 1163–1174

Reigelman S 1960 The effect of surfactants on drug stability. I. Journal of the American Pharmaceutical Association (Scientific Edition) 49: 339–343

Savello D R, Shangraw R F 1971 Stability of sodium ampicillin solutions in the frozen and liquid states. American Journal of Hospital Pharmacy 28: 754

Uekama K, Narisawa S, Hirayama F, Otagiri M, Kawano K, Ohtani T, Ogino H 1983 Improvement of thermal and photochemical stability of benzaldehyde by cyclodextrin complexation. International Journal of Pharmacy 13: 253–261

8. Containers and closures for dispensed products

J. A. Rees

A pharmaceutical formulation cannot exist as a product and have a shelf-life without a suitable container and/or package. According to the Pharmaceutical Codex (1979), 'the function of a container for a medical preparation is to maintain the quality, safety and stability of its contents'. Packs for all types of pharmaceutical products are discussed by Dean in Chapter 12 of the companion volume (Aulton 1988), who defines packaging as 'an economical means of providing presentation, protection, identification/information, containment, convenience and compliance for a product during storage, carriage, display and use until such time as the product is used or administered'.

The containers and closures likely to be used by the pharmacist in hospital or community practice for dispensing or small-scale manufacture of non-sterile dosage forms are described below.

Although the final choice of a pack is inevitably a compromise between various requirements, the ideal container or package should:

1. *protect the contents from physical and mechanical hazards*. These include:
a. Vibration — usually due to transportation. The vibrations may vary in both amplitude and frequency.
b. Compression — this includes pressure applied during stacking or storage.
c. Shock — such as impact, drops or rapid deceleration.
d. Puncture — penetration from sharp objects or during handling operations.
e. Abrasion — this may create electrostatic effects.
2. *not interact with the product*. Equally importantly the product should not interact with the container. Interactions include migration, absorption, adsorption or extraction whereby ingredients either from the product or container are lost or gained. Examples include loss of preservative from aqueous solutions by absorption into rubber closures, softening of plastic containers by esters of salicylic acid, leaching out of plasticizers from plastic containers into pharmaceutical formulations and permeation of volatile substances from the formulation through plastic-walled containers.

3. *protect the contents from the effects of atmospheric gases*, such as oxygen and carbon dioxide. In other words, the container should be impervious to these and other gases. Oxygen has the ability to support the growth of micro-organisms, as well as being involved in oxidation processes. Carbon dioxide may cause pH shifts or occasionally a chemical reaction if absorbed by a liquid formulation.

4. *be capable of withstanding extremes of temperature and humidity*. There can be wide variations in temperature and humidity between seasons or between different latitudes. Containers may experience low temperatures during transportation in the winter months and products for domiciliary use may be stored in damp, hot bathrooms.

5. *protect the contents from both water loss and gain*. Moisture gain from the atmosphere may cause chemical reactions, encourage or initiate microbial growth or cause physical changes such as the softening of gelatin capsules. Moisture loss from a product may cause creams to contract and develop a rubbery feel, and solutions to concentrate.

6. *protect the contents from loss of volatile materials*. The amount of a volatile drug present in a formulation may be reduced, e.g. methyl salicylate, or the loss of excipients such as alcohol and chloroform will concentrate the product or reduce its preservative content.

7. *protect the contents from light*. Many drugs are photosensitive and degraded in the presence of light

8. *be sufficiently transparent to permit the inspection of the contents*. This may be impractical for drugs sensitive to light.

9. *protect the contents from airborne particulate contamination*. This contamination can be microbiological (bacteria, moulds or yeasts) or it can be solid matter such as dirt, dust, hair, fibres, etc.

10. *protect the product from animal contaminations*, e.g. rodents and insects.

11. *not shed particles into the contents*. Examples include spicules from glass bottles and metal flakes from metal ointment tubes.

12. *have a 'pharmaceutically elegant' appearance*. The appearance of a product may vary to some extent depending whether it is generic, proprietary or an over-the-counter product, and whether it is intended for sale or for dispensing.

13. *be easy to label and thus to identify the product*. In certain cases the label may be large relative to the package and cover most of the package.

14. *be convenient and easy to use*. It should be easy for the user to extract the contents or empty the container. When necessary the closure should be easily removed and replaced. However, child-resistant containers may not always satisfy this criteria. If the package is easy and convenient to use then patient compliance may be increased.

15. *be cheap and economical*.

Not all the above criteria can be met by the packages and containers currently available, but the pharmacist should select the container which seems to comply with most of the required properties.

Closures

With respect to closures, the Pharmaceutical Codex defines four types of container:

Airtight container. This container protects the contents from contamination with extraneous solids, liquids and vapours, from loss of volatile constituents, and from changes due to efflorescence, deliquescence and evaporation under ordinary conditions of handling, storage and transport.

Security closed container. This is an airtight container fitted with some means of preventing the unintentional displacement of the closure.

Hermetically sealed container. This container is impervious to air and other gases under ordinary conditions of handling, storage and transport. It is usually a glass ampoule sealed by fusion of the glass.

Child-resistant container. A container designed to prevent children gaining access to its contents. Such containers may be used when supplying medicines for domiciliary use, especially for substances known to be dangerous to children.

PACKAGING MATERIALS

There is an apparently infinite variety of containers for pharmaceutical products. Some containers are suitable for a number of products, e.g. glass bottles for oral medicines including solutions, suspensions, syrups and emulsions, whereas other containers are designed for one particular product, e.g. inhaler devices for bronchodilators. The pharmacist must use his or her professional judgement to select a suitable container and closure for each particular pharmaceutical product. In the following section the materials used to manufacture containers and closures will be described as well as giving typical examples and their uses.

Glass

Glass is a traditional packaging material which has been widely used for both liquid and solid dose forms. Its *advantages* are:

1. It can be moulded to a rigid construction in a variety of shapes and sizes.
2. It is available in clear or amber (light-resistant) forms.
3. It can be sealed hermetically or by removable closures.
4. It is impermeable to moisture and atmospheric gases.
5. It is cheap and readily available.
6. It is easily labelled.

The *disadvantages* of glass are:

1. It is fragile — easily breaking when dropped or knocked.
2. It is heavy, which means transportation costs are high.
3. It may release alkali to aqueous contents.

Types of glass containers

Bottles

These can be amber medicine bottles (Figs 8.1, 8.2) or fluted (ribbed) oval bottles (Fig. 8.3). Both types of bottles come in a variety of sizes (50 ml up to 500 ml) and are supplied with a screw closure.

Amber medicine bottles are used for all oral medicines including mixtures, elixirs, syrups, emulsions and linctuses. A paper label is fixed to the curved front surface.

Ribbed oval bottles have flutes down the back. The characteristic feel of the flutes warns the user, even in the dark or if blind or partially sighted, that the contents are not to be taken. This is further emphasized by a 'Not To Be Taken' label on the bottle. Ribbed oval bottles are used for mouthwashes, gargles, throat paints, liniments, lotions, inhalations and antiseptic solutions. A paper label is fixed to the plain front surface.

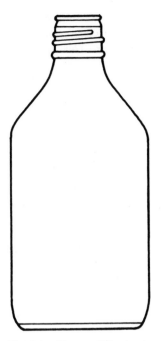

Fig. 8.1 Glass medicine bottle

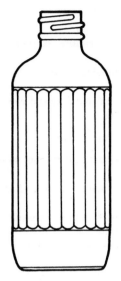

Fig. 8.3 Ribbed oval glass bottle

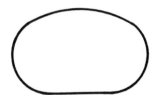

Fig. 8.2 Section of medicine bottle

Ear and nasal dropper bottles

These are generally hexagonal in shape, fluted on four sides, amber coloured and fitted with a rubber teat and glass dropper as the closure. They are similar to the eye dropper bottle (Fig. 28.3). The label is fixed to the plain sides of the bottle.

Containers for semi-solid preparations

These are wide-mouthed, squat, cylindrical pots made of clear or amber glass and fitted with a screw closure, which usually requires a paper board or polymer liner. They are used for packing extemporaneously prepared ointments and pastes as well as commercial products where contamination by the patient's fingers is not too detrimental.

Containers for tablets and capsules

These are manufactured in amber glass and fitted with a conventional screw closure (Fig. 8.4) or child-resistant screw closure. They are available in a number of sizes. Tablets and hard and soft capsules are adequately protected from crushing, puncture, etc. by packaging in glass tablet bottles.

Plastics

Plastics is a collective term used for a variety of polymeric materials used for containers and closures. They include such substances as polyvinyl chloride (PVC), low-density and high-density polyethylene and polystyrene. The actual properties of plastics differ between the various materials used. However, the *advantages* of plastics (in general) are:

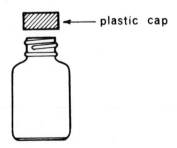

plastic cap

Fig. 8.4 Rectangular glass tablet bottle

1. Flexible nature.
2. Less brittle than glass.
3. Lightweight — therefore transportation costs are cheaper than glass.
4. They can be moulded into a multitude of shapes and sizes.
5. Suitable for both container and closure.
6. Readily available.

The general *disadvantages* are:

1. Few will withstand heat without softening or distorting.
2. Permeability to water vapour and atmospheric gases.
3. May interact with certain chemicals to cause softening or distortion.
4. May sorb substances, particularly preservatives, from solution.
5. Leaching out of plasticizers and stabilizers into solutions.
6. Relatively expensive.

Types of plastic containers

Bottles

Plastics are used to make medicine bottles; e.g. rigid amber PVC bottles of the same shape and design as glass medicine bottles, as well as bottles for external preparations such as lotions. In the latter case, the bottle will be opaque not ribbed, and it may be flexible enough to squeeze the lotion out through a small orifice at the top.

Containers for tablets and capsules

These can be plastic replicas of a conventional tablet bottle with a screw-cap or a plastic vial with either a press-in or slip-over closure. Bellamy et al (1980) have evaluated several plastic containers for solid dose forms and reported that several of the available containers on the market have a poor resistance to moisture ingress and a tendency to fracture on impact.

Containers for semi-solid preparations

These can be plastic vials with slip-over plastic lids or plastic replicas of glass ointment pots.

Alternatively, plastic tubes may be used. Tubes considerably reduce contamination of the unused contents since only a narrow orifice is presented to the patient. Tubes are considered to reduce wastage by the patient, but this is a debatable point. However, plastic tubes do not collapse after squeezing some of the contents out, but return to their original shape replacing the contents by the same volume of air. This disadvantage, normally termed 'suck back', may result in microbial contamination, oxidation, hydrolysis or dehydration of the contents.

Closures

Plastics are the main materials used for closures. They can be in the form of screw-on, child-resistant, push-on or slip-over caps. Some types, such as the black thermosetting plastic used on medicine bottles, will require a suitable liner which is strong enough to resist distortion or fracture on repeated tightening of the cap. White polypropylene caps are moulded to contain a crab claw sealing ring that compensates for irregularities in the bottle lip and does not require a liner. Closures consisting of a winged cap make removal easier for the arthritic patient.

Specialist containers

These are used mainly for manufactured products rather than extemporaneously dispensed ones. They include plastic squeeze bottles incorporating a dropper or spray device for drops (ear, eye, nose) (see Fig. 28.2) or nasal sprays, tubes with specially adapted nozzles for insertion into body cavities and plastic delivery devices, e.g. Rotahaler®, Spinhaler®, for administration of dry powder to the respiratory tract. Plastics are also used for unit dose packaging (see later in this chapter).

Metals

Metals used as pharmaceutical packaging materials include aluminium, tin and tin-coated lead. The *advantages* of metals are:

1. Lightness.
2. Robustness.
3. Impermeability to light, moisture and gases.
4. Can be made into rigid, unbreakable containers by impact extrusion or into collapsible tubes or foil.
5. Labels can be printed directly on to their surface.

The main *disadvantages* of metals are:

1. Their chemical and electrochemical activity.
2. They may shed metal particles in to the pharmaceutical product.
3. Expensive.
4. Not generally available for extemporaneous dispensing.

Types of metal containers

1. *Collapsible tubes for semi-solid preparations.* These tend to shed metal particles near their screw-threads. Aluminium tubes are often coated with lacquer or heat-cured epoxy resins to prevent attack by acids, alkalis and ethyl alcohol as well as amalgam formation by mercury compounds. The crimped end may well be further sealed to prevent leakage by coating the inside of the tube with a pressure-sensitive latex.

2. *Metal containers for tablets and capsules.* These are made from aluminium thus producing a light, robust and unbreakable container. If an aluminium cap is used then the screw action may be gritty and difficult. It is usual to lacquer the inside of the container to prevent grey marks due to abrasion appearing on tablets.

3. *Metal foil may be used for wrapping individual moulded suppositories or pessaries.* However, its main use is in strip packaging or blister packs.

Paper and paperboard

Paperboard is used extensively as an outer container to provide additional mechanical protection to other containers. For example, strip and blister packs of tablets, capsules, suppositories and pessaries may be packed in an outer paperboard carton (Fig. 8.5). Also tubes of ointments, creams and gels, as well as liquid medicines in sizes 500 ml and below, may be packed by the manufacturer in an outer paperboard carton. Slide paperboard boxes may be used, suitably lined, for extemporaneous dispensed suppositories, pessaries and powders.

Paper may be used to wrap individual powders and to line, if necessary, paperboard boxes.

CHILD-RESISTANT CONTAINERS

Child-resistant containers (CRCs) for pharmaceuticals have been introduced in response to public demands for greater protection of children from accidental, as opposed to deliberate poisoning. Accidental ingestion of poisons including medicines usually occurs most commonly in the under-five age-group. There is demonstrable evidence that child-resistant containers are effective in preventing accidental poisoning (Sibert & Craft 1981). However, it must be emphasized that child-resistant containers are not child proof and are only intended as a last line of defence when other precautions have failed. The commonsense rule that all medicines should be kept out of the reach of children should still apply.

Recloseable CRCs or unit packaging of the strip or blister type should be used for dispensing of all solid dosage forms, unless:

1. They are in a manufacturer's original pack so designed that transfer to a recloseable child-resistant container would be a retrograde or unnecessary procedure, e.g. tins or tubes of throat lozenges or effervescent tablets, sachets of powder or insufflation capsules. Attention should be paid to the special requirements for glyceryl trinitrate tablets, or

2. The patient is elderly or handicapped and will have difficulty in opening a child-resistant container, or

3. The patient specifically asks that a product shall not be dispensed in such a container.

In the last two cases, the pharmacist should make a particular point of advising that the medicines be kept well out of the reach of children.

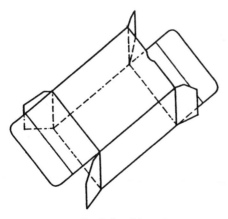

Fig. 8.5 Collapsible carton

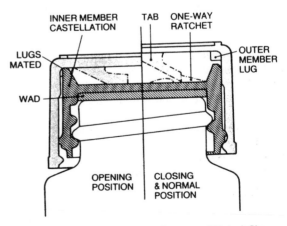

Fig. 8.6 The Clic-Loc closure. (Courtesy of United Closures & Plastics)

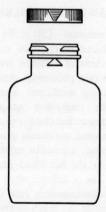

Fig. 8.7 The Snap-Safe closure. (Courtesy of Cope Allman Plastics Ltd)

All container/closure systems marketed as child resistant must comply with *current* British Standard (BS 6652). Such child-resistant containers basically consist of a glass or plastic vial or bottle with a specially designed closure. The most commonly marketed ones are Clic loc®. (Fig. 8.6), and Snap-safe® (Fig. 8.7). A detailed description of them can be found in Sibert & Craft (1981).

A comparison of some of the properties of child-resistant containers, such as moisture vapour penetration, the fit of the closures and removal force required, have been reported by Bellamy et al (1981).

UNIT DOSE PACKAGING

In recent years unit dose packaging has become increasingly common. The *advantages* of unit dose packaging are:

1. Hygienic.
2. Tamper evident.
3. Lightweight.
4. Child resistant.
5. Protects solid dose forms from moisture and abrasion.
6. Available as calender packs to aid patient compliance.
7. Wastage is reduced.
8. Accurate volumes can be administered.

The *disadvantages* are:

1. Expense.
2. Patients may experience difficulty in use.
3. Machinery is required which may be suitable for industrial or hospital use only.

Types of unit dose packaging for oral medicines include strip packaging, blister packaging and oral liquid containers and dispensers.

Blister packs

These consist of a lid and a blister (usually transparent). The lid material has to satisfy certain criteria:

1. Protect the pack contents.
2. Seal to the blister material and retain the medicament within the blister.
3. Act as a barrier to moisture and atmospheric gases.
4. Accept printing to label and identify the product.
5. Tear easily when the blister content is pushed through it.

The blister material has to:

1. Adequately protect the medicament from abrasion.
2. Be flexible enough to allow removal of the contents.
3. Act as barrier to moisture and atmospheric gases.
4. Be easy to machine, that is, it must soften without shrinking but stay soft without melting.

The materials used for the construction of the lid consist of three layers:

1. A printed paper, or printing and lacquer.
2. Aluminium foil (20–40 μm thick).
3. A sealing lacquer layer.

Blister materials include polyvinyl chloride (PVC), polyvinylidene chloride on PVC, polypropylene and many other new laminates as well as aluminium. Figure 8.8 shows a 10-capsule blister strip.

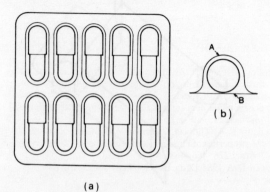

(a)

(b)

Fig. 8.8 Blister pack. (**a**) From above; (**b**) vertical section of a single blister (A, heat-formed blister; B, heat-sealed lid)

Strip packaging

Flexible packaging materials can be produced from laminates formed from combinations of paper, foil, plastics and cellulose films. These laminates can be readily sealed into units to contain simple doses of tablets or capsules. Strip packaging is invariably flexible, as opposed to blister packs which are rigid.

Oral liquid dispensers

Oral liquids can be unit packaged in two ways at the present time:

1. In a plastic syringe-type dispenser. The syringe is available in a number of sizes. The lip of the syringe is sealed by a small plastic ring.
2. A plastic pot sealed with a laminate. The laminate is torn off before use.

Other non-parenteral types of products which may be unit packaged include:

1. Suppositories.
2. Enemas in plastic packs with rectal nozzles.
3. Unit-packaged eye ointments and drops for hospital use.
4. Topical products packed in small sachets and tubes.

ORIGINAL PACK DISPENSING (OPD)

Definition

Original pack (OP) dispensing of prescription pharmaceuticals, whether branded or generics, is the process whereby a package of predetermined size is prescribed by the doctor and dispensed by the pharmacist in the original form in which it was produced by the manufacturer. In other words the pharmacist does not measure or count out manufactured products for repacking in another container.

Advantages of OPD

1. All the packs bear complete product identification data, including the batch number and source of manufacture. This aids batch identification in case of product recall, in relation to strict product liability and in cases of accidental or intentional overdosage.
2. The pack remains closed until opened by the patient. The product is therefore less likely to become contaminated or mislabelled and there is less risk of fulfilling a prescription with a product from a mixture of batches.
3. The manufacturer's pack allows for the inclusion of more information for the patient which should lead to improved compliance.
4. The dispensing process becomes more efficient thus allowing the pharmacist greater opportunity for counselling patients.
5. The dispensing process should be cheaper.

Disadvantages of OPD

1. Standardization of treatment pack size across a range of medicines may be inconvenient (Shaw 1985).
2. Pack design and manufacture may be more costly.
3. Storage space required for OPs may be greater than for an equivalent amount of stock in bulk packs. However, the total stock required to be held may well be significantly reduced with little change in overall storage space required.
4. Emergency supplies of small quantities may be a problem.
5. Some patients, particularly the elderly and infirm, may find the packaging of OPs difficult to open. However there is evidence that strip packaging may be especially helpful to partially sighted patients.

BIBLIOGRAPHY

Aulton M E (ed) 1988 Pharmaceutics: the science of dosage form design. Churchill Livingstone, Edinburgh
Bellamy K A, Thomas S, Barnett M I 1980 Evaluation of plastic containers for solid dosage forms. Pharmaceutical Journal 224: 459–462
Bellamy K A, Thomas S, Barnett M I 1981 Comparison of the properties of child resistant containers. Pharmaceutical Journal 226: 466–468
Dean D A 1984 Drug Development and Industrial

Pharmacy 10: 1463–1495
Pharmaceutical Codex 1979 Pharmaceutical Press, London
Royal Pharmaceutical Society of Great Britain 1982 Council statement on containers for dispensing. Pharmaceutical Journal 228: 107–108
Shaw J G 1985 Original pack dispensing by 1987? Pharmaceutical Journal 235
Sibert J R, Craft A W 1981 CRCs: Proof of the pudding? Pharmaceutical Journal 226: 164–168

9. Responding to the prescription

M. G. Aiken   A. L. G. Pugh

Introduction

Dispensing may be defined as the supply of a medicine to an individual patient in accordance with a prescription given by a practitioner and should be undertaken by or under the direct supervision of a pharmacist.

This chapter describes the activities of the pharmacist related to responding to the prescription. The general format of the prescription is illustrated by different types of prescription form. The procedures to be followed when dispensing a prescription are then listed.

All the activities of the pharmacist must be in accordance with current legislation. Details of the legal requirements current at the date of publication for prescriptions written in the UK are given in Appendix 1. Additional details of the various types of UK National Health Service (NHS) prescriptions are given in Appendix 2.

THE PRESCRIPTION

A prescription is an order from a doctor, dentist or veterinary practitioner or veterinary surgeon for the supply of a medicine, dressing or appliance to a patient (or to the owner of an animal). It is usually given in a written form (i.e. written in indelible ink, type written or computer printed), but may on occasion involve the pharmacist taking verbal instructions from the prescriber by telephone.

Prescriptions should be written or printed legibly. For medicines in some legal categories the prescription must be written in the prescriber's own hand writing (see Appendix 1).

In accordance with current legislation. National Health Service (NHS) prescriptions must be written on a form supplied by the area authority (see Fig. 9.1 and Appendix 2).

A prescription for a medicine to be used by the patient at home should contain the following information. For certain classes of medicine some of these requirements are mandatory (see Appendix 1):

1. The patient's name, address and age if under 12 years.
2. The names and quantities of the medicaments to be supplied.
3. Instructions for the patient.
4. The prescriber's profession, address and signature.
5. The date on which the prescription was written or signed.
6. Proper name labelling requirement (NP).

A request for repeat dispensing may be included (but not for NHS prescriptions). These requirements are discussed in more detail below.

1. The patient's name, address and age if under 12 years

The title of the patient, e.g. Mr, Mrs, Miss, Ms, together with the surname. Initials and/or one full forename are particularly useful when dealing with prescriptions for different members of the same family. These details will be included on the label of the medicine.

The age of a child under 12 years should also be included (and is a legal requirement for some medicines). This will help when the pharmacist is checking the prescribed dose. In some cases the weight of the patient or animal may also be required in order to calculate the appropriate dose.

The address should be clear and unambiguous — this is a legal requirement for some medicaments, and is also essential if the medicine is to be delivered to elderly or infirm patients in their own home and when records are to be made of the supply.

2. The names and quantities of the medicaments to be supplied

Prescribers are recommended to write the names of medicines in full (British National Formulary) but many use abbreviations and the pharmacist must take care that these abbreviations are not misinterpreted. A medicament may be prescribed as:

61

a. An official preparation — that is a preparation prescribed by non-proprietary title and complying with a standard in an appropriate specified publication (e.g. European Pharmacopoeia, British Pharmacopoeia, or British Pharmaceutical Codex 1973).

b. A preparation prescribed by non-proprietary (generic) title which may not be defined in an official publication.

c. A proprietary product prescribed by brand name.

d. A special or individual formula, in which case the quantity of each ingredient will be stated together with a description of the type of preparation, e.g. cream, mixture, lotion. Sometimes only the active ingredients are stated by the prescriber and the pharmacist is expected to use skill and experience in order to formulate a suitable product.

Prescribers in the UK are recommended to prescribe by generic name whenever possible. The pharmacist may then dispense any suitable product. However, in some instances (e.g. lithium carbonate tablets) the tablets from different manufacturers have such different bioavailability characteristics that the brand name or manufacturer should be stated by the prescriber.

Many medicines are available in more than one dosage form, e.g. liquid, tablet, capsule, suppository. The pharmaceutical form of the product should be written on the prescription to avoid ambiguity and is a legal requirement for controlled drugs prescribed in the UK (see Appendix 1).

The strength of the preparation should also be stated by the prescriber and is essential when various strengths of a product are available.

The quantity of the medicament supplied may be expressed as:

a. A weight (e.g. 5 g, 30 g) or volume (e.g. 50 ml, 300 ml)

b. A number of dosage units (e.g. 20 tablets, 50 capsules, 12 suppositories)

c. In terms of a number of manufacturer's original packs (e.g. 1 OP, 6 × OP). Packaging of medicines in unit packs containing a full course of treatment or sufficient medicine for 1 week or 1 month is becoming increasingly common.

d. As a daily dose together with the number of days or months of treatment (e.g. 5/7 indicating 5 days' supply, 1/52 indicating 7 days' (e.g. 1 weeks') supply, 1/12 indicating 28 days' (1 months') supply. In this case the pharmacist requires a precise dose to be stated by the prescriber in order to calculate the total quantity to supply. It would not be possible to calculate a suitable quantity to supply if the dosage was 'one to be taken when required'.

3. Instructions for the patient

Instructions may include:

a. The quantity to be taken or amount to be used.

b. The frequency and timing of administration or application.

c. The route of administration or method of use.

d. Special instructions such as dilution directions.

4. The prescriber's profession, address and signature

There should be some indication on the prescription whether the prescriber is a doctor, dentist, veterinary surgeon or veterinary practitioner. For some classes of medicines this is a legal requirement (Appendix 1).

It is often difficult to decipher a prescriber's signature but the pharmacist should be satisfied that it is genuine, especially before supplying medicines subject to the stricter forms of legal control.

5. The date on which the prescription was written or signed

There is a legal requirement for prescribers to date prescriptions for some classes of medicines. There may also be a time limit after which the prescription ceases to be valid (see Appendix 1).

6. Proper name labelling requirement (NP)

NP (N.P.) is an abbreviation for the Latin 'nomen proprium' which literally means the proper name. It is now common practice for dispensed medicines to be labelled fully with the name of the product. Should the prescriber wish to conceal from the patient the identity of the medicine he must indicate the fact on the prescription. The letters 'NP' are printed on NHS prescription forms and may be cancelled by deletion. The medicine is then labelled 'The Mixture', 'The Tablets' as appropriate.

A request for repeat dispensing

A repeatable prescription is a prescription which contains a direction that it may be dispensed on more than one occasion. Repeatable prescriptions are not acceptable under the NHS but a prescriber may request more than one supply to be made on a private prescription except for controlled drugs. See Appendix 1 for more details.

Bulk prescriptions

Prescriptions are usually written for one named patient. Certain items may be ordered in bulk for schools or institutions for 20 or more patients on NHS prescription forms. The name of the institution and number of patients replaces the patient's name. See Appendix 2 for more details.

Incomplete prescriptions

Before dispensing the prescription the pharmacist must be sure that all the legal requirements are fulfilled. These requirements will vary according to the category of medicine prescribed (see Appendix 1). Prescriptions not legally complete should be referred back to the prescriber before dispensing.

In the case of an incomplete prescription for a preparation other than a controlled drug the pharmacist may consider it inappropriate for the patient to return to the prescriber. If the prescriber is contacted by telephone, missing details such as strength, quantity and dosage may be added by the pharmacist and the prescription endorsed 'prescriber contacted' (p.c.). The endorsement should be initialled and dated by the pharmacist.

If the prescriber cannot be contacted and the pharmacist has sufficient information to make a professional judgement he may obtain details of the strength of the preparation and dosage from the patient or patient's record card. If there is any doubt as to the correct dosage the patient must be referred back to the prescriber. For NHS prescriptions from which the quantity has been omitted the pharmacist may supply sufficient to complete up to 5 days' treatment or supply the smallest original pack. The prescription is then endorsed 'prescriber not contacted' (p.n.c.) together with the quantity, strength and dosage supplied where applicable. The prescription is then initialled and dated by the pharmacist.

DIFFERENT TYPES OF PRESCRIPTION FORMS

The main types of prescription form encountered by the pharmacist currently practising in Britain are as follows.

Community

1. NHS prescriptions of various types
2. Private prescriptions from doctors, dentists or veterinary practitioners.

Hospital (NHS)

3. Prescriptions for hospital inpatients.
4. Prescriptions for medicines to be taken home by patients discharged from a hospital ward.
5. Hospital outpatient prescriptions.

1. NHS prescriptions

Medical and dental practitioners contracted to the NHS may prescribe a range of drugs, medicines and listed appliances on NHS prescription forms. Details of items that may be prescribed are listed in the Drug Tariff (current edition).

A facsimile of a standard FP10 prescription form is shown in Figure 9.1. These forms are issued by general practitioners in England and Wales. Similar forms are issued by dentists and by prescribers in other parts of the UK (see Appendix 2).

The front of the FP10 form consists of three main parts:

A. The prescription with details of the names and quantities of the medicament to be supplied and instructions for the patient, the signature of the prescriber and the date. There is a box at the top of this section for the number of days treatment which may be used to calculate the quantity to supply. Proper name labelling may be cancelled by the prescriber by deletion of the letters NP.

B. The name and address of the patient and age if under 12 years.

C. Endorsement sections for completion by the pharmacist.

The top left-hand corner is stamped with the name and address of the pharmacy together with the date of dispensing when the prescription has been dispensed.

Details of the medicaments supplied are entered in the left margin under 'Pharmacist's pack and quantity endorsement' (Appendix 2). The current endorsement requirements are given in the Drug Tariff. Since the requirements are regularly revised the reader should always refer to the most recent edition of the Drug Tariff. The pharmacist should endorse with as much relevant information as possible, especially if the prescription is difficult to interpret.

Patients do not pay for medicaments prescribed on NHS prescriptions but may be charged a levy in respect of each item dispensed. This levy is collected by the pharmacist on behalf of the NHS.

The number of items on the form is entered in the box marked 'No. of Prescns. on form'

FRONT

BACK

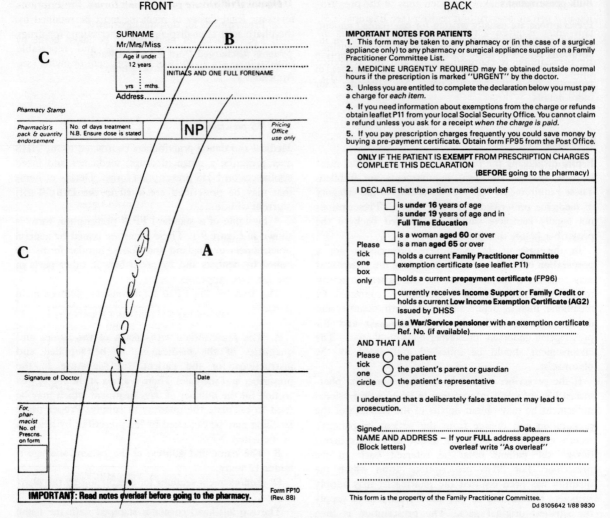

IMPORTANT NOTES FOR PATIENTS
1. This form may be taken to any pharmacy or (in the case of a surgical appliance only) to any pharmacy or surgical appliance supplier on a Family Practitioner Committee List.
2. MEDICINE URGENTLY REQUIRED may be obtained outside normal hours if the prescription is marked "URGENT" by the doctor.
3. Unless you are entitled to complete the declaration below you must pay a charge for *each item*.
4. If you need information about exemptions from the charge or refunds obtain leaflet P11 from your local Social Security Office. You cannot claim a refund unless you ask for a receipt *when the charge is paid*.
5. If you pay prescription charges frequently you could save money by buying a pre-payment certificate. Obtain form FP95 from the Post Office.

ONLY IF THE PATIENT IS **EXEMPT** FROM PRESCRIPTION CHARGES
COMPLETE THIS DECLARATION
(BEFORE going to the pharmacy)

I DECLARE that the patient named overleaf

☐ is **under 16** years of age
is **under 19** years of age and in **Full Time Education**

Please tick one box only
☐ is a woman **aged 60** or over
is a man **aged 65** or over
☐ holds a current **Family Practitioner Committee** exemption certificate (see leaflet P11)
☐ holds a current **prepayment certificate** (FP96)
☐ currently receives **Income Support** or **Family Credit** or holds a current **Low Income Exemption Certificate (AG2)** issued by DHSS
☐ is a **War/Service pensioner** with an exemption certificate Ref. No. (if available)...

AND THAT I AM

Please tick one circle
○ the patient
○ the patient's parent or guardian
○ the patient's representative

I understand that a deliberately false statement may lead to prosecution.

Signed.......................................Date.........................
NAME AND ADDRESS – If your **FULL** address appears
(Block letters)　　　　　　overleaf write "As overleaf"

....
....

This form is the property of the Family Practitioner Committee.
Dd 8105642 1/88 9830

Fig. 9.1 NHS FP10 prescription form. (Reproduced with permission from the Family Practitioner Committee)

Remuneration to the pharmacist is paid monthly after the prescription forms, suitably endorsed, have been submitted to the prescription pricing authority. Examples of NHS endorsement are shown in Appendix 2.

Disposal of NHS forms. After dispensing, stamping and dating and endorsement, the prescriptions are sent to the Processing Division of the Prescription Pricing Authority as soon as possible after the first day of each month. Details of prescription sorting are shown in Appendix 2. In the future, 'on-line' pricing is likely to become widely available. This process uses a direct computer link between the pharmacy and the pricing authority.

2. Private prescriptions

A typical private prescription for human medication is shown in Example 9.1a and for animal treatment in Example 9.2a. The prescription is usually handwritten by the prescriber on headed notepaper. The dispensing of private prescriptions differs from NHS dispensing in several respects.

The patient pays the full cost of the medicine to the pharmacist, together with appropriate additional charges for the container and for professional service. A guide to 'Pricing of private prescriptions' has been published by the Pharmaceutical Society of Great Britain.

The pharmacist makes a written copy of the prescription in a private prescription register (see Example 9.3). This entry is given a reference number which is included on the label of the medicine. After dispensing, the prescription is stamped, dated and the reference number written near to the pharmacy stamp (see Examples 9.1b, 9.2b).

Disposal of private prescription forms. Prescriptions for some legal classes of medicine must be retained by the pharmacist after dispensing. Prescriptions for drugs not subject to strict legal control and repeatable prescriptions are given back to the patient or owner (see Appendix 1).

Example 9.1

a. Private prescription

```
                        A. J. Henderson MB BS
                        10 Grand Drive
                        Storringwell

Mr J. Smith
Old Rectory
Storringwell

        20 Ativan tablets 1 mg
        1 at bed time
        Repeat twice
                    H. J. Henderson
                      1.8.89
```

b. Prescription endorsement

```
                        A. J. Henderson MB BS
                        10 Grand Drive
                        Storringwell

Mr J. Smith
Old Rectory
Storringwell

        20 Ativan tablets 1 mg

    1 at bed time       ACHEM PHARMACY
                            2.8.89
                        Main Street Lewes
    Repeat twice         Ref  R238·1
                        1st disp.

                    H. J. Henderson
                      1.8.89
```

Example 9.2

a. Veterinary prescription

```
                        A. Vero MRCVS
                        Carean Veterinary
                        Group
                        Hove
This prescription is for an animal under my
care

Mrs J. Jones (for Domino)
1, High Street
Hove

        30 Tabs. Oxytetracycline 50 mg
        1 three times daily

        10 ml Gentamicin eye drops
        use four times daily
                            A. Vero
                            1.8.89
```

b. Prescription endorsement

```
                        A. Vero MRCVS
                        Carean Veterinary
                        Group
                        Hove
This prescription is for an animal under my
care

Mrs J. Jones (for Domino)
1, High Street
Hove

        30 Tabs. Oxytetracycline 50 mg
        1 three times daily      Ref. 238.2

        10 ml Gentamicin eye drops
        use four times daily
            Ref. 238.3      ACHEM PHARMACY
                                2.8.89
                            Main Street Lewes

                        A. Vero
                        1.8.89
```

Example 9.3

Prescription records

Prescription book identification letter R

		Page 238	
1.	Mr J. Smith Old Rectory Storringwell	2.8.89 A. J. Henderson MB BS 10 Grand Drive Storringwell 1.8.89 20 Ativan tablets 1 mg 1 at bed time Repeat twice 1st disp ·	£. . . .
2. 3.	Mrs J. Jones 1, High Street Hove For Domino (5 kg dog) for an animal underhis care 30 Tabs Oxytetracycline 50 mg 1 three times daily 10 ml Gentamicin eye drops use four times daily	A. Vero MRCVS Carean Veterinary Group Hove 1.8.89	 £. . . . £. . . .

3. Prescriptions for hospital inpatients

Most hospitals use a combined prescription and record of administration form. Details included are patient identification, name of drug, route of administration, dose and frequency or time of administration and the prescriber's signature (Figs 9.2, 9.3). Forms for long-stay patients may vary slightly from those for short-stay patients. A typical form for short-stay patients is divided into sections (Figs 9.2, 9.3). Drugs to be given on a single occasion, often prior to surgery, are written as 'Once only or pre-medication drugs'. Drugs to be administered at regular intervals are written in a second section which may also contain 'As required prescriptions' (Fig. 9.2). The latter are used when a patient requires or requests medication, postoperative analgesics, night sedation, laxatives, etc. It is usual for each ward to have a stock of commonly used drugs for administration to any patient for whom they are prescribed. The stock may be supplied from the pharmacy in response to a written request by the nurse in charge of the ward or ward stocks may be regularly 'topped up' by members of the pharmacy staff to an agreed level. If a medicine not held as ward stock is prescribed for an individual patient a temporary stock may be provided.

Disposal of inpatient prescription forms. When the patient is discharged from the ward the prescription form is filed with the patient's medical records.

AFFIX ADDRESSOGRAPH, IF AVAILABLE

Patients name	
Ward	
Hospital No.	

Known Drug HYPERSENSITIVITIES

ONCE ONLY & PREMED. DRUGS

DATE	TIME	DRUG (Approved Name in BLOCK LETTERS)	DOSE	ROUTE	DR'S SIGNATURE	TIME GIVEN	GIVEN BY	PHARM. USE

REGULAR AND AS REQUIRED PRESCRIPTIONS

DATE		DRUG (Approved Name in BLOCK LETTERS)	DOSE	ROUTE	TIME OF ADMIN.				OTHER DIRECTIONS	DR'S SIGNATURE	DATE CANCELLED with (Dr's Initials)	PHARM. USE
					9	13	17	22				
	A											
	B											
	C											
	D											
	E											
	F											
	G											
	H											
	I											
	J											
	K											
	L											
	M											
	N											
	O											
	P											
	Q											
	R											
	S											
	T											
	U											

Fig. 9.2 Inpatient prescription form showing sections for 'Once only', 'Regular' and 'As required' medication. (Reproduced by kind permission of the District Pharmaceutical Officer, Worthing District Health Authority)

ONCE ONLY & PREMED. DRUGS

DATE	TIME	DRUG (Approved Name in BLOCK LETTERS)	DOSE	ROUTE	DR'S SIGNATURE	TIME GIVEN	GIVEN BY	PHARM. USE

ADMINISTRATION RECORDS

DATE				DATE				DATE				DATE				DATE				DATE				DATE			
9	13	17	22	9	13	17	22	9	13	17	22	9	13	17	22	9	13	17	22	9	13	17	22	9	13	17	22

Fig. 9.3 Inpatient prescription form. Showing section for 'Administration records' corresponding to prescribing information in Figure 9.2. The nurse's initials are entered in the appropriate box. (Reproduced by kind permission of the District Pharmaceutical Officer, Worthing District Health Authority)

4. Prescriptions for medicines to be taken home by patients discharged from a hospital ward (known as TTO — To Take Out)

These may be written in a form similar to an outpatient prescription or may be written on the inpatient form in a separate section (Fig. 9.4). There may be a hospital policy on the quantity of medicine to be supplied, e.g. 1 or 2 weeks' supply. If necessary, the patient then obtains further supplies from the general practitioner.

These prescriptions are also filed with the patient's medical record.

....Hospital

In-patient PRESCRIPTION Sheet

Sheet Number

AFFIX ADDRESSOGRAPH, IF AVAILABLE

Surname Mr/Mrs/Miss		Ward	
Fore Names		Date of Birth	Weight (Kg)
Address			
		Date of Admission	
Hospital Number	Consultant		

Relevant previous medication	Duration		**?**	
			Monoamine Oxidase Inhibitors	
			Digoxin/Anti-Arrythmics	
		Steroids	Anti-Coagulants	
		Cytotoxics	Anti-Convulsants	
			Anti-Diabetic Drugs	

Any Additional information, e.g. Special Diet

Please PRINT in FULL (no abbreviations), in ENGLISH (not Latin), ALL treatment details

DRUGS TO TAKE HOME	(Normal maximum of 14 days supply)	Discharge Date ....

N.P. Prescription

Signature ....

Fig. 9.4 Inpatient prescription form showing patient details and prescription section for 'drugs to take home' (TTO). (Reproduced by kind permission of the District Pharmaceutical Officer, Worthing District Health Authority)

5. Hospital outpatient prescriptions

For hospitals which provide a dispensing service for outpatients special prescription forms valid only within the hospital are used (Fig. 9.5). Details on the form include the patient's identification, name, address, date of birth and hospital registration number. Medicines are invariably prescribed by approved name and there may be a hospital policy on the quantity to be supplied, e.g. 2 weeks' supply or sufficient to last until the next outpatient appointment.

Disposal of outpatient prescriptions. A record of the prescription is usually included with the patient's records and a copy is retained in the pharmacy. If the hospital is unable to provide a full dispensing service for outpatients, a special type of NHS prescription form may be issued to the patient for dispensing in a local community pharmacy (see Appendix 2).

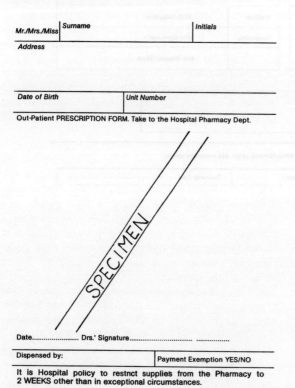

Fig. 9.5 Outpatient prescription form. (Reproduced by kind permission of the District Pharmaceutical Officer, Worthing District Health Authority)

GENERAL DISPENSING PROCEDURE

Guidelines for good pharmaceutical practice in dispensing are given in ch. 5.

To ensure safety and efficiency it is sensible to adopt a strict set of procedures in dispensing.

1. Read the prescription carefully and check that it is complete and valid.
2. Check that the dosage and directions are appropriate.
3. Dispense the medicine.
4. Counsel the patient.
5. Endorse the prescription and collect any fee.
6. Dispose of the prescription.
7. Make the appropriate records.

1. Read the prescription

The prescription must be read carefully to ensure that all the necessary information is present. Some prescriptions are difficult to read because of illegible writing by the prescriber. The prescriber should be contacted if there is any doubt as to his/her intention. Many medicines have very similar names but very different actions. *Confusion may be fatal.*

Where possible, prescriptions should be dispensed in the order in which they are received. Some patients prefer to wait while others will leave the prescription for collection later. It is good practice to check that the prescribed item is in stock so that the patient can be warned of any possible delay.

Preparing extemporaneous preparations may take time and this should be explained to the patient.

2. Check that the dosage and directions are appropriate

Details of the posology or dosage schemes of medicines may be found in the information sources detailed in Appendix 8. It should be remembered that dosages quoted in the literature are based on expert opinion and are for guidance, they are not intended to be binding on the prescriber. Unusually high or low doses should be queried with the prescriber although an unusual dose may be prescribed quite intentionally and may indeed be underlined or endorsed in some other way by the prescriber.

Paediatric dosage may present a particular problem and the pharmacist is strongly recommended to consult one or more of the guides to paediatric posology (see Appendix 8).

It is also essential to check that there are no pharmaceutical or therapeutic incompatibilities in a prescribed preparation and that different medicines

RESPONDING TO THE PRESCRIPTION 71

prescribed for the same patient do not interact with each other to the detriment of the patient.

Contacting the prescriber. If any delay is anticipated because of the need to contact the prescriber, the patient should be informed. It is important that the confidence of the patient in the prescriber is not undermined.

Before contacting a prescriber it is essential to have all the necessary information to hand. The full name and address of the patient and the name and telephone number of the pharmacy should be stated. Concise details of the query should be given and the pharmacist must be prepared to quote recommended doses if querying a dose, suitable alternatives if querying a product and likely problems if querying an unsuitable combination of drugs.

Prescribers are usually busy and may be difficult to contact. It may be possible on occasion to clarify a query with a receptionist or medical secretary who has access to the patient's medical record. However, if direct access to the prescriber is considered to be essential the pharmacist must be politely insistent.

The pharmacist must be satisfied that the prescription represents the prescriber's wishes but also that the medicine in the amount prescribed will not adversely affect the patient. *The pharmacist has the ultimate professional responsibility to decide whether or not to dispense the prescription.*

3. Dispense the medicine

a. Check any calculations.
b. Check the storage requirements.
c. Collect the container.
d. Write the label.
e. Prepare or select the medicine.
f. Pack the medicine into the container.
g. Fix the label.
h. Check the finished preparation.

a. Check any calculations. The calculation for the quantity of medicine to be supplied should be checked, particularly if ordered by number of days of treatment. Due note should be made of the expiry date so that quantities in excess of the shelf-life are not supplied. This is particularly important for diluted products which may frequently need to be supplied in instalments.

For extemporaneously prepared products the calculations should be checked against the master formula (on the prescription or from an appropriate reference source). It is essential to use the correct units, the correct ingredients and where necessary the correct diluent.

b. Check the storage requirements. This information will determine the choice of container and labels.

c. Collect the container. Details of appropriate containers may be found in Chapter 8 and in Part 2. A 5 ml plastic measuring spoon should be supplied with liquid oral medicines unless an alternative measure, e.g. a pipette, is required.

d. Write the label. All labels should be typewritten or printed and should be prepared before dispensing the medicine as an additional check of dosage and frequency. This procedure also avoids the potentially dangerous situation of having several unlabelled containers on the dispensing bench. Details of labelling procedures for dispensed medicines are described in Chapter 10.

e. Prepare or select the medicine. Ensure that the dispensing bench is tidy and clear from previous prescriptions in order to reduce the risk of errors. Select the prescribed medicine if available from stock, taking care to obtain the correct dosage form, strength and size as applicable. At the same time check the expiry date of the product. For extemporaneously prepared medicines ensure that the product is carefully and accurately made and the ingredients thoroughly mixed.

f. Pack the medicine into the container. The container should be of an appropriate size and the product should be packed neatly. Glass bottles should be polished and all containers should be clean and pharmaceutically elegant.

g. Fix the label. The label should be placed so that it fits neatly onto the container. For small containers the standard size of label may need to be trimmed neatly, taking care not to remove any of the information. Wherever possible labels should be fixed to one face only of the container. For products dispensed in a manufacturer's original pack the dispensing label should be fixed to the actual container, not to any outer packaging; it should not obscure important information already on the container.

h. Check the finished preparation. As the label is fixed to the patient's container it should be re-checked against the prescription and the stock container. This double-checking system reduces errors to a minimum.

4. Counsel the patient

The completed medicine is handed to the patient (except for hospital inpatient medicines which are usually supplied to the ward staff). It is good practice to check the patient's name and address against that written on the prescription before handing over the medicine.

The pharmacist may reinforce the information given on the label and give any necessary additional verbal advice or information (see Ch. 37).

5. *Endorse the prescription and collect any fee*

NHS prescriptions are endorsed with the number of items dispensed, the details of medicaments supplied, the pharmacy stamp and the date of dispensing.

Private prescriptions are also stamped and dated and the reference number corresponding to the prescription record added. If the prescription is repeatable the number of times the prescription has been dispensed is also usually noted.

Hospital inpatient prescriptions may be initialled by the pharmacist on the ward or in the pharmacy to indicate that the relevant checks have been made. For outpatient prescriptions the quantities supplied may be recorded for internal records and the prescription form is usually initialled by the dispenser and by the person checking the dispensing.

6. *Dispose of the prescription*

The procedures for disposal of the different types of prescription forms are summarized in Table 9.1.

7. *Make the appropriate records*

A written copy of all private prescriptions is made in the prescription register (see Example 9.3). It may be useful to record any unusual formulations prescribed on NHS forms. For details of other records legally required see Appendix 1.

Table 9.1 Prescription disposal

Type of prescription form	Disposal
NHS form	Retain until end of month Sort and send for pricing
Private form for prescription-only medicine or controlled drug	Retain 2 years
Private form for prescription-only medicine, repeats allowed	Return to patient Retain after final repeat
Private form for Pharmacy or General Sales List medicine	Return to patient
Hospital inpatient form	Return to ward
Hospital outpatient form (for use within the hospital)	Retain in pharmacy (usually 2 years)

To summarize

Dispensing involves the interpretation and clarification of the prescriber's wishes and the preparation and labelling of the medicine. The dispensing process includes the handing of the medicine to the patient (or the patient's representative) and the giving of any necessary advice, and concludes when the appropriate records have been made.

BIBLIOGRAPHY

ABPI Data Sheet Compendium current edition. Datapharm Publications, London (updated annually)
British National Formulary 1988 16th edn. British Medical Association and Royal Pharmaceutical Society of Great Britain, London (updated twice yearly)
British Pharmacopoeia 1980 HMSO, London (and addenda 1982, 1983 and 1986)
British Pharmacopoeia 1988 HMSO, London
British Pharmaceutical Codex 1973 Pharmaceutical Press, London
Drug Tariff current edition. HMSO, London (updated monthly)
European Pharmacopoeia, 2nd edn. First cycle (1980–82), Second cycle (1983–84), Third cycle 1985. Maisonneuve St Ruffine, S. A., France
Martindale, see Reynolds J E F
Medicines, ethics and practice — A guide for pharmacists 1988 No. 1. Royal Pharmaceutical Society of Great Britain, London (updated twice yearly)
Monthly Index of Medical Specialities (MIMS). Medical Publications, London
NPA Guide to the Drug Tariff 1987/88 National Pharmaceutical Association, St Albans
Pearce M E (ed) 1984 Medicines and poisons guide, 4th edn (with cumulative amendments in the *Pharmaceutical Journal*). Pharmaceutical Press, London
Pharmaceutical Codex 1979 11th edn, incorporating the British Pharmaceutical Codex. Pharmaceutical Press, London
Pharmaceutical Society 1979 Guide to good dispensing practice. Pharmaceutical Journal 223: 157–158
Pricing Private Prescriptions 1985 Pharmaceutical Society of Great Britain, London
Reynolds J E F (ed) 1989 Martindale, The Extra Pharmacopoeia, 29th edn. Pharmaceutical Press, London
Wade A (ed) 1980 Pharmaceutical handbook, 19th edn. Pharmaceutical Press, London

10. Labelling of dispensed medicines

M. G. Aiken   A. L. G. Pugh

Introduction

The label on a dispensed medicine should provide the patient with all the information necessary so that the medicine may be taken or used appropriately.

This chapter describes the various categories of information to be communicated to the patient via the label:

1. General labelling requirements for dispensed medicines.
2. Cautionary and advisory labels.
3. Special instructions for different types of product.

The information on the labels of dispensed medicines should be:

1. Accurate. The label should be checked immediately after writing and again prior to fixing to the container.

2. Legible. Labels should be typewritten or printed. The use of label writers is discussed further in this chapter.

3. Intelligible. The information should be completely unambiguous and arranged to avoid confusion. The terms used should be readily understandable by the lay person.

4. Adequate and relevant. Care should be taken to avoid causing confusion or anxiety. Too much information on the label may mean that none of it is noted.

The label must comply with the requirements specified in current legislation and with current professional opinion.

THE INFORMATION ON THE LABEL

The labels on dispensed medicines should:

1. Indicate clearly the patient for whom it has been prescribed.
2. Include the name and address of the supplier and the date of supply.
3. In most cases give precise details as to the contents of the container when dispensed.

4. State the storage conditions and shelf-life of the medicine.
5. Give the patient clear and complete instructions on how and when to take or use the preparation.

1. Indicate clearly the patient for whom it has been prescribed

The patient's title, forename(s) or initial(s) and surname should appear on the label of each medicine dispensed. This is to minimize confusion with other members of the same family with similar medicines. The address of the owner should also be included on the label of a dispensed veterinary medicine.

2. Include the name and address of the supplier and the date of supply

The name and address of the pharmacy may be preprinted on the dispensing labels. Some labelling systems allow this information to be printed when producing the label. Most labelling systems also automatically include the date which is re-set daily. For private prescriptions the reference number of the prescription register entry is also added to the label (see Ch. 9 and Appendix 1).

3. Give precise details as to the contents of the container when dispensed

a. The quantity in the container. It is recommended that the labels of all dispensed medicines should indicate the total quantity of the product dispensed in the container to which the label refers. If more than one container with the same medicine is dispensed the amount on the label should be the amount in each container.

b. The name of the medicine. This should be included unless otherwise requested by the prescriber, i.e. NP deleted (see Ch. 9).

In community pharmacy the name written by the prescriber is the name that should appear on the label. This applies to medicines prescribed by proprietary name, by generic or non-proprietary name, by approved name or by a title given in the BP, BPC, BNF or DPF.

If the prescriber uses a non-proprietary name for a preparation, then that name should appear on the label even if the medicine is only available as a proprietary product. If a prescribed product has a special formula with several ingredients and has no official or proprietary name, then the product may be labelled by its pharmaceutical form, e.g. 'The Ointment', 'The Application'. However, it is good practice to include the names and quantities of the active ingredients on the label and wherever possible the names of the excipients. In some cases an apparently inert ingredient such as lactose or white soft paraffin may evoke a reaction in susceptible individuals.

In a few cases the prescriber may not wish to disclose the name of the medicine to the patient. This is indicated to the pharmacist by deletion of the letters NP (nomen proprium) on the prescription form and the medicine is then labelled by its pharmaceutical form, e.g. 'The Tablets', 'The Ointment' as appropriate. Alternatively the prescriber may request a descriptive title such as 'The Sedative Tablets'.

In hospital pharmacy, generally only non-proprietary names are used on labels even if a proprietary product is supplied. Some hospitals do include both proprietary and non-proprietary names on the label for outpatient prescriptions.

c. The strength of the medicine. This is essential for preparations that are available in different strengths.

The strength of a medicine designed for internal use is usually expressed as the amount of active ingredient in each dosage unit, e.g. the amount in each tablet, capsule, metered aerosol inhalation, etc. The amount in each unit of dose volume should be stated for liquid oral medicines. This will usually be in terms of a 5 ml spoonful but may be in terms of a smaller volume for paediatric formulations intended to be measured by pipette.

The strength of a medicinal product for external use is usually expressed in terms of the percentage of active ingredient(s) present although the quantity of each active ingredient in the container may be stated.

For rectal and vaginal preparations the amount of active ingredient in each suppository or pessary is usually given.

If the strength of an official product is defined in the monograph a reference to the official publication (and the date of the edition if not current) is sufficient (e.g. Aqueous Calamine Cream BP 1988, Magnesium Carbonate Mixture BPC 1973, Compound Bismuth Subgallate Suppositories BP 1980).

The strength must be included on the label of an official product for which no strength is defined in the monograph (e.g. Aminophylline Suppositories BP, Chloramphenicol Oral Suspension BP and Chlorhexidine Cream BP).

Units. Whenever possible quantities should be expressed as whole numbers of units, e.g. 100 mg rather than 0.1 g, 6 μg rather than 0.006 mg. When decimals are unavoidable a zero should be written before the decimal point where there is no other figure, e.g. 0.5% not .5%.

Batch identification. The inclusion of a batch reference is a standard labelling requirement for medicines packed for sale in the UK (see Appendix 1). Although dispensed medicines are presently exempt from this requirement, medicines packed by the manufacturer for dispensing to an individual patient (original packs) usually carry a batch reference. Likewise, products prepared within a hospital pharmacy production department usually carry a batch number which may appear on the label.

Diluted products. Particular care should be taken when labelling medicines prepared by the dilution of more concentrated products. Since diluted preparations generally have a reduced shelf-life, it is useful to include the word 'diluted' in the title of the medicine together with the degree of dilution or the strength of the diluted product. For example:

e.g. 1.

> Diluted Chloral Mixture BP
> 50% v/v

or 2.

> Diluted Chloral Mixture BP
> Half Strength

or 3.

> Diluted Chloral Mixture BP
> containing 250 mg/5 ml
> Chloral Hydrate

Options 1 or 2 may be used if the preparation has a number of ingredients but option 3 is preferred for medicines with one active ingredient.

A similar policy may be adopted for ointments and creams:

e.g. 1.

> Diluted Calmurid Cream
> Half Strength

e.g. 2.

> Diluted Propaderm Ointment
> containing beclomethasone
> dipropionate 0.0125%

4. State the storage conditions and shelf-life of the product

Wherever possible packaging should protect medicines against inappropriate storage in a domestic situation. Furthermore, ideally medicines should be prescribed and dispensed in sufficiently small quantities so as to be used by the patient before significant deterioration occurs. However, it is often necessary to indicate special storage requirements to the patient. Guidance for the pharmacist may be found in the monographs for official products or for the individual ingredients of unofficial products. For proprietary products the manufacturer's data sheet will provide the necessary information.

a. Temperature. A number of products need to be stored in a cool place, preferably below 15°C. Preparations such as moulded pessaries or suppositories which are intended to melt at body temperature may be spoilt if placed near heat sources. Insulin injections are usually required to be stored between 2°C and 8 or 10°C (in a refrigerator but not in the freezing compartment).

Antibiotic suspensions, products with volatile ingredients and some creams also require cool storage conditions, while syrup-based medicines should be stored so as to avoid fluctuations in temperature. Formaldehyde solutions should be stored in a moderately warm place.

b. Humidity. Most solid unit dose forms should be protected from moisture. Such products should be supplied in air- and moisture-proof containers and the patient should be encouraged to replace the cap after use. Divided powders packed in the traditional paperboard boxes should be stored in a dry place.

c. Light. The use of amber containers will assist in keeping light from a light-sensitive product. Further protection can be obtained by storing the container inside a box. A few substances, e.g. paraldehyde, must be stored in complete darkness. Containers should not be exposed to direct sunlight even if they are light resistant.

d. Sources of ignition. Products that contain large proportions of flammable solvents should be labelled 'flammable, keep away from naked flames'. Preparations such as Salicylic Acid Lotion BP which is used as a scalp lotion requires further advice to avoid drying the hair near a fire or naked flame.

Shelf-life. This is the period during which the quality of a medicine may be expected to remain within acceptable limits and the patient should be given some indication of the time after which the preparation should be discarded. The expiry date should reflect stability data from various sources, possible poor domestic storage and the need to discourage the hoarding of medicines.

Proprietary medicines dispensed in an original package may be expected to have a shelf-life which approaches that given by the manufacturer, providing that the advice given on storage conditions is heeded by the patient. However, transfer from an original pack to another container, particularly if the product is modified or diluted, will significantly reduce shelf-life. An arbitrary shelf-life of 14 days after preparation is usually assigned to diluted preparations dispensed in a community pharmacy. Guidance on the stability of pharmacopoeial preparations is usually included in the monograph and information on the shelf-life of proprietary products is given in the manufacturer's data sheet. Other products should be treated as unresearched and given an arbitrarily short shelf-life. Recommended maximum storage times for preparations extemporaneously prepared or diluted are listed in Chapter 5 (see Table 5.2)

Although many patients may understand what is meant by 'expiry date', it is preferable to give the information in the least ambiguous way. 'Any unused to be discarded on (date)' or 'do not use after (date)', leaves little room for confusion.

It may be assumed that patients receiving a medicine for the first time will open the container immediately. However, patients receiving regular medication, e.g. with eye drops, may require the container to be labelled with an 'opened' as well as an 'unopened' expiry date. 'To be discarded 4 weeks after first opening' may be accompanied by 'date opened . . . .'. The inclusion of a space for the patient to enter the date first opened provides a useful reminder.

5. Give the patient clear and complete instructions on how to take or use the preparation

a. Directions. These include the quantity to be taken or the amount to be used, the frequency and timing of administration or application and the route of administration or the method of use. The prescriber normally includes instructions on the prescription form although the pharmacist may need to amplify or clarify the directions given by the prescriber.

In the absence of complete instructions from the prescriber, for non-systematically administered medicines and for antacid preparations the guide-lines given in the BNF may be followed. These should be qualified with the phrase 'unless otherwise directed' to avoid conflict with any verbal instructions the prescriber may have given the patient. The phrases 'to be taken', 'to be given' or 'to be used' are preferred to the alternative 'take', 'give' or 'use'. Any instruction written on the label of a dispensed medicine should be simple and preferably open to a single interpretation. 'One to be taken before breakfast' may be confusing to a patient who does not eat in the morning. If a dose is to be taken at bedtime, 'To be taken at night' should be further qualified. 'Three tablets to be taken daily' may be interpreted as three tablets to be taken on one occasion or one tablet to be taken on three occasions each day and should be clarified.

Numbers, except where they occur in statements of strength or in the term '5 ml spoonful', should be given in words. 'Two 5 ml spoonfuls' is preferable to '2 5 ml spoonfuls' to avoid possible misinterpretation.

b. *Shake the bottle*. Liquid medicines that are disperse systems need to be shaken immediately prior to use to ensure that the preparation is homogenous. This instruction must appear on the label of all suspensions, liquid emulsions, foams and aerosols whether for internal or external use in order to ensure accuracy of dosage.

c. *Take with water.* Mixtures for adult patients with a dose volume of 10 ml or more should be diluted with water before taking. For mixtures which are likely to cause gastrointestinal irritation, e.g. Potassium Citrate Mixture BP, the need for the dose to be 'well diluted' must be emphasized. Paediatric medicines with a 5 ml dose volume are generally given undiluted except for potentially irritant preparations, e.g. Chloral Elixir, Paediatric BP.

Most patients take oral solid-dose preparations with water or other liquid to aid swallowing. If tablets or capsules are allowed to remain in the oesophagus severe irritation may result. It is therefore important to ensure that sufficient liquid is taken to wash the medicine into the stomach, especially for elderly or supine patients.

CAUTIONARY AND ADVISORY LABELS

For external use only

This label must be applied to liquid preparations or gels formulated for external application (for definitions see Ch. 1). The label is also usually applied to all semi-solid and solid medicinal products for external use, e.g. ointments, creams and dusting powders.

Not to be taken

This label may be used on preparations that are neither administered by mouth nor used on the skin. It may also be used on preparations which appear to be used 'internally' on which the words 'for external use' might worry a patient, e.g. medicines for rectal, vaginal or nasal application. 'For nasal use only', 'For rectal use only', 'For vaginal use only' labels may be preferred.

'Not to be swallowed in large amounts' is a better label for mouthwashes and gargles where swallowing of a small amount is inevitable but swallowing large quantities is undesirable.

Hexachlorophane warning

Products containing hexachlorophane should not be used indiscriminately in very young children or in certain animals because of possible serious toxicity. A warning to this effect should be included on the labels of products containing this substance.

Keep out of the reach of children

All medicines should be stored in a place inaccessible to children and must be so labelled.

For animal treatment only

A clear distinction must be made between medicines intended for human use and those intended for veterinary use.

RECOMMENDED CAUTIONARY AND ADVISORY LABELS

It is generally recognized that patients require adequate information so that they will take their medicine safely and effectively. Guidance for pharmacists on the cautionary and advisory labels to be applied to dispensed medicines is provided by the Royal Pharmaceutical Society of Great Britain. Pharmacists may use their discretion in applying standard labels and in using verbal counselling as an alternative. Occasionally a prescriber may not wish additional cautionary labels to be used and will endorse the prescription 'N.C.L.' — no cautionary labels.

The recommended label wordings are published in the BNF and are divided into two sections. Labels 1 to 19 are usually given as separate warnings and labels 21 to 28 may be incorporated into the directions for dosage or administration. The BNF also shows under many products the numbers of any labels recommended for application by the pharmacist. In the paragraphs below, the numbers printed on the labels refer to the 'Cautionary advisory label warnings' listed in the BNF.

The following label wordings and numbers are those recommended in Appendix 4 of the BNF No. 16 1988. The BNF is constantly updated and the reader is recommended at all times to use the current edition.

Drowsiness warnings

Patients should be warned if their medicine is likely to cause drowsiness, dizziness, blurred vision or may impair their ability to drive or operate machinery safely, especially in combination with alcohol. Drowsiness warning labels may be worded to suit different circumstances.

> Warning. May cause
> 1   drowsiness

This label is to be used for children's medicines which may cause sedation and where driving or alcohol intake warnings would be inappropriate. For children of school age an additional warning about cycling may be appropriate.

> Warning. May cause
> drowsiness. If affected do not
> drive or operate machinery.
> 2   Avoid alcoholic drink

Many preparations can cause drowsiness particularly in combination with alcohol. Driving under the influence of drink or drugs is an offence in many countries including the UK.

> Warning. Causes drowsiness
> which may persist the next
> day. If affected do not drive
> or operate machinery. Avoid
> 19   alcoholic drink

Hypnotics taken at bedtime are expected by the patient to induce sleep. However, drowsiness persisting the next day may be less expected. The patient should therefore be warned of the possibility.

> Warning. May cause
> drowsiness. If affected do not
> drive or operate machinery
> 3

For patients who have had separate counselling on alcohol intake this label is more appropriate.

Potential interactions with food or drink

> Warning. Avoid alcoholic drink
> 4

Alcohol may provoke a reaction such as flushing when taken in combination with substances like metronidazole or chlorpropamide and should therefore be avoided when taking such medication.

> 21 . . . with or after food

Products that are liable to cause gastrointestinal irritation and substances that are better absorbed with food should carry this label. The patient should be counselled that 'food' does not necessarily mean a full meal.

> . . . half to one hour before
> 22   food

Some medicines should be allowed to exert an effect on the gastrointestinal tract prior to food being taken. For other preparations the absorption is improved if taken before food.

> . . . an hour before food or
> 23 on an empty stomach

To be used for oral antibiotics where the absorption is significantly decreased by the presence of food and acid in the stomach.

Potential interactions with other medicines

> Do not take remedies
> containing aspirin while
> 12 taking this medicine

For drugs whose activity is reduced by aspirin or for drugs with a similar action to aspirin (see also label 10)

> Do not take iron preparations
> or indigestion remedies at the
> same time of day as this
> 6   medicine

> Do not take milk, iron preparations or indigestion remedies at the same time of
> 7   day as this medicine

Some drugs chelate with calcium, magnesium and iron and are less well absorbed in the presence of these ions. The problem may be avoided by giving incompatible preparations about 2 hours apart.

> Do not take indigestion remedies at the same time of
> 5   day as this medicine

To be used for enteric-coated preparations coated to resist gastric acid and to disintegrate at alkaline pH in the small intestine. Raising the gastric pH may result in premature release of the drug.

Special dosage instructions

> Do not stop taking this medicine except on your
> 8   doctor's advice

> Take at regular intervals. Complete the prescribed course unless otherwise
> 9   directed

> Warning. Follow the printed instructions you have been
> 10 given with this medicine

To be used for preparations where separate instructions are provided, e.g. oral anticoagulant or monoamine-oxidase inhibitor treatment cards.

> To be applied sparingly . . .
> 28

To be used with external products where excessive use may produce local side-effects or unwanted absorption through the skin.

Warnings not to exceed a recommended dose

> Not more than . . . in 24 hours
> 17

This label is recommended for use on preparations for the treatment of acute migraine (except for ergotamine-containing preparations — see label 18). It may also be useful for medicines prescribed on an 'as required basis' where a recommended total daily dose should not be exceeded.

> Not more than . . . in 24 hours or . . . in any one week
> 18

To be used on preparations of ergotamine tartrate.

> Do not take more than 2 at any one time. Do not take
> 29 more than 8 in 24 hours

To be used on solid unit dose preparations containing paracetamol for adults. The warning should be modified for children's doses.

Special methods of administration

> Dissolve or mix with water
> 13   before taking.

To be used on soluble preparations or for powders or granules to be dispersed in water prior to taking.

> 27 . . . with plenty of water

To be used on preparations likely to cause gastrointestinal irritation unless well diluted. Also where a high fluid intake is desirable.

> . . . swallowed whole, not
> 25   chewed

To be used for enteric-coated, sustained-release or unpleasantly tasting preparations

> . . . dissolved under the
> 26   tongue

To be used on preparations formulated for absorption through the sublingual mucosa.

Allow to dissolve under the tongue. Do not transfer from this container. Keep tightly closed. Discard 8 weeks after 16 first opening

To be used on sublingual glyceryl trinitrate tablets. The additional comments reflect the volatility of glyceryl trinitrate.

24 ... sucked or chewed

For preparations like pastilles and lozenges formulated to dissolve in the mouth and for large or chewable tablets.

Cautions in use

Avoid exposure of skin to direct sunlight or sun lamps 11

To be used on preparations that may induce photosensitization.

This preparation may colour the urine or stools 14

This label should be qualified by verbal advice on the likely effect.

Caution flammable: keep 15 away from naked flames

To be applied to preparations containing a high proportion of flammable solvent

Pharmacists must use professional discretion in the use of recommended labels. Although many labelling systems are programmed to generate the BNF labels automatically, indiscriminate use may not be in the best interests of the patient. In some cases one or more of the labels may be omitted and the patient counselled. In some cases additional written information may be supplied in the form of manufacturer's package inserts or other advisory leaflets (see Ch. 37).

Advisory statements for patients are also included in many of the monographs of the Pharmaceutical Codex 1979. These are particularly useful for older formulations which may no longer be included in the BNF.

SPECIAL LABELLING INSTRUCTIONS FOR PARTICULAR TYPES OF DISPENSED DOSAGE FORM

The following is a summary of the guidance given in the Pharmaceutical Codex 1979 and the British Pharmacopoeia

Pressurized inhalations (Aerosol inhalations)

Pressurized container, keep away from heat sources including the sun. Do not puncture or burn even when empty

Shake before using

Follow the instructions and do not exceed the prescribed dose

Applications

For external use only

Cachets

Immerse the cachet in water for a few seconds, place on the tongue and swallow with a draught of water

Capsules

Swallow whole with a draught of water

Collodions

For external use only

Flammable

Creams

> For external use only

> Store in a cool place but do not freeze

'Sterile' only if appropriate,

> Sterile

Dusting powders

> For external use only

> Not to be applied to open wounds or to raw or weeping surfaces

'Sterile' only if appropriate,

> Sterile

Ear drops

> For external use only

Emulsions

> Shake the bottle

Enemas

> For rectal use only

> Shake before use

(for large volumes)

> Warm to body temperature before use

Eye drops

> Avoid contamination in use

> Discard 28 days after first opening

Eye lotions

If unpreserved,

> Discard 24 hours after first opening

Gargles and mouthwashes

Dilution directions if appropriate and unless intended to be swallowed after use.

> Not to be swallowed in large amounts

Gels

> For external use

If appropriate,

> Sterile

Granules

> To be dissolved or dispersed in water before taking

or

> To be placed on the back of the tongue and swallowed with a draught of water

Inhalations

> Not to be taken

> Shake the bottle

If volatile at room temperature,

> Add a small quantity to an absorbent pad and inhale the vapour

or if intended to be added to hot water,

> One teaspoonful to be added to one pint of hot, not boiling water and the vapour inhaled for 5 to 10 minutes

Insufflations

> Not to be swallowed

Linctuses

> To be sipped and swallowed slowly without the addition of water

Liniments and lotions

> For external use only

> Shake the bottle

> Avoid broken skin

Mixtures

> Shake the bottle

Most adult mixtures should be taken with water, some should be

> . . . well diluted

Paediatric mixtures with a 5 ml dose volume should be given undiluted unless stated in the monograph.

Nasal drops

> For nasal use only

or

> Not to be taken

Usually, for decongestant preparations,

> Avoid prolonged or excessive use

Ointments

> For external use only

If appropriate,

> Sterile

Paints

> For external use only

If appropriate,

> Flammable

Pastes

> For external use only

Pessaries

> For vaginal use only

or

> Not to be swallowed

> Store in a cool place

If appropriate,

> To be unwrapped before insertion

Powders (oral)

Single-dose powders should be stirred into water before swallowing or placed on the back of the tongue and swallowed with a draught of water.

Effervescent powders should be dissolved in water before taking.

Bulk powders may be measured in level 5 ml spoonfuls and dissolved or dispersed in a little water before swallowing.

Solutions

If for external application,

> For external use only

If not to be taken orally nor to be applied externally,

> Not to be taken

If sterile,

> Sterile — not to be used for injection

Suppositories

> For rectal use only

or

> not to be swallowed

> Store in a cool place

If appropriate,

> To be unwrapped before insertion

Tablets

For soluble or dispersible tablets,

> Dissolve or disperse in water before taking

For chewable tablets,

> Chew before swallowing

for sustained-release, enteric-coated or unpleasant-tasting tablets.

> Do not crush or chew

Other tablets are intended to be swallowed whole with a draught of water, preferably while sitting or standing.

PREPARATION OF LABELS FOR DISPENSED MEDICINES

The use of a typewriter or mechanical printer to produce dispensing labels has been recommended by the Royal Pharmaceutical Society of Great Britain since January 1984. Although printed labels are to be preferred to poorly handwritten labels, it should be remembered that faint print, particularly of small size, may be difficult for the elderly and those with impaired sight to read. Traditionally, gummed labels were purchased ready printed with the name and address of the pharmacy together with other standard information. Internal preparations carried labels with black printing and external preparations carried labels with red printing. Many modern printers use only one type of label and use only black ink, the name and address of the pharmacy being printed on each label at the same time as the other information for the patient. All the information required by the patient may be printed onto the main label, if there is sufficient space. The use of computerized systems allows the automatic inclusion of standard advisory statements on the main label. Alternatively, separate preprinted additional labels may be used. These should be arranged neatly, preferably on the 'front' of the container where they will be obvious to the patient. For preparations supplied in manufacturer's original packs which already bear complete instructions to the patient, care should be taken to avoid obscuring these instructions when additional labels are added. When the product is supplied in a paperboard outer package, the label should be attached to the inner container since the outer packaging may be discarded immediately by the patient.

Computer labelling

The availability of relatively inexpensive computer systems has provided a major advance in label writing in the pharmacy. The ability to generate labels is usually combined with a stock control function including automatic re-ordering. Patient medication profiles may also be automatically stored. Telephone links between computers allow access to wholesalers and on-line information sources such as PINS (Pharmacy News and Information Service) and Martindale On Line. Progress in this field is rapid and current awareness is essential.

BIBLIOGRAPHY

ABPI Data Sheet Compendium current edition. Datapharm Publications, London (updated annually)
British National Formulary 1988 16th edn. British Medical Association and Royal Pharmaceutical Society of Great Britain, London (updated twice yearly)
British Pharmacopoeia 1980 HMSO, London (and addenda 1982, 1983 and 1986)
British Pharmacopoeia 1988 HMSO, London
British Pharmaceutical Codex 1973 Pharmaceutical Press, London
Dental Practitioners Formulary (DPF) 1986–88 with British National Formulary 1986 12th edn
Martindale, see Reynolds J E F
Martindale On Line: Drug information Thesaurus and User Guide 1984 Pharmaceutical Press, London
Medicines, Ethics and Practice — A Guide for Pharmacists

1989 No 3. Royal Pharmaceutical Society of Great Britain, London (updated twice yearly)
Pearce M E (ed) 1984 Medicines and poisons guide, 4th edn. (with cumulative amendments in the *Pharmaceutical Journal*). Pharmaceutical Press, London
Pharmaceutical Codex 1979 11th edn, incorporating the British Pharmaceutical Codex. Pharmaceutical Press, London
Pharmaceutical Society 1979 Guide to good dispensing practice. Pharmaceutical Journal 223: 157–158
Reynolds J E F (ed) 1989 Martindale, The Extra Pharmacopoeia, 29th edn. Pharmaceutical Press, London
Wade A (ed) 1980 Pharmaceutical handbook, 19th edn. Pharmaceutical Press, London

PART 2

Pharmaceutical preparations

INTRODUCTION

The chapters in this part of the book are concerned with the preparation on a small scale of different types of dosage form and the dispensing of extemporaneously prepared or commercially manufactured products. The products are grouped according to their physical nature: solutions, suspensions, emulsions, semi-solid preparations suppositories and pessaries, bulk powders and granules, oral unit dosage forms and aerosols.

The chapters have a common format. For each class of product the following aspects are described:

Formulation

Brief reference is made to the fundamental principles underlying the practical aspects of the formulation of the different product types. The reader is referred to the companion volume (Aulton 1988), in which the principles of dosage form design are fully discussed.

Compounding

The practical aspects of compounding on a small scale are described for each class of product. Examples of tried and tested traditional formulations are included at the end of each chapter in order to illustrate the application of the general principles. The reader should then be able to apply the general principles to any particular product. The methods described have been found to be suitable for bench-scale extemporaneous compounding.

Types of dosage form

The special features of the dosage forms associated with each class of product are described, together with an indication of special storage, packaging and labelling requirements. These notes are for general guidance only; requirements for individual products will depend on the legal and professional regulations currently applicable.

Examples

The examples also have a common format:

Instruction
Ingredients and master formula
Formulation
Compounding
Storage and shelf-life
Container
Advice for patients when dispensed
Actions and uses

It is hoped that the student will be encouraged to develop a systematic approach to compounding and dispensing as described in Chapter 5. Although a brief indication of storage, packaging and special labelling requirements are given for the examples chosen these are not intended to be exhaustive and the reader should use a range of current reference sources for further information (see Appendix 8).

11. Solutions

D. M. Collett

Solutions are homogeneous liquid preparations containing one or more dissolved ingredients and are used as a variety of dosage forms for internal and external use. The reader is referred to the companion volume (Aulton 1988) for further details on solutions.

FORMULATION

Vehicles

The vehicle is the medium in which the ingredients of a medicine are dissolved or dispersed — for solutions this is the solvent. Water is the vehicle of choice for the majority of pharmaceutical solutions. Water is generally available, relatively inexpensive, palatable and non-toxic for oral use and non-irritant for external use. It also acts as a solvent for a wide range of substances.

An important advantage of the formulation of a medicament in solution rather than in suspension, particularly for oral dosage forms, is the uniformity of dosage without the necessity to shake the bottle. For substances with low aqueous solubility it is often preferable to use a mixture of water with other solvents to give a complete solution rather than to make a suspension. Water acts as a solvent for a wide range of substances, although its use is limited by their solubility and by their resistance to degradation by hydrolysis (see Ch. 7).

Types of water

Potable water

This is drinking water freshly drawn from the public mains supply (it does not include water from a local storage tank which may be heavily contaminated with micro-organisms). If available, potable water is suitable for the preparation of pharmaceutical preparations for internal and external use (but not for parenteral purposes).

Purified water

This is prepared by deionization or distillation of potable water. If allowed to stand it may gain a high content of vegetative organisms and must always be freshly boiled and cooled before use in a pharmaceutical product.

Water for preparations

This may be either freshly drawn potable water or, if this is unavailable, freshly boiled and cooled Purified Water.

Potable water from some areas may be unsuitable for certain pharmaceutical products because of 'hardness' (high content of dissolved minerals) or pH. In such cases freshly boiled and cooled Purified Water should be used. Boiling has the additional advantage of removing dissolved oxygen and carbon dioxide from solution in the water.

Water for injections

This is pyrogen-free distilled water, sterilized immediately after collection and is used for parenteral preparations (see Part 3).

Solubility

Before attempting to formulate a solution, the solubilities of any ingredients must be determined. The pharmacopoeias state solubilities as the number of parts of solvent (by volume) that will dissolve one part (by weight of a solid or volume of a liquid) of the substance. For example, the statement that proflavine hemisulphate is soluble in 300 parts of water means that 1 g will dissolve in 300 ml of water at 20°C. The volume of such a solution will be more than 300 ml but less than 301 ml since the 1 g of proflavine hemisulphate will occupy a volume of less than 1 ml in the solution.

Solution of medicaments of low water solubility

Cosolvency

The phenomenon of cosolvency is discussed in detail in the companion volume (Chapter 14, Aulton 1988).

For oral solutions ethanol, glycerol and propylene glycol may be used in variable combinations with water as cosolvents (Example 11.1). The amount of ethanol in oral medicines is kept to a minimum because of its pharmacological effect, burning taste in high concentration and cost.

Solubilization

An alternative method for increasing the solubility of poorly water-soluble medicaments is by the use of a surface active agent and is called *solubilization*. The surface active agent must be present in solution at or above the critical micelle concentration (CMC). The increase in solubility of the solubilized material is explained in terms of partition between the aqueous phase and the micelles. For a detailed account of micelles and other interfacial phenomena see the companion volume (Chapters 4 and 6, Aulton 1988). Soaps have been used for many years to solubilize phenolic antiseptic substances (Example 11.2). For oral preparations, non-toxic surface active agents, such as polysorbates, many be used (see also Ch. 13).

Other pharmaceutical vehicles for solutions

Syrup (sucrose solution)

This is used alone or as a cosolvent for a number of oral medicines, particularly in elixirs and linctuses. Whilst acting as a sweetening agents, syrup has the disadvantage of promoting dental decay and being unsuitable for diabetic patients.

Ethanol

Ethanol is rarely used alone for internal preparations but is a useful solvent for substances to be applied externally to unbroken skin, particularly where fairly rapid evaporation is required. For example, insecticide lotion for application to hair infested with head lice. In the formulation of products intended solely for external use Industrial Methylated Spirit (IMS) may be substituted for ethanol provided that the statutory regulations are observed (Examples 11.2 and 11.3). IMS, which is 'denatured' by the addition of methyl alcohol, is free from excise duty and is less expensive than Ethanol BP.

Because of the toxicity of methyl alcohol, IMS must never be administered internally. IMS may contain a little acetone which reacts with iodine to produce irritating vapours. An acetone-free grade must be used for the preparation of alcoholic solutions of iodine.

Glycerol

Glycerol is used as a vehicle for some external preparations, such as ear drops, and as a cosolvent with water in solutions for internal use. Glycerol acts additionally as a sweetening agent and, in concentrations above 20%, as a preservative.

Propylene glycol

This has similar uses to glycerol. It is also used as a vehicle for ear drops (Example 11.4) and as a cosolvent in aqueous solutions. In some instances it is a better solvent than glycerol and produces less viscous solutions. It inhibits mould growth and fermentation. It may be included in spray solutions to stabilize the droplet size.

Arachis oil

This is a bland oil used as the solvent for Methyl Salicylate Liniment BP (see Example 3.10).

Acetone

Acetone is used as a cosolvent in some external preparations.

Solvent ether

This has been used as a cosolvent in external preparations for pre-operative skin preparation. The extreme volatility of ether and the risk of fire and explosion limit its usefulness.

Other additives

The gastrointestinal tract will tolerate solutions with a wide range of pH values. Solutions formulated for application to mucous membranes or broken skin may need to be adjusted to a neutral pH by the addition of a phosphate buffer or similar non-toxic substance.

Hypertonic solutions such as Potassium Citrate Mixture BP should be well diluted before taking orally. Solutions prepared for application to mucosal surfaces such as nasal drops usually include sodium chloride to increase the tonicity to that of body fluids.

Stabilizers

Oxidation is a common route of degradation of substances included in pharmaceutical solutions. Ascorbic acid is a useful antioxidant (Example 11.5) since it is non-toxic and palatable. Sodium metabisulphite is a permitted reducing agent.

Preservatives

Microbial contamination of medicinal products should be minimized by choice of suitable raw materials and by good dispensing practice. The inclusion of a preservative makes conditions in the solution less favourable to microbial growth.

For solutions designed for oral administration chloroform (0.25% v/v) included as Chloroform Water BP or benzoic acid (0.1% w/v) are suitable preservatives. Solutions for external use may include chlorocresol (0.1% w/v), chlorbutol (0.5% w/v, Example 11.6) and the parahydroxybenzoates (parobens).

Colours and flavours

Colour may be included in solutions for external use as an identification or warning. Solutions for oral administration may be sweetened or flavoured to disguise an unpleasantly tasting medicament and coloured appropriately (see Chapter 6).

COMPOUNDING

The basic techniques for preparation of pharmaceutical solutions are weighing, measuring of liquids, dissolution and filtration. These are described in Chapter 4.

SOLUTIONS AS ORAL DOSAGE FORMS

Elixirs, linctuses, mixtures and oral solutions

Elixirs are solutions for oral administration. The vehicle usually contains syrup, ethanol or other cosolvents to give a clear solution and a pleasant taste.

Linctuses are formulated with syrup as the vehicle and are designed to soothe sore mucous membranes in the treatment of cough (Example 11.7).

Mixtures are liquid preparations for oral administration and contain medicaments dissolved and/or suspended in water.

Oral solutions contain one or more ingredients dissolved in a suitable vehicle.

Advantages of solutions as an oral dosage form

— Absorption of the medicine from the gastrointestinal tract is rapid.
— Easy to swallow for children and some adults, especially the elderly.
— Uniform distribution of medicament, no need to shake.

Disadvantages of solutions as an oral dosage form

— Medicaments are less stable in solution than in a dry dosage form.
— Unpleasant flavours may be difficult to mask.
— Bulky to carry around.
— Vulnerable to loss by breakage of the container.
— A means of measuring the dose is required.
— Measurement depends on the accuracy and reliability of the patient.

Preparing dilutions of solutions for oral administration

If a dose less than 5 ml is prescribed, an oral liquid is usually diluted so that the patient can measure the dose in 5 ml spoonfuls. Exceptions include some preparations with cosolvent vehicles, e.g. Paediatric Digoxin Oral Solution BP 1988 and Paediatric Paracetamol Oral Solution BP 1988.

Choice of diluent

Dilution of a mixture, elixir or linctus may adversely affect its flavour, appearance or stability, therefore choice of the most appropriate diluent is crucial. For proprietary preparations which may be diluted the diluent to be used is that recommended by the manufacturer. The relevant information may usually be found in the manufacturer's data sheet, in the BNF or in the NPA diluent directory.

Extemporaneously dispensed products are usually diluted with the vehicle which is often water or syrup and usually appears as the last line in the formula (Examples 11.7 and 11.8). It should be noted that if the penultimate line in the formula for a mixture is 'Chloroform Water Double Strength' then the vehicle is actually single strength Chloroform Water BP and this should be used as the diluent (Example 11.5). In this circumstance the use of water as the diluent would effectively halve the preservation concentration in the preparation. For some 'official' preparations the appropriate diluent is stated in the BNF formulary and may not be the vehicle (Example 11.9).

Shelf-life of elixirs, linctuses, mixtures and oral solutions

Most 'official' mixtures and some oral solutions should be freshly or recently prepared and have a relatively short shelf-life (see Table 5.2). 'Official' elixirs, linctuses and manufactured products are generally more stable unless diluted — the appropriate monograph or data sheet should be consulted for details.

Diluted liquid oral products generally have a shorter shelf-life than the original preparation — usually a maximum of 14 days after dilution (see Table 5.2). The dilution should be freshly prepared.

Supply of liquid oral preparations with a short-shelf-life

The quantity of any medicine supplied to a patient must not exceed that which would be expected to be used within the shelf-life. If more than 2 weeks' supply of a product with a 2-week shelf-life is prescribed the medicine must be supplied in installments (see Example 11.5). The patient or the patient's representative should be asked to call back for further supplies at appropriate intervals. Whenever possible the supply should be made in filled rather than partly filled containers but the patient should be asked to call back on the minimum number of occasions practicable (see Example 11.5).

Containers for elixirs, linctuses, mixtures and oral solutions

Amber medicine bottles should be used. A 5 ml measuring spoon should be supplied to the patient.

Special labels and advice for patients

Linctuses should be sipped and swallowed slowly, without the addition of water.

Mouthwashes and gargles

Mouthwashes are used to clean and refresh the buccal cavity. They contain antiseptics or astringents in a pleasantly flavoured vehicle (Example 11.10).

Gargles are used to relieve soreness in mild throat infections and contain antiseptic, analgesic and weak astringents.

Gargles and mouthwashes are usually diluted by the patient with warm water before use and most are not intended to be swallowed in significant amounts.

Shelf-life of mouthwashes and gargles

Commercial products usually have a long shelf-life and the 'official' examples are generally stable preparations which may be prepared for stock (see Table 5.2).

Containers for mouthwashes and gargles

Extemporaneously prepared or poured preparations are supplied in amber fluted bottles although manufacturer's original bottles are often non-fluted. Medicine bottles may be used for products intended to be swallowed.

Special labels and advice for patients

Dilution directions should be in terms that the patient can understand (see Example 11.10).

For preparations not intended to be swallowed

> not to be swallowed in large amounts

is the appropriate warning.

SOLUTIONS INSTILLED INTO BODY CAVITIES

Nasal drops and sprays

Solutions of medicaments designed to be applied to the nasal mucosa in a small volume are usually formulated to be iso-osmotic with nasal secretions and if necessary buffered slightly to the acid side of neutral (pH 6.5) in order to minimize damage to the nasal cilia. Nasal solutions are used commonly to relieve nasal irritation and congestion, although antimicrobial substances may also be included. The nasal route can be used to introduce drugs required to produce a systemic effect, e.g. the peptide hormones of the posterior lobe of the pituitary gland and their synthetic analogues. Most nasal preparations are supplied in manufacturer's original packs. Ephedrine nasal drops may be prepared extemporaneously (Example 11.6).

Shelf-life of nasal preparations

Manufacturer's data sheets should be consulted for information on the shelf-life of commercial preparations.

The 'official' monographs provide guidance for products prepared extemporaneously

Containers for nasal preparations

Extemporaneously prepared nasal drops are supplied in hexagonal, amber fluted glass bottles with a rubber teat and dropper closure. Some commercially produced nasal drops are also supplied in glass dropper bottles which may or may not be fluted.

Single-application containers of nasal drops are also produced.

Nasal sprays may be packed in flexible plastic bottles designed to deliver a fine spray through a small orifice when the bottle is squeezed or may be packed in pressurized containers designed to deliver a metered dose of medicament.

Special labels and advice for patients

For decongestant nasal drops patients should

> Avoid excessive use

and

> Avoid use in very young babies unless under medical advice

Counselling in the use of the different types of applicator should be given.

Patients receiving systemic medication via the nasal route (e.g. for enuresis) require special counselling.

Ear drops

Ear drops are usually simple solutions of medicaments designed to exert a local effect in the ear, to soften wax, to treat local inflammation and infection, or to relieve pain. The vehicle may be water although glycerol and propylene glycol may also be used (Example 11.4).

Shelf-life of ear drops

Most products are stable but preparations containing antibiotics may require special storage.

Containers for ear drops

Ear drops are supplied in containers similar to those used for nasal drops, i.e. glass bottles with a teat and dropper closure or plastic squeeze bottles.

Special labels and advice for patients

The method of use of the ear drops should be explained to the patient.

Enemas

Enemas are aqueous or oily solutions or suspensions that are introduced into the rectum for cleansing, therapeutic or diagnostic purposes.

Cleansing preparations are used to evacuate faeces in constipation or before surgery or childbirth. They act by stimulating peristalsis because they are introduced in a large volume (0.5–1 litre) in the case of plain water or because, in the case of e.g. magnesium sulphate retention enema, they are introduced in a smaller volume (130 ml) and cause the osmotic retention of water in the bowel.

Cleansing preparations may also act by lubricating impacted faeces in constipation, e.g. enemas containing glycerol, sodium citrate and sodium lauryl sulphoacetate.

Therapeutic enemas may contain medicaments required to exert a local effect in the large bowel, e.g. anti-inflammatory agents.

The rectum may also be used as a route of administration for drugs to exert a systemic effect in a patient who is unconscious, vomiting or otherwise unable to tolerate the drug by mouth, e.g. diazepam, paraldehyde (Example 11.11). X-ray contrast media may be administered in the form of an enema to aid diagnostic investigation of the large bowel.

Shelf-life of enemas

See manufacturer's data or monograph. Paraldehyde is very unstable especially if exposed to light.

Containers for enemas

Amber fluted glass bottles.

Commercially produced enemas are usually packed in disposable polythene or polyvinyl chloride bags sealed to a rectal nozzle.

Special labels and advice for patients

> For rectal use only

Large volume enemas should be warmed to body temperature before use. For enemas to be self-administered by the patient special counselling is required.

SOLUTIONS FOR EXTERNAL USE

Liniments, lotions and paints

Liniments that are solutions are formulated with an alcoholic or an oily vehicle and are intended for rubbing into unbroken skin.

Lotions are also intended to be applied to unbroken skin but without friction. For lotions intended to evaporate quickly on the skin surface the vehicle is usually alcoholic and acetone may also be included (Example 11.3).

Paints are usually applied to the skin with a brush. The solvent may be water or an organic solvent where rapid evaporation is required.

Shelf-life of liniments, lotions and paints

These preparations are usually stable but packaging and storage must protect against evaporation of volatile constituents.

Containers for liniments, lotions and paints

Solutions for external use should be dispensed in fluted amber containers. A brush may be required for application of a paint and commercially packed products often incorporate a brush or applicator in the closure of the container.

Special labels and advice for patients

Liniments and lotions should not be applied to broken skin. Flammable products must carry a warning to avoid naked flames.

Antiseptic and disinfectant solutions

These contain antimicrobial substances and may be used to reduce the numbers of micro-organisms on the skin surface or on inanimate objects such as equipment or work surfaces. Aqueous solutions of antiseptics are easily contaminated with resistant micro-organisms and only concentrated solutions should be stored if not sterilized on preparation. Examples include benzalkonium chloride solution (Example 3.12), cetrimide solution (Example 3.13), potassium permanganate solution (Examples 3.14 and 11.12) and proflavine solution (Example 3.15).

Chloroxylenol is only slightly soluble in water and is prepared as a solution solubilized with a potassium ricinoleate soap (Example 11.2).

Shelf-life of antiseptic and disinfectant solutions

Non-sterile aqueous solutions of antiseptics that are not concentrates should be discarded within 7 days of preparation. Concentrated solutions of cetrimide (40% w/v), benzalkonium chloride (50% w/v) or chlorhexidine gluconate (20% w/v) are commercially available and carry pack expiry dates.

Containers for antiseptic and disinfectant solutions

Solutions for external use are supplied to patients in fluted amber containers. Commercially produced solutions are often supplied in plastic containers which may not be fluted.

Special labels and advice for patients

Dilution directions are required for some antiseptic solutions (Examples 3.14, 3.15 and 11.12).

Patients should be warned to discard the stock solution after 7 days and to discard any diluted solution immediately after use.

EXAMPLES

Example 11.1

Prepare 100 ml phenobarbitone elixir to the following formula:

Ingredients	Master formula
Phenobarbitone	400 mg
Ethanol (90%)	40 ml
Compound Orange Spirit	2.5 ml
Glycerol	40 ml
Amaranth Solution	1 ml
Water	to 100 ml

Label: 10 ml to be given at night.
(Dosage confirmed as suitable for a paediatric patient).

Formulation
Ethanol (90%) and glycerol are included as cosolvents for the phenobarbitone.

Compound orange spirit is used with the glycerol for flavour and the amaranth solution for colour.

Suggested diluent: Syrup BP.

Compounding
Dissolve the phenobarbitone in the ethanol (90%) and

add the compound orange spirit before adding the glycerol, amaranth solution and water to volume.

Addition of water to the compound orange spirit displaces some of the oil from alcoholic solution. The excess oil may be removed by adding approximately 25 g sterilized purified talc per litre of elixir as an adsorbent. The product is allowed to stand for a few hours with occasional shaking before the talc is filtered off.

Storage and shelf-life
The preparation is light sensitive.

This is an 'unofficial' preparation therefore treat as unstable until researched.

Container
Amber medicine bottle.

Advice for patients when dispensed
Phenobarbitone causes drowsiness, alcohol should be avoided — use appropriate warning for a child.

Anticonvulsant therapy should not be discontinued without medical advice.

Actions and uses
Anticonvulsant.

Label (for dispensing)

---

100 ml PHENOBARBITONE ELIXIR

containing in each 5 ml dose
Phenobarbitone 20 mg, Ethanol (90%) 2 ml
Compound Orange Spirit 0.125 ml, Glycerol 2 ml
Amaranth Solution 0.05 ml

TWO 5 ml spoonfuls to be given at night

Store in a dark place
and do not use after (state date)

Warning. May cause drowsiness

Patient's name   date
Name and address of Pharmacy
Keep all medicines out of reach of children

Example 11.2

Prepare 200 ml Chloroxylenol Solution BP 1988

Ingredients	Master formula	
Chloroxylenol	50.0	g
Potassium hydroxide	13.6	g
Oleic Acid	7.5	ml
Castor Oil	63.0	g
Terpineol	100	ml
Ethanol 96%	200	ml
Purified Water, freshly boiled and cooled sufficient to produce	1000	ml

Formulation
Chloroxylenol is only slightly soluble in water (1 in 3000). Solubilization of the chloroxylenol in micelles is

achieved by means of a castor oil soap, mainly potassium ricinoleate produced during preparation from the castor oil and potassium hydroxide. Oleic acid is used to neutralize excess alkali by forming potassium oleate soap because the antimicrobial action of chloroxylenol is reduced in alkaline solutions which may also cause smarting. Chloroxylenol is very soluble in ethanol and terpineol. The terpineol helps to prevent separation of the chloroxylenol on dilution and also contributes to the characteristic odour of the preparation. Since the preparation is for external use Industrial Methylated Spirit BP (IMS) may be substituted for the Ethanol 96% BP.

Compounding
The soap is first prepared by dissolving the potassium hydroxide in a little water, adding a solution of castor oil in part of the IMS, mixing well and setting aside for about an hour until a small portion gives a clear solution with 19 times its volume of purified water. Saponification occurs more quickly in alcoholic solution and, therefore, it is very important not to exceed the volume of water recommended for dissolving the alkali. Oleic acid is then added to neutralize the soap solution.

Chloroxylenol is dissolved in the remaining alcohol (IMS), the solution is mixed with the terpineol and the mixture added to the neutralized soap solution. Finally the volume is adjusted with water with constant stirring. The preparation should remain clear because the chloroxylenol is solubilized by the soap micelles. On further dilution with water a fine white emulsion is produced.

Storage and shelf-life
The preparation should be kept in well-closed containers and contamination in use avoided. Cool storage is appropriate for volatile ingredients.

Container
Amber fluted bottle, well cleaned before filling. The solution should not be allowed contact with cork, a polyethylene liner is appropriate.

Advice for patients when dispensed
To be diluted before use (a 5% v/v (1 in 20) dilution is suitable for general use in the treatment of abrasions, cuts and wounds). Wet dressings should not be left in contact with the skin.

Actions and uses
Antiseptic for the skin.

Example 11.3

Prepare 500 ml Salicylic Acid Lotion BP 1988

Ingredients	Master formula
Salicylic Acid	20 g
Castor Oil	10 ml
Ethanol 96% sufficient to produce	1000 ml

Formulation
Since the preparation is for external use only the Ethanol 96% BP may be replaced with Industrial Methylated Spirit BP.

Compounding
The castor oil is very viscous, the measure should be well rinsed with the vehicle.

Storage and shelf-life
The preparation should be stored in a cool place away from naked flames.

Container
Amber fluted bottle.

Advice for patients when dispensed
The preparation should not be used nor the hair dried near a fire or naked flame.

Actions and uses
Keratolytic scalp lotion.

Example 11.4

Prepare 20 ml ear drops containing chloramphenicol 5% w/v in propylene glycol

Ingredients
Chloramphenicol
Propylene Glycol

Formulation
Chloramphenicol is only sparingly soluble in water. Propylene glycol may be used to prepare solutions of higher concentration than could be achieved with water but may not be used if the solution is to be applied to mucous membranes, e.g. eye drops or nasal drops, because of irritation.

Note that although a standard is given for Chloramphenicol Ear Drops in BP 1988 Addendum 1989 neither the strength nor the vehicle is specified. The product label therefore must state clearly the concentration of the ingredients.

Compounding
Propylene glycol is a viscous vehicle — all measures used should be well drained.

Storage and shelf-life
Chloramphenicol should be protected from light.

Container
Amber fluted dropper bottle.

Advice for patients when dispensed
The prescribed course should be completed.

Actions and uses
Antibiotic.

Example 11.5

Respond to a prescription for 150 ml Paediatric Ferrous Sulphate Oral Solution BP 1988 for a 4-month-old child.

Ingredients	Master formula
Ferrous Sulphate	12 g
Ascorbic Acid	2 g
Orange Syrup	100 ml
Double-strength, Chloroform Water	500 ml
Water sufficient to produce	1000 ml

Label: 2.5 ml to be given twice daily.

Formulation
Ascorbic acid is included as an antioxidant for the ferrous sulphate. Orange syrup masks the unpleasant taste and chloroform water acts as flavouring, preservative and vehicle.

The use of 'hard' tap water may lead to discoloration of the product and the use of purified water, freshly boiled and cooled is recommended.

Dilution The product should be diluted to give a 5 ml dose volume. No special diluent is specified so the vehicle should be used. The penultimate line in the formula is double-strength chloroform water and therefore the vehicle is chloroform water single strength.

Diluting the product reduces the shelf-life of the mixture and the amount to be issued to the patient on one occasion should be a maximum of 14 days' supply.

Calculation of the amount to send The prescriber has ordered 150/2.5 ml = 60 doses. Therefore 60 × 5 ml doses (300 ml) or 30 days' supply of the diluted preparation must be dispensed in total. Two weeks supply = 10 × 14 = 140 ml in this case. The patient's representative will need to return twice to the pharmacy to collect further supplies. Whilst they could be given 140 ml followed by 140 ml and 20 ml, it would be more sensible to supply the medicine in three instalments each of 100 ml in filled containers. 50 ml of the mixture would be prepared on each occasion and diluted to 100 ml with the diluent.

Compounding
Dissolve the ascorbic acid in the double-strength chloroform water and use this solution to dissolve the ferrous sulphate, add the orange syrup and adjust to volume.

Storage and shelf-life
Ferrous sulphate in solution oxidizes rapidly on exposure to air. The undiluted mixture should be recently prepared.

Container
Amber medicine bottle.

Advice for patients
To be given well diluted with water.

Actions and uses
Haematinic.

Example 11.6

Prepare 20 ml Ephedrine Nasal Drops BPC 1973

Ingredients	Master formula
Ephedrine Hydrochloride	0.5 g
Chlorbutol	0.5 g
Sodium Chloride	0.5 g
Water	to 100 ml

Formulation
The active ingredient is the ephedrine hydrochloride, chlorbutol acts as a preservative and sodium chloride is present to make the drops iso-osmotic with nasal secretions.

Compounding
Chlorbutol is a volatile substance that dissolves very slowly in the cold. In order to achieve rapid solution the method described in Chapter 4 should be used:

1. Powder a slight excess of the chlorbutol prior to weighing accurately.
2. Select a small conical flask with a suitable stopper.
3. Heat as much water as the formula allows to 60°C in the open conical flask.
4. Add the chlorbutol to the hot water.
5. Quickly insert the stopper and shake until solution is complete.

The solution should then be cooled before dissolving the other ingredients and adjusted to volume at room temperature.

The solution is to be used in the nasal cavity in contact with mucous membranes and should be clarified by passing through filter paper before making up to volume through the filter (see Ch. 4).

Storage and shelf-life
Ephedrine hydrochloride should be protected from light. The preparation should be stored cool in a well-closed container to avoid loss of volatile preservative.

Container
Amber fluted dropper bottle.

Advice for patients when dispensed
Avoid excessive use.

Actions and uses
Nasal decongestant.

Example 11.7

Prepare 500 ml Simple Linctus BP 1988

Ingredients	Master formula
Concentrated Anise Water	10 ml
Amaranth Solution	15 ml
Citric Acid Monohydrate	25 g
Chloroform Spirit	60 ml
Syrup sufficient to produce	1000 ml

Formulation
The anise, citric acid and chloroform act as flavouring, the amaranth as colouring and the syrup as a demulcent vehicle.

Dilution For diluted preparations the diluent specified is Syrup BP (see BNF).

Compounding
The citric acid should be dissolved in the chloroform spirit, concentrated anise water and amaranth solution before adding the syrup to volume.

Storage and shelf-life
The storage temperature should not exceed 25°C and marked fluctuations should be avoided.

Container
Amber medicine bottle.

Advice for patients when dispensed
To be sipped and swallowed slowly undiluted.

Actions and uses
Demulcent in the treatment of cough.

Example 11.8

Prepare 200 ml Paediatric Chloral Elixir BP 1988. Label for dispensary stock

The BNF lists many BP formulae. The master formulae for most children's liquids, linctuses and elixirs are given in terms of a 5 ml dose volume. The following is an example of scaling *up* from a master formula for 5 ml.

Ingredients	Master formula (from BNF*)	Scaled quantities
Chloral Hydrate	200 mg	8 g
Water for Preparations	0.1 ml	4 ml
Black Currant Syrup	1.0 ml	40 ml
Syrup	to 5.0 ml	to 200 ml

Formulation
Black currant syrup and syrup are used as sweetening and flavouring agents to mask the unpleasant taste of the chloral hydrate and make the preparation palatable for children.

Chloral hydrate dissolves readily in the small amount of water included in the formula.

For diluted preparations the diluent is syrup (see Example 3.21).

Compounding
Dissolve the chloral hydrate in the water before adding the viscous vehicle.

Add the black currant syrup (drain measure well and rinse with syrup).

Make up to volume with syrup in a tared container because of the problem of draining the viscous preparation from a measure (see Ch. 4).

Storage and shelf-life
Chloral hydrate is volatile and sensitive to light. The preparation should be recently prepared

Container
Amber medicine bottle.

Advice for patients (not applicable until dispensed)
Chloral hydrate is corrosive to skin and mucous membranes unless well diluted.

Chloral hydrate causes drowsiness.

Actions and uses
Hypnotic and sedative.

Label (for stock)

> 200 ml CHLORAL ELIXIR, PAEDIATRIC BP
> BN ex11   date prepared
> Keep well closed and store in a cool dark place
> Discard if not issued before   (*state date)
> Name and address of Pharmacy

*Two weeks after preparation.
This allows for 2 weeks' shelf-life in the hands of the patient, thus a total shelf-life of 4 weeks.

Example 11.9

Prepare 200 ml Potassium Citrate Mixture BP 1988

Ingredients	Master formula
Potassium Citrate	300 g
Citric Acid Monohydrate	50 g
Lemon Spirit	5 ml
Quillaia Tincture	10 ml
Syrup	25 ml
Double-strength, Chloroform Water	300 ml
Water sufficient to produce	1000 ml

Formulation

The active ingredients are citric acid and potassium citrate. Lemon spirit is the flavouring agent and consists of lemon oil in alcoholic solution. The oil tends to be displaced from solution in an aqueous medium especially in the presence of the high concentration of salts. The quillaia tincture is a surfactant included to emulsify any displaced lemon oil. Syrup is also included to improve the taste of the mixture. Because of the large quantities of medicaments and adjuncts in this mixture the amount of double-strength chloroform water is less than half the total volume of the preparation (300 ml per litre instead of the usual 500 ml per litre).

Dilution   For diluted preparations the preferred diluent specified is Syrup BP (see BNF).

Compounding

The product requires a large quantity of salts to be completely dissolved in a mixture of the syrup and double-strength chloroform water. Dissolution may be hastened by prior size reduction of the solids and by vigorous agitation but heat should be avoided because of the volatility of the chloroform (see Ch. 4).

The quillaia tincture should be added prior to the lemon spirit with constant agitation in order to achieve adequate emulsification of the oil.

Storage and shelf-life

The product should be recently prepared.

Container

Amber medicine bottle.

Advice for patients when dispensed

To be taken very well diluted with water. Shake the bottle.

Actions and uses

Alkalinization of urine in mild urinary tract infections.

Example 11.10

Prepare 200 ml Zinc Sulphate and Zinc Chloride Mouthwash BPC 1973

Ingredients	Master formula
Zinc Sulphate	20 g
Zinc Chloride	10 g
Compound Tartrazine Solution*	10 ml
Dilute Hydrochloric Acid	10 ml
Chloroform Water, Double-strength	500 ml
Water	to 1000 ml

*For tartrazine-sensitive patients, this may now be omitted (see Ch. 6).

Formulation

The active ingredients are the astringent zinc salts. Zinc chloride usually contains some oxychloride which makes the solution turbid; this disappears when the hydrochloric acid is added. Tartrazine provides colour and chloroform acts as a flavouring and preservative.

Compounding

Zinc chloride is very deliquescent and should be stored in a dessicator. A small quantity should be crushed in a mortar before weighing.

The solution is to be used in the oral cavity in contact with mucous membranes and should be free from irritant particles. Zinc chloride reacts with filter paper and therefore a sintered glass filter should be used to clarify the solution before making up to volume, preferably through the filter (see Ch. 4).

Storage and shelf-life

No special requirements.

Container

Amber fluted bottle.

Advice for patients when dispensed

The preparation should be diluted with 20 times its volume of warm water before use (i.e. 15 ml with 300 ml). Suitable directions are

> Three 5 ml spoonfuls to be
> added to a tumblerful of
> warm water before use

The mouthwash is

> not to be swallowed in large
> amounts

Actions and uses

Astringent solution.

Example 11.11

Prepare an enema containing a dose of paraldehyde suitable for a child aged 5 years

Ingredients	Formula
Paraldehyde	4 ml
Benzyl Alcohol	1 ml
Sodium Chloride Solution (0.9% w/v)	to 40 ml

Formulation

A suitable dose of paraldehyde for a 5-year-old child is 4 ml. For rectal administration a 10% enema in physiological saline is recommended (i.e. sodium chloride solution 0.9% w/v, which is iso-osmotic with body fluids). Benzyl alcohol is included to reduce the local irritation caused by the paraldehyde in the rectal mucosa.

Compounding

Paraldehyde decomposes on storage to form acetic acid

and the administration of partly decomposed paraldehyde is dangerous. Paraldehyde should be stored in small (50 ml) containers fully protected from light. Once opened the contents should be discarded within 24 hours and immediately if discolored or if an odour of acetic acid is detected.

The sodium chloride solution should be freshly prepared and chilled since paraldehyde is more soluble in the cold. The paraldehyde may be measured into the final container previously tared to the appropriate final volume and the chilled vehicle added almost to volume. The paraldehyde is near to its maximum solubility and vigorous shaking is required to effect dissolution. It is important to distinguish between air bubbles and undissolved globules of paraldehyde when checking the solution.

Storage and shelf-life
Paraldehyde should be stored in complete darkness in a cool place. The enema should be discarded 2 days after preparation if unused.

Container
Amber fluted glass bottle. Contact with cork and some plastics should be avoided. A polyethylene liner is suitable.

Advice for nursing staff
Discard any unused after administration.

Actions and uses
Hypnotic and sedative with anticonvulsant effects.

Example 11.12

Prepare 500 ml potassium permanganate solution 0.2% and label with directions for preparing 2 litre quantities of a 1 in 8000 solution for use as an antiseptic footbath

Ingredients	Formula
Potassium Permanganate	1 g
Water for Preparations	to 500 ml

Formulation
Since the solution is used as a mild antiseptic the vehicle should be freshly boiled and cooled.
Calculation of dilution factor (see Examples 3.14 and 3.15)

Strength of concentrate = 0.2%
Strength of dilute solution required is 1 in 8000 = 0.0125%

$$\frac{\text{strength of concentrate}}{\text{strength of dilute solution}} = \text{dilution factor}$$

$$\frac{0.2\%}{0.0125\%} = 16$$

The dilute solution is obtained by diluting 1 part of the original solution with 15 parts of water (to produce a total volume of 16 parts) before use, i.e. diluting 125 ml of the concentrated solution with 1875 ml to produce 2 litres.

Compounding
Potassium permanganate will react with any oxidizable residues and turn brown with loss of strength. The use of the preparation as an antiseptic indicates that it should be free from contamination and therefore all the apparatus used should be scrupulously clean. The solute dissolves slowly in water and since it may not be heated the use of an electric stirrer is recommended. As an alternative a glass mortar may be used, grinding the crystals with small quantities of water and pouring off the resulting supernatant solution into a measure. The solution should be clarified before issue and, since potassium permanganate will oxidize filter paper, a sintered glass filter should be used. The solution should be adjusted to volume preferably by passing the appropriate quantity of vehicle through the filter.

Storage and shelf-life
The preparation should be prepared just before use. Antiseptic solutions should not be stored for longer than 7 days. Cool storage is advisable.

Container
Amber fluted bottle with a closure that resists oxidation, e.g. polyethylene liner.

Advice for patients when dispensed
The solution should be diluted before use. In this case a household measuring jug would be adequate to measure 125 ml to be diluted to produce 2 litres. The diluted solution should be discarded after use. The solution stains skin, hair and fabric.

Actions and uses
Mild disinfectant and deodorant.

BIBLIOGRAPHY

ABPI Data Sheet Compendium current edition Datapharm Publications, London (updated annually)
Aulton M E (ed) 1988 Pharmaceutics: the science of dosage form design. Churchill Livingstone, Edinburgh, C
British National Formulary 1988 16th edn. British Medical Association and Royal Pharmaceutical Society of Great Britain, London (updated twice yearly)
British Pharmacopoeia 1980 HMSO, London (and addenda 1982, 1983 and 1986)
British Pharmacopoeia 1988 HMSO, London and addendum
British Pharmaceutical Codex 1973 Pharmaceutical Press, London

Diluent Directories (Internal and External) current edn National Pharmaceutical Association (NPA). St Albans, UK
Martindale, see Reynolds J E F
Pharmaceutical Codex 1979 11th edn (incorporating the British Pharmaceutical Codex). Pharmaceutical Press, London
Pharmaceutical Society 1979 Guide to good dispensing practice. Pharmaceutical Journal 223: 157–158
Reynolds J E F (ed) 1989 Martindale, the extra pharmacopoeia, 29th edn. Pharmaceutical Press, London
Wade A (ed) 1980 Pharmaceutical handbook, 19th edn. Pharmaceutical Press, London

12. Suspensions

D. M. Collett

A pharmaceutical suspension is a type of disperse system in which one substance (the disperse phase) is distributed in particulate form throughout another (the continuous phase). Suspensions may be classified into coarse suspensions in which the particles are larger than 1 μm in diameter and colloidal suspensions in which the particles may be considerably less than 1 μm in diameter. For more detailed information, see the companion volume (Chapters 6 and 15, Aulton 1988).

FORMULATION

Vehicles

The vehicle is the medium in which the ingredients of a medicinal suspension are dispersed and as for pharmaceutical solutions, water is usually the vehicle of choice. The density of an aqueous vehicle may be increased by adding glycerol or sucrose and the viscosity may be modified as described below. Non-aqueous vehicles, eg. fractionated coconut oil, may occasionally be used for drugs that are unstable in the presence of water.

Other additives

The additives that are included in some pharmaceutical solutions (see Ch. 11) may also be required for suspensions, i.e. buffers, stabilizers, preservatives, colours and flavours.

Properties of a good pharmaceutical suspension

1. After shaking, the medicament stays in suspension long enough for a dose to be accurately measured.
2. The suspension is easily removed from the container, i.e. it is pourable.
3. The sediment formed on standing is bulky and easily redispersed.
4. The particles in suspension are small and relatively uniform in size so that the product is free from a gritty texture.

Factors affecting the properties of a pharmaceutical suspension

The physical properties of disperse systems and the design of suspensions as drug delivery systems are discussed in detail the companion volume (Chapters 6 and 15, Aulton 1988). A brief description only of the factors affecting the formulation of pharmaceutical suspensions is included in this chapter.

Diffusible solids

Some insoluble powders are light and easily wettable. They mix readily with water and on shaking diffuse evenly through the liquid and remain distributed for long enough for a dose to be measured. Such substances are known as diffusible or dispersable solids, e.g. light kaolin (Example 12.1), magnesium trisilicate (Example 12.2) and light magnesium carbonate (Example 12.3).

Stokes' law

The rate of settling or sedimentation of particles in a suspension can be described by Stokes Law which gives the velocity, v, of a spherical particle, radius a and density σ falling in a liquid of density ρ and viscosity η where g is the acceleration due to gravity.

$$v = \frac{2a^2g\,(\sigma-\rho)}{9\eta}$$

It follows that a decrease in settling rate in a suspension may be achieved by reducing the size of the particles, by increasing the density of the liquid continuous phase and by increasing the viscosity of the continuous phase.

Control of particle size

On a small scale a mortar and pestle may be used to grind down any ingredients not already in fine powder.

Deflocculated suspensions

In a completely deflocculated system all the particles remain separate as very small individual units and settling is therefore slow. The repulsion between particles prevents the formation of larger aggregates during sedimentation. However, the sediment that forms eventually is very hard to redisperse and is described as a 'cake' or 'clay'.

Flocculated suspensions

Flocculation involves the aggregation of individual small particles to form larger groups, clumps or floccules. Settling of these larger aggregated particles is much faster than in the deflocculated state because the size is greater. However, the sediment formed is loose and easily redispersible. If excessive flocculation occurs vehicle trapped inside the floccules can cause the suspension to become very viscous and unpourable.

In practice controlled flocculation is desirable so that a suitable combination of rate of sedimentation, type of sediment and pourability is achieved.

Flocculating agents include electrolytes, ionic surfactants and some polymeric materials, e.g. starch and cellulose derivatives. This phenomenon is discussed in detail in the companion volume (Aulton 1988).

Poorly wettable solids

Some substances are both insoluble in water and poorly wetted by it. When dispersions in water are prepared it is difficult to disperse clumps and the foam produced by shaking tends to persist because it is stabilized by the film of unwettable solid at the liquid/air interface. To ensure satisfactory wetting, the interfacial energy between the solid particles and the liquid must be reduced. This may be achieved by adding a suitable wetting agent which is adsorbed at the solid/liquid interface in such a way that the affinity of the particles for the surrounding medium is increased while the interparticular forces are decreased, i.e. deflocculation occurs.

Surface active agents used as wetting agents for external applications include quillaia tincture (Example 12.4) and sodium lauryl sulphate. For oral administration the less toxic polysorbates and sorbitan esters are preferred. Hydrophilic colloids, such as acacia, tragacanth and the alginates, will also act as wetting agents by coating solid hydrophobic particles and imparting a hydrophilic character. These substances also cause deflocculation of particles in suspension, especially at low concentration.

Indiffusible solids

These insoluble powders will not remain evenly distributed in a vehicle long enough to ensure uniformity of dose, e.g. chalk (Example 12.5), zinc oxide and calamine (Example 12.6). The simplest way of correcting the problem is to increase the viscosity of the vehicle by adding a thickening agent. This delays sedimentation by impeding the fall of particles under gravity and by obstructing those particle collisions which lead to the formation of aggregates that settle quickly.

Thickening agents

Polysaccharides

Acacia gum. This is a natural material obtained from some species of *Acacia* tree and occurs as colourless or amber tears of exudate or as a white powder. Solutions of acacia in water (4 parts by weight of gum to 6 parts by volume of water) form a viscous mucilage.

Acacia is a poor thickener compared with other natural gums and semisynthetic compounds but is a good protective colloid and its value as a suspending agent is largely due to this. It is used in combination with tragacanth and starch in Compound Tragacanth Powder BP for internal preparations but is generally too sticky for external products. Since it is a natural product, acacia may be contaminated with micro-organisms and may need to be sterilized before use. It also contains peroxidase enzymes which may affect susceptible products but which are destroyed by heating to 100°C.

Tragacanth. This is a dried extract from some species of *Astralagus* shrub and occurs as thin, whitish, ribbon-like flakes or as a white powder. With water it forms viscous solutions or gels depending on concentration and is therefore a much better thickener than acacia. It is also less sticky than acacia and may be used for external preparations. Tragacanth is used to suspend heavy indiffusible powders. Appropriate quantities are 0.2 g of tragacanth powder for 100 ml of suspension. Compound Tragacanth Powder BP 1980 consists of acacia (20%), tragacanth (15%), starch (20%) and sucrose (45%) and is used in quantities of about 2 g per 100 ml of product. As an alternative, a mucilage may be prepared and used in quantities of about 25 ml per 100 ml suspension. For the method of preparing the mucilage see Example 12.7. Tragacanth contains a soluble and an insoluble fraction; the latter hydrates slowly and the maximum viscosity of mucilages prepared from tragacanth is achieved after several days.

Outside the pH range 4–7.5 tragacanth mucilages lose viscosity quickly. They must be preserved if prepared for long storage.

Sodium alginate. This consists mainly of the sodium salt of alginic acid and is derived from seaweed. It is a white or buff powder. It forms a viscous solution with water, about 1% giving a product with about the same suspending power as Tragacanth Mucilage BP. In preparing alginate mucilage, lumps are prevented by using 2–4% of alcohol, glycerol or propylene glycol as dispersing agent. Alternatively the vehicle may be mechanically stirred and the powder sprinkled into the vortex. Warming the vehicle hastens solution but temperatures above 70°C cause depolymerization with consequent loss of viscosity. The mucilage should be allowed to stand overnight before use in order to attain a stable viscosity. Maximum viscosity is at pH 7 although there is little change between pH 4 and pH 10. At pH 3 the alginic acid is precipitated. Sodium alginate is an anionic compound and is therefore incompatible with cationic substances. It is also incompatible with heavy metals, calcium salts and phenyl mercuric salts.

Starch. Starch is a constituent of Compound Tragacanth Powder BP and has also been used in combination with carboxymethycellulose. A mucilage containing 2.5% starch in water produces a viscous product (Example 12.8).

Xanthan gum. Xanthan gum is a semisynthetic polysaccharide consisting of the sodium, potassium or calcium salts of a partially acetylated polysaccharide of high molecular weight. It is a cream-coloured powder and is soluble in hot or cold water. A concentration of 0.5% produces a viscous product that shows little change in viscosity over a wide temperature and pH range. It may be convenient to prepare a 1% stock solution with appropriate preservatives which can be then be used as required (Bumphrey 1986).

Water-soluble celluloses

Methylcellulose. These are methyl ethers resulting from the methylation of cellulose. The varying degrees of methylation and chain length produce various characteristics and the name is usually followed by a number that gives an indication of the viscosity of a 2% aqueous solution at 20°C. The high-viscosity grades (2500 and 4500) are used as thickening and dispersing agents. They are white or creamy-white powders that disperse in water forming viscous solutions. They are soluble in the cold but insoluble in hot water. A mucilage may be prepared by adding about a third of the water, heated to boiling and allowed to stand for 30 minutes. The remainder of the water is then added, either ice-cold or as ice, and the product stirred until homogeneous.

Methylcellulose mucilages are clear or opalescent, colourless, tasteless, inert and neutral. They are non-ionic

and stable over a wide pH range. On heating, these mucilages first decrease in viscosity and then, as the temperature rises, the methylcellulose molecules gradually become dehydrated until, at about 50°C, the dispersion gels. On cooling, the gel reverts to a sol and the viscosity returns to normal.

Methylcellulose is used in both external and internal preparations. The concentration used depends on the polymer but is usually between 0.5% and 2%. Details of substances that are incompatible with methylcellulose are given in Martindale (Reynolds 1982).

Hydroxyethylcellulose. This substance has hydroxyethyl instead of methyl groups but the substitution is less precise than in methylcellulose. It is soluble in cold and hot water, producing solutions that are clearer than methylcellulose solutions and do not gel on heating. Mucilages are made by sprinkling the powder into the vortex while the vehicle is mechanically stirred. They are used for the same purposes as methylcellulose when freedom from gel formation and clarity are an advantage.

Sodium carboxymethylcellulose. Also called carmellose sodium, this differs from methylcellulose in having one of the hydrogen atoms of the methyl group replaced by a carboxy group. Grades with different degrees of polymerization producing aqueous solutions of differing viscosities are available. Carmellose sodium dissolves in the cold and to a greater extent in hot water producing clear solutions.

Carmellose sodium mucilages are usually prepared by the method described under hydroxyethylcellulose while heating the vehicle. Stock solutions should contain a preservative. Carmellose sodium is more sensitive to pH than methylcellulose, being stable in the range pH 5–10. It is used in concentrations between 0.25% and 1% as a suspending agent. It is incompatible with strong acids and heavy metal ions.

Clays

Several natural clays are used as thickening agents. These are native colloidal hydrated silicates, bentonite, hectorite and aluminium magnesium silicate. Pharmaceutical grades should be free from gritty particles. These clays hydrate readily, absorbing many times their volume of water to produce sols or gels depending on the concentration. The sols are most suitable for suspending indiffusible powders in aqueous suspensions. They do not support but do not inhibit microbial growth and therefore a preservative is necessary. Because of their source they may be contaminated with microbial spores and should preferably be sterilized before use in pharmaceutical products, especially if for application to broken skin.

Bentonite. This is a very fine pale buff or cream hygroscopic powder with a faint earthy taste. Its colour is a disadvantage for some preparations. A dispersion containing 7% is just pourable and one containing 25% has the consistency of wool fat.

About 2% is used for suspending indiffusible solids in external preparations (Example 12.6). A sol containing 5% is convenient for dispensing and may be prepared by sprinkling the bentonite on the surface of hot water and allowing to stand for 24 hours with occasional stirring. Dispersions are flocculated by strong electrolytes and positively charged particles or solutions.

Aluminium magnesium silicate. This occurs as creamy-white, odourless and tasteless powder or small flakes. It is used mainly in industry, as a thickening agent in internal or external preparations, either alone, in a concentration of 0.5–2%, or partially to replace other suspending agents.

Hectorite. This is a white powder. It contains traces of lithium or fluorine but fluorine-free grades are available. It is used industrially in suspensions for external use. Hectorite absorbs more water then bentonite and a 1% or 2% dispersion is a clear, highly thixotropic gel.

Synthetic thickeners

These were introduced to overcome the problems arising from the variable quality of natural products.

Carbomer (carboxyvinyl polymer). This is a very high molecular weight polymer of acrylic acid with crosslinkages of allyl sucrose. It is a white fluffy hygroscopic powder. Its solutions are acidic because it has a high proportion of carboxy groups. They are also of low viscosity but when neutralized with sodium hydroxide (0.4 parts by weight to 1 part of carbomer) are converted to highly viscous gels. Less than 1% of the sodium salt will produce a gel with water. An important advantage of carbomer as a suspending agent is the low concentration needed (generally 0.1–0.4%).

Gels are produced by first adding the powder in small amounts to water while agitating with a high-speed stirrer; then the alkali solution is added and the dispersion is slowly stirred with a broad paddle-like stirrer taking care not to incorporate air bubbles. Carbomer is sensitive to oxidation when exposed to light and stability is improved by the incorporation of an antioxidant and a chelating agent to sequester heavy metal ions that catalyse the breakdown. The viscosity of the gels is highest within the pH range 6–11 and is markedly reduced above pH 12 or below pH 3 and by oxidation or strong electrolytes. The effects of weak ionic agents are less predictable. Stock gels require a preservative.

Colloidal silicon dioxide. This is a form of silicon dioxide with a particle size of colloidal dimensions. It is a very light, white, non-gritty powder. It acts as a thickening agent because when suspended in a liquid the particles associate, due to hydrogen bonding and produce a network that obstructs sedimentation. About 12% gives a soft gel with water but 1.5–4% is enough to stabilize suspensions. It can be used to gel nonpolar liquids. Suspensions can be made in a mortar but the lightness of the powder is a nuisance. Products of greater stability and viscosity are obtained by high-speed stirring. Because of the fineness of the particles, sediments tend to cake causing difficulties in redispersion.

COMPOUNDING

The basic techniques for preparation of pharmaceutical suspensions are weighing, measuring of liquids, size reduction and mixing. These are described in Chapter 4.

SUSPENSIONS AS ORAL DOSAGE FORMS

Mixtures

Mixtures are liquid preparations for oral administration and contain medicaments dissolved and/or suspended in water.

Advantages of suspensions as oral dosage forms

— Suspended insoluble medicaments are easy to swallow.
— Insoluble derivatives in suspension may be more palatable than soluble derivatives in solution.
— Bulky insoluble powders, such as kaolin and chalk, may be administered in suspension in order to act as adsorbents of toxins or to reduce excess acidity in the gastrointestinal tract.

Disadvantages of suspensions as oral dosage forms

— The preparation must be shaken prior to measuring a dose.
— Accuracy of dosage is less reliable than with solutions.
— Storage may lead to changes in the disperse system, particularly if there are fluctuations in temperature.

Preparing dilutions of suspensions for oral administration

As with oral solutions dilution of a suspension may be necessary if a fractional dose is prescribed. For a discussion on the choice of the appropriate diluent, see the section on oral solutions in Chapter 11.

Shelf-life of oral suspensions

Most 'official' mixtures have a relatively short shelf-life and should be recently or freshly prepared (see Table 5.2).

For ready-made proprietary suspensions the manufacturer's literature should be consulted. Some proprietary suspensions are packed and stored as dry powders for reconstitution by the pharmacist immediately prior to issue to the patient. The reconstituted product usually has a short shelf-life after issue (see Table 5.2). Diluted products also have a reduced shelf-life, usually a maximum of 14 days.

Containers for oral suspensions

Amber medicine bottles. A 5 ml measuring spoon should be supplied to the patient

Special labels and advice for patients

> Shake the bottle

SUSPENSIONS FOR EXTERNAL USE

Lotions

Lotions containing suspended solids evaporate when applied to the skin leaving a light deposit of medicament on the surface. Suspensions made with some types of thickening agent, such as the semisynthetic polysaccharides, leave a fairly strong, non-sticky film that holds the medicament in contact with the skin and gives protection, but is easily removed by washing. Preparations for use on broken or inflamed skin should be free from harmful micro-organisms.

Containers for lotions

Amber fluted glass bottles are used for extemporaneously prepared lotions. If the preparation is particularly viscous a wide-mouthed jar may be used.

Special labels and advice for patients

> Shake the bottle

> Not to be applied
> to broken skin

Inhalations

One class of inhalation consists of one or more volatile oils in water and, to ensure uniform dispersion of the oil on shaking, light magnesium carbonate, a diffusible solid, is added to adsorb some of the oil and finely divide the remainder. Unlike emulsification (see Ch. 13) the powder does not interfere with the free vaporization of the oil when the inhalation is added to water at about 65°C for use. If the quantity is not included in the formula, 1 g of light magnesium carbonate for each 2 ml of oil (e.g. eucalyptus and pumilio pine oils) or 2 g of volatile solid (e.g. menthol and thymol) gives satisfactory results (Example 12.3).

Containers for inhalations

Amber fluted glass bottles.

Special labels and advice for patients

> Shake the bottle

> Not to be taken

Other types of dispensed product

Some ear drops and enemas are formulated as suspensions. For a general description of these products see Chapter 11.

Every dosage form designed as a suspension requires a

> Shake the bottle

label.

Suspensions as 'emergency' formulations

Medicaments that are available commercially in solid dosage form may be prescribed for a patient able only to swallow liquids. In the absence of a commercially available liquid preparation the pharmacist is requested to prepare a liquid dosage form from the commercial material to hand. This usually involves crushing tablets or opening capsules to prepare a suspension which will also contain unknown excipients together with the nominal quantity of drug. Suitable suspending agents are Compound Tragacanth Powder BP or xanthan gum mucilage. The bioavailability of the resulting preparation will be unknown and the products must be considered as unstable until researched. Such preparations should be replaced by more conventional formulations if powdered drug can be obtained.

EXAMPLES

Example 12.1

Prepare 100 ml Paediatric Kaolin Mixture BP 1980

Ingredients	Master formula
Light Kaolin or Light Kaolin (Natural)	200 g
Amaranth Solution	10 ml
Benzoic Acid Solution	20 ml
Raspberry Syrup	200 ml
Double-strength Chloroform Water	500 ml
Water, freshly boiled and cooled sufficient to produce	1000 ml

Formulation
Light kaolin contains a dispersing agent and is used in dispensing unless the natural form is particularly required. The kaolin should preferably be sterilized to remove any contaminating soil pathogens. Note that the record should state the ingredients actually used and not the alternatives which may be used. Kaolin is a diffusible solid and therefore no additional suspending agent is required, although the raspberry syrup increases the viscosity of the vehicle.

Benzoic acid solution and chloroform water act as preservatives. The raspberry syrup provides a flavour and amaranth solution colour which is attractive to children.

Compounding
First tare the final container because if the preparation is made up to volume in a measure it is difficult to transfer it satisfactorily to a bottle (see Ch. 4). The preparation should be made in a mortar of sufficient size to allow for adequate mixing of the product. Add the kaolin to the mortar and prepare a paste with the raspberry syrup and a little of the chloroform water. Add the amaranth solution and mix well.

If the dye is added at a later stage in the preparation it will not penetrate into the powder and white specks will be visible in the final product. Dilute the suspension until pourable and transfer to the bottle. Although it is desirable to add volatile ingredients such as chloroform water to the bottle rather than the mortar, care should be taken to incorporate all the chloroform water before making up to volume with water. Add the benzoic acid solution to the bottle and make up to final volume.

Storage and shelf-life
Unless the kaolin has been sterilized the preparation should be recently prepared.

Container
Amber medicine bottle.

Advice for patients when dispensed
Shake the bottle. Maintain fluid intake in diarrhoea. If the product is counter-prescribed the patient should seek medical advice if the condition persists.

Actions and uses
Antidiarrhoeal mixture for children.

Example 12.2

Prepare 200 ml Magnesium Trisilicate Mixture BP 1988

Ingredients	Master formula
Magnesium Trisilicate	50 g
Light Magnesium Carbonate	50 g
Sodium Bicarbonate	50 g
Concentrated Peppermint Emulsion	25 ml
Double-strength Chloroform Water	500 ml
Water sufficient to produce	1000 ml

Formulation
Magnesium trisilicate and magnesium carbonate act as antacids and adsorbents in the gastrointestinal tract. Sodium bicarbonate is a rapidly acting antacid. Peppermint provides flavouring and acts as a carminative and chloroform water acts as flavouring, preservative and vehicle. Both the magnesium powders are diffusible and no extra thickening agent is required.

Compounding
First tare the final container and select a mortar of sufficient size to allow for adequate mixing of the product. Add the sodium bicarbonate to the mortar and mix with the two insoluble powders by doubling the bulk on each addition. This method is to be preferred to making a separate solution of the sodium bicarbonate which is time consuming. Add enough vehicle to make a smooth paste and dilute with the vehicle until sufficiently pourable to transfer to the bottle. The volatile peppermint emulsion should be added to the bottle before making up to final volume.

The mixture may also be prepared from a pre-packed mix of the three powdered ingredients with the addition of the appropriate amounts of peppermint emulsion and chloroform water.

Storage and shelf-life
The mixture should be recently prepared.

Container
Amber medicine bottle.

Advice for patients when dispensed
Shake the bottle. The mixture may be taken alone or with water or other fluid between meals. If counter-prescribed, the patient should seek medical advice if the condition persists.
Note: This mixture contains a relatively high concentration of sodium ions which may be inappropriate for some patients.

Actions and uses
Antacid used to treat dyspepsia.

Example 12.3

Prepare 50 ml inhalation to the following formula: menthol 3%, eucalyptus 8%.

Ingredients	Master formula	Scaled quantities
Menthol	3 g	1.5 g
Eucalyptus Oil	8 ml	4.0 ml
Light Magnesium Carbonate	—	2.75 g*
Water	to 100 ml	50.0 ml

Formulation
Light magnesium carbonate, a diffusible solid, is used to adsorb the volatile ingredients to ensure a uniform dispersion. The appropriate quantity is calculated:
   1 g for each 2 g of menthol and 1 g for each 2 ml of eucalyptus oil.

Quantity of magnesium carbonate required:
For menthol	= 0.75 g
For oil	= 2.00 g
	2.75 g*

Compounding
Finely powder the menthol in a glass mortar and dissolve in the oil. Add the light magnesium carbonate in small amounts and mix well. Gradually add the vehicle to produce a pourable cream.
   Transfer to a previously tared container and adjust to final volume.

Storage and shelf-life
The preparation is chemically stable but should be stored cool because of the volatile ingredients.

Container
Amber fluted bottle.

Advice for patients when dispensed

> Shake the bottle.
> Not to be taken.
> One teaspoonful to be
> added to 1 pint of hot,
> not boiling water and
> the vapour inhaled for 5 to
> 10 minutes.

Actions and uses
Relief of nasal congestion.

Example 12.4

Prepare 200 ml Sulphur Lotion. Compound BPC 1973

Ingredients	Master formula
Precipitated Sulphur	40 g
Quillaia Tincture	5 ml
Glycerol	20 ml
Alcohol (95%) or IMS	60 ml
Calcium Hydroxide Solution	to 1000 ml

Formulation
Quillaia tincture is used as a wetting agent for the poorly wettable sulphur. Glycerol is an emollient and with the alcohol helps to wet the sulphur and promote dispersion. Since this preparation is for external use Industrial Methylated Spirit may be used in place of the alcohol.

Compounding
Mix the quillaia tincture, IMS and glycerol and triturate the mixture with the sulphur in a mortar. Gradually dilute with the lime water and transfer to the previously tared container to make up to final volume.

Storage and shelf-life
The preparation is stable.

Container
Amber fluted bottle.

Advice for patients when dispensed
Clean the skin before use and apply sparingly to the affected area. The treatment should be discontinued if excessive dryness or irritation occurs.

Actions and uses
Mild antiseptic used in the treatment of acne.

Example 12.5

Prepare 100 ml Paediatric Chalk Mixture BP 1988

Ingredients	Master formula
Chalk	20 g
Powdered Tragacanth	2 g
Concentrated Cinnamon Water	4 ml
Syrup	100 ml
Double-strength Chloroform Water	500 ml
Water sufficient to produce	1000 ml

Formulation
Chalk is an indiffusible solid and tragacanth is included as a suspending agent. Cinnamon provides flavouring and also acts as a carminative. Syrup provides sweetening and adds to the viscosity of the product and chloroform water acts as flavour, preservative and vehicle.

Compounding
First tare the final container and select a mortar of sufficient size to allow for adequate mixing of the product. Mix the chalk and tragacanth in the mortar and prepare a paste with the syrup and a little of the vehicle. Dilute until pourable and transfer to the bottle. Add the other ingredients to the bottle and shake well before making up to final volume.

Storage and shelf-life
The preparation should be recently prepared.

Container
Amber medicine bottle.

Advice for patients when dispensed
Shake the bottle.
   Maintain fluid intake in diarrhoea. If the product is counter-prescribed the patient should seek medical advice if the condition persists.

Actions and uses
Antidiarrhoeal mixture for children.

Example 12.6

Prepare 200 ml Calamine Lotion BP 1988

Ingredients	Master formula
Calamine	150 g
Zinc Oxide	50 g
Bentonite	30 g
Sodium Citrate	5 g
Liquefied Phenol	5 ml
Glycerol	50 ml
Purified Water, freshly boiled and cooled sufficient to produce	1000 ml

Formulation
Calamine and zinc oxide are mildly astringent and soothing to the skin. Both are indiffusible solids and therefore bentonite is included as a thickening agent which causes marked flocculation of the calamine and makes it very difficult to pour from the bottle. Sodium citrate is included to cause partial deflocculation of the calamine and so make the preparation more pourable. Liquefied phenol acts as a preservative and glycerol as an emollient miscible with the aqueous vehicle.

Compounding
First tare the final container and select a large mortar. Mix the dry powders in the mortar until evenly dispersed. It is important that the bentonite is well distributed in the indiffusible powders.
   Dissolve the sodium citrate in 140 ml water (70%) and add this solution to the mortar to make a smooth paste and to dilute it for transfer to the bottle. Add the glycerol and liquefied phenol to the bottle and make up to final volume with the vehicle.
   Note that liquefied phenol is very caustic.

Storage and shelf-life
The preparation is stable, cool storage is advised because of the volatile preservative.

Container
Amber fluted bottle.

Advice for patients when dispensed
Shake the bottle. For external use only.
   The lotion should be applied to the skin as required and allowed to dry.

Actions and uses
Cooling lotion useful for treating mild sunburn.

Example 12.7

Prepare 100 ml Tragacanth Mucilage BPC 1973

Ingredients	Master formula	Scaled quantities
Tragacanth, finely powdered	12.5 g	1.25 g
Alcohol (90 per cent)	25 ml	2.5 ml
Chloroform Water	to 1000 ml	to 100 ml

Formulation
The alcohol is used as a dispersing agent because it is poorly absorbed by the gum. The chloroform water acts as a preservative.

Compounding
On a small scale the mucilage is conveniently made by shaking the ingredients together in a jar calibrated to 100 ml. Measure 95 ml of the vehicle and have to hand. Put the alcohol into the jar and then add the tragacanth powder. (The order of addition is important). Mix and spread the resulting suspension around the inside of the jar. Pour in the 95 ml of the vehicle as quickly as possible, put on the closure and shake without delay. Success depends on speed. Any vehicle spilled on the outside of the jar can be replaced when making to volume. A product that appears lumpy at first will become homogeneous on standing for a few days.

Storage and shelf-life
If the preparation is to be stored, freedom from contamination with micro-organisms should be assured.

Container
Amber bottle.

Advice for patients when dispensed
Not applicable.

Actions and uses
Suspending and thickening agent.

Example 12.8

Prepare 100 ml Starch Mucilage BPC 1973

Ingredients	Master formula	Scaled quantities
Starch	25 g	2.5 g
Water	to 1000 ml	to 100 ml

Formulation
Note that the mucilage is unpreserved and must be prepared as required for use in dispensed products.

Compounding
Triturate the starch with 20 ml of the cold water in a small beaker or small mortar. Heat the remaining 80 ml water to boiling in a wide-mouthed conical flask or beaker. Pour the cold suspension into the centre of the boiling water and reheat to boiling with constant stirring. The resulting gelatinized mucilage should be free from lumps. Immediate rapid cooling prevents the formation of a skin. The cooled preparation may be transferred to a measure and the water lost by evaporation replaced to volume.

Storage and shelf-life
The preparation should be used at once.

Container
Amber bottle.

Advice for patients when dispensed
Not applicable.

Actions and uses
Suspending and thickening agent.

BIBLIOGRAPHY

ABPI Data Sheet Compendium current edition Datapharm
  Publications, London (updated annually)
Aulton M E (ed) 1988 Pharmaceutics: the science of dosage
  form design. Churchill Livingstone, Edinburgh,
  Chs 6, 15
British National Formulary 1988 16th edn. British Medical
  Association and Royal Pharmaceutical Society of Great
  Britain, London (updated twice yearly)
British Pharmacopoeia 1980 HMSO, London (and addenda
  1982, 1983 and 1986)
British Pharmacopoeia 1988 HMSO, London
British Pharmaceutical Codex 1973 Pharmaceutical Press,
  London
Bumphrey G 1986 Extremely useful resuspending agent.

Pharmaceutical Journal 237: 665
Diluent Directories (Internal and External) current edition.
  National Pharmaceutical Association (NPA)
Martindale, see Reynolds J E F
Pharmaceutical Codex 1979 11th edn (incorporating the
  British Pharmaceutical Codex). Pharmaceutical Press,
  London
Pharmaceutical Society 1979 Guide to good dispensing
  practice. Pharmaceutical Journal 223: 157–158
Reynolds J E F (ed) 1982 Martindale, the extra
  pharmacopoeia, 28th edn. Pharmaceutical Press,
  London
Wade A (ed) 1980 Pharmaceutical handbook, 19 edn.
  Pharmaceutical Press, London

13. Emulsions and creams

D. M. Collett

An emulsion is a disperse system consisting of two immiscible liquids, one of which (the disperse phase) is finely divided and distributed through the other (the continuous phase). Since this type of dispersion is inherently unstable, an emulsifying agent (emulgent) is usually required to maintain the dispersion. In pharmaceutical emulsions, one phase is usually aqueous and the other oily. When the continuous phase is aqueous the system is described as oil-in-water (o/w) and when the continuous phase is oily the system is described as water-in-oil (w/o). Factors affecting the type of emulsion produced include the relative proportions of the two phases present and the type of emulsifying agent chosen. In addition to the relatively simple two-phase systems, so-called multiple emulsions are also possible. The reader is referred to companion volume (Chapters 6, 16 and 22, Aulton 1988) for more information on emulsions.

Determination of emulsion type

Several tests may be used to distinguish between o/w and w/o emulsions:

1. Miscibility tests —
   o/w emulsions are miscible with water
   w/o emulsions are miscible with oil
2. Microscopic examination after staining with an oil-soluble dye —
   coloured droplets indicate o/w emulsion
   coloured background indicates w/o emulsion
3. Microscopic observation under ultraviolet radiation —
   o/w emulsions only the droplets fluoresce
   w/o emulsions show continuous fluorescence
4. Conductivity measurements —
   o/w emulsions act as conductors of electricity
   w/o emulsions are poor conductors of electricity

FORMULATION

Emulsifying agents

The mechanisms of emulsion stabilization are discussed in detail in the companion volume (Chapter 6, Aulton 1988). Briefly, emulsifying agents facilitate the production of a dispersion by reducing interfacial tension and then maintain the separation of the droplets of the dispersed phase by forming a barrier at the interfaces. Effective emulgents are surface active agents (surfactants) which have both hydrophilic polar groups that are orientated towards the water and lipophilic non-polar groups that are orientated towards the oil. The balance between the hydrophilic and lipophilic properties of the emulgent will affect the type of emulsion produced. The ideal pharmaceutical emulsifying agent should be colourless, tasteless and odourless, non-toxic and non-irritant and produce stable emulsions at low concentration.

For oral or parenteral administration, o/w emulsions are required, while for external use both o/w and w/o systems may be used to achieve different therapeutic effects.

Types of emulsifying agent

For convenience these are classified into three groups, synthetic or semisynthetic substances, natural products and finely divided solids. Many of the substances described as thickening agents in Chapter 12 also act as emulgents.

Synthetic emulgents

Depending on their ionization in aqueous solution these are further classified as anionic, cationic, non-ionic or ampholytic (amphoteric) emulgents or surfactants.

Anionic surfactants

Alkali metal and ammonium soaps. These are the sodium, potassium or ammonium salts of long-chain fatty acids, such as oleic, stearic and ricinoleic. They produce o/w emulsions that can be prepared with either:

1. A preformed soap, such as soft soap used in Turpentine Liniment BP (Example 13.1), or
2. A soap formed during preparation of the emulsion, such as the ammonium soap used in White Liniment BP (Example 13.2).

In addition, fixed oils and fats, because they contain traces of free fatty acid, can be emulsified with solutions of alkali hydroxides or ammonia alone. Substances without free acid, e.g. turpentine and liquid paraffin, cannot be emulsified in this way. Alkali soap emulsions are stable above pH 10 but are very sensitive to acids: even weak organic acids precipitate free fatty acid and break the emulsion.

High concentrations of electrolyte salt out the soap. They are incompatible with polyvalent cations such as $Al^{3+}, Ca^{2+}, Mg^{2+}$ and Zn^{2+}, which cause phase reversal. Their toxicity and unpleasant taste make them unsuitable for internal emulsions and, because of their alkaline pH, they should not be applied to broken skin. They are resistant to attack by micro-organisms.

Soaps of divalent and trivalent metals. Although calcium, magnesium, aluminium and zinc salts of fatty acids are w/o emulsifying agents, only the calcium salts are commonly used as such.

Calcium salts are made during the preparation of the emulsion by the interaction of a fatty acid with calcium hydroxide, e.g. Zinc Cream BP and Oily Calamine Lotion BP 1980 (Example 13.3). Wool fat may be used as an emulsion stabilizer and to improve emollience. Like alkali soap emulsions, these soaps cannot be used internally, but they are less alkaline and less sensitive to acid.

Amine soaps. A number of amines form salts with fatty acids. Triethanolamine is the most widely used in pharmaceutical products. Triethanolamine soaps produce fine-grained, almost neutral (pH 7.5–8) o/w emulsions. They can be applied to broken skin but are unsuitable for internal use. They are incompatible with acids and high concentrations of electrolyte. They darken on storage, especially in the light, and in contact with heavy metals.

Alkyl sulphates and phosphates. These are esters of fatty acids with sulphuric or phosphoric acids. The most important are sodium lauryl sulphate and sodium cetostearyl sulphate. Alkyl sulphates and phosphates alone produce o/w emulsions of low stability but, when used in combination with fatty alcohols, products of excellent stability and quality are obtained.

Emulsifying Wax BP is a mixture of sodium lauryl sulphate or similar sodium salts of sulphated higher primary aliphatic alcohols (10%) and cetostearyl alcohol (90%) Emulsifying Ointment BP contains 30% of Emulsifying Wax with soft and liquid paraffins (see Example 14.4). This anhydrous ointment can absorb considerable quantities of water or aqueous solutions to form stable o/w creams (e.g. Aqueous Cream BP, Example 13.4).

Emulsions prepared with anionic emulsifying waxes are compatible with calcium and magnesium ions (and therefore hard water), because the alkyl sulphates of these metals are water soluble. They are neutral and tolerate fairly large changes in pH. When heated (e.g. for sterilization) they become acid due to hydrolysis of the ester linkage. Anionic emulsifying waxes are incompatible with cationic emulsifying agents such as cetrimide and with cationic medicaments.

Cationic surfactants

The most important group of cationic surfactants are the quaternary ammonium compounds. They are o/w emulsifying agents also used for their disinfectant and preservative properties.

If used alone their emulsifying power is poor but, like the alkyl sulphates and phosphates, they produce emulsions of great stability when combined with fatty alcohols.

The most useful quaternary ammonium compound is cetrimide which is included in a cationic emulsifying wax comparable with anionic Emulsifying Wax BP (10% cetrimide and 90% cetostearyl alcohol). The corresponding ointment contains 30% Cetrimide Emulsifing Wax BP with soft and liquid paraffins. This ointment will absorb at least an equal quantity of aqueous solution to form stable o/w cetrimide creams (Example 13.5). Cationic wax emulsions are most stable within the pH range 3–7 and, since the skin pH is about 5.5, are very suitable for dermatological purposes. Because of their antimicrobial activity no additional preservative is required. They are compatible with cationic compounds and with calcium and magnesium ions, but are extremely sensitive to anionic surfactants, including soaps and to non-ionic compounds.

Non-ionic surfactants

The hydrophilic and hydrophobic (lipophilic) groupings tend to be equally balanced in the non-ionic emulsifying agents.

Since they do not ionize to any great extent in solution they are generally compatible with both anionic and cationic substances. They are highly resistant to electrolytes, pH changes and polyvalent cations. However, they do tend to inactivate preservatives with phenolic or carboxylic acid groups.

Glycol and glycerol esters. The glycol and glycerol esters of certain fatty acids are used as emulgents and emulsion stabilizers but because of their strongly hydrophobic nature they produce poor (w/o) emulsions when used alone. However, when mixed with a soap or other primary o/w emulgent the mixture is self-emulsifying and can itself be used as primary emulgent for o/w creams and lotions, e.g. self-emulsifying glyceryl monostearin.

Sorbitan esters. Sorbitan esters are amber or yellow oily liquids or amber or tan waxy solids in which hydrophobic groups slightly predominate and confer oil solubility and w/o emulsifying power. They are insoluble in water but can be dispersed in cold or warm water. They are used to prepare emulsions, creams and ointments, either alone when they produce w/o emulsions, or with polysorbates when either o/w or w/o products can be obtained. Sorbitan creams are fine textured and relatively insensitive to high concentrations of electrolytes and changes in pH.

Polysorbates. These are polyethylene glycol derivatives of sorbitan esters. Polysorbates may be oily liquids, ranging from pale yellow to orange in colour, or waxy solids, yellow to tan in colour. They have a disagreeable bitter soapy taste that complicates their use in oral preparations. They are neutral, non-volatile and thermostable. Most are soluble or dispersible in water. Their properties may vary slightly from batch to batch because they are not pure compounds — the composition of the mixtures are defined in the BP and Eur. P. Like the sorbitan esters they produce fine-textured o/w emulsions that have a long shelf-life and are stable to high concentrations of electrolytes and to changes in pH. They are suitable for internal emulsions of mineral, vegetable and fish liver oils. They are also useful for creams and ointments that are water soluble or readily removed by washing. Frequently they are used with a sorbitan ester and, by careful choice from these two groups of compounds, mixtures with o/w or w/o emulsifying properties and products with different textures and consistencies can be obtained.

Emulsions can be made by dissolving the sorbitan ester in the oil and the polysorbate in the water and then shaking or mixing the two solutions together.

In general, polysorbates are compatible with anionic, cationic and non-ionic compounds but their emulsions are difficult to preserve because of complex formation between the polyethylene groups and many preservatives.

Macrogol ethers (fatty alcohol polyglycol ethers). These are condensation products of polyethylene glycol and fatty alcohols, usually cetyl or cetostearyl. The macrogol that is used most widely as a pharmaceutical emulsifying agent is cetomacrogol 1000. It is a cream-coloured waxy, greasy solid that melts at not less than 38°C. It is soluble in water and aqueous solutions are best prepared by sprinkling the wax on hot water, stirring and leaving to cool.

Like sodium lauryl sulphate and cetrimide, it is too hydrophilic to produce very stable emulsions when used alone, but gives excellent products when combined with the hydrophobic emulgent cetostearyl alcohol. Corresponding to the anionic emulsifying wax, containing sodium lauryl sulphate and the cationic emulsifying wax containing cetrimide, there is a non-ionic emulsifying wax which contains 80% cetostearyl alcohol and 20% macrogol 1000. The corresponding emulsifying ointment (Cetomacrogol Emulsifying Ointment BP) contains 30% of the wax with soft and liquid paraffins. This will emulsify considerable amounts of water to form stable o/w cetomacrogol creams (Example 13.6). Because of their non-ionic nature, these emulsions are compatible with many anionic, cationic and non-ionic medicaments. They are stable over a wide pH range because the ether linkages in the macrogol ethers, unlike the ester linkages in the macrogol esters (below), are not susceptible to hydrolysis. Moderate levels of electrolytes are also tolerated but they are incompatible with phenolic preservatives and may reduce the antimicrobial activity of quaternary ammonium compounds.

Macrogol esters (fatty alcohol polyglycol esters). These have fairly well-balanced hydrophilic and hydrophobic properties and are good o/w emulsifying agents. The stearate esters are most often used but because of the ester linkage they are susceptible to hydrolysis, particularly if the pH is not neutral. Emulsions are stable to electrolytes but incompatible with phenolic preservatives.

Poloxalkols. These are polyoxyethylene derivatives of polyoxypropylene. They are used in low concentrations (less than 1%) as o/w emulgents* in intravenous fat emulsions.

Higher fatty alcohols. These are higher members of the series of aliphatic monohydric alcohols mostly derived from the hydrogenation of fatty acids. The higher fatty alcohols used in pharmacy are white- or cream-coloured solids. They are weak w/o emulgents and are used either to replace part of another w/o emulgent or as stabilizers for o/w emulsions. Their stabilizing action is due partly to their ability to increase the viscosity of the preparations. They also improve the texture and emollient quality of w/o emulsions. The substances used include cetyl alcohol, stearyl alcohol and cetostearyl alcohol. The main application of the latter is as an emulsion stabilizer in the three emulsifying waxes.

Ampholytic (amphoteric) surfactants

These are not widely used as emulsifiers in pharmacy.

Natural products

Many traditional emulsifying agents used in extemporaneous dispensing are derived from plant or animal sources. As with all naturally derived products the quality may vary from batch to batch. Microbial contamination may also cause problems and natural products tend to deteriorate to a greater extent than their synthetic counterparts.

Polysaccharides

Most of the natural polysaccharides act as emulsion stabilizers rather than primary emulgents.

Acacia. This is the best emulsifying agent for extemporaneously produced oral emulsions. Preparations of good quality and appearance and of adequate stability can be made by hand with a mortar and pestle. This is because the concentrated emulsion formed in the initial stage of the preparation is very viscous and sticky and therefore the oil cannot escape the vigorous shearing action of the pestle and is easily reduced to fine globules (Example 13.7).

Because of the low viscosity of acacia emulsions, creaming occurs rather quickly and often thickening agents, such as tragacanth, are used as stabilizers.

Acacia emulsions are palatable and they are stable over a wide pH range (2–10), but they are too sticky for external use.

Tragacanth. The emulsifying ability of tragacanth is due largely to the high viscosity of its mucilages. Its emulsions are coarse and therefore it is used mainly as an emulsion stabilizer, particularly for acacia emulsions. A suitable proportion is 1 part to 10 parts acacia.

Sodium alginate. As with tragacanth, the emulsifying ability of sodium alginate is due largely to the high viscosity of its solutions. A 1% mucilage will produce satisfactory emulsions of fish liver and vegetable oils but not mineral oils. Its chief use is as an emulsion stabilizer for acacia emulsions.

Other natural polysaccharides. Starch, chondrus, pectin and agar have been used but have been largely replaced by synthetic emulgents.

Semisynthetic polysaccharides. The use of the water-soluble celluloses as suspending agents is described in Chapter 12. Low-viscosity grades of methylcellulose are suitable as emulgents and emulsion stabilizers. Methylcellulose 20 in a concentration of 2% is used in Liquid Paraffin Oral Emulsion BP (Example 13.8). Methylcellulose emulsions are very stable to pH changes and alcohol but are coagulated by high concentrations of electrolytes.

Medium-viscosity grades of carmellose sodium (sodium carboxymethylcellulose) are used in a concentration of 0.5–1% as emulsion stabilizers.

Sterol-containing substances

Beeswax. Beeswax consists mainly of myricyl palmitate, an ester of a higher alcohol, and its emulsifying properties are partially due to this constituent. In addition, it contains small amounts of esters of cholesterol and free cerotic acid which can be used to form a soap.

Beeswax is not a very good emulgent but is a useful stabilizer for w/o creams in which it facilitates the incorporation of water.

It occurs in yellow or white discs or blocks. The white form which has been bleached is preferred when ingredients are colourless, white or pale.

Wool fat. This is a type of wax. It consists chiefly of fatty acid esters of cholesterol and other sterols together with fatty alcohols. It is a pale yellow, greasy, very sticky material with a melting point of 36–42°C.

Wool fat can absorb about 50% of water but when mixed with other fatty substances it can emulsify several times its own weight of aqueous or hydro-alcoholic liquid. The emulsions are w/o in type. It is used in creams and ointments and as an emulsion stabilizer in lotions (see Example 13.3). Attempts have been made to modify the physical characteristics of wool fat while retaining its advantageous properties.

Wool alcohols. This is obtained by relatively crude fractionation of wool fat. It is a golden-brown solid with a fainter odour than the parent substance and a melting point of not less than 58°C.

It contains at least 30% of cholesterol together with other alcohols. It is susceptible to oxidation and an antioxidant is incorporated.

Like wool fat, wool alcohols is a good w/o emulsifying agent and is used with hydrocarbons to produce hydrophilic bases such as Wool Alcohols Ointment BP which is used for preparing creams (Example 13.9).

Small amounts (up to 2.5%) are used to stabilize o/w emulsions and to add emollience. High concentrations cause phase inversion.

Finely divided solids

Finely divided solids with suitably balanced hydrophilic and hydrophobic properties are adsorbed at an oil–water interface forming a coherent film that prevents coalescence of the dispersed globules. If the solid particles are preferentially wetted by the oil w/o emulsions are formed while preferential wetting by the water results in o/w products. In pharmacy the solids that produce o/w emulsions are most important. These include the natural clays, bentonite, aluminium magnesium silicate and hectorite described as suspending agents in Chapter 12. The hydrated dispersions resulting from the high affinity of these substances for water are viscous, and this contributes to the stability of the emulsions. The clays are mainly used as emulsion stabilizers for external lotions and creams.

For internal preparations the colloidal aluminium and magnesium hydroxides may be used as emulsifying agents.

Choice of an emulsifying agent

Some of the many types of emulsifying agent available have been described above. Selection of an appropriate emulsification system depends on the active ingredients to be incorporated into the product and on the use of the final product and will be based on theoretical considerations and on experience. Emulgents for o/w emulsions are listed in Table 13.1 and emulgents for w/o emulsions are listed in Table 13.2.

Formulation by the HLB method

The balance between the hydrophilic and lipophilic (hydrophobic) properties of the emulgent will affect the type of emulsion produced and this tends to be indicated by the relative solubility of the emulgent in polar and non-polar solvents. This 'hydrophile-lipophile balance' (HLB) can be used to select the appropriate emulsifying

Table 13.1 Emulgents for oil-in-water emulsions

Alkali metal and ammonium soaps
Amine soaps
Anionic, cationic and non-ionic emulsifying waxes
Glycol and glycerol esters containing a soap
Polysorbates
Macrogol ethers
Macrogol esters
Poloxalkols
Polysaccharides
Finely divided clays and colloidal hydroxides

Table 13.2 Emulgents for water-in-oil emulsions

Soaps of divalent and trivalent metals
Glycol and glycerol esters alone
Sorbitan esters
Macrogol esters
Higher fatty alcohols

Table 13.3 HLB ranges and their applications

HLB range	Application
3–6	Emulsifying agent (w/o)
7–9	Wetting agent
8–18	Emulsifying agent (o/w)
13–15	Detergent
15–16	Solubilizing agent

Table 13.4 HLB values of emulsifying agents

Emulsifying agent	HLB value
Acacia	8.0
Glyceryl monostearate (pure)	3.8
Glyceryl monostearate (self-emulsifying)	5.5
Sorbitan monolaurate	8.6
Sorbitan mono-oleate	4.3
Sorbitan monostearate	4.7
Polysorbate 20	16.7
Polysorbate 60	14.9
Polysorbate 80	15.0
Potassium oleate	20.0
Sodium lauryl sulphate	40.0
Sodium oleate	18.0
Tragacanth	13.2
Triethanolamine oleate	12.0

Table 13.5 'Required HLB' values of oils and waxes

	HLB values	
	w/o	o/w
Beeswax	4	12
Cetyl alcohol	—	15
Liquid paraffin	5	12
Soft paraffin	5	12
Wool fat	8	10

agents for a particular system and is described in detail in the companion volume (Chapters 6 and 16, Aulton 1988). A brief summary of the practical aspects of formulation by the HLB method are included in this chapter.

Each surfactant is allocated a HLB number representing the relative proportions of lipophilic and hydrophilic parts of the molecule. High numbers indicate hydrophilic (lipophobic) properties while low numbers represent hydrophobic (lipophilic) properties. Generally, emulgents with high numbers (8–18) produce o/w emulsions and those with low numbers (3–6) give w/o emulsions. These and other properties that can be correlated with HLB numbers are listed in Table 13.3.

This system was originally devised for non-ionic emulsifiers but has been extended to include anionic and cationic substances. A list of HLB values of some emulsifying agents is given in Table 13.4. In addition 'required HLB' values for the different emulsion types have been determined for some oils, fats and waxes (Table 13.5). When several oils and fats are included in a formula the total 'required HLB' may be calculated and an emulgent or blend of emulgents chosen accordingly (Example 13.10). Further details are included in the companion volume (Chapter 16, Aulton 1988).

Other additives

Antioxidants

Fats, oils and some emulgents of animal and vegetable origin are subject to oxidation by atmospheric oxygen and by enzymes produced by micro-organisms. Atmospheric oxidation is controlled by adding approved antioxidants, e.g. butylated hydroxyanisole (BHA) or butylated hydroxytoluene (BHT). Ethyl, propyl or dodecyl gallate may also used.

Preservatives

Micro-organisms can grow rapidly in emulsions with a high water content, particularly if substrates such as carbohydrates, proteins and steroids are present. Contamination may include bacteria, moulds and yeasts and therefore preservatives that are both fungicidal and bactericidal are required.

Desirable properties of a preservative for emulsions

These include:

— A broad spectrum of activity over a wide range of conditions of temperature and pH.
— Rapidly effective even in the presence of large numbers of micro-organisms.
— Effective in the presence of the other ingredients of the product.
— Free from toxicity and sensitizing effects at the concentrations used.
— Free from objectionable odour, taste and colour.
— A low oil/water partition coefficient, i.e. higher concentration in the aqueous phase.

Although preservatives may be selected on theoretical grounds it is important that their efficacy in a particular emulsion system be tested by microbial challenge. A combination of preservatives may prove most effective.

Preservatives commonly used in emulsions

Organic acids. Benzoic acid is effective at a concentration of 0.1% at a pH below 5.

Sorbic acid is similarly used at a concentration of 0.1–0.2% in acid conditions.

Parahydroxybenzoic acid esters. Mixtures of methyl, ethyl, propyl and butyl esters are used to give a total concentration of 0.1–0.2% preservative in the final product. They are most effective in the pH range 7–9.

Chlorocresol. A concentration of 0.1% is a suitable preservative for aqueous creams and other external preparations. Its activity may be reduced in the presence of vegetable oils and at high pH.

Phenethyl alcohol. This has antimicrobial properties and is more active against Gram-negative than Gram-positive organisms. It may be used at concentrations of 0.025–0.5%, usually in combination with another bactericide.

Phenoxyethanol. This substance is particularly useful against *Pseudomonas aeruginosa* at a concentration of 0.5–1% and is used in combination with other broader spectrum compounds, such as the hydroxybenzoates.

Bronopol. At concentrations of 0.02–0.05% this substance is also active against *Pseudomonas aeruginosa* and a range of other bacteria. It is less effective against moulds and yeasts and therefore is used in combination with other preservatives.

Quaternary ammonium compounds. Cetrimide is used as a primary emulsifying agent and is occasionally used as a preservative at a concentration of 0.002–0.01%. These compounds are relatively ineffective against Gram-negative bacteria and bacterial spores.

Organic mercurial compounds. Phenylmercuric nitrate and acetate are sometimes used in concentrations of 0.004–0.01% to preserve emulsions containing non-ionic emulgents.

Chloroform. This is a traditional preservative for extemporaneously prepared oral emulsions (see Example 13.7).

Colour and flavour

Most pharmaceutical emulsions have an attractive white appearance and additional colour is rarely necessary. Emulsions for oral administration are usually flavoured to mask the taste of the ingredients (see Ch. 6). Medicinal creams and lotions, unlike cosmetic products, are rarely perfumed.

Texture

Factors affecting the rheological properties, consistency and texture of products for external use are discussed in the companion volume (Aulton 1988).

Factors affecting the physical stability of emulsions

The stability of emulsions is discussed in the companion volume. The main difficulties encountered in practice are listed here.

Creaming

This is the separation of the emulsion into two regions, one containing more of the disperse phase, e.g. cream on milk.

The phases can be redispersed by shaking, but the phenomenon is undesirable because it is inelegant, may lead to inaccurate dosage if shaking is not thorough and indicates a lack of stability in the system which may result in cracking of the emulsion.

Creaming is less likely to occur if the droplets are of small (1–3 μm) size and if the size distribution is small, i.e. the product is homogeneous.

Increasing the viscosity of the continuous phase will also tend to reduce creaming.

Cracking

This involves the coalescence of the dispersed globules and separation of the disperse phase as a separate layer. Redispersion cannot be achieved by shaking and the preparation is no longer an emulsion. Cracking may result from adding an incompatible emulsifying agent, e.g. anionic to cationic, by chemical or microbial decomposition of the emulsifying agent, by addition of a solvent common to both phases, by addition of electrolytes or by a significant change in pH or storage temperature.

Phase inversion

The most stable range of disperse phase concentrations is 30–60%. If the amount of disperse phase is increased until it approaches or exceeds the theoretical maximum of 74% of the total volume then phase inversion may occur, i.e. from o/w to w/o, or from w/o to o/w. The factors described above that cause cracking may alternatively cause phase inversion without total separation of the two phases.

COMPOUNDING

The basic techniques for the preparation of pharmaceutical emulsions are weighing, measuring of liquids and mixing. These are discussed in detail in Chapter 4.

Good emulsions can be prepared on a small scale using a pestle and mortar although its efficiency is limited and globule size may be larger than 10 μm. Electric mixers may also be used on a small scale although entrapped air may be a problem. Since the quality and stability of the product is improved by decreasing globule size and by reducing the size range of globules in the disperse phase the use of homogenizers is to be recommended. All homogenizers embody the same principle, that is to force the emulsion through fine apertures to apply shearing forces in order to reduce the size of the globules. Small, hand-operated homogenizers, marketed as domestic 'cream makers', are useful for extemporaneously prepared emulsions. The manufacture of emulsions on a large scale is described in Chapter 16 of the companion volume (Aulton 1988).

EMULSIONS AS ORAL DOSAGE FORMS

In pharmacy it is generally accepted that the term 'emulsion' as a dosage form refers only to products for oral administration.

Emulsions for oral use are almost invariably o/w and are a convenient means of administering oils and fats or oily solutions of unpalatable drugs of low aqueous solubility (Examples 13.7 and 13.8). For more details, see Chapter 16 of the companion volume (Aulton 1988).

Acacia emulsions

Unless otherwise specified, extemporaneously prepared emulsions for internal use are made with acacia gum. To prepare acacia emulsions using a pestle and mortar, a thick (primary) emulsion must be made first. The quantities for primary emulsions have been determined by experience and are given in Table 13.6.

'Parts' is interpreted as parts by volume for fixed, mineral and volatile oils, and water, and parts by weight for oleo-resins and acacia (Example 13.7).

Table 13.6 Quantities for primary emulsions

Type of oil	Examples	Quantities for primary emulsion (parts)		
		Oil	Water	Gum
Fixed	Almond oil Arachis oil Castor oil Cod-liver oil	4	2	1
Mineral	Liquid paraffin	3	2	1
Volatile	Turpentine oil Cinnamon oil Peppermint oil	2	2	1
Oleo-resin	Male fern extract	1	2	1

When an emulsion contains two or more oily liquids the quantity of acacia for each is calculated separately and the sum of these quantities used.

The method is as follows:

1. Measure the oil very accurately in a dry measure, pour it into the bottom of a large, perfectly dry, flat-bottomed mortar and allow the measure to drain by resting it against the head of a dry flat-headed pestle, placed in the mortar.

2. While the oil is draining, measure the quantity of water or aqueous vehicle required for the primary emulsion in a clean measure and place this within easy reach.

3. Weigh the acacia powder.

4. Remove the oily measure from the mortar, place the gum on the oil and mix lightly for just long enough to disperse the lumps. Take care to keep the suspension in the bottom of the mortar. Do not over mix.

5. Immediately add all the previously measured water and stir continuously but lightly in one direction until the mixture thickens under the pestle. Then triturate vigorously (i.e. stir and mix vigorously in the mortar) to produce a thick cream.

6. When the primary emulsion is well formed there is usually a characteristic 'cracking' sound. Continue to triturate for a further 2–3 minutes to produce a white, stable emulsion. The finer the dispersion the whiter the product.

7. Gradually dilute the primary emulsion with small volumes of the vehicle ensuring complete mixing between additions.

8. Transfer to a measure and make up to final volume.

9. If necessary decant through a muslin strainer into a calibrated bottle.

Problems

Sometimes the primary emulsion does not form properly and the contents of the mortar become oily, thin and translucent. This is due to *phase inversion*, the product which has become a w/o emulsion cannot be diluted with water and must therefore be discarded. Possible causes are:

— Insufficient shear between the mortar base and the pestle head.
— Inaccurate measurement of water or oil.
— Cross contamination of oil and water.
— Use of a wet mortar.
— Excessive mixing of oil and gum.
— Too early or too rapid dilution of the primary emulsion.
— Poor quality acacia.

Shelf-life of oral emulsions

Unpreserved emulsions deteriorate rapidly but stabilized and preserved systems may be stored.

Containers for oral emulsions

Emulsions should be supplied in well-filled containers with airtight closures. Metallic closures should be avoided. For viscous preparations wide-mouthed amber glass bottles are most appropriate.

Special labels and advice for patients

> Shake the bottle

> Store in a cool place but avoid freezing

EMULSIONS FOR EXTERNAL USE

Applications, liniments and lotions

These are liquid or semi-liquid emulsions designed for application to the skin. Preparations intended for use on broken skin should be free from microbial contamination. (Examples 13.1, 13.2, 13.3 and 13.11).

Shelf-life of applications, liniments and lotions

These are generally stable preparations. Diluted lotions should not be stored for long periods (maximum 1 month).

Containers for applications, liniments and lotions

Amber fluted bottles or jars are used for extemporaneously prepared products. Some manufactured products may be packed in plastic containers.

Special labels and advice for patients

> Shake the bottle

Advise the patient that the product should not be applied to broken skin.

Creams

Creams are viscous semisolids for external use. They are usually either o/w emulsions, i.e. aqueous creams (Examples 13.4, 13.5 and 13.6) or w/o emulsions, i.e. oily creams (Example 13.9). The possibility of microbial contamination of creams during preparation must be minimized since they provide suitable substrates for the growth of micro-organisms which may cause spoilage or pathogenicity. The preservative systems used are usually a compromise between clinical acceptibility, formulation stability and efficacy and may be inadequate to cope with heavy microbial contamination. Creams should therefore be prepared under conditions of strict hygiene or better still using aseptic technique. As a minimum, all apparatus used in the preparation and the final containers should be thoroughly cleaned before use and rinsed with freshly boiled and cooled purified water before drying. Swabbing of working surfaces, spatulas and other equipment with 70% ethanol will reduce the possibility of microbial contamination. The operator must maintain the highest standards of hygiene. The aqueous component should always be prepared with freshly boiled and cooled purified water and the purity and freedom from contamination of all ingredients assured.

General compounding procedure for creams

Emulsified creams are prepared by heating the components of the oily phase (usually including the emulgent) until molten and then cooling to 60°C.

The components of the aqueous phase are mixed in a separate vessel and also heated to 60°C. The aqueous phase is then added to the oily phase at the same temperature. This is important and a thermometer should be used. The resulting emulsion should be stirred until cool. Rapid cooling may result in separation of high melting point components. Excessive aeration caused by vigorous stirring may also lead to a granular product. If necessary the product may be homogenized after cooling.

Creams may contain one or more medicaments in solution in one or other of the phases. Finely powdered insoluble medicaments may be dispersed in a cream base (Example 13.12).

Diluted creams

The pharmacist may be asked to prepare extemporaneous dilutions of proprietary creams. Choice of the appropriate diluent is crucial since dilution may impair the preservative system in the cream and significantly affect the bioavailability of any active ingredients. Furthermore, the risk of microbial contamination is great and the practice should not be encouraged unless considered by the prescriber to be essential.

Dilutions should be made only if the diluent to be used is stated in the manufacturer's data sheet (the information is usually also quoted in the BNF). Diluted creams must be freshly prepared without the application of heat and with strict hygienic precautions (Example 13.13).

Shelf-life of creams

Extemporaneously prepared creams should generally be given a short shelf-life unless freedom from micro-organisms can be assured. Proprietary products in original packs carry an expiry date suggested by the manufacturer, assuming appropriate storage. Diluted creams should be freshly prepared and should not be used for more than 2 weeks after issue.

Containers for creams

Wide-mouthed squat jars may be used for creams where the risk of contamination in use is considered to be minimal, e.g. oily creams. The containers must be well closed and prevent water evaporation. The mouth of the jar should be covered with a disc of greaseproof paper.

Collapsible metal or flexible plastic tubes are to be preferred since these reduce the risk of contamination in use and most proprietary products are packed in tubes. Aluminium tubes may interact with the ingredients of some creams and are usually coated internally with a lacquer of heat-cured epoxy resin. A method for filling collapsible tubes in extemporaneous dispensing is described in Example 13.14.

Special labels and advice for patients

> Store in a cool place

The labels for collapsible tubes should be fixed to the upper (nozzle) end of the tube.

Sterilized products should be labelled

> Sterile until opened

EXAMPLES

Example 13.1

Prepare 100 ml of Turpentine Liniment BP 1988

Ingredients	Master formula
Soft Soap	75 g
Camphor	50 g
Turpentine Oil	650 ml
Purified Water, freshly boiled and cooled	225 ml

Note that in order to prepare 100 ml of this product the total number of formula 'units' must be in excess of 100. 120 units is a convenient quantity (see Example 3.5).

Formulation

This is an alkali soap type of emulsion. The soap is preformed soft soap, an appropriate proportion being 10% of the weight of the oil for a fixed oil or 20% of the weight of the oil for a fat. The turpentine oil and camphor act as rubefacients and counter-irritants.

Compounding

Finely powder the camphor in a fairly large mortar, add the soap and mix well. Add the oil in small amounts, mixing well after each addition. When all the lumps have been dispersed and a smooth suspension produced, the rest of the oil may be added quickly.

Transfer the suspension to a beaker for ease of pouring. Place all of the water in the formula into a bottle at least 50% larger than the final volume of the product. Add the oily suspension in small quantities, shaking vigorously after each addition. Note that, if the oily suspension is placed in the bottle and the water added, the emulsion will invert. It is necessary to wait for the air generated by shaking to disperse before transferring the appropriate quantity to a calibrated bottle.

Storage and shelf-life

The preparation should be stored cool but not allowed to freeze. Turpentine should be protected from light.

Container

Amber fluted bottle, preferably glass since turpentine reacts with some plastics.

Advice for patients when dispensed.

Shake the bottle.

The liniment should be applied to the skin with considerable friction; it should not be applied to broken or inflamed skin or near the eyes or mucous membranes.

Actions and uses

Counter-irritant and rubefacient.

Example 13.2

Prepare 200 ml of White Liniment BP 1988

Ingredients	Master formula
Oleic Acid	85 ml
Turpentine	250 ml
Dilute Ammonia Solution	45 ml
Ammonium Chloride	12.5 g
Purified Water	625 ml

Note that 20% of the BP quantities will produce slightly more than 200 ml.

Formulation

This is an ammonium soap type of emulsion. The soap is prepared by the interaction of a fatty acid (oleic acid) and ammonia during preparation of the emulsion which is made by shaking.

Ammonium oleate is an o/w emulsifying agent but the ammonium chloride causes suppression of the ionization of the soap by the common ion effect. This together with the high percentage of turpentine in the liniment causes phase inversion to occur producing a w/o emulsion.

Compounding

Mix the turpentine oil and oleic acid in a bottle 50% larger than the final volume of the product.

Add an equal volume of warm water (approximately 50°C) to the dilute ammonia solution and add this dilution in small quantities with shaking to the oily liquid, shaking vigorously after each addition.

Dissolve the ammonium chloride in the rest of the water and add to the bottle in small amounts, again shaking vigorously after each.

Transfer the appropriate quantity to a tared bottle.

Storage and shelf-life

The preparation should be stored cool but not allowed to freeze. Turpentine should be protected from light.

Container

Amber fluted bottle, preferably glass since turpentine reacts with some plastics.

Advice for patients when dispensed

Shake the bottle.

The liniment should be applied to the skin with considerable friction; it should not be applied to broken or inflamed skin or near the eyes or mucous membranes.

Actions and uses

Counter-irritant and rubefacient.

Example 13.3

Prepare 100 ml of Oily Calamine Lotion BP 1980

Ingredients	Master formula
Calamine	50 g
Oleic Acid	5 ml
Wool Fat	10 g
Arachis Oil	500 ml
Calcium Hydroxide Solution sufficient to produce	1000 ml

Formulation

This is a 'lime' cream type of lotion. The emulgent for the arachis oil is a soap produced from the calcium hydroxide and the oleic acid. Wool fat is included as an emulsion stabilizer.

Compounding

Warm the wool fat, oleic acid and arachis oil together in an evaporating basin on a water-bath until the wool fat has melted. Mix well.

Sieve and weigh the calamine and place on a warm tile. Add a little of the oily mixture and rub with a large spatula until smooth.

Dilute the paste until it is fluid and transfer it as completely as possible to the basin. Stir, if necessary, with a small glass pestle to distribute the suspension evenly.

Pour into a calibrated bottle previously warmed

slightly on the water-bath and add the lime water in small amounts, shaking vigorously after each addition.

Storage and shelf-life
This is an 'official' preparation but may separate on storage. It is unpreserved and therefore should not be stored for long periods. Store in a cool place but do not allow to freeze.

Container
Amber fluted bottle.

Advice for patients when dispensed
Shake the bottle.

Actions and uses
Soothing lotion for the treatment of eczema.

Example 13.4

Prepare 30 g of Aqueous Cream BP 1988

Ingredients	Master formula
Emulsifying Ointment	300 g
Phenoxyethanol	10 g
Purified Water, freshly boiled and cooled	690 g

Formulation
This is a cream made with anionic emulsifying wax. Phenoxyethanol, a viscous water-soluble liquid, acts as preservative.

Compounding
Dissolve the phenoxyethanol in hot purified water and adjust the solution to weight. Maintain the solution at 60°C.
  Melt the emulsifying wax and warm to 60°C.
  Check that the temperature of both phases is 60°C then add the aqueous phase to the melted ointment and stir continuously until cold.

Storage and shelf-life
The preparation should be stored cool but not allowed to freeze.

Container
Collapsible metal tube (see Example 13.4).

Advice for patients when dispensed
Not applicable. Usually used as a diluent or cream base.

Actions and uses
Emollient cream base.

Example 13.5

Prepare 25 g of Cetrimide Cream BP 1988

Ingredients	Master formula
Cetrimide	5 g or a sufficient quantity
Cetostearyl Alcohol	50 g
Liquid Paraffin	500 g

Purified Water, freshly boiled and cooled sufficient to produce	1000 g

Note that the BP formula suggests a suitable concentration of cetrimide (0.5%) but allows flexibility in the choice of strength. The product must be labelled with the concentration actually incorporated.

Formulation
This is a cream made with cationic emulsifying wax. Cetrimide also acts as preservative.

Compounding
Melt the cetostearyl alcohol, add the liquid paraffin and warm to 60°C.
  Dissolve the cetrimide in the freshly boiled and cooled water and warm to the same temperature.
  Check that the temperature of both phases is 60°C and then add the aqueous phase to the oily mixture and stir continuously until cold.

Storage and shelf-life
The preparation should be stored cool but not allowed to freeze.

Container
Collapsible metal tube (see Example 3.14).

Advice for patients when dispensed
The cream should not be applied repeatedly. Wet dressings should not be applied.

Actions and uses
Antiseptic cream.

Example 13.6

Prepare 50 g of Cetomacrogol Cream (Formula B) BP 1988

Ingredients	Master formula
Cetomacrogol Emulsifying Ointment	300 g
Benzyl Alcohol	15 g
Propyl Hydroxybenzoate	0.8 g
Methyl Hydroxybenzoate	1.5 g
Purified Water, freshly boiled and cooled sufficient to produce	1000 g

Note that there are two formulae for Cetomacrogol Cream BP differing only in the preservative system used.

Formulation
Formula A uses chlorocresol as the preservative and for Formula B, the preservatives are the hydroxybenzoate esters and benzyl alcohol.
  A better product is obtained if the emulsifying ointment is replaced by the appropriate quantities of its ingredients, i.e. liquid paraffin, white soft paraffin and cetomacrogol emulsifying wax.

Compounding
Make an excess of the product which enables the small amount of propyl hydroxybenzoate required to be weighed on an analytical balance.

Melt the cetomacrogol emulsifying wax, liquid paraffin and white soft paraffin and warm to 60°C.

Dissolve the preservatives in the freshly boiled and partly cooled water (benzoic acid is volatile in steam) and adjust to weight.

Check that the temperature of both phases is 60°C and then add the aqueous phase to the oily mixture and stir continuously until cold.

Adjustment to temperature is particularly critical for this product.

Storage and shelf-life
The preparation should be stored cool but not allowed to freeze. It should be freshly prepared unless the microbiolial quality can be assessed.

Container
Collapsible metal tube (see Example 3.74). If not freshly prepared it is recommended that a readily breakable seal should cover the closure or the tube be enclosed in a sealed plastic envelope or sealed carton. If aluminium tubes are used the inner surface should be coated with a suitable lacquer.

Advice for patients when dispensed
Not applicable (rarely dispensed alone)

Actions and uses
Emollient and diluent cream.

Example 13.7

Prepare 200 ml of an emulsion containing: arachis oil 50 ml, concentrated peppermint emulsion 5 ml, in a chloroform water vehicle

Ingredients	Formula
Arachis Oil	50 ml
Peppermint Emulsion, Concentrated	5 ml
Double-strength Chloroform Water	100 ml
Water	to 200 ml

Formulation
Peppermint is included as flavouring and chloroform water as preservative. The vehicle is prepared by using half the volume of double-strength chloroform water.

Acacia is a suitable emulgent for an internal preparation. Arachis oil is a fixed oil and from Table 13.6 the proportions for the primary emulsion are oil: water: gum — 4:21.

Therefore the quantities for the primary emulsion are:

Arachis oil	50 ml
Water	25 ml
Acacia powder	12.5 g

Compounding
The dry gum method for making acacia emulsions has been described in this chapter.

1. Accurately measure the oil and place in a large perfectly dry mortar allowing the measure to drain.
2. Measure the 25 ml water from the vehicle and have to hand.
3. Weigh the acacia powder.
4. Disperse the acacia powder lightly in the oil.
5. Add the 25 ml water at once and triturate until the primary emulsion is well established.
6. The emulsion may now be diluted and the remaining ingredients added before making up to final volume.

Storage and shelf-life
A short shelf-life would be appropriate for an 'unofficial' preparation (see Table 5.2).

Store in a cool place but do not allow to freeze.

Container
Amber medicine bottle with a wide mouth.

Advice for patients when dispensed
Shake the bottle.

Actions and uses
Nutritious, demulcent and mildly laxative.

Example 13.8

Prepare 200 ml of Liquid Paraffin Oral Emulsion BP 1988

Ingredients	Master formula
Liquid Paraffin	500 ml
Vanillin	500 mg
Chloroform	2.5 ml
Benzoic Acid Solution	20 ml
Methylcellulose 20	20 g
Saccharin Sodium	50 mg
Water	a sufficient quantity

Formulation
The emulgent for the liquid paraffin is methylcellulose 20, present in a concentration of 2%. Chloroform and benzoic acid act as preservatives and saccharin sodium and vanillin are present as sweetening and flavouring agents.

Compounding
To prepare the mucilage Mix the methylcellulose 20 with about six times its weight of boiling water and allow to stand for 30 minutes to hydrate the powder. Add an equal weight of ice and stir mechanically until the mucilage is homogeneous.

Dissolve the vanillin in a mixture of the benzoic acid solution and chloroform because it is more soluble in organic solvents. Add the solution to the mucilage and stir for 5 minutes.

The small quantity of saccharin sodium may be obtained by trituration in water and the appropriate volume of solution added to the mucilage which may then be made up to 100 ml volume. It may be necessary to allow the mucilage to stand to eliminate entrapped air before adjusting to volume.

To prepare the emulsion Add together equal volumes of liquid paraffin and the mucilage with constant stirring. The emulsion is more stable if passed through a hand homogenizer.

Storage and shelf-life
This is an 'official' preparation with an effective preservative system and therefore should remain stable on storage. Store in a cool place but do not allow to freeze.

Container
Amber medicine bottle with a wide mouth.

Advice for patients when dispensed
Shake the bottle.
    The mixture should not be taken within 30 minutes of meal times and preferably on an empty stomach.
    If the product is counter-prescribed the patient should seek medical advice if the condition persists.

Actions and uses
Laxative.

Example 13.9

Prepare 50 g of oily cream (Hydrous Ointment BP 1988)

Ingredients	Master formula
Wool Alcohols Ointment	500 g
Phenoxyethanol	10 g
Dried Magnesium Sulphate	5 g
Purified Water, freshly boiled and cooled	485 g

Formulation
Wool Alcohols Ointment contains wool alcohols, liquid paraffin, hard paraffin and yellow or white soft paraffin. If the oily cream is to be used for products with pale ingredients then the ointment made with white soft paraffin is to be preferred.
    The wool alcohols acts as a w/o emulgent. The addition of the magnesium sulphate enhances the stability and appearance of the product. Phenoxyethanol is a preservative. It is a liquid at room temperature and is best dissolved by shaking in hot water.

Compounding
Melt the wool alcohols ointment and allow to cool to about 60°C.
    Boil the purified water, dissolve the phenoxyethanol and magnesium sulphate and cool to 60°C.
    Gradually add the water to the ointment with constant stirring until a smooth cream is formed. It is important to maintain the temperature at 60°C until the cream has formed to avoid the higher melting point constituents of the ointment solidifying out.

Storage and shelf-life
The preparation should be stored cool but not allowed to freeze. If on storage some aqueous liquid separates it may be re-incorporated by stirring.

Container
Collapsible metal tube (see Example 3.14) or wide-mouthed jar.

Advice for patients when dispensed
Not applicable.

Actions and uses
Emollient cream base.

Example 13.10

Example of the formulation of an o/w lotion using the HLB method

Formula

Liquid paraffin	35
Wool fat	1
Cetyl alcohol	1
Emulgent	7
Water	to 100

'Required HLB' values of the first three ingredients are respectively 12, 10 and 15 for an o/w emulsion.
    The total percentage of oil phase is $35 + 1 + 1 = 37\%$, and the proportions of the oil phase ingredients are:

Liquid paraffin $\dfrac{35}{37} = 94.6\%$

Wool fat $\dfrac{1}{37} = 2.7\%$

Cetyl alcohol $\dfrac{1}{37} = 2.7\%$

The total 'required HLB' value is obtained as follows:

Liquid paraffin $\dfrac{94.6}{100} \times 12 = 11.4$

Wool fat $\dfrac{2.7}{100} \times 10 = 0.3$

Cetyl alcohol $\dfrac{2.7}{100} \times 15 = 0.4$

Total 'required HLB' $= 12.1$

Assume that a mixture of sorbitan mono-oleate (HLB value = 4.3) and polysorbate 80 (HLB value = 15) is to be used as the emulgent blend. The proportion of these two substances that will provide the 'required HLB' value of 12.1 is calculated as follows:
    Let x = the percentage of sorbitan mono-oleate in the mixture.
    Then $100 - x$ = the percentage of polysorbate.
    Contribution from sorbitan mono-oleate

$$= 4.3 \times \frac{x}{100}$$

Contribution from polysorbate 80 $= 15 \times \dfrac{(100 - x)}{100}$

Since the total contribution must = 12.1, the expression for calculating x is

$$4.3 \times \frac{x}{100} + 15 \times \frac{(100 - x)}{100} = 12.1$$

$$4.3x + 1500 - 15x = 1210$$
$$290 = 10.7x$$
$$x = 27\%$$

Hence, the percentages of the emulsifying agents in the mixture are:

Sorbitan mono-oleate	27
Polysorbate 80	73

Since the total percentage of the mixed emulgents in the formula is 7, the percentages of the individual substances are

Sorbitan mono-oleate $7 \times \dfrac{27}{100} = 1.89$

Polysorbate 80 $7 - 1.89 = 5.11$

Example 13.11

Prepare 100 ml of Benzyl Benzoate Application BP 1988

Ingredients	Master Formula
Benzyl Benzoate	250 g
Emulsifying Wax	20 g
Purified Water, freshly boiled and cooled sufficient to produce	1000 ml

Formulation
In this preparation 25% of benzyl benzoate is emulsified with 2% Emulsifying Wax BP (an anionic emulgent).
  Note the benzyl benzoate is a liquid.

Compounding
First calibrate the container and place on the water-bath to warm.
  Weigh the benzyl benzoate into an evaporating basin and put to warm.
  Melt the emulsifying wax (m.p. about 52°C) in a separate dish, add the benzyl benzoate, mix and allow the mixture to cool to about 60°C.
  Warm an excess of the water to 60°C.
  Transfer the oily mixture to the jar and quickly add (in one amount) a sufficient quantity of the warmed water up to the tare mark. It is difficult to make any additions accurately once the jar has been shaken because the preparation froths when shaken.
  Either replace the closure and shake until cold or alternatively use an electric stirrer to stir gently until cold. Avoid placing the container on a cold surface until fully cooled because this may cause separation of the wax.

Storage and shelf-life
The preparation should be stored cool but not allowed to freeze.

Container
Amber fluted wide-mouthed jar.

Advice for patients when dispensed
Shake the bottle. The application should not be applied to broken or inflamed skin and contact with the eyes, ears and lips should be avoided.
  Detailed instructions for the use of the application in the treatment of scabies and pediculosis are given in the Pharmaceutical Codex.

Actions and uses
Ascaricide.

Example 13.12

Prepare 25 g of Salicylic Acid and Sulphur Cream BP 1980

Ingredients	Master formula
Salicylic Acid, finely sifted	20 g
Precipitated Sulphur	20 g
Aqueous Cream sufficient to produce	1000 g

Formulation
Aqueous cream is used as a base for the dispersion of the solid ingredients.

Compounding
The salicylic acid should be sifted before weighing using a 180 μm stainless steel sieve. The powder is very irritant to the respiratory tract and precautions should be observed to avoid inhalation.
  The preparation should be made under conditions of strict hygiene.
  Working surfaces, balances, tiles, spatulas and all equipment should be spotlessly clean and swabbed with 70% ethanol before use to minimize microbial contamination. The powders should be mixed lightly on a large tile with a large flexible spatula and the base incorporated. The product should remain uncovered as little as possible and the container filled as hygienically as possible.

Storage and shelf-life
The preparation should be stored cool but not allowed to freeze.

Container
Collapsible metal tube (see Example 3.14).

Advice for patients when dispensed
The cream should not be applied to broken or inflamed skin: contact with the eyes should be avoided.
  Detailed advice for use in scalp or skin disorders is given in the Pharmaceutical Codex.

Actions and uses
Keratolytic with bacteriostatic and fungicidal properties.

Example 13.13

Supply 25 g of a cream containing beclomethasone diproprionate 0.0125%
A cream containing beclomethasone diproprionate 0.025% w/w is available.

Formulation
The recommended diluent for proprietary beclomethasone cream is Cetomacrogol Cream, Formula A (BP 1988) (see BNF).
  Calculation (see Example 3.20).
Prepare 5 g excess to allow for manipulative losses

$$\frac{\text{weight required} \times \text{\% required}}{\text{\% of concentrated}} = \frac{\text{weight of concentrated}}{\text{cream to be used}}$$

$$= \frac{30 \text{ g} \times 0.0125\%}{0.025\%} = 15 \text{ g}$$

Formula
Beclomethasone diproprionate
cream (0.025% w/w)   15 g
Cetomacrogol Cream (Formula A)   15 g

Compounding
The preparation should be made under conditions of strict hygiene to minimize microbial contamination.

The creams should be mixed on a large tile with a large flexible spatula. The product should remain uncovered as little as possible and the container filled as hygienically as possible.

Storage and shelf-life
The preparation should be stored cool but not allowed to freeze.
Shelf-life 14 days.

Container
Collapsible metal tube (see Example 3.14).

Advice for patients when dispensed
Apply sparingly as directed.

Action and uses
Topical steroidal anti-inflammatory cream.

Example 13.14

Method for extemporaneous filling of collapsible metal tubes

Individual tubes may be filled as follows:

1. Cut a piece of greaseproof paper to a length about 50 mm longer than the tube and wide enough to encircle it comfortably twice. Place this on a clean tile and turn up one of the long edges.
2. Place the cream in the centre, parallel to the turn up, leaving very little uncovered paper at one end and keeping the cream well within the length of the tube at the other (Fig. 13.1).
3. Turn the near edge of the paper over to the bottom of the turn-up as if wrapping a powder (see Figure 16.1).

Fig. 13.1 Filling a collapsible tube

Hold the edges together and, placing a spatula with its blade parallel to the turn-up, bring it towards the cream gently, shaping the mass into a cylindrical form. When the diameter is slightly smaller than the internal diameter of the tube, roll the cylinder over the rest of the paper and then slide it into the tube.

Close the tube by placing the edge of the spatula at right angles to its length and about 2.5 mm from its end; and pressing down with the left hand. Release the pressure just enough to allow gradual withdrawal of the paper with the right hand. If the pressure is correct the paper will come out easily without removing cream.

Turn over 2.5 mm of the tube with the spatula and press down with tube-sealing pliers. Repeat so that the end of the tube is turned inside the second fold.

It is difficult to avoid some loss of cream and it is advisable, unless very experienced, to put an excess on the paper (e.g. 30 g when 25 g is ordered) to ensure that the patient does not receive short weight. The weight can be checked before issue.

As the patient may roll up the end of the tube as it is used, the label should be placed as near to the top of the tube as possible.

BIBLIOGRAPHY

ABPI Data Sheet Compendium current edition Datapharm Publications, London (updated annually)
Aulton M E (ed) 1988. Pharmaceutics: the science of dosage form design. Churchill Livingstone, Edinburgh
British National Formulary 1988 16th edn. British Medical Association and Royal Pharmaceutical Society of Great Britain, London (updated twice yearly)
British Pharmacopoeia 1980 HMSO, London (and addenda 1982, 1983 and 1986)
British Pharmacopoeia 1988 HMSO, London
British Pharmaceutical Codex 1973 Pharmaceutical Press, London
Diluent Directories (Internal and External) current edition. National Pharmaceutical Association (NPA)

European Pharmacopoeia 2nd edn. First cycle 1982, Second cycle 1983–84; Third cycle 1985. Maisonneuve S.A., St Ruffine, France
Martindale, see Reynolds J E F
Pharmaceutical Codex 1979 11th edn (incorporating the British Pharmaceutical Codex). Pharmaceutical Press, London
Pharmaceutical Society, 1979 Guide to good dispensing practice. Pharmaceutical Journal 223: 157–158
Reynolds J E F (ed) 1989 Martindale, The Extra Pharmacopoeia, 29th edn. Pharmaceutical Press, London
Wade A (ed) 1980 Pharmaceutical handbook, 19th edn. Pharmaceutical Press, London

14. Ointments, pastes and gels

D. M. Collett

Ointments, pastes and gels are semi-solid preparations for application to the skin. Ointments are greasy preparations, the base is usually anhydrous and immiscible with skin secretions. Gels are transparent or translucent, non-greasy, aqueous preparations. Pastes contain a higher proportion of finely powdered medicament than ointments or gels but have similar bases. The factors influencing the design of dermatological preparations are discussed in detail in the companion volume (Chapter 22, Aulton 1988). Practical aspects of the formulation and compounding of semi-solid ointments, pastes and gels are described in this chapter.

FORMULATION OF OINTMENTS AND PASTES

Bases for ointments and ointment-type pastes

These may be classified into four main groups: hydrocarbon bases, absorption bases, water-miscible bases and water-soluble bases.

Hydrocarbon bases

These bases are immiscible with water and are not absorbed by the skin. They are almost inert and absorb very little water from a formulation or from skin exudate. However, they inhibit water loss from the skin by forming a waterproof film and by improving hydration, may encourage absorption of the medicaments through the skin.

The constituents of hydrocarbon bases include:

Soft paraffin. This is a purified mix of semi-solid hydrocarbons from petroleum or heavy lubricating oil. There are two varieties, one is yellow and the other (bleached) form is white. Both have a melting point range of 38–56°C although there may be some batch variation in properties. Pharmaceutically, the white form is used for products with colourless, white or pale ingredients and the yellow form for products with

dark-coloured ingredients. However, the unbleached form is less likely to elicit an adverse skin reaction in sensitive patients.

Hard paraffin. This is a mixture of solid hydrocarbons obtained from petroleum or shale oil. It is a colourless or white, odourless, translucent, wax-like substance that feels slightly greasy and often appears to have a 'crystalline' structure. It solidifies between 50°C and 57°C and is used to stiffen ointment bases.

Liquid paraffin. This is a mixture of liquid hydrocarbons obtained from petroleum. It is a transparent, colourless, almost odourless oily liquid. On long storage it is liable to oxidation with production of peroxides and therefore it may require an antioxidant, e.g. tocopherol or butylated hydroxytoluene (BHT). It is used to soften ointment bases and to reduce the viscosity of creams.

Paraffin substitute. A soft ointment base is produced by dissolving polythene (mol. wt 21 000) in liquid paraffin with the aid of heat and cooling the resulting solution rapidly to form a gel. The consistency of the base varies little over a wide temperature range (−15 to 60°C). The base is compatible with most medicaments and is readily applied to the skin.

Paraffin Ointment BP. This is an 'official' hydrocarbon ointment base.

Absorption bases

A. Non-emulsified. These bases absorb water and aqueous solutions to produce water-in-oil (w/o) emulsions. They consist of a mixture of a sterol-type emulgent (see Ch. 13) with one or more paraffins.

The constituents include:

Wool fat (anhydrous lanolin). This is a type of wax that can absorb about 50% of its weight of water and is used in ointments in which the proportion of aqueous fluid is too large for incorporation into a hydrocarbon base. Some patients become sensitized to products containing lanolin. Wool fat is a major constituent of Simple

Ointment BP (Example 14.1) and Eye Ointment Basis BP.

Wool alcohols. This is the emulsifying fraction of wool fat used in Wool Alcohols Ointment BP.

Beeswax and cholesterol. Beeswax consists mainly of myricyl palmitate with small amounts of cholesterol. Beeswax and cholesterol are included in some ointment bases to increase water-absorbing power (see Example 14.2).

B. Water-in-oil emulsions. These are similar in properties to the previous group and are capable of absorbing more water. The constituents of emulsified absorption bases include Hydrous Wool Fat BP (lanolin) and Oily Cream BP (see Examples 13.9, 14.2 and 14.3).

Absorption bases are less occlusive than the hydrocarbon bases and are easier to spread. They are good emollients.

Water-miscible bases

Despite their hydrophilic nature, absorption bases are difficult to wash from the skin. Although they can emulsify a large quantity of water they are immiscible with an excess. Ointments made from water-miscible bases are easily removed after use. The three emulsifying ointments form water-miscible bases, i.e. Emulsifying Ointment BP (anionic), Cetrimide Emulsifying Ointment BP (cationic) and Cetomacrogol Emulsifying Ointment BP (non-ionic). These contain paraffins and an o/w emulgent and have the general formula:

anionic, cationic or non-ionic emulsifying wax	30%
White Soft Paraffin	50%
Liquid Paraffin	20%

They are used for preparing o/w creams (see Ch. 13) and as ointment bases when easy removal from the skin is advantageous (Example 14.4). Other advantages of this type of base include, miscibility with exudates, good contact with the skin, high cosmetic acceptibility and easy removal from the hair. These are therefore useful for scalp ointments.

Water-soluble bases

Completely water-soluble bases have been developed from the macrogols (polyethylene glycols). The macrogols are mixtures of polycondensation products of ethylene oxide and water and they are described by their average molecular weights. Like the paraffin hydrocarbons, they vary in consistency from viscous liquids to waxy solids. The liquids are clear and colourless, have a faint characteristic odour and are miscible with water,

alcohol and other glycols. The solids are white or cream solid lumps or flakes, soluble 1 in 3 of water or 1 in 2 of alcohol and their solidifying points range from 40°C to 60°C depending on molecular weight. They are remarkable in being both wax-like and water soluble.

Macrogols are non-toxic and non-irritating to the skin unless it is badly inflamed. The liquid and semi-liquid forms are hygroscopic and 5% solutions have a pH within the range 4–7.5.

Products with ointment-like consistency can be obtained by mixing liquid and waxy forms in suitable proportions. The water-soluble bases have the advantages of being non-occlusive, miscible with exudates, non-staining and easily removed by washing.

The macrogol bases, being water-soluble, have the disadvantage of having a very limited capacity to take up water without a physical change. They are less bland than the paraffins and reduce the activity of a number of antimicrobial substances for example, phenols, hydroxybenzoates and quaternary ammonium compounds. They may also react with plastic closures.

Other ingredients of ointment bases

Vegetable oils

Arachis, castor, coconut and olive oils are examples of oils used in ointment bases. All are liquid except coconut oil which liquefies readily on heating and generally has a melting point range of 20–26°C. These oils are used as emollients and softening agents. They have the disadvantages of natural products, i.e. variation in composition and susceptibility to oxidation requiring the inclusion of antioxidant stabilizers which may cause sensitization in some patients.

Synthetic esters of fatty acids

Esters such as isopropyl myristate, linoleate, palmitate and palmitate-stearate are more consistent in composition than the vegetable oils and are more resistant to oxidation. They may be used as substitutes for the vegetable oils in ointment bases.

Higher fatty alcohols

Cetyl, stearyl and cetostearyl alcohols, described in Chapter 13 as emulgents, are used in ointment bases. They have good emollient properties but are not greasy, they do not rancidify and they facilitate the incorporation of water for example, by the absorption of water by the macrogol bases.

Silicones

Dimethicones or dimethyl polysiloxanes are used in barrier ointments to protect the skin against water-soluble irritants.

Propylene glycol

This may be used as a polar organic solvent to disperse very small quantities of active medicament through a relatively large quantity of ointment base.

Other additives for ointments and pastes

Antioxidants

The antioxidants that are used in ointment bases are similar to those listed for emulsions in Chapter 13 and include butylated hydroxyanisole (BHA), butylated hydroxytoluene (BHT), and ethyl, propyl or dodecyl gallates. Chelating agents such as ethylene-diaminetetra-acetic acid (EDTA) may also be used. The antioxidant chosen must be compatible with the medicaments incorporated into the base.

Preservatives

Preservatives may not be required in anhydrous ointments because the substrate is generally unfavourable to the multiplication of any contaminating micro-organisms. Ointments with an aqueous component require effective antimicrobial agents to prevent the growth of organisms that may cause spoilage and pathogenicity.

The preservatives described in Chapter 13 for emulsions are also suitable for hydrous ointment bases. Those used most commonly are mixtures of hydroxybenzoate esters, sorbic acid, phenethyl alcohol, organic mercurials and quaternary ammonium compounds. The effectiveness of the preservative system should be established by challenge tests with appropriate organisms.

FORMULATION OF GELS

Gels as bases

Gelling agents are either organic hydrocolloids or hydrophilic inorganic substances. These substances may also act as suspending agents (see Ch. 12) and emulsifying agents (see Ch. 13). The viscosity of the gel produced may be varied to suit the requirements of the final product. Slightly viscous gels may be used as replacement solutions for body secretions, e.g. artificial saliva and artificial tears. Slightly more viscous gels may

be used as lubricants for catheters, examination gloves and surgical instruments. Gels may also be used as dermatological bases. All gels should be free from microbial contamination and those designed for ophthalmic or surgical use must be supplied sterile.

Tragacanth. Tragacanth gels are susceptible to microbial degradation, to changes in pH outside the range pH 4.5–7 and to the variation typical of a natural product.

The formulation must contain a dispersing agents such as alcohol (see Example 12.7), glycerol or a volatile oil to prevent lumpiness. Concentrations of tragacanth from 2% to 5% produce gels of increasing viscosity.

Sodium alginate. The viscosity of alginate gels is more standardized than that of tragacanth. A concentration of 1.5% produces fluid gels and 5–10% gels are suitable as dermatological vehicles. Alginate gels also require a dispersing agents such as glycerol in the formulation.

Pectin. Pectin gels are suitable for acid products. They are prone to microbial contamination and to water loss by evaporation and may require the inclusion of a humectant. Pectin may be used in combination with other gelling agents such as sodium carboxymethylcellulose (carmellose sodium) and gelatin.

Starch. Starch gels are little used as dermatological bases. Mucilages prepared with water alone lose water by evaporation and are prone to microbial contamination. Glycerol concentrations of 50% or greater combine humectant and preservative functions.

Gelatin. Gelatin forms gels at concentrations of 2–15% or more. Gelatin gels are rarely used alone as a dermatological base but may be combined with other ingredients such as pectin and carmellose sodium.

Cellulose derivatives. These are widely used because they produce neutral gels of stable viscosity, good resistance to microbial attack, high clarity and a good film strength when dried on the skin. Methylcellulose 450 at a concentration of 3–5% produces satisfactory gels. Carmellose sodium (i.e. sodium carboxymethylcellulose) is easier to dissolve and the medium viscosity grade produces lubricant gels at a concentration of 1.5–5% and dermatological gels at greater concentrations.

Hypromellose (hydroxypropyl methylcellulose) forms exceptionally clear gels which are used in ophthalmic products.

Carbomer. Neutralized carbomer gels are also used as the bases for lubricants (0.3–1%) and in dermatological preparations (0.5–5%). These gels are clear provided that an excessive amount of air is not incorporated during preparation.

Polyvinyl alcohols. Polyvinyl alcohols (PVAs) have been used to prepare gels that dry very quickly. The residual film is strong and plastic, giving good contact between the skin and the medicament. The required concentration is usually between 10% and 20% depending on the grade of PVA and the desired viscosity.

Clays. Gels containing 7–20% of bentonite are used as dermatological bases. They are opalescent and lack the attractive clear appearance of many other types of gel. The powdery residue left on drying may make them more acceptable than some other gels for use on the face. Uniform distribution of solids is comparatively easy although the pH (about 9) is not ideal for application to the skin and the viscosity is modified by changes in pH.

Gels containing about 10% of aluminium magnesium stearate are also suitable bases for medicated gels.

Other additives for gels

Humectants

Loss of water can quickly lead to skin formation in gels and humectants such as glycerol, propylene glycol or sorbitol solution may be added to retain water.

Preservatives

All gels have a high water content and therefore are liable to support microbial growth unless a suitable preservative is added. The chosen preservative must be compatible with the gelling agent.

Methyl and propyl hydroxybenzoates either alone or in combination are suitable for gels containing tragacanth, sodium alginate, pectin, carmellose sodium, hypromellose and carbomer. Suitable concentrations for the methly ester are 0.1–0.2% and for the propyl ester 0.02–0.05%.

Pectin and alginate gels may be preserved with chlorocresol (0.1–0.2%) or benzoic acid (0.2%), providing that the product is acid. Benzalkonium chloride (0.01% w/v) is used for methylcellulose and hypromellose gels and phenylmercuric nitrate (0.001%) may be used for methylcellulose. Chlorhexidine acetate (0.02%) has been used with polyvinyl alcohol gels.

Chelating agents

Bases and medicaments sensitive to heavy metals are sometimes protected by a chelating agent such as EDTA.

COMPOUNDING OF OINTMENTS AND PASTES

The basic techniques for the preparation of ointments and pastes are weighing, measuring of liquids, size reduction and size separation, and mixing. These are described in Chapter 4. Two mixing techniques are used in making ointments.

Mixing by fusion

In this method the ingredients are melted together and stirred to ensure homogeneity.

On a small scale, fusion is usually carried out in an evaporating basin over a water-bath. Glazed porcelain or stainless steel basins are to be preferred. Stainless steel vessels offer good heat transfer but react with a few ingredients, e.g. iodine. Glazed porcelain is less reactive but also less conductive of heat. Nickel vessels react badly with phenolic compounds that are common ingredients of ointments, e.g. resorcinol and salicylic acid.

Preparation of the ointment base by fusion

The constituents of the base should be placed together in the basin and allowed to melt together. Melting time is shortened if high melting point ingredients, such as hard paraffin and the emulsifying waxes, are grated into the basin and heated while other ingredients are being weighed.

After melting the ingredients should be stirred gently until cool. Vigorous stirring causes excessive aeration and should be avoided. Localized cooling, such as by the use of a cold spatula, may result in separation of hard lumps of high melting point ingredients.

Any foreign particles from the ingredients that are visible on melting may be removed by decantation or by passage through a warmed muslin strainer into a clean vessel.

If the product is granular after cooling due to separation of some of the high melting point ingredients, it may be remelted with the minimum of heat and re-stirred until cold.

Stock bases such as Paraffin, Simple or Wool Alcohols Ointments of the BP can be made successfully by pouring the melted mixture into a warmed jar, covering and allowing to stand undisturbed on a non-conducting surface (not a cold bench) until set (Examples 14.1 and 14.4).

Preparation of medicated ointments and pastes by fusion

Solids that are completely or partially soluble in the base should be added in fine powder to the molten base at as low a temperature as possible and the mixture stirred until cold.

Liquids such as methyl salicylate (Example 14.2) and coal tar solutions (Example 14.3) and semi-solids such as ichthammol (Example 14.5) should be added just as the base is thickening (i.e. at about 40°C). When a solid is soluble in a liquid ingredient, for example, menthol in methyl salicylate, it may be more convenient to add it in solution.

Insoluble solids, such as calamine, zinc oxide and starch, should be passed through a 180 μm sieve and added in small amounts, with stirring, to the melted base when it first shows signs of thickening. The product must be stirred until thick enough to prevent sedimentation (Examples 14.3 and 14.6).

If the product contains liquid paraffin or a fixed oil, a small amount can be used to levigate the powder before adding to the base to produce a smoother product.

Mixing by trituration

This method is applicable when the medicament is a solid insoluble in the base or a liquid present in small amount. Solids should be finely powdered and passed through a sieve of appropriate size. Since the particle size may be further reduced by the process of trituration it is possible to use less fine powders than are required for the fusion method. A 250 μm mesh is suitable unless the formula specifies a *fine powder* (180 μm mesh) or a *very fine powder* (125 μm mesh).

Trituration may be carried out with an ointment tile and spatula or using a mortar and pestle (Examples 14.1 and 14.4).

Trituration using a tile and spatula

Tiles are of glazed porcelain or glass and should be large enough for the quantity of ointment to be prepared. For small-scale work 300 mm square is a useful size. The spatula should be flexible and have a broad, non-tapering long blade (e.g. 25 mm by 200 mm) to provide a large rubbing surface.

Another smaller spatula may be useful for removing accumulated material from the large one. Stainless steel spatulas are preferred except for the few medicaments that react with stainless steel (e.g. iodine and mercurial compounds). For these corrosive substances a vulcanite spatula should be used.

The powders for incorporation by trituration are placed on the tile and gently mixed. Unless the base is very soft it may be helpful to warm the tile, but overheating should be avoided or the base will become too fluid for efficient levigation and may run off the edge of the tile. The powders should be levigated with only about two or three times their weight of the base until the mixture is smooth and homogeneous. The dispersion is then diluted with increasing amounts of base, doubling the quantity each on the tile of each addition. Finally any liquid ingredients are incorporated, taking care to avoid splashing.

Trituration using a mortar and pestle.

A mortar with a fairly flat base and a pestle with a flat head will give best results. Porcelain or composition mortars are usually used. As in the previous method, warming the equipment is helpful if the base is very stiff but the mortar should not be too hot. The sequence of mixing is as in the tile method, i.e. powders mixed then gradually incorporated into the base and finally any liquid ingredients added. The mortar method is more suitable for larger quantities of product and splashing of liquids is more easily controlled in a mortar.

The beginner is advised to try both methods and to compare the products produced. Many pharmacists develop a personal preference for one or other of the methods.

COMPOUNDING OF GELS

Most of the gelling agents listed in this chapter are also used as suspending agents and the methods for producing solutions of these substances are described in Chapter 12.

OINTMENTS, PASTES AND GELS AS DOSAGE FORMS

Ointments

Ointments are used for their emollient effect on the skin, for the protection of lesions and for topical medication.

Pastes

Pastes differ from ointments in containing a large amount of finely powdered solids and in consequence are very stiff. They are emollient but porous and absorb exudate.

Gels (jellies)

Gels may be used as dermatological bases (Example 14.7) or as lubricants for catheters and examination gloves (Example 14.8). Gels for introduction into body cavities or the eye should be sterilized.

Shelf-life of ointments, pastes and gels

Ointments and pastes are generally stable preparations. Dilutions of proprietary ointments may sometimes be prescribed. As for dilution of creams (see Ch. 13), the appropriate diluent should be chosen with reference to the product data sheet. Ointments are less vulnerable to microbial contamination than creams but the recommended shelf-life for diluted ointments is usually 14 days. Gels have a high water content and therefore are liable to microbial growth. They must be used immediately unless an adequate preservative system is included. Care should be taken to avoid contamination in use.

Containers for ointments, pastes and gels

Ointments and pastes prepared extemporaneously are usually packed in screw-capped amber glass or plastic pots. Some medicaments, e.g. methyl salicylate, are incompatible with plastic containers. The ointment should be packed tidily and the top surfaces should be smoothed neatly. The container should be well filled if possible. The mouth of the jar should be covered with a greaseproof-paper disc. Ointments may also be packed into collapsible metal tubes as described under 'Con-

tainers for creams' (see Ch. 13). Ointments packed by manufacturers for dispensing are usually supplied in collapsible metal or plastic tubes. Lubricant gels should be packed in collapsible tubes and may need to be sterilized. Stiffer gels for application to the skin may be supplied in ointment pots. Containers should be well filled and airtight to prevent evaporation.

Special labels for ointments, pastes and gels

> Store in a cool place

The labels for collapsible tubes should be fixed to the upper (nozzle) end of the tube.

Sterilized products should be labelled

> Sterile

EXAMPLES

Example 14.1

Prepare 50 g Simple Ointment BP 1988 and use to prepare 50 g Sulphur Ointment BP 1980

For Simple Ointment BP 1988

Ingredients	Master formula
Wool Fat	50 g
Hard Paraffin	50 g
Cetostearyl Alcohol	50 g
White Soft Paraffin or Yellow Soft Paraffin*	850 g

*Note: Use white soft paraffin for white ointments and yellow soft paraffin for coloured ointments.

For Sulphur Ointment BP 1980

Ingredients	Master formula
Precipitated Sulphur, finely sifted	100 g
Simple Ointment prepared with White Soft Paraffin	900 g

Formulation
Simple Ointment is an absorption base prepared by fusion. Sulphur is an insoluble solid incorporated by trituration.

Compounding
Grate the hard paraffin and weigh out the ingredients for the base. Place to melt in an evaporating dish on a water-bath. Stir gently to aid melting and to mix the ingredients. When homogeneous, remove from the heat and stir until cold. If for stock, the molten base could be poured into a warm pot and allowed to cool slowly and undisturbed on a non-conducting surface.

Weigh the sulphur after sifting (180 μm sieve) and place on a large ointment tile. Levigate the powder

(i.e. mix in the powder to form a smooth paste) with two or three times its weight of base, gradually incorporating more base until homogeneous.

Storage and shelf-life
Store in a cool place.

Container
Wide-mouthed amber jar with a greaseproof paper disc.

Advice for patients when dispensed
The skin should be cleansed prior to application and the ointment applied sparingly to the affected area.

Actions and uses
Mild antiseptic.

Example 14.2

Prepare 30 g Methyl Salicylate Ointment BP 1988

Ingredients	Master formula
Methyl Salicylate	500 g
White Beeswax	250 g
Hydrous Wool Fat	250 g

Formulation
Methyl salicylate is a volatile liquid and should be added to the base at as low a temperature as possible. Beeswax helps to stiffen the base which would otherwise be made very soft by the large proportion (50%) of liquid methyl salicylate.

Compounding
Melt the grated beeswax and hydrous wool fat in an evaporating dish on a water-bath. Remove from the heat

and cool until about to solidify. Add the methyl salicylate and stir until cool.

Storage and shelf-life
Store in a cool place.

Container
Wide-mouthed amber glass jar with a greaseproof paper disc and well-fitting closure. Note that methyl salicylate reacts with some plastics.

Advice for patients when dispensed
The ointment should be massaged well into the skin. It should not be applied to broken or inflamed skin or near to the eyes or mucous membranes. The container should be kept tightly closed.

Actions and uses
Relief of pain in rheumatic conditions.

Example 14.3

Prepare 50 g Calamine and Coal Tar Ointment BP 1988

Ingredients	Master formula
Calamine, finely sifted	125 g
Zinc Oxide, finely sifted	125 g
Strong Coal Tar Solution	25 g
Hydrous Wool Fat	250 g
White Soft Paraffin	475 g

Formulation
The ointment contains two insoluble solids and a volatile liquid. The various forms of tar products used in medicinal products are described in Table 14.1.

Compounding
Sift the zinc oxide and calamine through separate 180 μm sieves and weigh the required amounts.

Melt the soft paraffin and hydrous wool fat at as low a temperature as possible. Add small amounts of each powder alternately to the molten base and stir in thoroughly until homogeneous. Continue to stir until the temperature falls to 40°C before adding the strong coal tar solution and stirring until cold.

Note that because the coal tar solution is volatile it should not be weighed in advance and left uncovered on the bench to evaporate.

Storage and shelf-life
Store in a cool place.

Container
Wide-mouthed amber jar with a greaseproof paper disc.

Advice for patients when dispensed
The ointment should not be applied to broken or inflamed skin or near to the eyes. It stains skin, hair and fabrics

Actions and uses
Mild astringent and anti-pruritic.

Example 14.4

Prepare 50 g Emulsifying Ointment BP 1988 and use to prepare 50 g Whitfield's ointment

For Emulsifying Ointment BP 1988

Ingredients	Master formula
Emulsifying Wax	300 g
White Soft Paraffin	500 g
Liquid Paraffin	200 g

For Compound Benzoic Acid BP 1988
Whitfield's ointment is Compound Benzoic Acid Ointment BP 1988.

Ingredients	Master formula
Benzoic Acid, in *fine powder*	60 g
Salicylic Acid, in *fine powder*	30 g
Emulsifying Ointment	910 g

Table 14.1 Tar preparations used in medicinal products. Tar preparations are frequently included as ingredients of products for the treatment of eczema, psoriasis and other skin diseases. The information summarized in this table is intended to aid the selection of the appropriate ingredient for tar containing products

Form	Source	Examples of use
Tar BP 1988 (Stockholm Tar)	Destructive distillation of pine wood	Proprietary bath additive
Coal Tar BP 1988 (crude coal tar)	Destructive distillation of coal	Coal Tar and Salicylic Acid Ointment BP 1988 Zinc and Coal Tar Paste BP 1988 Coal Tar Solution BP 1988 Strong Coal Tar Solution BP 1988
Prepared Coal Tar BPC 73	Heating coal tar at 50°C for 1 hour	Proprietary shampoo
Strong Coal Tar Solution BP 1988	40% solution of coal tar in ethanol with 5% polysorbate 80	Calamine and Coal Tar Ointment BP 1988 Coal Tar Paste BP 1988
Coal Tar Solution BP 1988	20% solution of coal tar in ethanol with 5% polysorbate 80	Can be applied undiluted to the skin

Formulation
Emulsifying Ointment BP 1988 is a water-miscible base prepared by fusion.
  Salicylic and benzoic acids are incorporated by trituration.

Compounding
Place ingredients for the base in an evaporating dish on a water-bath and allow to melt. It is most convenient to weigh the liquid paraffin directly into the dish and to add the other ingredients. Stir gently to aid melting and to mix the ingredients. When homogeneous, remove from the heat and stir until cool. If for stock, the molten base could be poured into a warm pot and allowed to cool slowly and undisturbed on a non-conducting surface.
  Sift the medicaments through separate 180 μm sieves (using stainless steel for the salicylic acid). Note that salicylic acid is very irritant to the respiratory tract and precautions should be observed to avoid inhalation. Weigh the powders after sifting and place on a large ointment tile. Levigate the powders (i.e. mix in the powders to produce a smooth paste) with two or three times their weight of base, gradually incorporating more base until homogeneous.

Storage and shelf-life
Store in a cool place.

Container
Wide-mouthed amber jar with a greaseproof-paper disc.

Advice for patients when dispensed
The ointment should be applied sparingly to the affected area. It should not be applied to broken or inflamed skin.

Actions and uses
Topical antifungal preparation.

Example 14.5

Prepare 30 g Ichthammol Ointment BP 1980

Ingredients	Master formula
Ichthammol	100 g
Wool Fat	450 g
Yellow Soft Paraffin	450 g

Formulation
Ichthammol is a black viscous liquid consisting of the ammonium salts of the sulphonic acids of an oily substance from bituminous schist or shale. Wool fat aids the incorporation of the water-soluble ichthammol.

Compounding
Place the ingredients for the base in an evaporating dish on a water-bath and allow to melt. Stir gently to aid melting and to mix the ingredients. When homogeneous, remove from the heat and cool to about 40°C. Add the ichthammol and stir until cool.

Storage and shelf-life
Store in a cool place.

Container
Wide-mouthed amber jar with a greaseproof-paper disc.

Advice for patients when dispensed
The ointment should be rubbed lightly on the affected area. It should not be applied to broken skin.

Actions and uses
Mild antibacterial and anti-inflammatory.

Example 14.6

Prepare 50 g Zinc and Coal Tar Paste BP 1988

Ingredients	Master formula
Emulsifying Wax	50 g
Coal Tar	60 g
Zinc Oxide, finely sifted	60 g
Starch	380 g
Yellow Soft Paraffin	450 g

Formulation
The preparation contains a high proportion of powders. The emulsifying wax is present as a dispersing agent for the tar. The various forms of tar preparations used in medicinal products are described in Table 14.1.

Compounding
Sift the zinc oxide (180 μm sieve) and weigh the required amounts of zinc oxide and starch.
  Mixing by fusion (BP method)
— Melt the emulsifying wax at 70°C
— Add the coal tar and half of the soft paraffin
— stir at 70°C until melted
— add the remainder of the soft paraffin
— cool to 30°C and add the zinc oxide and starch with constant stirring until cold.
  Mixing by fusion and trituration (alternative method)
Coal tar constituents precipitate readily on heating. The following method reduces the risk of over heating of the tar:
— Melt the soft paraffin and emulsifying wax at as low a temperature as possible.
— Mix well and stir until just setting.
— Incorporate the powders on a warm tile.
— Finally incorporate the tar.

  Coal tar is a very viscous preparation and should be weighed by difference.

Storage and shelf-life
Store in a cool place

Container
Wide-mouthed amber jar with a greaseproof-paper disc.

Advice for patients when dispensed
The paste should be applied liberally and carefully to the lesions with a suitable applicator. It should not be applied to broken or inflamed skin. It stains the skin, hair and fabrics.

Actions and uses
Antipruritic preparation.

Example 14.7

Prepare 100 g Zinc Gelatin BP 1968 (Unna's paste)

Ingredients	Master formula
Zinc Oxide, finely sifted	150 g
Gelatin	150 g
Glycerol	350 g
Water	350 ml, or a sufficient quantity

Note: This preparation is included as an example of a paste with a gelatin base. Its use in the UK has been superseded by newer types of dressing, although similar preparations remain in many pharmacopoeias.

Formulation
The preparation is designed to be re-melted before application as dressing for varicose ulcers and similar lesions. The gel reforms on cooling and the zinc oxide acts as an absorbent and mild astringent.

Compounding
Heat the water to boiling, remove from the heat, add the gelatin and stir gently to dissolve. Add the glycerol, previously heated to 100°C but no higher, and stir gently to avoid incorporating air bubbles until solution is complete.

Maintain the base at 100°C for 1 hour to remove contaminant micro-organisms (see Ch. 15 for heat treatment of glycero-gelatin base).

Adjust the base to weight by evaporation or by adding hot water as required.

Sift the zinc oxide (180 μm) and add in small amounts to the molten base. Continue stirring without aeration until the preparation is viscous enough to hold the powder in suspension but still pourable.

Pour into a suitable vessel (usually a shallow tray) and allow to set.

Storage and shelf-life
Store in a cool place.

Container
Traditionally the preparation is divided into small pieces before packing in a jar so that the patient can melt an appropriate number for each treatment.

Advice for patients when dispensed
The paste is melted, cooled and applied with a brush to the affected part before covering with a gauze bandage. Several layers are applied and the dressing left in place for 3 days or more before removing with the aid of warm water.

Actions and uses
Protective and supportive dressing.

Example 14.8

Prepare 50 g lubricating jelly to the following non-official formula

Ingredients	Formula
Carmellose Sodium	1.0 g
Propylene Glycol	12.0 ml
Methyl Hydroxybenzoate	0.05 g
Purified Water, freshly boiled and cooled	to 50.0 ml

Formulation
Carmellose sodium is the gelling agent, methyl hydroxybenzoate acts as a preservative and propylene glycol as humectant.

Compounding
Dissolve the methyl hydroxybenzoate in the propylene glycol and add the carmellose sodium.

Heat the water to boiling and add the propylene glycol mixture with constant stirring until cold.

Storage and shelf-life
Store in a cool place. The preparation should be freshly prepared unless sterilized.

Container
Collapsible metal tube.

Advice for patients when dispensed
Not applicable.

Actions and uses
Non-sterile lubricating gel.

BIBLIOGRAPHY

ABPI Data Sheet Compendium current edition Datapharm Publications, London (updated annually)

Aulton M E 1988 Pharmaceutics: the science of dosage form design. Churchill Livingstone, Edinburgh

British National Formulary 1988 16th edn. British Medical Association and Royal Pharmaceutical Society of Great Britain, London (updated twice yearly)

British Pharmacopoeia 1968 HMSO, London

British Pharmacopoeia 1980 HMSO, London (and addenda 1982, 1983 and 1986)

British Pharmacopoeia 1988 HMSO, London

British Pharmaceutical Codex 1973 Pharmaceutical Press, London

Diluent Directories (Internal and External) current edition. National Pharmaceutical Association (NPA)

Martindale, see Reynolds J E F

Pharmaceutical Codex 1979 11th edn (incorporating the British Pharmaceutical Codex). Pharmaceutical Press, London

Pharmaceutical Society 1979 Guide to good dispensing practice. Pharmaceutical Journal 223: 157–158

Reynolds J E F (ed) 1989 Martindale, The Extra Pharmacopoeia, 29th edn. Pharmaceutical Press, London

Wade A (ed) 1980 Pharmaceutical Handbook, 19th edn. Pharmaceutical Press, London

15. Suppositories and pessaries

D. M. Collett

Suppositories are solid medicated preparations designed for insertion into the rectum where they melt, dissolve or disperse and exert a local or systemic effect. Suppositories that are produced extemporaneously are usually prepared by pouring molten mass into suitable moulds to produce rounded cone, bullet or torpedo shapes suitable for retention by the rectum. Extemporaneous methods of compression moulding are rarely used in the UK.

Commercially produced solid rectal dosage forms include soft gelatin rectal capsules and compressed tablets, in addition to the more commonly produced moulded suppositories.

Pessaries are similar solid medicated preparations designed for insertion into the vagina, usually to exert a local effect. Moulded pessaries are prepared in a similar way to suppositories and are usually cone shaped with a rounded tip. Commercially, pessaries are often produced by compression in the form of diamond, wedge, disc or other shaped, vaginal tablets.

Factors affecting the design of rectal and vaginal dosage forms as drug delivery systems are discussed in detail in Chapter 23 of the companion volume (Aulton 1988). Practical aspects of formulation and compounding of suppositories and pessaries are described in this chapter.

FORMULATION OF SUPPOSITORIES AND PESSARIES

There are two main classes of suppository base:

I. Fatty bases designed to melt at body temperature.
II. Water-soluble or water-miscible bases designed to dissolve or disperse within the body.

The properties of an ideal suppository base are:

1. Melts at body temperature or dissolves in body fluids.
2. Non-toxic and non-irritant.
3. Compatible with any medicament.
4. Releases any medicament readily.
5. Easily moulded and removed from the mould.
6. Stable to heating above the melting point.
7. Resistant to handling.
8. Stable on storage.

I. Fatty bases

Theobroma oil (cocoa butter)

This is a yellowish-white solid with an odour of chocolate and is a mixture of the glyceryl esters of stearic, palmitic, oleic and other fatty acids.

Advantages of theobroma oil include:

a. A melting point range of 30–36°C (i.e. solid at normal room temperatures but melts in the body).
b. Readily melted on warming, rapid setting on cooling.
c. Miscible with many ingredients.
d. Bland and non-irritating.

Disadvantages of theobroma oil include:

a. *Polymorphism.* When melted and cooled it solidifies in different crystalline forms, depending on the temperature of melting, rate of cooling and the size of the mass.

If melted at not more than 36°C and slowly cooled it forms stable beta crystals with normal melting point, but if over-heated it may produce, on cooling, unstable gamma crystals which melt at about 15°C or alpha crystals melting at about 20°C. These unstable forms eventually return to the stable condition but this may take several days and in the meantime the product is not suitable for issue to a patient.

b. *Adherence to the mould.* Oil of theobroma does not contract sufficiently on cooling to loosen the suppositories in the mould. Sticking is a problem which may be overcome by adequate lubrication.

c. *Softening point too low for hot climates.*

d. *Melting point reduced by soluble ingredients.* Additives such as beeswax may be incorporated to raise the melting point sufficiently to counteract the effects of medicaments and/or climate.

e. *Rancidity on storage.* Due to oxidation of unsaturated glycerides.

f. *Poor water-absorbing ability.* Improved by the addition of emulsifying agents.

g. *Leakage from the body.* Sometimes melted base escapes from the rectum or vagina, for this reason, oil of theobroma is rarely used as a pessary base.

h. *Expense.*

Synthetic hard fat

Oil of theobroma is the only natural fat with suitable properties for a suppository base.

Synthetic hard fat bases are prepared by first hydrolysing the vegetable oil, then hydrogenating the resulting fatty acids and finally re-esterifying the acids by heating with glycerol. Controlled modifications of the process yield a wide range of materials containing mixtures of mono-, di- and try-glycerides of saturated fatty acids with chain lengths C_9 to C_{17}.

Advantages of these bases over theobroma oil:

a. Their solidifying points are unaffected by overheating.

b. They have good resistance to oxidation because their unsaturated fatty acids have been reduced.

c. The difference between melting and setting points is small; generally only 1.5–2°C and seldom over 3°C. Hence they set quickly, the risk of sedimentation of suspended ingredients is low and they are easier to administer. When the setting point of a base is well below the melting point, the suppositories soften quickly when handled and become too slippery to administer.

d. Most manufacturers market a series of grades with slightly different melting point ranges and degrees of hardness which can be chosen to suit particular products and climatic conditions.

e. They usually contain a proportion of partial glycerides some of which, e.g. glyceryl monostearate, are w/o emulsifying agents and, therefore, their water-absorbing capacities are good.

f. No mould lubricant is necessary because they contract significantly on cooling.

g. They produce suppositories that are white and almost odourless and have an attractive, clean, polished appearance.

Disadvantages of synthetic bases include:

a. Low viscosity when melted allows sedimentation of suspended ingredients at the melted stage (but see the advantage of rapid setting); sedimentation problems may be overcome by the use of thickeners.

b. Brittle if cooled rapidly, avoid refrigeration during preparation.

Proprietary hard fat bases include:

Coberine
Massa Estarinum
Massuppol
Suppocire
Witepsol Suppository Bases

For details of manufacturers and suppliers see 'Martindale, the extra pharmacopoeia' (Reynolds 1989).

Fractionated Palm Kernel Oil BP

This is a white, brittle, odourless, solid fat with a melting point of 31–36°C, obtained from palm kernel oil by selective solvent fractionation and hydrogenation.

II. Water-soluble and water-miscible bases

Glycero-gelatin

This is a mixture of glycerol and water gelled by the addition of gelatin. The mixture in varied proportions is used for dermatological bases and for suppositories and pessaries.

Glycerol suppository mass usually contains 70% glycerol and a minimum of 14% gelatin. Higher concentrations of gelatin may be required for use in hot countries or to counteract the softening effect of any liquid ingredients included in the product.

Gelatin. Gelatin consists of colourless or pale-yellowish or amber-coloured translucent sheets, shreds or powder. The powder is to be preferred for most pharmaceutical uses. Gelatin is derived from the partial hydrolysis of animal collagenous tissue including skins and bones and although pharmaceutical grades should be free from pathogens, preparations for application to abraded skin or mucous membranes should be heat treated during their preparation.

Gelatins vary widely in quality and are usually graded by 'jelly strength' or 'Bloom' gelometer rating. Acceptible limits for these parameters are stated in the Pharmacopoeial monographs.

Two types of gelatin are available for pharmaceutical use:

Type A is prepared by acid hydrolysis, has an iso-electric point between 7 and 9 and on the acid side of this range behaves as a cationic agent, being most effective at pH 3.2.

Type B is prepared by alkali hydrolysis, has an iso-electric point between 4 and 7 and on the alkaline side of the range behaves as an anionic agent being most effective at pH 7–8.

Cationic or anionic medicaments or preservatives should be formulated with bases of the appropriate type.

Disadvantages of glycero-gelatin base include:

a. *A physiological effect*. Glycerol suppositories have a laxative action.

b. *Unpredictable solution time*. This varies with the batch of gelatin and the age of the base.

c. *Hygroscopic*. The base requires protection from heat and moisture and also has a dehydrating effect on the rectal or vaginal mucosa leading to irritation.

d. *Microbial contamination likely*. The base may require preservatives leading to problems of incompatibility.

e. *Long preparation time*. The base is more time consuming to prepare than the fatty bases and may be difficult to remove from the mould. Lubrication of the mould is essential.

Macrogols (polyethylene glycols)

Mixtures of macrogols may be used as bases for suppositories and pessaries. Their physical properties can be varied by suitable mixtures of high and low polymers. High polymers yield products that disintegrate and release their drug slowly. Softer, less brittle preparations that disperse and liberate their drug more quickly are obtained by mixing high with either medium or medium and low polymers, or by adding plasticizers (e.g. hexane-1,2,6 triol). Examples of recommended mixtures are given in Table 15.1.

Table 15.1 Examples of macrogol bases

	I	II	III	IV	V
Macrogol 400	—	—	20	—	—
Macrogol 1000	—	—	—	—	75
Macrogol 1540	—	33	33	94	—
Macrogol 4000	33	—	—	—	25
Macrogol 6000	47	47	47	—	—
Water	20	20	—	—	—
Hexane-1,2,6 triol	—	—	—	6	—

Variations in the mixture may also be made to allow for the depression of melting point caused by soluble medicaments.

Advantages of macrogol bases include:

a. *No laxative effect*.

b. *Microbial contamination less likely*.

c. *Preparation is convenient*. The base contracts slightly on cooling and no lubricant is necessary.

d. *Melting point generally above body temperature*. Cool storage is therefore not so critical, they are suitable for hot climates and less likely to melt on handling. The high melting point also means that the bases do not melt in the body but dissolve and disperse the medication slowly, providing a sustained effect.

e. *Produce high-viscosity solutions*. This means that after dispersing in the body, leakage is less likely.

f. *Good solvent properties*.

g. *Give products with clean smooth appearance*.

Disadvantages of macrogol bases include:

a. *Hygroscopic*. Like glycero-gelatin base, macrogol bases may cause irritation to the mucosae. This can be partly overcome by incorporation of 20% water in the mass or by instructing the patient to dip the preparation in water prior to insertion.

b. *Poor bioavailability of medicaments*. The good solvent properties may result in retention of the drug in the liquefied base with consequent reduction in therapeutic effect.

c. *Incompatibilities*. Macrogol bases are incompatible with some medicaments, e.g. bismuth salts, ichthammol, benzocaine and phenol, and reduce the activity of quaternary ammonium compounds and hydroxybenzoates. They also interact with some plastics which limits the choice of container.

d. *Brittleness*. Macrogol suppositories may be brittle unless poured at as low a temperature as possible. The addition of surface active agents or plasticizers may reduce brittleness. Products sometimes fracture on storage, particularly if they contain water. One cause is the high solubility of the macrogols which can lead to a supersaturated solution in the water and subsequent crystallization. This in turn makes the mass granular and brittle.

e. *Crystal growth of certain medicaments may occur*, particularly if they are partly in solution and partly in suspension in the base. In addition to making the product brittle, the crystals may be irritant and, because they are large, take longer to dissolve.

Other additives

Antioxidants

Bases or medicaments susceptible to deterioration by oxidation may require the inclusion of an antioxidant. Suitable antioxidants are those described in Chapter 13 for emulsions. The antioxidant chosen must be compatible with the medicament and not produce any adverse change in the base.

Preservatives

Anhydrous fatty bases provide a poor substrate for micro-organisms. The water-miscible, water-soluble bases may require a preservative system if formulated for a long shelf-life. A list of preservatives suitable for pharmaceutical products is given in Chapter 13. As with all preservative systems the base should be challenged with appropriate organisms to test the efficacy of the preservative chosen.

Emulsifiers

Emulsifying agents, such as emulsifying wax, wool fat, wool alcohols, macrogol stearates and polysorbates, may be included in suppository bases to facilitate incorporation of aqueous solutions or polar liquids. They should be used with extreme caution since their effects on bioavailability of the medicaments may not be predictable (see the companion volume, Aulton 1988). Surfactants may also cause problems of foaming when preparing the base and bubbles in the product.

Hardening agents

These are substances added to the base to raise the melting point. This may be necessary for hot countries or when the melting point is depressed by medicaments dissolved in the base.

The use of different blends of hard fats and different combinations of macrogols to achieve bases of particular hardness has been described.

Additional gelatin may be added to increase the gel strength of glycero-gelatin base.

White beeswax is used to increase the melting point of theobroma oil. However, beeswax also acts as an emulsifier and may modify the release of medicament from the base.

Furthermore, raising the melting point to cope with changes outside the body may result in different melting characteristics within the rectum or vagina and again alter the bioavailability of incorporated medicament.

Viscosity modifiers

Increasing the vicosity of the molten base may be desirable to reduce the sedimentation rate of insoluble medicaments of high density suspended in the base. Magnesium stearate, bentonite and colloidal silicon dioxide have been used for this purpose. However, the creation of a gel-like system on melting in the body is likely to slow the release rate of the medicament.

Choice of a suppository or pessary base

The factors affecting the choice of a base for suppositories and pessaries are discussed in Chapter 23 of the companion volume (Aulton 1988) and by Florence and Attwood (1981). One of the main factors to consider is the solubility of the drug in the vehicle. For effective release from the base a fat-soluble drug is best formulated in a water-miscible base and a water-soluble drug in a fatty base.

For extemporaneously produced products a hard fat base such as Witepsol (45 grade) is suitable for fatty suppositories. The macrogols are suitable water-miscible bases. Glycero-gelatin base is used rarely for medicated suppositories because of the stimulant action that justifies its use as a laxative preparation.

Fatty bases are rarely used for extemporaneously prepared pessaries; a water-miscible base is more suitable for this purpose.

COMPOUNDING OF SUPPOSITORIES AND PESSARIES

The basic techniques for the compounding of suppositories and pessaries are weighing, measuring of liquids, size reduction and size separation and mixing. These are described in Chapter 4.

Suppository and pessary moulds

The moulds used for small-scale preparation of suppositories and pessaries are made of metal and usually have six (occasionally twelve) cavities. By removing a screw they can be opened longitudinally for lubrication, extraction of the contents and careful cleaning.

The nominal capacities of the commonly used moulds are 1 g, 2 g, 4 g and 8 g.

Proprietary suppositories may be prepared in similar moulds or in strips of plastic moulds which also function as packaging for supply.

The nominal capacity of the mould implies a calibration using oil of theobroma and will vary with different bases. The capacity of each mould should be confirmed by filling the mould with base alone, weighing the

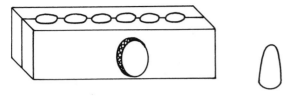

Fig. 15.1 Dispensing suppository mould

products and taking the mean weight as the true capacity. The data should be recorded for future use. In the examples given at the end of this chapter nominal mould capacities are assumed to be correct to simplify the illustrative calculations.

Displacement values

The *volume* of suppositories from a particular mould will be constant but the *weight* will vary because the densities of the medicaments usually differ from the density of the base with which the mould was calibrated.

The density of the medicament affects the amount of base required for each suppository. One part by weight of a medicament with density equal to the base will 'displace' an equivalent volume of the base. A medicament with twice the density of the base will 'displace' half the volume, while a medicament with five times the density of the base will 'displace' only one-fifth of the volume of base. It is necessary therefore to make an allowance for each medicament in terms of the particular base, this allowance is the '*displacement value*'.

The displacement value may be defined as 'the number of parts by weight of medicament that displaces one part by weight of the base'. Table 15.2 lists displacement values with respect to a fatty base for a number of substances prescribed in suppositories and pessaries. Displacement values in the literature are usually quoted with respect to oil of theobroma but the same figure may be used for other fatty bases. For glycero-gelatin suppository base about 1.2 g occupies the same volume as 1 g of oil of theobroma (see later). The displacement value for a medicament may be calculated as shown in Example 15.1.

The use of displacement values is illustrated in Examples 15.2 and 15.3. Note that when the amount of medicament is prescribed as a percentage the displacement value is irrelevant; to use it would make the percentage incorrect (Example 15.4).

Mould lubrication

It is usually unnecessary to lubricate the mould when synthetic fat or macrogol bases are used. Lubrication is necessary for oil of theobroma suppositories and for glycero-gelatin bases.

The chosen lubricant must be immiscible with the base and compatible with the medicament and any other formulation additives. For theobroma oil, an alcoholic solution of soft soap and glycerol is the traditional lubricant although silicones and solutions of sodium lauryl sulphate in water or propylene glycol have also been used. Liquid paraffin is a suitable lubricant for the water-miscible bases.

Preparation of suppositories with a fatty base

1. *Calculate the quantities required.* Take the displacement value into account if required. There are inevitable manipulation losses in the preparation of suppositories. It is usual to prepare for at least two more suppositories than are ordered. Beginners may find a greater excess necessary, thus, in order to send six suppositories, prepare the quantities for ten.

2. *Prepare the mould.* Select a clean dry mould and have to hand. If lubrication is necessary, lubricant should be applied with gauze or muslin (not cotton wool because this leaves fibres) to all the inner surfaces including the flat faces of the mould. After lubrication, close the mould and invert on a clean tile to allow any excess lubricant to drain.

3. *Prepare the base.* Shredding the base speeds melting and helps to avoid over-heating. A domestic fine food grater is suitable for the purpose. Weigh the shredded base into an evaporating basin. Porcelain basins are to be preferred for fatty bases since their relatively poor heat conductivity reduces the risk of over-heating.

4. *Prepare the medicament.* Insoluble solids should be powdered if necessary and sieved before weighing

Table 15.2 Displacement values with respect to fatty bases

Medicament	Displacement value
Aminophylline	1.3
Aspirin	1.1
Bismuth subgallate	3.0
Castor oil	1.0
Chloral hydrate	1.5
Cinchocaine hydrochloride	1.0
Cocaine hydrochloride	1.4
Dimenhydrinate	1.3
Hamamelis dry extract	1.5
Hydrocortisone acetate	1.5
Ichthammol	1.0
Liquids	1.0
Morphine hydrochloride	1.6
Resorcinol	1.5
Zinc oxide	5.0

(180 μm). Other ingredients should be weighed or measured.

5. *Melt the base*. Place the dish containing the shredded base on the water-bath and heat until melting is almost complete. Remove from the heat source and stir gently with a small spatula to allow the residual heat in the dish to melt the remainder of the base.

6. *Incorporate the medicament*. Immiscible liquids and insoluble solids are incorporated into the base by levigation (i.e. mixing to produce a smooth paste) with a little of the melted base on a warm tile. The dispersion is returned to the dish and mixed with the rest of the base. Soluble solids, semi-solids and miscible liquids may be incorporated directly into the base which may need to be modified to compensate for the resulting depression in melting point (see above).

7. *Fill the mould*. The homogeneous mixture in the dish should be stirred until the base begins to thicken. Then fill each cavity in the mould to overflowing to allow for contraction on cooling. If the consistency of the base is correct the 'overflow' should remain above each cavity. If the 'overflows' merge or worse still run down the side of the mould, the base has been poured at too high a temperature and more patience is required. If setting occurs during pouring, the base can be very briefly re-heated to restore flow. The base should be stirred throughout to prevent sedimentation of insoluble solids.

8. *Remove the excess*. When the mass has set (2–3 minutes under normal circumstances) contraction of the base will have occurred and the excess may be removed. This is best achieved by the process of cold compression. Place the blade of a firm spatula on the excess at one end of the mould, draw it across the mould pressing down at the same time. This process will tend to fill any holes in the suppositories which may have resulted from pouring too cold. Reserve the excess together with the surplus mass in case there is a need to remelt and repour any failures.

9. *Open the mould*. After 10 minutes' standing in a cool place the suppositories may be removed from the mould, inspected and packed.

Preparation of suppositories with a macrogol base

These are prepared in essentially the same way as the fatty suppositories. No lubrication of the mould is required. If the base contains water, this should be warmed separately and added to the melted base. Water-soluble ingredients are dissolved in the water before it is added. Insoluble ingredients are incorporated by the method described for fatty bases.

The mass is poured as cool as possible and the mould overfilled to allow for significant contraction on cooling.

Preparation of suppositories with a glycero-gelatin base (see Example 15.5)

1. *Calculate the quantities required*. Since the nominal capacity of the mould refers to theobroma oil, multiply the total quantity of base required to fill the nominal capacity by 1.2 to take into account the greater density of glycero-gelatin. When appropriate, use the displacement values in the normal way and after the amount of base has been calculated multiply by the density factor 1.2. Prepare an excess to allow for manipulation losses.

2. *Prepare the mould*. Lubricate the mould including the internal flat surfaces with liquid paraffin or arachis oil. Invert and cool.

3. *Prepare the medicament*. Thermostable soluble medicaments should be dissolved in the water before heating. Insoluble solids should be sifted (180 μm).

4. *Prepare the base*. Weigh the glycerol into a suitable dish and heat to 100°C, but not higher.

Weigh the water into a second tared dish (the weight of the dish will be required for adjustment of the product to weight). Use approximately 30 ml per 100 ml base. Although the calculated amount of water for 100 g Glycero-gelatin base is 16 g, the use of an excess helps the dissolution of the gelatin and is easily adjusted if necessary by evaporation.

Bring the water to the boil and remove the source of heat to prevent undue evaporation.

Add the gelatin powder to the water taking care to avoid the sides of the dish and stir gently to dissolve.

The gelatin solution may be cautiously heated intermittently over the bunsen taking care to avoid charring. The hot glycerol is then added and the solution stirred until homogeneous. As an alternative slower method the hot glycerol may be added to the wetted gelatin and the mixture placed on a water-bath until solution is complete, usually about 15 minutes.

For both methods the solution should be stirred frequently but gently to avoid incorporating air bubbles.

5. *Heat treatment of the base*. Because of its origin, gelatin may be contaminated with pathogenic microorganisms. Although pharmaceutical grades of gelatin should not contain any pathogens the base may, as a precaution, be heat treated by maintaining it at a temperature of 100°C for 1 hour in an electric steamer. This is particularly important for products for application to abraded skin (Example 14.7) or to the vaginal mucosa (Example 15.4). The heat treatment is carried out before

adjustment to weight and before the addition of thermolabile ingredients (Example 15.4).

6. *Adjustment of base to weight.* The base is adjusted to weight by adding sufficient hot water or by evaporation, whichever is necessary. After adjustment to weight any large air bubbles can be removed by passing the molten mass through a warm muslin strainer into a second hot dish.

7. *Incorporate any medicament.* Soluble thermolabile medicaments are dissolved in a little water before adding to the molten mass. Insoluble substances are rubbed down on a tile with a little of the glycerol (not the base because of problems in remelting solidified base).

8. *Fill the mould.* The molten mass should be poured down a glass rod to fill each cavity in the mould. Overfilling is undesirable since the base does not contract significantly on cooling. Aim for a slightly convex or flat top. Allow to set for about half an hour for small size suppositories, longer for larger size suppositories and pessaries.

9. *Open the mould.* Watch carefully for any tendency to split in the centre line. If this occurs invert the mould and attempt to open from the bottom. After removal from the mould and inspection, the products may be very lightly lubricated with liquid paraffin before packing.

SUPPOSITORIES AND PESSARIES AS DOSAGE FORMS

Suppositories

Medicaments are prescribed in the form of suppositories for three reasons:

a. *To exert a local effect on the rectal mucosa.* Substances used are usually anti-inflammatory, antibacterial or analgesic.

b. *To promote evacuation of the bowel.* The effect may be mainly physical (e.g. glycero-gelatin) or pharmacological (e.g. bisacodyl).

c. *To provide a systemic effect.* This is of value for the administration of drugs which cause irritation of the upper gastrointestinal tract and for patients who are unconscious, vomiting or for some other reason are not able or willing to take oral medication.

The factors affecting the partitioning of the drug between the base and the rectal secretions and the factors affecting the absorption or otherwise of drugs from the rectal mucosa are discussed in Chapter 23 of the companion volume (Aulton 1988).

Pessaries

Medicaments are prescribed in the form of pessaries mainly to exert a direct effect on the vaginal mucosa. The substances used are anti-infective, anti-inflammatory, anti-pruritic and hormonal. Spermicides may also be formulated as pessaries. Occasionally drugs intended for absorption are introduced into the vagina, e.g. prostaglandin preparations. The possibility of unintentional absorption from the vaginal mucosa should be remembered. The factors affecting absorption from this site are also discussed in Chapter 23 of the companion volume (Aulton 1988).

Shelf-life of suppositories and pessaries

Provided that the packaging provides adequate protection and that the storage temperature is low, most suppositories and pessaries are stable preparations. Commercially packed products carry an expiry date recommended by the manufacturer for products stored appropriately.

Containers for suppositories and pessaries

Extemporaneously prepared suppositories and pessaries should be individually wrapped in metal foil (or waxed paper if the medicament interacts with metals). Glass or plastic screw-cap jars are suitable containers, particularly for products that are hygroscopic.

Traditionally suppositories were supplied in divided paperboard boxes, but these offer little protection from the atmosphere.

Commercially prepared products are often supplied in strips of sealed semi-rigid moulds prepared from polyvinyl chloride or polyethylene. A paperboard carton is an adequate dispensing container for such products since the plastic mould should provide adequate protection against the atmosphere.

Special labels and advice for suppositories and pessaries

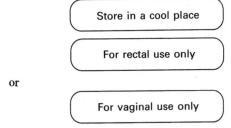

Store in a cool place

For rectal use only

or

For vaginal use only

If appropriate, the patient should be advised to unwrap the product before use.

EXAMPLES

Example 15.1

Use of displacement values

Method for determining displacement value
Using a nominal 1 g mould
Prepare and weigh six suppositories of unmedicated base

$= a$ g

Prepare base containing 30% medicament, fill six moulds and weigh six suppositories

$= b$ g

Calculate the amount of base, c g and medicament d g in the six suppositories

$c = 70\% \, b$ and $d = 30\% \, b$

Therefore the amount of base displaced by

d g $= a - c$ g

$$\text{displacement value} = \frac{d}{a - c}$$

For example:

Weight of six unmedicated suppos.	= 6.0 g
Weight of six suppos. containing 30% drug	= 7.5 g
Base = 70% of 7.5	= 5.25
Drug = 30% of 7.5	= 2.25
Base displaced by 2.25 g = 6 – 5.25	= 0.75 g

Therefore the displacement value of the drug $= \dfrac{2.25}{0.75} = 3$

Method for using displacement value
Required: to prepare for 8 suppositories each containing 300 mg drug of displacement value 3 using a nominal 1 g mould.

Total amount of drugs required = 8 × 300 mg = 2.4 g

This will displace $\dfrac{2.4}{3} = 0.8$ g of base

Therefore amount of base required = 8 – 0.8 = 7.2 g

Example 15.2

Send six Compound Bismuth Subgallate Suppositories BP 1980

Ingredients and formula	for each suppository	for 10
Bismuth Subgallate	200 mg	2.0 g
Resorcinol	60 mg	0.6 g (600 mg)
Zinc Oxide	120 mg	1.2 g
Castor Oil	60 mg	0.6 g (600 mg)
Suitable fatty base such as Theobroma oil BP	sufficient to fill a 1 g mould	

Calculation Prepare for 10 suppositories to allow for manipulation losses.

Displacement values (from Table 15.2)

Bismuth Subgallate	3.0
Resorcinol	1.5
Zinc Oxide	5.0
Castor Oil	1.0

Amount of base required

$(10 \times 1) - \left(\dfrac{2}{3} + \dfrac{0.6}{1.5} + \dfrac{1.2}{5} + \dfrac{0.6}{1} \right)$

$= 10 - (0.67 + 0.4 + 0.24 + 0.6)$

$= 10 - 1.91$

$= 8.09 \ (8.1 \text{ g})$

Compounding
Use Witepsol base as a preferred alternative to theobroma.

Use the general method for preparation of suppositories with a fatty base and shred and weigh the appropriate amount of Witepsol. Powder the bismuth subgallate and resorcinol (if necessary) and sieve the powders (180 μm mesh stainless steel sieve for resorcinol) before weighing and mixing on a warm tile. Levigate the powders with the castor oil and a little of the melted base. Return the dispersion to the rest of the melted base, stir until homogeneous and pour into a 1 g mould. Allow to set, remove from the mould, wrap and pack.

Storage and shelf-life
Store in a cool place.

Container
Amber glass screw-capped jar or plastic pot.

Advice for patients when dispensed
After unwrapping, insert the suppository as high as possible in the rectum. Use one night and morning and after defaecation unless otherwise directed.

If counter-prescribed prolonged use should be discouraged without medical advice.

Actions and uses
Mildly astringent, mildly antiseptic soothing preparation for the treatment of haemorrhoids.

Example 15.3

Send six suppositories each containing dimenhydrinate 50 mg in a suitable base

Ingredients	for each suppository	for 8
Dimenhydrinate	50 mg	400 mg
Suitable base	sufficient to fill a 1 g mould	

Calculation Prepare for 8 suppositories to allow for manipulation losses.

Displacement value (from Table 15.2) of Dimenhydrinate is 1.3, assuming chosen base has a density similar to oil of theobroma. Check if necessary.

Amount of base required:

$(8 \times 1) - \dfrac{0.4}{1.3}$

$= 8 - 0.3 = 7.7$ g

Formulation
Dimenhydrinate is an antinausea drug for which systemic absorption is required. It is sparingly soluble in water and therefore should be formulated in a water-miscible macrogol base.

Compounding
Use the general method for preparation of suppositories with a macrogol base and treat the medicament as insoluble.

Storage and shelf-life
Store in a cool place.

Container
Amber glass screw-capped jar on plastic pot.

Advice for patients when dispensed
After unwrapping, insert the suppository as high as possible in the rectum.
    This preparation may cause drowsiness.

Actions and uses
Antihistamine used to relieve nausea and vertigo.

Example 15.4

Send six pessaries containing 5% lactic acid w/w

Ingredients and formula for the base
Gelatin   14 g
Glycerol   70 g
Purified Water   a sufficient quantity
                                (to produce 100 g)

Ingredients and formula for the pessaries
Lactic Acid   5% w/w
Base   95% w/w

Formulation
The usual size of lactic acid pessary is 8 g. A glycero-gelatin base is most appropriate.

Calculation
Prepare sufficient base for 10 pessaries to allow for manipulative losses.
    The quantity of mass for 10 pessaries is:

$10 \times 8 \times 1.2 = 96$ g

    In this case make 100 g for convenience.

Compounding
Use the method for preparation of glycero-gelatin suppositories.
    When the gelatin has dissolved the base should be heated for 1 hour at 100°C in a suitable steamer to kill possible contaminating viable micro-organisms that could be pathogenic in the vagina.
    Adjust the base to weight after steaming (100 g). 95 g base is required for the pessaries, therefore 5 g of the base should be removed from the dish using a metal spatula or spoon and the base allowed to cool slightly.
    5 g lactic acid may then be added to the 95 g base and thoroughly mixed.

Note:
— That in the case of a medicament included by percentage, the displacement value is irrelevant.
— That 5 g of base is replaced by the lactic acid. It would not be correct to adjust by evaporation to 95 g before adding the lactic acid since this would then be incorrectly replacing water.

Pour into a chilled mould and delay opening the mould as long as possible because lactic acid lowers the setting point of the mass.

Storage and shelf-life
Store in a cool place. The pessaries are very hygroscopic.

Container
Airtight amber glass screw-capped jar or plastic pot.

Advice for patients when dispensed

> After unwrapping, insert the pessary as high as possible in the vagina.

After unwrapping, insert the pessary as high as possible in the vagina.

Actions and uses
Treatment of leucorrhoea in vaginal candidiasis.

Example 15.5

Send six child's size Glycerol Suppositories BP 1988

Ingredients	*Master formula*
Gelatin	14 g
Glycerol	70 g
Purified Water	a sufficient quantity (to produce 100 g)

Calculation
The usual size of a glycerol suppository for a child is 2 g (for infants 1 g size and for adults 4 g size).
    Prepare sufficient base for 10 suppositories to allow for relatively large manipulative losses.
    The quantity of mass for 10 suppositories is:

$10 \times 2 \times 1.2 = 24$ g

    In this case make 25 g because that is a more convenient fraction of the master formula quantities.

Compounding
Use the method for preparation of glycero-gelatin suppositories using 7.5 ml of water initially.

Storage and shelf-life
Store in a cool place.

Container
Amber glass screw-capped jar or plastic pot.

Advice for patients when dispensed
After unwrapping, moisten with a little water and insert the suppository as high as possible in the rectum. Retention in the rectum may be helped by crossing the legs or lying on one side.

Actions and uses
Promotes peristalsis and bowel evacuation in the treatment of constipation.

BIBLIOGRAPHY

ABPI Data Sheet Compendium current edition. Datapharm Publications, London (updated annually)

Aulton M E 1988 Pharmaceutics: the science of dosage form design. Churchill Livingstone, Edinburgh,

British National Formulary 1988 16th edn. British Medical Association and Royal Pharmaceutical Society of Great Britain, London (updated twice yearly)

British Pharmacopoeia 1980 HMSO, London (and addenda 1982, 1983 and 1986)

British Pharmacopoeia 1988 HMSO, London

British Pharmaceutical Codex 1973 Pharmaceutical Press, London

Florence F T, Attwood D 1989 Physiochemical principles of pharmacy 2nd edn. Macmillan, London

Martindale, see Reynolds J E F

Pharmaceutical Codex 1979 11th edn (incorporating the British Pharmaceutical Codex). Pharmaceutical Press, London

Pharmaceutical Society 1979 Guide to good dispensing practice. Pharmaceutical Journal 223: 157–158

Reynolds J E F (ed) 1989 Martindale, the extra pharmacopoeia, 29th edn. Pharmaceutical Press, London

Wade A (ed) 1980 Pharmaceutical handbook, 19th edn. Pharmaceutical Press, London

16. Powders and granules

D. M. Collett

Undivided oral powders usually contain non-potent medicaments such as antacids where the accuracy with which the patient measures the dose is not critical.

Divided oral powders are packaged individually, each dose is separately wrapped in paper or sealed in a sachet. Granules for oral administration are small irregular particles (0.5–2 mm in diameter) often supplied in single-dose sachets.

Dusting powders for external use are free-flowing very fine powders for application to the body surfaces but not to open wounds unless sterilized.

FORMULATION

Oral undivided powders

These are usually a simple mixture of the prescribed medicaments without additional ingredients. The substances prescribed in this form are bulky powders such as light magnesium carbonate, heavy magnesium carbonate and magnesium trisilicate (Example 16.1).

Oral divided powders

This form of powder may contain one or more active ingredients together with an inert diluent to produce a minimum quantity (120 mg) that can be weighed by the dispenser and handled by the patient (Example 16.2).

The usual diluent is lactose because it is colourless, soluble and generally harmless. For patients unable to tolerate lactose an alternative inert diluent may be used. Light kaolin is useful for powders into which a liquid is incorporated. In the past, effervescent preparations were produced by wrapping separately a powder containing sodium bicarbonate and one containing tartaric acid for the patient to mix in water before taking.

Granules

Granulation of a powder allows the addition of flavouring and colouring agents and produces an easily handled attractive product. On a small scale, the ingredients are moistened with a granulating agent such as water, starch mucilage, gelatin or sucrose solutions or dilutions of alcohol. The mass is then pressed through a sieve of appropriate size and the resulting granules dried. The granules should be as uniform in size as possible

Dusting powders

These may contain one or more medicaments mixed with an inert diluent, such as talc, starch or kaolin powders.

COMPOUNDING

The basic techniques for the compounding of powders and granules are weighing, size reduction, size separation and mixing. These are described in Chapter 4.

Preparation of undivided oral powders

On a small scale the powdered ingredients may be mixed using a mortar and pestle. The ingredient of the smallest bulk is placed in the mortar and the other ingredients are added in order of increasing bulk so that the amount in the mortar is approximately doubled at each addition.

After mixing the powders should be passed through a 250 μm sieve and lightly re-mixed using a spatula since sieving may cause partial separation of the ingredients. The powder may then be packed.

Preparation of divided oral powders

Manipulative losses are inevitable when small quantities are weighed from bulk, therefore it is necessary to prepare for at least one powder extra to requirement. The medicament is powdered if necessary in a small mortar and appropriate quantities of lactose or other inert diluent added to raise the weight of each powder to a convenient amount, minimum 120 mg. If the total amount of medicament is very small (less than 50 mg), the minimum weighable quantity should be diluted by trituration to give the required amount (Examples 3.23 and 16.2). The final powder mix is passed through a 250 μm sieve and lightly remixed before 120 mg aliquots are weighed and wrapped.

Method for wrapping divided powders

White glazed paper (known as demy) is generally used for wrapping. A suitable size is 120 mm × 100 mm. Carry out the wrapping on a clean tile or large sheet of demy to protect the product.

Arrange the papers with their long edges parallel to the front of the bench and turn up the long edge of each paper to about one-seventh of its width (Fig. 16.1(**a**)).

Weigh out the powder and place towards the front of the paper.

Carry the front of the paper over to the turned-up edge (Fig. 16.1(**d**), (**c**)), bring the turn-up down and then fold this edge forward until it covers about two-thirds of the distance to the near edge of the packet (Fig. 16.1(**c**), (**e**)). Turn the edges of the packet under, using a powder folder (Fig. 16.1(**g**)) if available, so that the overlap is equal at both ends (Fig. 16.1(**f**)). Firm the creases using a clean flexible spatula but avoid excessive pressure which would cause caking of the enclosed powder.

The packets are best packed in pairs, flap to flap and restrained with an elastic band.

In a well-wrapped product there should be no powder within the flaps or folds. When opened by the user the powder should appear in the centre of the paper, easily available for administration.

Preparation of granules

On a small scale, granules are made with a mortar and pestle and suitable sieves.

The ingredients are moistened with a granulating agent until they are coherent but not too damp.

The coherent material is passed through a suitable sieve (2.8 mm).

The resulting granules are shaken gently on a finer sieve (710 μm) to remove loose powder and dried in an oven at not more than 60°C.

Preparation of dusting powders

These are prepared using the method described for undivided oral powders but the sieve size should be 180 μm.

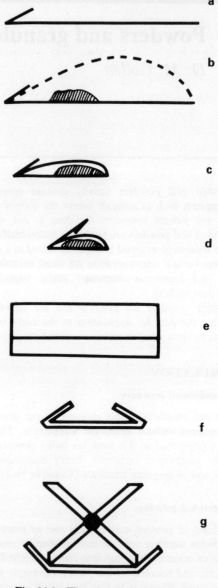

Fig. 16.1 Wrapping divided powders

ORAL POWDERS AS DOSAGE FORMS

Undivided powders as oral dosage forms

Relatively few medicaments are formulated as undivided powders. An example of an indigestion remedy is given in Example 16.1. Similar proprietary products are available.

Advantages of undivided powders:

1. Useful for bulky drugs with a large dose, e.g. indigestion powders.
2. Absorption is faster than from corresponding tablets or capsules.
3. Dry powders are more stable than liquid preparations.

Disadvantages of undivided powders:

1. Inconvenient to carry.
2. Measurement of dose may be inaccurate.
3. Difficult to mask unpleasant tastes.

Shelf-life of undivided powders

Suitably packaged and stored, the powders remain stable over a long period.

Containers for undivided powders

Plain glass jars with close-fitting closures. A 5 ml measuring spoon should be supplied when dispensed.

Special labels and advice for patients

Patients should be advised that the powders should be dissolved or dispersed as appropriate in a little water before taking.

Divided powders as oral dosage forms

Relatively few medicaments are formulated as divided powders although this may be a useful dosage form for children (Examples 16.2 and 16.3). The advantages of divided powders are similar to those of undivided powders, i.e. rapid absorption after administration and relative stability of dry ingredients. Divided powders have the additional advantage that the dose has been accurately measured by the pharmacist. The disadvantage of unpleasant taste remains.

Cachets

These are now rarely used but are a dosage form in which a quantity of powder (minimum 200 mg) is enclosed inside a rice-paper shell. Although cachets offer a means of administering comparatively large amounts of disagreeable powders they offer very little protection from light, moisture or mechanical handling. They are also large to swallow and must be moistened by immersion in water immediately prior to swallowing with a draught of water.

Shelf-life of divided powders

Extemporaneously prepared divided powders are best not stored for long periods unless the exclusion of atmospheric moisture can be assured. Packaging for commercially prepared powders may be fully protective against the atmosphere and the shelf-life will be correspondingly longer.

Containers for divided powders

Traditionally divided powders were supplied in paperboard boxes but these provide little protection against the atmosphere. For extemporaneously prepared powders a screw-capped jar or plastic container is preferable. Proprietary powders packed in moisture-proof sachets may be dispensed in an outer paperboard carton.

Special labels and advice for patients

Patients should be instructed that individual powders should be dispersed in a little water or placed on the back of the tongue before swallowing.

GRANULES AS ORAL DOSAGE FORMS

Like undivided powders, bulk granules can be used to deliver bulky medicaments of low potency. Granules packed commercially in individual sachets have the advantages of more accurate dosage and protection from the atmosphere. Granules are rarely produced extemporaneously but an example of a bulk granule preparation is included as Example 16.4.

Shelf-life for granules

As for undivided powders.

Containers for granules

Bulk granules should be packed in plain glass jars with close-fitting closures. A measuring spoon should be supplied.

A paperboard carton is a suitable dispensing outer container for commercially packed sachets.

Special labels and advice for patients

Effervescent granules should be dissolved in water before taking. Otherwise granules may be dispersed in water or placed on the back of the tongue before swallowing.

Granules for mixtures

Some of the antibiotics that are unstable in solution or suspension are formulated by manufacturers as dry granules containing the medicament and various adjuncts such as buffering, preservative, colouring, flavouring and suspending agents. They are packed in bottles large enough to hold the water that is added when a prescription is received. The granules are formulated to dissolve or disperse rapidly and the pharmacist should ensure that satisfactory suspension or complete solution has occurred before issue to the patient.

BULK POWDERS FOR EXTERNAL USE

Dusting powders that are intended for application to open wounds or raw surfaces must be sterilized. For unbroken skin, freedom from pathogenic organisms should be assured and the individual ingredients may require sterilization before incorporation into the preparation. An example of a dusting powder is included as Example 16.5.

Bulk powders used to be formulated as insufflations designed to be blown into various body cavities, e.g. ear, nose or throat. These are now rarely if ever prescribed for extemporaneous preparation. Commercial single-dose insufflations designed to deliver medicament to the respiratory tract are described with hard gelatin capsules in Chapter 17.

Shelf-life of dusting powders

Providing the container gives adequate protection against moisture the products may be stored for long periods.

Containers for dusting powders

Coloured glass or plastic jars, preferably with a recloseable perforated lid. Manufactured products are usually packed in plastic or metal containers with the appropriate closure.

Special labels and advice for patients

> Store in a dry place.

A clear distinction must be made between sterilized and non-sterilized products.

EXAMPLES

Example 16.1

Prepare 100 g Compound Magnesium Trisilicate Oral Powder BP 1988

Ingredients	Master formula
Magnesium Trisilicate	250 g
Chalk, in powder	250 g
Sodium Bicarbonate	250 g
Heavy Magnesium Carbonate	250 g

Formulation
The ingredients are all 'active' ingredients.

Compounding
Mix the powders in a mortar in order of increasing bulk volume. Pass the resulting mix through a 250 μm sieve, lightly re-mix and pack.

Storage and shelf-life
Store in a dry place.

Container
Amber glass screw-capped jar or plastic pot.

Advice for patients when dispensed
The powder should be taken mixed with a little water or other fluid between meals. If counter-prescribed prolonged use should be discouraged without medical advice.

Actions and uses
Adsorbent and antacid for the treatment of dyspepsia.

Example 16.2

Send three powders each containing 8 mg propranolol hydrochloride for a child weighing 8 kg

Ingredients and formula	for one powder	for four powders
Propranolol hydrochloride	8 mg	32 mg*
Lactose	112 mg	448 mg
Total	120 mg	480 mg

Notes: *Delivered as 160 mg triturate, see below. Prepare for one extra powder to allow for manipulation losses.

Formulation
Lactose is used as an inert diluent to raise the weight of each powder to 120 mg. The 32 mg of propranolol is unweighable, therefore make a trituration in the lactose and subtract the amount of lactose used in the trituration from the total to be added.

Trituration

Propranolol Hydrochloride	100 mg
Lactose	400 mg
Total	500 mg

Thus each 100 mg of triturate contains 20 mg propranolol and therefore 160 mg of triturate contains the required 32 mg*.

Compounding
Mix the powders in a mortar. Pass the resulting mix through a 250 μm sieve and lightly remix. Weigh out

120 mg aliquots and check that the remainder weighs approximately 120 mg. Wrap the powders and pack.

Storage and shelf-life
Store in a cool dry place. Since the product has been prepared extemporaneously a short shelf-life is appropriate.
Propranolol should be protected from light.

Container
Amber glass screw-capped jar or plastic container.

Advice for patients when dispensed
To be given before feeds.

Actions and uses
Beta-adrenoceptor antagonist.

Example 16.3

Prepare a sufficient quantity of Oral Rehydration Salts (Formula A) BP 1988 for three separate 200 ml doses of solution. Pack the powder for each dose separately.

Ingredients	Master formula
	(sufficient for 1 litre solution)
Sodium Chloride	1.0 g
Potassium Chloride	1.5 g
Sodium Bicarbonate	1.5 g
Anhydrous Glucose	36.4 g

Formulation
The ingredients are all 'active'. The preparation may be flavoured if required.

Compounding
Make a small excess to allow for losses in the mortar. Mix the powders in a mortar in order of increasing bulk. Pass the resulting mix through a 250 μm sieve, lightly re-mix and pack.

Storage and shelf-life
Store in a dry place.

Container
Supply each dose (8.08 g) in an individual amber glass screw-capped jar on plastic pot.

Advice for patients when dispensed
Each dose of the powder should be dissolved in sufficient freshly boiled and cooled water to make 200 ml of solution taking hygienic precautions. After reconstitution any unused solution should be discarded after 1 hour unless refrigerated when it may be kept for 12–24 hours.

Actions and uses
Rehydration and electrolyte replacement in the treatment of diarrhoea.

Example 16.4

Prepare 250 g Methylcellulose Granules BP 1988

Ingredients	Master formula
Methylcellulose	64 g
Amaranth, food grade of commerce	20 mg
Saccharin Sodium	100 mg
Vanillin	200 mg
Acacia	4 g
Lactose sufficient to produce	100 g

Formulation
High-viscosity grades of methylcellulose (such as 2500 or 4000) are used as intestinal bulking agents (the compounding record should indicate the variety actually used). Vanillin and saccharin are used to sweeten and flavour the granules and amaranth is a permitted colour. Acacia helps to bind the granules.

Compounding
Mix the powders in a mortar in order of increasing bulk, taking care to distribute the dye evenly.
Add sufficient water to form a coherent mass. If the mass is too wet the granules will be too large, if too dry there will be too much ungranulated powder.
Press the mass through a 2.8 mm sieve and collect the resulting granules on the mesh of a 710 μm sieve. Fine granules and powder will fall through the lower sieve leaving uniform granules on its surface.
Spread the granules to dry on a tray in a drying oven at a temperature of 60°C.

Storage and shelf-life
Store in a dry place.

Container
Amber glass screw-capped jar or plastic pot.

Advice for patients when dispensed
The granules should be placed on the back of the tongue and swallowed with water. For the treatment of constipation the granules should be taken well diluted with water. For the treatment of diarrhoea, the minimum of fluid should be taken.

Actions and uses
Intestinal bulking agent used as a laxative, appetite depressant or in the treatment of diarrhoea.

Example 16.5

Prepare 100 g Zinc, Starch and Talc Dusting Powder BPC 1973

Ingredients	Master formula
Zinc Oxide	250 g
Starch, in powder	250 g
Purified Talc, sterilized	500 g

Formulation
The ingredients are all 'active' ingredients.

Compounding
Mix the powders in a mortar in order of increasing bulk. Pass the resulting mix through a 180 μm sieve, lightly re-mix and pack.

Storage and shelf-life
Store in a dry place.

Container
Amber glass screw-capped jar or plastic pot with recloseable perforated lid.

Advice for patients when dispensed
The powder should be dusted lightly onto the affected area. It should not be applied to broken skin or to raw surfaces of large area.

Actions and uses
Absorbent dusting powder.

BIBLIOGRAPHY

ABPI Data Sheet Compendium current edition. Datapharm Publications, London (updated annually)

Aulton M E 1988 Pharmaceutics: the science of dosage form design. Churchill Livingstone. Edinburgh, Ch 17

British National Formulary 1988 16th edn. British Medical Association and Royal Pharmaceutical Society of Great Britain, London (updated twice yearly)

British Pharmacopoeia 1980 HMSO, London (and addenda 1982, 1983 and 1986)

British Pharmacopoeia 1988 HMSO, London

British Pharmaceutical Codex 1973 Pharmaceutical Press, London

Martindale, see Reynolds J E F

Pharmaceutical Codex 1979 11th edn (incorporating the British Pharmaceutical Codex). Pharmaceutical Press, London

Pharmaceutical Society 1979 Guide to good dispensing practice. Pharmaceutical Journal 223: 157–158

Reynolds J E F (ed) 1989 Martindale, The Extra Pharmacopoeia, 29th edn. Pharmaceutical Press, London

Wade A (ed) 1980 Pharmaceutical handbook, 19th edn. Pharmaceutical Press, London

17. Oral unit dosage forms

D. M. Collett

These are dosage forms in which an accurately measured amount of medicament is presented in a single dosage unit which is easily handled by the patient. The major unit oral dosage forms are tablets and capsules which between them account for the vast majority of prescription items presently dispensed in the UK.

These products are rarely produced extemporaneously, being mass produced on a commercial scale at relatively low manufacturing cost. A detailed discussion of these processes is therefore more relevant to the companion volume (Aulton 1988) and details can be found therein.

Advantages of oral unit dosage forms include:

1. Accurate dosage.
2. Release characteristics of the drug can be controlled.
3. Uniform product.
4. Stable product.
5. Attractive product.
6. Easy to administer.
7. Unpleasant tastes can be masked.
8. Simple to pack.
9. Convenient to carry.

Disadvantages of oral unit dosage forms include:

1. May be difficult to swallow.
2. Unsuitable for the very young.
3. The excipients may produce unwanted effects.
4. Release characteristics may not be ideal.

TABLETS

The essential properties of tablets and their formulation requirements are discussed in detail in chapter 18 of the companion volume (Aulton 1988).

Dispensing of tablets

Most of the tablets prescribed in the UK are packaged by the manufacturer into unit packs suitable for issue to the patient without re-packing by the pharmacist (see Ch. 8). Providing that these packs are stored in accordance with the manufacturer's recommendations, the products generally have a long shelf-life and the appropriate expiry date will be printed on the package. The role of the pharmacist in the dispensing of these tablets is concerned mainly with the labelling of the pack for the individual patient (see Ch. 10) and counselling the patient about the medication (see Ch. 37).

Supply from a bulk pack

The required number of tablets must be counted from the bulk container. Several counting devices are available and include, a simple triangular tray with numbered rows, a funnel-type apparatus with an electronic counter and devices based on the detection of the weight of a predetermined number of tablets. In the absence of any counting aid the tablets may be counted by means of a spatula on a piece of clean demy paper.

Whichever method is used it is essential that the tablets remain untouched by hand. It is also essential that cross-contamination of different tablets does not occur. Counting devices should be cleaned after each usage since very small particles from a previous count adhering to tablets have been shown to evoke an allergic reaction in susceptible individuals.

Before and after counting, the label of the stock container should be checked against the prescription and the dispensing container labelled before returning the stock container to the shelf.

Containers for tablets

For tablets supplied in strip or blister packaging (see Ch. 8), a paperboard outer container is suitable. Tablets counted from bulk should be supplied in amber glass or plastic containers, preferably with child-resistant closures if for domestic use (see Ch. 8).

Special labels for tablets and advice for patients

Most tablets are designed to disintegrate in the stomach after swallowing and to release the medicament for absorption by the small intestine. These tablets should be swallowed with a draught of water.

Effervescent tablets are formulated to be dispersed in water before swallowing and should be so labelled.

Chewable tablets can be taken when water is unavailable and are useful for patients who find difficulty in swallowing whole tablets. Antacid tablets are often formulated for chewing.

Sublingual and buccal tablets are designed to dissolve in the mouth to allow absorption through the buccal mucosa.

Modified release tablets may be designed to release the medicament over a particular time period or in a selected part of the gastrointestinal tract. It is important that such tablets are swallowed whole. Tablets that are specially coated for release in the alkaline conditions of the small intestine should not be taken at the same time as antacid preparations which alter the pH of the stomach. Details of the labels to be applied to tablets of various types are explained in Chapter 10.

CAPSULES

These are dosage forms in which the medicament is enclosed within a hard or soft gelatin shell. Capsules as a dosage form (both soft gelatin and hard gelatin) are discussed in detail in Chapter 19 of the companion volume (Aulton 1988).

Soft gelatin capsules

These are formed, filled and sealed in one manufacturing operation and may contain powders, non-aqueous liquids, solutions, emulsions, suspensions and pastes.

Hard gelatin capsules

The shell is manufactured from gelatin with the addition of suitable plasticizers, preservatives and colouring agents. The shells are cylindrical with hemispherical ends and consist of a body and an overfitting lid. After filling, the two pieces are locked together. Hard gelatin shells are available in a range of sizes (Fig. 17.1, Table 17.1).

Table 17.1 Approximate capacities of hard gelatin capsule shells (based on lactose)

Capsule no.	000	00	0	1	2	3	4	5
Content (mg)	950	650	450	300	250	200	150	100

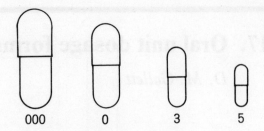

Fig. 17.1 Hard gelatin capsule shell sizes

In addition to the general advantages of oral unit dosage forms, hard gelatin capsules have a number of other advantages:

1. Unpleasant tastes readily masked.
2. Easy to swallow (suitable shape and slippery when moistened).
3. Fewer excipients required.
4. Rapid and uniform release of medicament.
5. Can be made light resistant.

FORMULATION

A detailed account of the formulation and large-scale manufacture of both hard and soft gelatin capsules is given in the companion volume (Chapter 41, Aulton 1988). *Soft* gelatin capsules are made only by an industrial process and not extemporaneously prepared.

On a small scale powdered medicament can be packed by hand into *hard* gelatin shells. If the required weight of medicament is small the weight should be raised to a recommended minimum weight of 100 mg by the addition of lactose or other suitable inert diluent such as magnesium carbonate, starch or kaolin. Glidants, lubricants and wetting agents can be included if necessary (see Chapters 19 and 41 of the companion volume, Aulton 1988, for details).

COMPOUNDING

Hand filling of hard gelatin capsules is rarely carried out in the community pharmacy but may be required on occasion in the hospital pharmacy. Two methods are suggested:

Filling from a powder mass

Place the sifted powder (250 μm sieve) on a clean, dry tile and holding the capsule on its side push powder into the shell with the aid of a spatula until the required weight has been enclosed. Alternatively invert the shell into a heap of powder to fill.

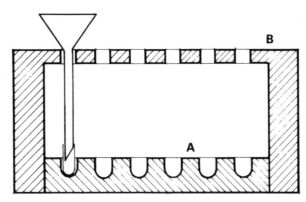

Fig. 17.2 Simple apparatus for capsule filling. A, Plastic block; B, plastic bridge

The latter procedure is less successful with free-flowing powders which tend to drop out. The use of surgical gloves is preferable to the use of forceps which may damage the shell.

Filling with weighed aliquots

The following method uses a simple apparatus (Fig. 17.2) consisting of a plastic block (A) with rows of cavities which hold the capsules and allow them to project slightly. Each row is designed to hold a different size of capsule.

A plastic bridge (B) contains a row of holes corresponding in position to the cavities in any row of the block. This is used to support a long-stemmed funnel so that the end of the stem of the funnel can pass into the mouth of the capsule below.

The capsule bodies are placed in the cavities in the block and a funnel of appropriate size (with a stem as wide as possible for the size of capsule) is passed through the hole in the bridge and down into the neck of the capsule. A weighed aliquot of powder is then tipped into the top of the funnel and passed down into the capsule. A thin glass or plastic rod or piece of non-corrodible wire is useful to break blockages and act as a plunger to loosely compress the material inside the capsule if necessary.

After filling the capsule, the top may be fitted loosely and the weight checked before sealing.

The capsule shell size should be chosen such that the shell is filled as completely as possible in order to produce a product of elegant appearance.

Table 17.1 may be used as a guide of fill capacities for powders of average bulky density. The size of capsule shell used should be recorded so that different batches will be of consistent size. For powders with poor

flow properties the addition of magnesium stearate (up to 1% w/w) may aid the filling process. There will be inevitable manipulative losses and, as for divided powders (see Ch. 16), it is necessary to prepare for one capsule extra to the number ordered (Example 17.1).

Shelf-life of capsules

Extemporaneously prepared capsules should not be stored for long periods without stability data. Commercially prepared and packed capsules, stored according to the manufacturers' recommendations, are generally very stable.

Containers for capsules

The containers in which capsules are supplied are similar to those recommended for tablets, i.e. amber glass or plastic containers — preferably with a child-resistant closure for domestic use (see Ch. 8). Protection from humidity is particularly important since this will cause softening of the gelatin.

Special labels for capsules

Capsules should generally be swallowed whole with a draught of water or other liquid. Details of any special labels to be applied to capsules containing medicaments of various types are explained in Chapter 10.

OTHER PRODUCTS IN CAPSULE SHELLS

Insufflations

These are fine powders prepared for inhalation from a suitable insufflator. The powders, together with inert diluents and other excipients, are packed into hard gelatin capsule shells. After insertion into the insufflator these shells are pierced or broken and the flow of released powder is controlled by the patient's own respiratory effort.

Shelf-life, packaging and storage requirements are similar to those for capsules intended for oral administration. The product must be labelled

> Not to be swallowed

or an equivalent warning. Special counselling and a demonstration of the use of the insufflator should be given.

Eye ointments, and rectal or vaginal dosage forms

These may sometimes be packed in capsule shells. These products should be labelled clearly with the appropriate route of administration.

OTHER ORAL UNIT DOSAGE FORMS

Lozenges

These are compressed tablets designed to be dissolved in the mouth by sucking. They are prepared in a similar manner to tablets but do not include a disintegrant since they are intended to diminish in size by friction and/or dissolution rather than to disintegrate in the mouth. Most lozenges are designed to produce a local action in the mouth and throat and their active ingredients include antiseptics and local anaesthetics. Lozenges are rarely prepared extemporaneously and are usually packed by the manufacturer in suitable containers for issue to patients.

Pastilles

These generally consist of a glycerol and gelatin base, similar to that used for glycero-gelatin suppositories but with a greater proportion of gelatin and other gelling agents, such as acacia and agar, to add hardness. They are sweetened, flavoured and medicated. Pastilles have been used to deliver antacids but are more commonly used for remedies to soothe sore throats or cough. The high sugar content tends to encourage dental decay and pastilles may not be suitable for diabetic patients unless suitably formulated. Pastilles are commercially produced and packaged and are more commonly supplied as over-the-counter medication than as prescribed items.

Example 17.1

Send five capsules each containing 10 mg chlordiazepoxide. Incorporate 1% w/w magnesium stearate

Ingredients	for one	for six
Chlordiazepoxide	10 mg	60 mg
Magnesium stearate	1 mg	6 mg*
Lactose	89 mg	534 mg

*Delivered as a triturate in lactose, see below.

Formulation
Lactose is used as an inert diluent to raise the weight of each capsule to 100 mg. Magnesium stearate is added to improve the flow properties of the powders.
  * The 6 mg is unweighable, therefore make a trituration in the lactose and subtract the amount of lactose used in the trituration from the total to be added.

Compounding
Prepare for one extra capsule.
  Mix the powders in a mortar. Pass the resulting mix through a 250 μm sieve and lightly remix. Weigh out 100 mg aliquots and fill into separate capsule shells (size 5 should be appropriate). Check the weight of each capsule before sealing.

Storage and shelf-life
Store cool and dry. Chlordiazepoxide should be protected from light.

Container
Amber glass or plastic tablet container.

Advice for patients when dispensed
This product may cause drowsiness. If affected do not drive or operate machinery. Avoid alcoholic drink.

Actions and uses
Anxiolytic.

BIBLIOGRAPHY

ABPI Data Sheet Compendium current edition Datapharm Publications, London (updated annually)

Aulton M E 1988 Pharmaceutics: the science of dosage from design. Churchill Livingstone, Edinburgh, C

British National Formulary 1988 16th edn. British Medical Association and Royal Pharmaceutical Society of Great Britain, London (updated twice yearly)

British Pharmacopoeia 1980 HMSO, London (and addenda 1982, 1983 and 1986)

British Pharmacopoeia 1988 HMSO, London

British Pharmaceutical Codex 1973 Pharmaceutical Press, London

Martindale, see Reynolds J E F

Pharmaceutical Codex 1979 11th edn (incorporating the British Pharmaceutical Codex). Pharmaceutical Press, London

Pharmaceutical Society 1979 Guide to good dispensing practice. Pharmaceutical Journal 223: 157–158

Reynolds J E F (ed) 1989 Martindale, The Extra Pharmacopoeia, 29th edn. Pharmaceutical Press, London

Wade A (ed) 1980 Pharmaceutical handbook, 19th edn. Pharmaceutical Press, London

18. Therapeutic aerosols

D. M. Collett

In pharmacy 'aerosols' are usually produced by means of pressurized containers. A solution or suspension of a medicament is made in a propellent gas, liquefied under pressure and retained in a closed container. When the valve on the container is opened the vapour pressure of the propellent forces the mixture out of the container. A dispersion of the medicament is created by the large expansion of the propellent at room temperature and pressure.

True aerosols are colloidal dispersions of liquids or solids in gases, i.e. the particles are 50 μm or smaller. Most so-called 'aerosols' produce particles of greater size and are more correctly described as 'pressurized dispensers'.

PRESSURIZED INHALATIONS

These are designed to deliver medicament to particular sites in the respiratory tract. The pressurized cannister is fitted with an adaptor which is designed to fit the mouth or the nostril depending on the route of inhalation. A high concentration of drug can thus exert a localized therapeutic action with a minimum of systemic effects. The particle size or droplet size of the delivered aerosol is adjusted so that the medicament deposits in the desired region of the airways.

The physicochemical properties, formulation and generation of aerosols are described fully in Chapter 20 of the companion volume (Aulton 1988).

The amount of drug delivered to the respiratory system is related to the amount released from the container when the valve is actuated and may be controlled by means of a metering device. When the valve is actuated the product, still under pressure, fills the 'metering chamber'. This measured volume of product is then released from the 'metering chamber' to form an aerosol dispersion for inhalation via the adaptor. The valve may be actuated by finger pressure on the base of the container held vertically in an inverted position. This type of device demands a degree of co-ordination between in-spiration and valve actuation which may not be achieved by all patients. One type of device which has been devised to overcome this problem has a breath-actuated valve in which the negative pressure created by the patient inhaling automatically applies pressure to the valve stem and releases the medicament. Another approach to the problem of lack of co-ordination is to release the dose into a 'spacer' chamber from which the patient inhales. This has the additional advantage that the velocity of the aerosol has slowed, and most of the propellent lost by evaporation, by the time it is inhaled by the patient.

Aerosol inhalations are packaged by the manufacturers and the role of the pharmacist in dispensing is mainly concerned with the labelling of the product for the individual patient (see Ch. 10) and counselling the patient about the medication (see Ch. 37).

Patient counselling

In order to obtain optimum benefit from the inhalation the patient must learn the appropriate technique. Clear instructions are supplied by the manufacturer with each package and may be supplemented with explanatory leaflets produced by the pharmacy (see Ch. 37). However, written information is no substitute for demonstration and the pharmacist should be prepared to instruct and to observe the patient's inhalation technique, advising and correcting where appropriate. Many manufacturers supply demonstration kits with placebo aerosol for this purpose.

Aerosol inhalations are used commonly to deliver bronchodilator drugs and corticosteroids to the respiratory tract in the treatment of asthma. It is essential that regular administration of the prescribed dose is carried out in order to produce effective control of symptoms. The dose should be stated explicitly in terms of the number of 'puffs' or inhalations to be taken at any one time and the frequency and daily maximum recommended. It is essential that the prescribed dose of bronchodilators is not exceeded and the pharmacist may be in a unique position to recognize excessive use which usually indicates poorly controlled asthma. Patients should be advised that if the recommended dose does not produce the usual amount of relief they should seek medical advice.

Storage and shelf-life of aerosol inhalations

These should be stored in a cool place but protected from frost. They should be protected from heat including the sun because they may explode on heating even when apparently empty.

AQUEOUS AEROSOLS (NEBULIZER THERAPY)

These devices utilize a stream of pressurized gas (either oxygen or compressed air) which passes through an aqueous solution of the drug and creates an aerosolized mist for inhalation via a suitable mask or mouthpiece. With an appropriate rate of gas flow, larger droplets are trapped in a baffle and returned to the reservoir of drug solution resulting in the output of droplets of 2–4 μm diameter. An alternative, less frequently used system utilizes an ultrasonic generator to create a nebulized liquid dispersion.

For the treatment of severe airways obstruction, a nebulized aerosol may be preferred to a pressurized inhaler. The latter is limited in the amount of drug that can be delivered in a single inspiration. The administration of large doses would therefore require repeated inhalations. Large doses of bronchodilator (up to 20 times the dose from an aerosol inhaler) are readily delivered by nebulizer. The problems of co-ordination of inspiration with valve actuation have been discussed above.

Such problems are compounded in the seriously ill patient with little inspiratory effort. The nebulized drug is delivered during normal tidal breathing and requires little effort from the patient. In some patients the use of the propellants used in pressurized aerosols may be undesirable, this problem is avoided with the use of an isotonic aqueous vehicle for the nebulized drug solution.

Nebulizers are used routinely in hospital to deliver bronchodilator therapy. The drug solution may be ready packed in single-dose units or in multi-dose containers for dilution before use. The preferred diluent is normal saline since hypotonic solutions may cause bronchospasm when inhaled. The dose is usually administered over a period of about 15 minutes.

The driving gas chosen depends on the condition of the patient, oxygen should be used for oxygen-dependent patients but should be avoided in those patients reliant on hypoxia to maintain their respiratory drive (i.e.

chronic bronchitics). For these patients air should be used as the driving gas.

The popularity of domestic nebulizer therapy is increasing. For domiciliary use an electric compressor, usually purchased by the patient, is used to supply compressed air as the driving gas. The prescriptions for the nebulizer solutions will be presented at the pharmacy and the patient will require counselling on loading and using the nebulizer. As with aerosol inhalers the patient should be reminded that if the recommended dose does not produce the expected relief they should seek medical advice.

AEROSOL SPRAYS (PRESSURIZED DISPENSERS)

A number of different pharmaceutical products are packaged in the form of pressurized dispensers.

Surface sprays

These deliver spray droplets (100–200 μm) that will wet the surface on which they fall. They have the advantage that contamination in use is unlikely and the product can be easily directed to the required site. Dosage forms packed in pressurized dispensers include antiseptic, antibiotic, local anaesthetic and protective film dressings which can be applied to wounds and burns without undue distress to the patient. Spray-on dusting powders are also available.

Aerosol foams

These may be produced by creating an emulsified system in the product. As the propellant evaporates, bubbles stabilized by surfactants are formed. Spermicidal preparations and some rectal dosage forms are formulated as aerosol foams.

Topical analgesics

A number of aerosol preparations containing rubefacient and counter-irritant preparations are available for over-the-counter sale in the treatment of rheumatic aches and pains and sports injuries. Sprays containing only propellants are used to produce pain relief by cooling on evaporation from the skin surface.

Propellants

A number of compressed and liquefied gases have been used as aerosol propellants. Then halogenated hydrocarbons (HFCs), dichlorodifluoromethane (propellant 12) and trichlorofluoromethane (propellant 11) have been implicated in the depletion of the ozone layer of the stratosphere and have fallen into popular disrepute. This has led to the reformulation of a large number of commercial products to include hydrocarbon and other propellants that are considered to be 'ozone friendly'. However, explosive accidents have occurred with cannisters pressurized with butane.

Propellant abuse and toxicity

The toxicity to humans of aerosol propellants appears to be slight if they are not abused. However, there have been a number of reported deaths as a result of the abuse of aerosol propellants causing hallucinogenic effects. These have included the abuse of topical pain-relieving preparations purchased from a pharmacy.

Storage and shelf-life of pressurized dispensers

These should be stored in a cool place but protected from frost. They should be protected from heat including the sun because they may explode on heating, even when apparently empty.

BIBLIOGRAPHY

ABPI Data Sheet Compendium current edition Datapharm Publications, London (updated annually)
Aulton M E 1988 Pharmaceutics: science of dosage form design. Churchill Livingstone, Edinburgh,
British National Formulary 1988 16th edn. British Medical Association and Royal Pharmaceutical Society of Great Britain, London (updated twice yearly)
British Pharmacopoeia 1980 HMSO, London (and addenda 1982, 1983 and 1986)
British Pharmacopoeia 1988 HMSO, London
British Pharmaceutical Codex 1973 Pharmaceutical Press, London

Horsley M 1988 Nebuliser therapy. Pharmaceutical Journal 240: 22–24
Martindale, see Reynolds J E F
Pharmaceutical Codex 1979 11th edn (incorporating the British Pharmaceutical Codex). Pharmaceutical Press, London
Pharmaceutical Society 1979 Guide to good dispensing practice. Pharmaceutical Journal 223: 157–158
Reynolds J E F (ed) 1989 Martindale, The Extra Pharmacopoeia, 29th edn. Pharmaceutical Press, London
Wade A (ed) 1980 Pharmaceutical handbook, 19th edn. Pharmaceutical Press, London

Sterile pharmaceutical preparations

INTRODUCTION

All pharmaceutical products should be prepared under hygienic conditions using materials from which gross microbial contamination has been eliminated. The principles of good pharmaceutical practice are described in Part 1 of this book.

Part 3 of the book is concerned with the compounding of pharmaceutical products from which viable micro-organisms must be totally absent, i.e. sterile products. The production of sterile products requires special care and attention in order to eliminate microbial and particulate contamination at all stages of manufacture and wherever possible also includes a terminal sterilization process.

Chapter 19 introduces the reader to the concept of sterility and to the principles of sterilization. The sterilization methods of choice utilize heat and these are described in Chapter 20, whilst alternative methods which may be employed for heat-labile materials are described in Chapter 21.

Basic environmental standards for clean preparation areas are listed in Chapter 23. The range of pharmaceutical activities that require clean room facilities include:

— Aseptic dispensing (Ch. 22).
— Manufacture of parenteral products (Ch. 24).
— Preparation of intravenous additives (Ch. 25).
— Dispensing of cytotoxic agents (Ch. 26).
— Preparation of parenteral nutrition (Ch. 27).
— Preparation of ophthalmic products (Ch. 28).

Quality assurance, introduced in Chapter 29, is an important aspect of the production of all pharmaceuticals and is particularly relevant to the preparation of sterile products. Testing for sterility (Ch. 30) is a specialized aspect of the total quality assurance of sterile products.

Throughout the text the reader is referred to additional material in Part 4 of the companion volume (Aulton 1988) which discusses further aspects of microbiology and sterilization.

The stages in the manufacture of a sterile medicinal product are summarized in the table opposite.

Steps in the manufacture of a medicinal product

Production		Quality control
Preparation and inspection ——→	**CONTAINERS** ←——	Component testing
Bottle		Closure system
Closure system		Compatability of container and
Washing		contents
Documentation ——————→	**PREPARATION** ←——	Stability
Formulation		Expiry date
Method, i.e. solubilities		
Compatabilities		
Assembly of Components		
pH ————————————→	**IN-PROCESS CONTROL AND** ←——	Trend sheets
Colour	**ENVIRONMENTAL MONITORING**	Viable counts
Conductivity of water		Pyrogen testing
		Microbial testing
Fill volumes ——————→	**FILLING** ←——	Product accountability
Capping		Bubble point test
Filtration		
Identification of batch ——→	**STERILIZATION** ←——	Thermocouple testing
Indicators — Brownes Tubes		Time and temperature of load
Autoclave Tape		Testing of cooling water
Chart records and gauges		
Maximum loads		
Sealing bottle		
Backing off of cap ————→	**INSPECTION** ←——	Product accountability
Particles		Trend sheets
Components failure		
Design ————————→	**LABELLING** ←——	Design
Batch number		
Expiry date		
Label reconciliation		
Packaging for bond ———→	**FINISHED PRODUCT** ←——	Sampling
		Bonded till release
		Sterility testing
		Analytical testing
		Checking of charts and documentation
Stock control —————→	**RELEASE** ←——	Recall

19. Principles of sterilization

R. M. E. Richards

Introduction

Pharmaceutical products are generally required to be free from contamination with micro-organisms (bacteria, viruses, yeasts, moulds, etc.). Such organisms may cause spoilage by adversely affecting the appearance or composition of a product and may cause serious adverse effects in the patient. Adverse effects are particularly likely if the preparation is introduced into the body via a route which bypasses some of the body's normal defence mechanisms, especially in a seriously ill or immunocompromised patient.

Dosage forms designed for parenteral, ophthalmic or surgical use, as well as irrigation solutions and topical preparations for application to large open wounds, must be free from microbial and particulate contamination. These products are required to be prepared and maintained in a sterile state until used. Some of the terms used in connection with 'sterile pharmaceutical products' are defined below.

Sterility. Sterility may be defined as the *total* absence of viable micro-organisms and is an *absolute* state. The production of sterile pharmaceutical products may be achieved by aseptic technique (see Ch. 22) or by means of a terminal sterilization process (see Chs 20, 21).

Sterilization. This is the subjection of products to a process whereby all viable life forms are either killed or removed. The sterilization process is usually the final stage in the preparation of the product. The fundamental properties of micro-organisms and the actions of chemical and physical agents upon them are discussed in the companion volume (Aulton 1988), which also discusses the principles and practice of sterilization. The methods of sterilization in regular use include exposure to: saturated steam under pressure, dry heat, ionizing radiation, ethylene oxide or passage through a bacteria-retaining filter. When possible, exposure to saturated steam under pressure is the sterilization method of choice.

Aseptic technique. This is the preparation of pharmaceutical products from sterile ingredients by procedures that exclude the access of viable micro-organisms into the products. It is used for those products that would be adversely affected by being subjected to a sterilization process.

Sterility testing. Tests for sterility of pharmaceutical products attempt to reveal the presence or absence of viable micro-organisms in a sample number of containers taken from a production batch. From the results of such tests an inference is made as to the sterility of the batch.

Disinfection. Disinfection is a process which aims to reduce the number of harmful (pathogenic) micro-organisms in a particular situation. Disinfection will destroy infective vegetative organisms but not necessarily resistant spores, i.e. it is not an absolute process. It often involves the use of chemicals although other means of disinfection may be employed, e.g. the pasteurization of milk is a disinfection process that uses heat.

Disinfectant. This is a chemical agent used to destroy harmful micro-organisms usually in inanimate objects.

Antiseptic. This is a chemical agent usually applied to living tissues in humans or animals in order to destroy harmful micro-organisms.

STERILIZATION CRITERIA

The bioburden

In order to select the appropriate parameters for any method intended to kill micro-organisms in a given product or associated with a given material, it is necessary to know the initial number of organisms, the 'bioburden' or 'bioload', and their resistance to the chosen process. For example, it has been the practice to choose the time and temperature relationship for steam sterilization to ensure that a large number of the known most resistant pathogen would be killed. This treatment would not necessarily be sufficient to kill a large number of the known most resistant non-pathogenic organism which, however, are extremely unlikely to be present and is greatly in excess of the treatment necessary to kill the small number of heat-sensitive contaminants likely to be present in pharmaceutical solutions.

Establishing microbial death

Death in a microbial population is determined by assessing the reduction in the number of viable micro-organisms resulting from contact with a given destructive force. Viable organisms are those which when transferred to a culture medium can form a colony. This places the onus on the investigator to provide suitable culture conditions for recovery and growth of any surviving micro-organisms.

Death rates

The kinetics of microbial cell inactivation are discussed in detail in the companion volume (Chapter 25, Aulton 1988). When a population of micro-organisms is subjected to a destructive sterilization procedure the order of death is generally logarithmic. That is a constant proportion of the microbial population is inactivated in any given time interval, approximating to first-order kinetics.

A typical survivor curve is shown in Figure 19.1.

If N_o is the initial number of organisms and N_t is the number of organisms surviving after time t, the death rate constant (inactivation constant) k can be calculated.

$$N_t = N_o e^{-kt}$$
$$\ln N_t = \ln N_o - kt$$
$$\log_{10} N_t = \log_{10} N_o - \frac{kt}{2.303}$$

The death rate constant can be calculated as follows from Figure 19.1

Let $N_o = 10^6$ $N_t = 10^2$ $t = 10$

Then, $k = 1/10 \ (\log_{10} 10^6/10^2)$
$= 1/10 \ (6 - 2) = 0.4$

The determination of death rate provides the facility to compare the resistance of the same organism at different temperatures or to compare the resistance of different organisms to the same lethal agent, e.g. temperature, ionizing radiation, chemical agent, etc. Death rates may also be used to give a quantitative measure of the effect of environmental factors such as pH, osmolarity and the presence of various chemicals on the sterilization process. Since the same percentage of bacteria die each minute, it is impossible in theory to reach a point of zero survivors. From Figure 19.1 an extension

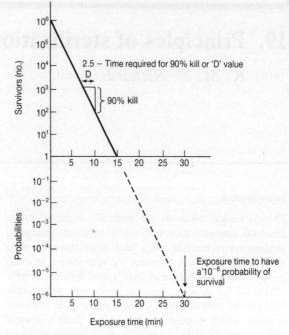

Fig. 19.1 Survivor curve

of the process to 30 minutes would give the assurance that the probability of survival of one member of the original population would be 1 in 10. In terms of containers of solution this would mean a probability of one container in a million being contaminated.

The concept of percentage reduction of a bacterial population reinforces the need for as small a bioburden as possible when a product is to be sterilized.

The methods that are used to prepare sterile fluids ensure that the bioburden is very low (see Chs 24, 29). If containers are filled through a bacteria-proof filter prior to sterilization the bioburden is effectively zero.

D value or decimal reduction time

The death rate can also be expressed as the decimal reduction time or D value. This is the time in minutes at any defined temperature to destroy 90% of viable organisms. In Figure 19.1 this is 2.5 minutes. Numerically it is also the reciprocal of the death rate constant. D values are often given a subscript to indicate the temperature at which they were measured, e.g. $D_{121°C}$. From the D value for a particular combination of organism/time/temperature an 'inactivation factor' (IF) can be calculated, e.g. if the D value of an organism exposed to a temperature of 121°C for 15 minutes was 2 minutes the IF would be $10^{15/2}$, i.e. $10^{7.5}$.

Z value or thermal destruction value

This relates the heat resistance of a micro-organism to changes in temperature. The Z value is the number of degrees of temperature change to produce a ten-fold change in D value. Bacterial spores have a Z value in the range 10–15°C while most non-sporing organisms have Z values of 4–6°C.

Q or temperature coefficient

This also gives a measure of the relative resistance of different micro-organisms and describes the change in the death rate over a 10°C change in temperature.

F values

The F value is a measure of the lethality of the total process of sterilization and equates heat treatment at any particular temperature with the time in minutes at a designated reference temperature that would be required to produce the same lethality in an organism of stated Z value. For a temperature of 121°C and organisms with a Z value of 10°C F becomes F_o. Annex 2 of Appendix XVIII of the BP 1988 contains the following description of F_o: 'The F_o value of a saturated steam process is the lethality expressed in terms of the equivalent time in minutes at 121°C delivered by that process to the product in its final containers with reference to micro-organisms possessing a Z value of 10°C'.

One F unit is equivalent to heating the load for 1 minute at 121°C. Mathematically F is defined as:

$$F_o = 10^{(T_c - 121/Z)} \, dt$$

where T_c = load temperature at time dt and $Z = 10°C$.

For many years it has been understood that both the heating up and cooling phases of a heat sterilizing cycle contribute to the total lethality of the process. The F principle allows an estimation of the overall lethality by integration of the lethal rates multiplied by the times at discrete temperature intervals (Fig. 19.2).

The total lethality (F_o) for the cycle is equal to the sum of the F_o values for each individual time/temperature segment. The accuracy of the estimated F_o is related to the time interval represented by each segment of the profile. Small intervals are conveniently handled by computer. The BP 1988 suggests the use of the F_o calculation for the overall lethality delivered to aqueous preparations for a microbiologically validated steam sterilization process and states that a total F_o value of not less than 8 applied to every container in the load would be considered satisfactory.

Where the product is especially heat sensitive an F_o of less than 8 is deemed justifiable so long as great care is taken to ensure that an adequate assurance of sterility is consistently achieved. That is: 'it is necessary not only to validate the process microbiologically, but also to perform continuous, rigorous, microbiological monitoring during routine production to demonstrate that microbiological parameters are within the established tolerances so as to give a theoretical level of not more than

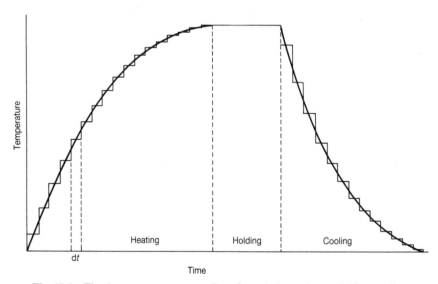

Fig. 19.2 The time–temperature recording of a typical autoclave cycle showing the method of integration by dividing the time axis into a series of segments (dt) (Kirk et al 1982)

one living organism in 10^6 containers of the final product' (BP 1988).

Kirk et al (1985) investigated the degradation under autoclaving conditions of 2,4-dihydroxybenzoic acid in aqueous phosphate buffer pH 7. They found that autoclave cycles delivering a standard process lethality ($F_o = 8$) by means of different holding temperatures caused different degrees of degradation of the chemical. That is high temperature, short time cycles ($121°C/F_o = 8$) caused approximately 12% degradation but prolonged exposure at a relatively low temperature ($112°C/F_o = 8$) caused approximately 30% degradation. Thus in the interest of stability these workers suggested that, where other factors permit, the optimum sterilization cycle would consist of the load being subjected to a temperature which continuously increased, no holding phase, until a prefixed F_o had been achieved. The load would then be cooled under controlled conditions and this cooling phase would provide the remaining F_o units required to achieve the predetermined level of sterility assurance.

There is further discussion on the use of the F_o concept in Chapter 26 of the companion volume (Aulton 1988).

STERILIZATION VALIDATION AND MONITORING

Tests for sterility of the products subjected to a sterilization procedure are discussed in Chapter 30. Whenever possible additional validation and monitoring of the sterilization process is carried out using indicators other than the product. Biological, chemical and physical indicators have all been used. (See also companion volume, Aulton 1988, Chapter 43).

Biological indicators

Biological indicators are supplied in one of two main forms, each of which incorporates a viable culture of a stated species of micro-organism. One form consists of spores added to a carrier such as a disc or strip of filter paper, glass or plastic, so packaged as to protect the contents before use but to allow the sterilizing agent to reach the spores and exert its effect during use. In the other form the spores are added to representative units of the product to be sterilized or to similar units if it is not practicable to add the spores to selected units of a particular product.

Choice of the biological indicator is critical if the indication given is to be a valid reflection of the efficacy of a sterilization cycle. The viability of the organisms, the storage conditions before use and the incubation and culture conditions after sterilization must be stand-

ardized for the result to be meaningful, especially for the less challenging protocols (e.g. F_o values of 8 or less).

The reader is referred to the monographs in the British Pharmacopoeia and United States Pharmacopeia for current recommendations.

The organisms used as biological indicators include:

Bacillus subtilis var. *niger* — dry heat
Bacillus stearothermophilus — steam
Clostridium sporogenes — steam
Bacillus subtilis var. *niger* — ethylene oxide
Bacillus pumulis — ionizing radiation

In order to use biological indicators effectively in the monitoring of a sterilization process a knowledge of the product bioburden in terms of numbers and resistance to the sterilization method is required. The biological indicator must be so chosen as to provide a greater challenge to the sterilization process than the natural bioburden of the product.

Sterilization by filtration

For the biological validation of sterilization by filtration see Chapter 22.

Chemical indicators

These are used to indicate whether a particular batch of product has been through a sterilization process, they do not generally indicate whether the process was successful. The indicator chosen undergoes some change in physical or chemical nature when exposed to the conditions of the sterilization process.

Browne's tubes

These are sealed glass tubes (manufactured by A. Browne, Ltd Leicester containing a red fluid which changes colour through yellow and brown to green on heating at the specified temperature for the appropriate length of time. Various types are available for different sterilization processes, e.g. moist heat and dry heat processes. They should not be used as quantitative indicators.

Heat-sensitive tape

The Bowie–Dick test is valuable for confirming that steam has displaced all the air from a porous load in a high vacuum autoclave (Bowie et al 1963). It consists of using autoclave tape which has heat-sensitive bars, at intervals of about 15 mm, which change colour after contact with steam. The tape is placed suitably wrapped at the centre of a test pack. All the bars on the tape should change colour to demonstrate full penetration of the steam. Duration of exposure or temperature attained is not indicated by this type of indicator.

Chemical degradation tests

Hoskins (1981) has described a test which follows the degradation kinetics of 2,4-dihydroxybenzoic acid by u.v. spectrophotometry. Bunn & Sykes (1981) were able to calibrate Thermalog S indicator strips in terms of F_o unit in the temperature range 115–123°C. Thermalog S (produced by Bio Medical Sciences, Fairfield, USA) would appear to be a useful monitor for moist heat sterilization.

Ethylene oxide sterilization

The Royce sachet contains an indicator which changes colour on exposure to a given time/concentration of ethylene oxide.

Chemical dosimeters

These are used to monitor the quantity of the radiation dose in the use of radiation sterilization. Qualitative indicators of exposure to radiation are also available.

Physical validation and monitoring

In the UK, guidelines on the acceptability of a sterilization cycle are given in the Health Technical Memorandum 10 on sterilizers (DHSS). A Master Temperature Record (MTR) is prepared as part of the validation procedure for a particular autoclave and for each specified product and load configuration. This is then used as a reference for the process record obtained from a single thermocouple placed in a strategic part of each load (Temperature Recording Chart, TRC).

In Scotland the MTR is established on the evidence of three successful sterilization cycles as recorded on a 12-point recorder monitoring the cycle in various fixed situations. For example, ten thermocouples could be placed separately in containers distributed throughout the load, one thermocouple could be left free in the centre of the autoclave and one thermocouple should be placed in the chamber drain which is expected to represent the coolest spot. The MTR should be checked at annual intervals and whenever significant changes occur in the TRC when compared with the MTR.

It is likely that microprocessor controlled sterilization cycles will replace the MTR approach to controlling sterilization cycles. This is because the microprocessor gives the possibility of a much tighter control and description of sterilization cycles than comparison of the TRC with the MTR as used at present in the UK.

Conclusion

From the foregoing it can be seen that the factors affecting sterilization include:

Factors relating to the bioburden. These are concerned with the initial number of organisms present, their heat resistance and in growth requirements.

Factors relating to the sterilization process. These are concerned with the method chosen, the probability of sterilization which is related to the overall lethality or efficiency of the process and the methods of validating and monitoring the sterilization processes.

Factors relating to the product to be sterilized. These are concerned with the physical and chemical properties of the product. That is its solubility, hydrogen ion concentration and nutritive properties and in particular its stability to heat and moisture.

In addition, it should be mentioned that the properties of the container are interrelated with the factors relating to the sterilization process and those relating to the product.

BIBLIOGRAPHY

Aulton M E (ed) 1988 Pharmaceutics: the science of dosage form design. Churchill Livingstone, Edinburgh
Block S S 1983 Disinfection, sterilization and preservation, 3rd edn. Lea and Febiger, Philadelphia
Bowie J H, Kelsey J C, Thompson G R 1963 The Bowie and Dick autoclave tape test. Lancet i: 586–587
British Pharmacopoeia 1988 London, HMSO
Buhlmann X, Gay M, Schiller I 1973 Test objects containing *Bacillus stearothermophilus* spores for the monitoring of antimicrobial treatment in steam autoclaves. Pharmacetica Acta Helvetiae 48: 223–244

Bunn J N, Sykes I K 1981 A chemical indicator for the rapid measurement of F values. Journal of Applied Bacteriology 51: 143–147
European Pharmacopoeia 1980 2nd edn. Maisonneuve S.A., Saint Ruffine, France
Health Technical Memorandum 1980 No. 10 London, HMSO
Heintz M T, Urban S, Schiller I, Gay M, Buhlmann X 1976 The production of spores of *Bacillus stearothermophilus* with constant resistance to heat and their use as biological indicators during the development

of aqueous solutions for injection. Pharmaceutica Acta
Helvetiae 51: 137–143

Hoskins H T 1981 Physical and chemical monitoring with
reliability techniques in steriliser management. Journal of
Parenteral Science and Technology 35: 285–292

Kirk B, Hambleton R, Everett M 1982 Computer aided
autoclave monitoring. Pharmaceutical Journal 299: 252–254

Kirk B, Hambleton R, Hoskins H T 1985 A model for
predicting the stability of autoclaved pharmaceuticals

using real time computer integration techniques. Journal
of Parenteral Science and Technology 39: 89–98

Perkins J J 1969 Principles and methods of sterilization, 2nd
edn. Thomas, Springfield, IL

Reich R R, Whitbourne J E, McDaniel A W 1979 Effect of
storage conditions on the performance of Bacillus
stearothermophilus biological indicators. Journal of the
Parenteral Drug Association 33: 228–234

United States Pharmacopeia 1985 XXI. Mack, Easton, PA

20. Heat sterilization

R. M. E. Richards

THERMAL DESTRUCTION OF MICRO-ORGANISMS

The killing of micro-organisms by heat is a function of the time-temperature combination used. If the temperature is increased then the time required for a given kill is decreased. The vital constituents of living matter such as proteins and nucleic acids are denatured with increasing rapidity as the temperature rises above 50°C. Although the mechanism of thermally induced death is not fully understood the traditional theory has been that death results from heat inactivation of vital enzyme systems within the cell.

The consensus of opinion in the literature indicates that bacterial death by moist heat is due to denaturation and coagulation of essential protein molecules, whereas dry heat appears to cause protein denaturation by oxidation processes. The mechanisms of action of dry and wet heat are certainly different. This is emphasized by the finding that *Bacillus subtilis* var. *niger* spores can resist dry heat at 121°C for nearly 2000 times longer than they resist moist heat at 121°C. However, moist heat only contains approximately seven times more energy than hot air at the same temperature. Thus the factor of 2000 cannot be adequately explained solely in terms of the extra energy content of moist heat.

MOIST HEAT STERILIZATION

The sterilization method of choice for aqueous preparations and for surgical dressings is heating in saturated steam under pressure. A number of time/temperature combinations have been proposed. The USP XX1 and BP 1988 recommended 121°C maintained throughout the load for 15 minutes as the preferred combination.

Principles of sterilization by steam under pressure

Pressure itself has no sterilizing power. Steam is used under pressure as a means of achieving an elevated temperature. It is important to ensure that steam of the correct quality is used in order to avoid the problems which follow incorrect removal of air, superheating of the steam, failure of steam penetration into porous loads, etc. A detailed account of the properties of steam is given in the companion volume (Chapter 30, Aulton 1988).

Steam production

This may be achieved in two ways. On a small scale, steam may be generated from water within the sterilizer and because water is present the steam is known as wet saturated steam. For large-scale sterilizers, dry saturated steam may be piped from a separate boiler.

Saturated and supersaturated steam

Steam is described as saturated when it is at a temperature corresponding to the liquid boiling point appropriate to its pressure. Important properties of saturated steam are illustrated by reference to Figure 20.1.

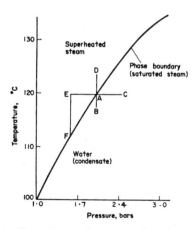

Fig. 20.1 Phase diagram for water and steam

The phase boundary is obtained by joining points representing saturated steam temperatures at different pressures, e.g. 115°C at 172 kPa (1.7 bar), 121°C at 202 kPa (2 bar) and 134°C 304 kPa (3 bar). If saturated steam at 'A' is isolated from water and heated without change of pressure 'A' to 'D', or the pressure is lowered without change of temperature 'A' to 'E', then the steam must become hotter because there is no water from which further evaporation can occur. Therefore it is no longer at the temperature corresponding to the liquid boiling point appropriate to its pressure and it is called *superheated* steam. Superheat is to be avoided because as steam becomes more superheated it becomes more like hot air and therefore less effective as a sterilizing medium. Very slight cooling will not make superheated steam condense. Before this can occur the temperature must be reduced to the temperature of the corresponding saturated steam point. That is 'D' to 'A' or 'E' to 'F' on the diagram. Superheated steam can arise from several sources but sterilizer jacket heat is the predominant source and the problem is caused when the jacket is hotter than the steam in the chamber. This is an example of a problem occurring similar to that involving point 'D' in Figure 20.1. Care should be taken to ensure that the jacket and the chamber temperatures are similar.

Now consider again the *saturated* steam at point 'A'. As soon as the steam is cooled at constant pressure, e.g. from 'A' to 'B', it will deposit water. (The same would happen if the pressure was raised to point 'C' without alteration of temperature.) The condensation of saturated steam on cooling liberates all of its latent heat immediately and this a very important property in sterilization.

Heat energy in steam is in the form of *sensible heat* and *latent heat*. Sensible heat is the heat required to raise the temperature of water and latent heat (of vaporization) is the amount of heat required to convert water at its boiling point to steam at the same temperature. Table 20.1 illustrates the high percentage of total heat that is latent heat at various temperatures.

Table 20.1 Heat content of steam at various pressures

Pressure (kPa) (bar)		Temperature (°C)	Heat		
			Sensible (kJ/kg)	Latent (kJ/kg)	Latent to total (%)
172	1.7	115	483	2216	82
202	2.0	121	505	2202	81
242	2.4	126	530	2185	80
304	3.0	134	561	2164	79

The advantages of saturated steam include:

Penetration. It flows quickly to every article in the load (and into porous articles). This is due to its contraction to a very small volume on condensation creating a low-pressure region into which more steam flows.

Rapid heating. It heats the load rapidly due to the release of its considerable latent heat.

Moist heat. The condensate produced on cooling contributes to the lethality by coagulating microbial protein.

No residual toxicity. The product is free from toxic contamination.

Presence of air

Air occupies the space in the sterilizer before steam is generated or admitted. Air is also present dissolved in water before its conversion to steam. Air allowed to remain in the sterilizer forms a thin layer which clings to every surface on which steam condensation occurs. Since air is a poor conductor it provides a barrier to heat penetration. In small sterilizers turbulence is likely to disperse the air film but in large sterilizers effective air removal is vital.

Wet steam

Wet steam contains less heat that dry saturated steam and is harmful to dressings.

THE DESIGN AND OPERATION OF AUTOCLAVES

The word autoclave means self-closing. Originally this referred to the closing of the lid by the excess pressure within the vessel. Modern usage of the word is rather wider and it is often used for modern sterilizing equipment which is not necessarily self-closing.

Portable autoclaves

These may be used for laboratory work and for small-scale production. They are generally of two types, pressure regulated and temperature regulated.

In a pressure-controlled type the pressure gauge is the sole indicator of the internal conditions and therefore all the air must be removed before the sterilizing exposure time begins.

In the temperature-controlled type shown in Figure 20.2 a thermometer or thermostat is used to indicate or ensure respectively that exposure temperature has been reached and it is less essential to expel the air. The recommended holding time/temperature relationship is 121°C for 15 minutes achieved at a pressure of 200 kPa

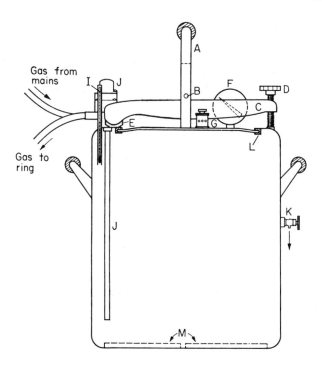

Fig. 20.2 Temperature-controlled portable autoclave (diagrammatic). A, Handle of lid; B, rivet; C, crossbar; D, thumbscrew; E, pad; F, pressure gauge; G, safety valve; I, thermometer; J, thermostat; K, air vent; L, gasket; M, semicircular plates.

(2.0 bar). Other recommended time/temperature relationships are listed in Table 20.2.

Large sterilizers

The essential features of a large sterilizer are shown diagrammatically in Figure 20.3 and will be used in the following general description. While the basic features are common to all types of sterilizer, the manufacturer's literature should be consulted for details of the features of a particular model.

Table 20.2 Possible time/temperature relationships for saturated steam sterilization

Temperature (°C)	Corresponding nominal pressure			Minimum (holding time (min)
	(kPa)abs	(lbf/in²)g	(bar) abs	
115–116	172	10	1.7	30
121–123	202	15	2.0	15
126–129	242	20	2.4	10
134–138	304	32	3.0	3

Note: Pressures expressed in kgf/cm² and lbf/in² are expressed as 'gauge' (g), i.e. in excess of atmospheric, and in kPa and bar as absolute (abs) pressures.

General procedure

1. Load material to be sterilized and close door.
2. Remove air.
3. Admit dry saturated steam (venting and condensate removal automatic).
4. Allow for heating up and expose for required duration.
5. Cut off steam supply.
6. Allow to cool (or spray cool if appropriate).

1. Loading. This should be carried out so that heat distribution within the load is optimal and will vary with the type of load, e.g. bottles, plastic containers, dressings, etc.

2. Remove air. This may be achieved by downward displacement by admitting steam at the top of the sterilizer and allowing air to escape through the discharge channel L in Figure 20.3. An alternative method is to apply a high vacuum (2.5 kPa, 25 mbar) to remove the air before the entry of the steam. This is particularly useful for porous loads since it aids steam penetration.

3. Admit dry saturated steam. In order to reduce the moisture content of steam delivered from the boiler the

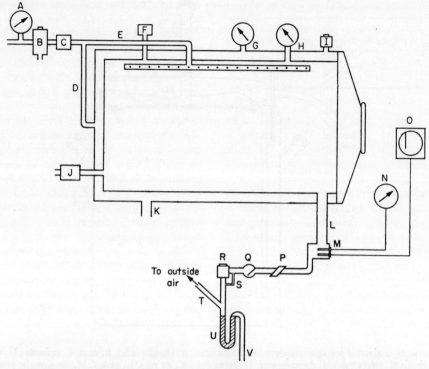

Fig. 20.3 Diagrammatic representation of the features of a large steam sterilizer (for simplicity, the control valves have been omitted). A, Mains pressure gauge; B, separator; C, reducing valve; D, steam supply to jacket; B, steam supply to chambers; F, air filter; G, jacket pressure gauge; H, chamber pressure gauge; I, jacket air vent; J, vacuum pump; K, jacket discharge channel (detail not shown); L, chamber discharge channel; M, thermometer pocket; N, direct-reading thermometer; O, recording thermometer; P, strainer; Q, check valve; R, balanced-pressure thermostatic trap; S, by-pass; T, vapour escape line; U, water seal; V, air-break

steam is passed through a separator (B in Fig. 20.3) which collects suspended condensate. The reducing valve C lowers the pressure to the required level and in doing so effects further drying.

Special requirements for plastic containers. For plastic containers there is an additional requirement for an over-pressure inside the autoclave chamber to prevent the containers from bursting during the sterilization cycle. The excess chamber pressure required will depend on the type and design of the container and the amount of residual air remaining inside the container after filling.

Automatic removal of condensate. Large volumes of condensate are produced, particularly during the heat-up cycle. Condensate runs down to the bottom of the chamber and drains through the same discharge channel as the air. A check valve and trap are incorporated to prevent suck-back contamination of the chamber on cooling.

4. Expose for required duration. At least two temperature-sensing devices should be used. One should be placed in the discharge channel and one in a container or in part of the load in a strategic place (i.e. that predicted to be the coolest) in the chamber (see Ch. 19).

5. Cut off steam supply.

6. Allow to cool. The method used for cooling depends on the type of load.

a. Fluid containers. Fluid containers cool very slowly because of the large heat capacity and because the containers may burst if the sterilizer is opened at too high a temperature. Cooling time may be reduced by using a very fine mist of cold water (50–100 μm diameter droplets) sprayed over the containers. Table 20.3 shows the time savings with forced cooling. Compressed air is admitted to the bottom of the chamber to compensate for the pressure drop caused by the condensation of steam. For plastic containers spray cooling must take place under air ballast to maintain an

Table 20.3 Time for contents to fall from 115°C to 95°C

Load	Without water cooling	With water cooling
24 × 500 ml bottles	3 h	10 min
200 × 1 litre bottles	22 h	17 min

excess pressure outside the bag in order to avoid bursting. Problems may arise if the spray water is contaminated and/or if the closures of the fluid containers are rendered ineffective by the sterilization process.

Autoclaves have recently been commissioned in Holland which are heated and cooled by the same re-circulating water passing through a suitable heat exchanger. The water is introduced through many small holes at the top of the autoclave and removed from the bottom of the autoclave. The pressure within the autoclave is maintained at a slightly higher pressure than the calculated pressure within the glass bottles or plastic containers. It is important with this type of autoclave to monitor the rate of water flow through the auto-

clave to check that it is maintained within the desired range.

Figure 20.4 represents the autoclave pressure (highest recorded line on the graph), hottest container temperature (second highest line), coldest container temperature (the lowest recorded line), together with the lethality for each of these temperatures. The record is produced in multicoloured graphical form by a linked micro-computer. This graph then forms the batch record.

b. Porous loads. Porous loads are wet at the end of the exposure period due to absorbed condensate and must be dried. This is best achieved by application of high vacuum. A vacuum pump is used to remove the steam and to reduce the pressure back to 2.5 kPa (25 mbar) in about 3 minutes. Under these conditions the moisture content of the dressings is only slightly greater than before sterilization.

The air used for breaking the vacuum after drying must be sterile.

Older methods of drying the load include radiation from the sterilizer jacket, low vacuum with no air and using a steam ejector to suck warm filtered air through the load.

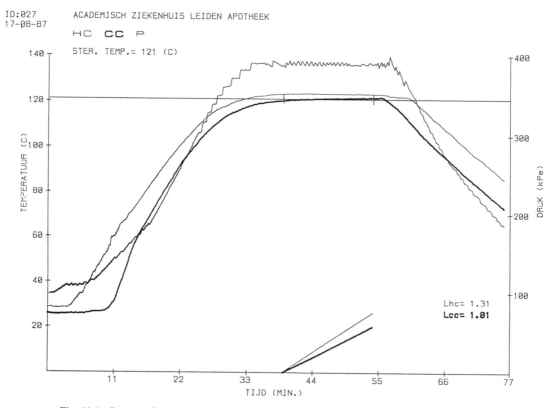

Fig. 20.4 Record of autoclave pressure and container temperature during a sterilization cycle

Hydrostatic continuous sterilizers

The need for the production of large batches of sterilized fluids has lead to the development of continuous sterilizers, represented diagrammatically in Figure 20.5. Containers are fed automatically onto an endless conveyor that carries them up and down a series of towers 17 m high. The containers are subjected in turn to preheating, sterilizing, water cooling and spray cooling before leaving the sterilizer.

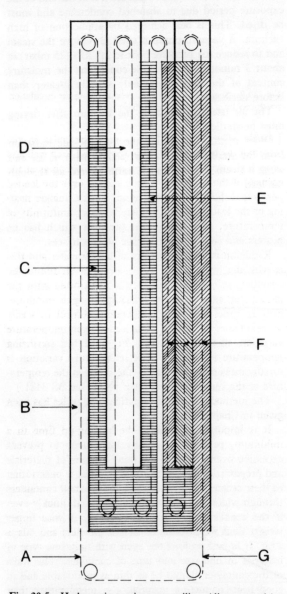

Fig. 20.5 Hydrostatic continuous sterilizer (diagrammatic). A, Infeed point; B, conveyor; C, hydrostatic preheating leg; D, sterilizing tower; E, hydrostatic cooling leg; F, spray cooling leg; G, discharge point

Automatic control of steam sterilizers

Most large sterilizers are operated under automatic control and may offer a series of 'programmes' for different types of load. It is essential that pressure and temperature recordings are checked for each cycle to ensure that no malfunction has occurred and that the selected conditions have been achieved.

Control by microprocessor

The microprocessor offers the facility to monitor and to control the steam sterilization process with a high degree of accuracy (Burrel et al 1979, Klieman 1982, Kirk et al 1982). A microprocessor can be used to control the steam inlet valve of a sterilizer in order to achieve a sterilization cycle profile which matches a 'model profile' chosen for a particular type of load.

The principles and practice of moist heat sterilization are also discussed in Chapters 25 and 43, respectively, of the companion volume (Aulton, 1988).

DRY HEAT STERILIZATION

This process may be used for heat-stable non-aqueous preparations, powders and certain impregnated dressings. It may also be used for some types of container.

Sterilization by dry heat is usually carried out in a hot-air oven in which heat is transferred from its source to the load by radiation, convection and to a small extent by conduction.

Published evidence on the temperature/time exposures necessary to kill pathogens by dry heat indicates that 90 min at 100°C will destroy all vegetative bacteria but that 3 hours at 140°C is needed for resistant spores.

Mould spores are of intermediate resistance and are killed by 90 minutes at 115°C. Most viruses have a resistance similar to vegetative bacteria but some viruses are known that are as resistant as bacterial spores, e.g. the virus that causes homologous serum jaundice.

Recommended time-temperature combinations

Different combinations are required for different products. Cycles recommended in the BP 1988 are:

— A minimum of 180°C for not less than 30 minutes.
— A minimum of 170°C for not less than 1 hour.
— A minimum of 160°C for not less than 2 hours.

Treatment at 250°C for 45 minutes is a useful method for preparation of glass containers intended for large-volume parenteral dosage forms since this is considered to be effective in denaturing pyrogens adsorbed onto the surface of the glassware.

In each cycle it is important to ensure that the whole of the contents of each container is maintained for an effective combination of time and temperature and especially to allow for temperature variations in hot-air ovens which may be considerable.

Design and operation of the hot-air oven

Ovens suitable for dry heat sterilization should be specially designed for the purpose and equipped with forced air circulation. The relevant British Standard is BS 3421:1961 and Figure 20.6 illustrates an appropriate type of hot-air oven. It consists of an aluminium or stainless steel chamber separated from the outer case by a thick layer of glass fibre insulation. The hollow, flanged door is also filled with insulation and carries an asbestos gasket that provides a tight seal. The reflecting inner surfaces, the lagging and the gasket all help to prevent heat losses. In the best designs of oven the electric heaters are fixed to the outside of the chamber in positions chosen to prevent cool spots anywhere inside. Only a small amount of the heat is transferred from the heat source to the articles in a hot-air oven by conduction because of the limited pathways and small areas of contact. Convection is responsible for more heat transfer but this is not a very efficient process. Maximum use of the heating capacity of the air is made by circulating with a fan in order to have the maximum number of air molecules collide with the load and hot chamber surfaces. In addition, pockets of stagnant cool air are prevented. Figure 20.7 shows the fan fitted to project from the back of the chamber and in front of the fan is

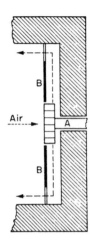

Fig. 20.7 Section of rear of an oven showing air circulation produced by a fan. A, Fan; B, false back

a baffle. The air is sucked through the holes in the centre of the baffle, passed over the heated back wall and propelled towards the door through the openings at the corners of the baffles. It is then sucked over the loaded perforated shelves to the fan again. Thus a quicker heating of the load is achieved, there is better uniformity of temperature, particularly near the door which has no heaters and so is cooler than the other surfaces.

Radiation is the chief source of heat transfer and this is why the heaters need to be arranged all round the chamber. It is useful to have the oven fitted with the facility for automatic boost heating to give minimum heat-up times. Accurate temperature control by easily set regulators is essential. The loaded oven temperature variation should not exceed 5°C once the sterilizing temperature is reached. (The temperature variation is usually measured as the difference between the temperature at the centre and any other point; see BS 3421.)

The method of validating sterilization cycles has been given in Chapter 20.

It is important to reduce the heating-up time to a minimum, partly for economy but chiefly to prevent excessive overheating of the outer regions of materials and preparations during the time that heat is penetrating to their centres. The best way is to use small containers through which the heat will be transferred quickly even if the containers are poor conductors. A wise upper weight limit for substances such as powders and oils is 25 g. It is best to load the oven with only one type of material in one size and type of container. The walls of the container should be as thin as practicable and of good heat-conducting material, e.g. metal rather than glass for powders. Tins should be blackened or dull to absorb and not reflect heat and, as a general rule, all containers should be either tall and narrow (e.g. a long

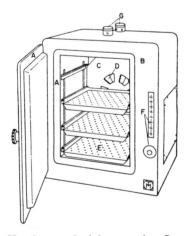

Fig. 20.6 Hot-air oven. A, Asbestos gasket; B, outer case containing glass-fibre insulation, and heaters in chamber wall; C, false wall; D, fan; E, perforated shelf; F, regulator; G, vents.

cylindrical tin) or shallow and very wide (e.g. a Petri dish) so that heat can penetrate rapidly in one direction. Glassware must be cleaned thoroughly because heat transfer will be impaired if the surface is coated with a greasy film.

Because articles sterilized by dry heat are not often used immediately, precautions must be taken to ensure that they are sterile when used. For example, glass pipettes, because they are dipped in sterile liquids, must be externally as well as internally sterile and therefore they are completely wrapped in paper or packed in tubes of card, metal or glass. Items such as glass vessels need protection at the mouth only and this can be given with a metal cap. Containers of products to be sterilized are sealed with a screw cap having a suitable liner.

After suitable packaging the containers are arranged on the oven shelves taking the following into account.

1. Spacing to allow air movement, radiation from the oven walls to reach the product and to prevent contact of articles with the sides of the oven.

2. Packing of small items in large tins should be avoided. The air inside the tin cannot easily escape and acts as an efficient insulator of the contents. It is better to wrap such things as Petri dishes in twos or threes.

3. Screw caps should be loosened half a turn to prevent distortion of the closure or bursting of the container.

Table 20.4 Advantages and disadvantages of saturated steam and hot air for sterilization processes

Saturated steam		Hot air	
Advantages	Disadvantages	Advantages	Disadvantages
1. High heat content plus rapid heat transfer	Unsuitable for anhydrous materials such as powders and oils	It can be used for substances that would be harmed by moisture, e.g. oily materials and powders	Low heat content and low heat transfer
2. Destroys micro-organisms more efficiently than dry heat (lethal action of water plus heat) and therefore a shorter exposure at a lower temperature is possible	It cannot be used for thermolabile substances	It causes less damage to glass and metal (except for sharp instruments) than moist heat	Most medicaments, rubbers and plastics are too thermolabile for sterilization by this method
3. It can be used for a large proportion of injections, ophthalmic solutions, irrigants dialysis fluids, etc.	It does not destroy pyrogens	It is suitable for sterilizing glass containers and equipment and can be used to destroy pyrogens on materials such as glass	It cannot be used for aqueous solutions
4. It rapidly penetrates porous materials and is therefore very suitable for sterilizing surgical dressings and materials		It does not contaminate materials with toxic substances	It cannot be used for surgical dressings
5. The process is adaptable for plastic containers and some other special dosage forms			Accurate control of the process parameters is more difficult than for dry saturated steam
6. It is more suitable than dry heat for sharp instruments			
7. Accurate control and monitoring of the process is possible			
8. No toxic contaminants are left in the materials sterilized			

The temperature recorders are checked, the vents on top of the oven closed, the door shut, the heaters and fan switched on. When the thermometer/temperature recorder shows that the oven air has reached the required temperature the appropriate exposure is given to include lag time and sterilization time. After switching off, the door is left closed until the temperature has fallen to 40°C in order to prevent breakages. The bottle caps are tightened.

A hot-air oven should have a door lock or accidental openings of the door may occur. Automatic control is easy to achieve consisting of a suitable device to start the timing when the required temperature is reached and to switch off the heating after the appropriate exposure including lag time has been given. A record of the temperature and time should be available for each sterilization cycle.

The infra-red conveyor oven

Infra-red radiation is thermal radiation, i.e. when absorbed its energy is converted to heat and therefore it is often known as radiant heat. The infra-red conveyor oven makes maximum use of this highly efficient means of heat transfer which is conveyed instantly and constantly from the source to the load and is virtually unaffected by the thermal resistance of static surface air films.

This type of oven can be used for small items such as glass syringes but, with the increased use of disposable plastic syringes, is becoming obsolete.

The principles and practice of dry heat sterilization are also discussed in Chapters 25 and 43, repectively, of the companion volume (Aulton 1988).

HEATING WITH A BACTERICIDE

This method has been used for sterilizing aqueous solutions that are too thermolabile to withstand normal autoclaving conditions but that can withstand heating to 98–100°C for 30 minutes in the presence of a bactericidal substance. A bactericide compatible with the product, container and closure was chosen and because of the potential toxic effects of the bactericide in the patient, the method was precluded for many parenteral and ophthalmic products. This method of sterilization is no longer recognized by the BP 1988.

APPLICATIONS OF HEAT STERILIZATION

Moist heat

Dry saturated steam under pressure is used in the sterilization of the following:

1. *Aqueous parenteral solutions and suspensions* — 121°C 15 min recommended, i.e. a total lethality (F_o, see Ch. 19) of not less than 8.
2. *Surgical dressings and fabrics* — 134°C 3 min recommended.
3. *Plastic and rubber closures* — if sterilized separately from the containers.
4. *Metal instruments* — immediate drying required to protect against corrosion.
5. *Glass apparatus and containers* — if unable to withstand dry heat, e.g. rubber parts.

Dry heat

Dry heat is used to sterilize:

1. *Glassware* — pre-washing in apyrogenic water is required.
2. *Porcelain and metal equipment.*
3. *Oils and fats* — including oily injections.
4. *Powders* — including natural products, e.g. talc, which may contain resistant spores. Severe heat treatment will destroy pyrogens, e.g. in sodium chloride.

Advantages and disadvantages of moist-heat and dry-heat sterilization

The relative advantages and disadvantages of saturated steam and hot air for sterilization processes are summarized in Table 20.4.

BIBLIOGRAPHY

Aulton M E (ed) 1988 Pharmaceutics: the science of dosage form design. Churchill Livingstone, Edinburgh
Block S S 1983 Disinfection, sterilization and preservation, 3rd edn. Lea and Febiger, Philadelphia
British Pharmacopoeia 1988. London, HMSO
British Standard 3421 1961 Performance of electrically heated sterilising ovens. British Standards Institution, London
Burrel R L, Wein R Z, Parisi A N 1979 SCOT (Sterilisation Computer Operating Terminal) for sterilisation control and monitor. Journal of the Parenteral Drug Association 33: 363–370
Coles J, Tedree R L 1972 Contamination of autoclaved fluids

with cooling water. Pharmaceutical Journal 209: 193–195

Higgins D 1972 Contamination of fluids in spray-cooled autoclaves. Pharmaceutical Journal 209: 306

Health Technical Memorandum 1980 No. 10. Sterilisers. HMSO, London

Kirk B, Hambleton R, Everett M 1982, Computer-aided autoclave monitoring. Pharmaceutical Journal 229: 252–254

Klieman L A 1982 Computer controlled sterilisation. Drug and Cosmetic Industry 130: 46–52, 106

Myers J A 1972 Faulty bottles for sterile fluids. Pharmaceutical Journal 208: 518

Myers J A, Keall A 1972 MRC bottles for sterile infusion fluids. Pharmaceutical Journal 209: 306–307

Perera R 1972 Autoclaving problems. Pharmaceutical Journal 208: 469

Perkins J J 1969 Principles and methods of sterilisation, 2nd edn. Thomas, Springfield, IL

Pharmaceutical Codex 1979, 11th edn (incorporating the British Pharmaceutical Codex). Pharmaceutical Press, London

Phillips I, Eykyn S, Laker M 1972 Outbreak of hospital infection caused by contaminated autoclaved fluids. Lancet i: 1258–1260

Raine G 1972 Contamination of bottled fluids. Pharmaceutical Journal 208: 568

United States Pharmacopeia 1985 XXI. Mack, Easton, PA

21. Non-heat methods of sterilization

R. M. E. Richards

Alternative methods to heat sterilization must be employed for heat-labile materials. Gaseous sterilization and sterilization by ionizing radiations are two possible alternatives. A third option is sterilization by filtration.

The latter is really an aseptic process and is discussed in Chapter 22. The principles and practice of non-heat methods of sterilization are discussed further in Chapters 25 and 43 of the companion volume (Aulton 1988).

GASEOUS STERILIZATION

Ethylene oxide

Ethylene oxide is the only gas that is successfully used on a large scale for industrial and medical applications. It is the simplest cyclic ether and has the formula

$$CH_2 \diagdown_{O} \diagup CH_2$$

At room temperature it is a colourless gas with a characteristic ethereal odour. It can be liquified easily and the liquid boils at 10.8°C. The main advantage of ethylene oxide is that many types of materials can be sterilized without damage. Another advantage is its diffusivity which gives it the ability to sterilize terminally the final product through packaging material and containers and afterwards to diffuse out of the material in a reverse process. However, there are complicating factors to the use of ethylene oxide such as toxicity, combustibility and the need for correct humidity of the gas–air mixtures. In addition, ethylene oxide is more expensive to use than heat. Toxicity includes inhalation toxicity, which causes nausea and vomiting, and skin toxicity as an irritant causing chemical burns. The latter occurs when materials have not been given a sufficient airing and are put into use too soon after sterilization has been completed, e.g. rubber gloves. This type of hazard is overcome by ensuring that those involved with the process are knowledgeable in using ethylene oxide. The inflammability is overcome by preparing special formulations of ethylene oxide mixed with inert gases such as carbon dioxide or various fluorinated hydrocarbons. The resulting mixtures can in turn be mixed with air in all proportions without any risk of explosion. A mixture known as Cryoxide is used in North America and contains 11% w/w ethylene oxide, 79% of trichlorofluoromethane (known in the UK as Arcton 11) and 10% of dichlorodifluoromethane (Arcton 12). In the UK Sterethox is available commercially and contains 12% ethylene oxide with 88% of Arcton 12.

Carbon dioxide has a high vapour pressure and consequently there is less ethylene oxide in the vapour when carbon dioxide is used compared with Arcton 11 and 12, which have vapour pressures approximately 1/50 and 1/10 of carbon dioxide respectively.

Antimicrobial activity

Ethylene oxide is active against all micro-organisms and there is only a relatively small difference between the concentrations necessary to kill vegetative bacteria and spores in the same exposure time. The ratio is 1:5 which is much less than the $1:10^3$ ratio for liquid disinfectants. *Bacillus subtilis* var. *niger* is one of the most resistant organisms to the action of ethylene oxide and is used in validating and monitoring ethylene oxide sterilization cycles (see Ch. 19).

Factors affecting sterilization

Sterilization efficiency is determined by (i) the humidity of the sterilizing atmosphere and in particular the state of hydration of the micro-organisms, (ii) the temperature of sterilization, (iii) the concentration of ethylene oxide and time of exposure and (iv) the penetrability of the load. These are discussed below in turn.

Relative humidity of sterilizing atmosphere

This is the most important parameter affecting the sterilizing efficiency of all gaseous sterilizing agents.

Under conditions which allow the materials to equilibrate with respect to the environment a relative humidity (r.h.) of 33% at 25°C was found to be optimal. In actual practice a higher r.h. is generally required. This is because sterilization processes are usually carried out at higher than normal room temperatures. If equilibrium with respect to r.h. has taken place at room temperature and the temperature of the materials to be sterilized is raised then conditions may be produced which are moisture deficient at the site of the microbial surfaces. Similar moisture-deficient conditions at the active sites may be produced if wrapping materials are used which present diffusion barriers to the moisture and optimum r.h. is produced only in the environment external to the packaging. Under such conditions the external r.h. must be in excess of 33% to provide a suitable driving force for the diffusion of moisture across the barrier in order to achieve optimum conditions at the surfaces of the micro-organisms. In practice the r.h. in the chamber atmosphere is usually raised to between 40% and 50%. This allows for absorption of moisture by materials in the load and creates a concentration gradient which increases the rate of diffusion through wrappings.

Moisture is also necessary during the pre-vacuum period of the sterilization cycle. Otherwise when the vacuum is applied dry spores could be dehydrated further and rendered resistant to the action of ethylene oxide.

Temperature of sterilization

Sterilization can be achieved at room temperature but a long exposure time is necessary. In practice, advantage is usually taken of the decrease in sterilization time with rise in temperature. Within the range 5–40°C this approximates to a halving of the sterilization time for each increase of 17°C. Since gas sterilization is used for thermolabile materials, very high temperatures are impracticable and 60°C can be regarded as the upper limit.

Concentration of ethylene oxide and time of exposure

Usually concentrations are expressed in mg/litre because the sterilization rate depends on the partial pressure of ethylene oxide which is determined by the amount in the specified volume of the chamber atmosphere. Concentrations used for sterilization range from 250 to 1000 mg/litre. If the concentration is doubled the exposure time necessary is approximately halved.

A manufacturer of ethylene oxide sterilizers recommends, for most purposes, exposure to 850–900 mg/litre for 3 h, or 450 mg/litre for 5 h, at 54°C.

Penetrability of ethylene oxide through the load

Ethylene oxide possesses the ability to penetrate paper, fabrics, a number of plastics and rubber. Therefore materials can be sterilized suitably packaged in appropriate containers. It is nevertheless important to ensure that the articles for gaseous sterilization are scrupulously clean. Organic matter reduces the efficiency of the process but does not prevent it. However, occlusion of organisms within crystals prevents the diffusion of moisture completely (Royce & Bowler 1961). Ernst & Doyle (1968) found that spores protected in this way resisted sterilization by exposure to steam, ethylene oxide or dry heat under conditions which would normally effect sterilization. Therefore care needs to be taken to prevent physical protection of micro-organisms in gas-impermeable deposits.

In addition to effectively penetrating many materials, ethylene oxide is also strongly absorbed by a wide variety of substances. This means that the sterilized articles should not be used until the absorbed gas has escaped or desorbed. Desorption can be achieved in several ways. Airing the materials in a well-ventilated room for a pre-determined time is commonly employed. An alternative is to apply a powerful vacuum immediately after sterilization, e.g. 1.5 kPa (15 mbar) for 2 hours. A third method is to apply a partial vacuum to about 20 kPa (0.2 bar) and then admit sterile air to atmospheric pressure as a flushing agent. This is repeated five or six times.

Ethylene oxide sterilizers

The following is a general outline of the more important features of sterilizer design and use.

Design

The features of suitable equipment include:

1. An exposure chamber that is gas tight and able to withstand high pressure and vacuum.

2. A means of heating the chamber, e.g. a steam or hot water jacket or heating elements clipped to the outside. In some types of sterilizer the load is heated and humidified by injecting steam into the chamber.

3. A baffled inlet of the gas mixture, usually at the bottom of the chamber. The baffle protects the contents from liquid ethylene oxide introduced accidentally. The liquid can badly damage certain plastics.

4. A method of completely vaporizing the gas mixture and warming it to the sterilizing temperature.

5. A means of extracting air before, and the gas mix-

ture after, sterilization. A high-efficiency pump is desirable. It should discharge to the open air.

6. A system for adding water to provide the right humidity. Also see 2 above.

7. Provision for the admission of sterile air at the end of the process.

8. A safety valve and suitable indicators and recorders of pressure and temperature. Automatic control is advisable because of the significant effects of alterations in temperature and humidity.

As with steam sterilization, the problem of accurate and sensitive measurement of humidity has not been satisfactorily solved.

Method of use

1. The chamber is loaded.

2. Sufficient water is introduced to prevent vacuum dehydration of micro-organisms. The sterilization time is significantly reduced if the load is humidified prior to gas admission. Hence, if gas and moisture are introduced together sterilization time is lengthened.

3. The door is closed and the temperature raised to sterilization level unless exposure is to be carried out at room temperature. When an increased temperature is used the load must be at the correct temperature throughout before the gas is admitted and timing of the sterilization exposure is begun. Steam injection rapidly raises the load to sterilization temperature, but heating up by a steam jacket or by external heaters is very slow.

4. The heat-exchanger is raised to a high temperature (about 100°C) because the gas mixture falls to well below room temperature as it leaves the cylinder.

5. A high-efficiency vacuum pump is used to reduce the air pressure in the chamber to about 1.5 kPa (15 mbar). On a small scale the gas may be used to displace the air but this method is wasteful and insufficiently reliable for large loads.

6. If necessary, more water is added to produce a satisfactory exposure humidity.

7. The warmed gas mixture is admitted until the correct pressure is reached.

8. The exposure time is allowed.

9. The gas is desorbed by one of the three methods mentioned previously and in each instance the vacuum is broken by admitting sterile air.

Control of the process

Methods similar to those for steam sterilization have been used — physical, chemical and biological monitoring of the actual process followed by sterility testing of random samples from each load of sterilized material. The temperature and pressure should be recorded on a chart throughout the sterilization cycle.

However, physical monitoring using conventional instrumentation is not able to provide assurance that each item of the load has been subjected to the predetermined conditions of r.h. and gas concentration. Chemical monitoring is also inadequate in monitoring the all-important parameter of r.h. Therefore the biological monitoring is of major importance. The monitor is in the form of either paper strips impregnated with, or aluminium foil coated with, known concentrations (e.g. 10^6) of *Bacillus subtilis* var. *niger* spores (USP XXI 1985, BP 1988). Usually at least ten test packages of biological indicator are placed in the least gas-accessible parts of a number of articles and containers situated in different regions of the sterilizer. After exposure they are tested for sterility. A recorded check is made to ensure that all biological indicators have been removed from the load.

Applications of ethylene oxide sterilization

Ethylene oxide is suitable for sterilizing those powders where it is known that the micro-organisms are on the surface of the particles and not embedded inside them.

Equipment, instruments and articles made from plastic, rubber, metal and other materials can be sterilized with ethylene oxide without causing damage. Commercial processes have been developed for catheters and syringes. Other articles which are suitable include intravenous sets, prostheses, blood oxygenators, bottles and vials and polythene-covered stirrers for magnetic mixers.

Some plastics may be damaged. The surface of polystyrene may become crazed if an ethylene oxide/Arcton(s) mixture is used. Damage does not occur with pure ethylene oxide or mixtures with carbon dioxide. Contact with liquid ethylene oxide must always be avoided.

Fragile rubber articles survive more treatments with ethylene oxide than with steam.

Equipment such as cystoscopes, bronchoscopes, ophthalmoscopes and Geiger–Müller counters can also be sterilized with ethylene oxide.

Advantages of ethylene oxide sterilization

1. It is suitable for thermolabile substances because it can be carried out at room temperature or only slightly above.

2. It does not damage moisture-sensitive substances and equipment because only a low humidity is required. However, humidification by steam injection, which

produces a higher than normal humidity, is inadvisable when such materials and articles are being sterilized.

3. Provided the container is made from one of the many materials that are permeable to the gas, it can be used for pre-packed articles, because of the great penetrating power of ethylene oxide.

4. Although ethylene oxide is a highly reactive compound comparatively few materials are damaged by the process.

Disadvantages of ethylene oxide sterilization

1. It is slow. Long exposures and desorption periods are necessary and, therefore, it is unsuitable in emergencies, or for expensive equipment that must be frequently used.

2. Although small batches of materials can be successfully sterilized with simple equipment, large batches require very expensive, elaborately instrumented sterilizers that need skilled and regular maintenance.

3. The running costs are high.

4. The hazards of inflammability, general toxicity and vesicant action necessitate special precautions.

5. Toxic substances, such as ethylene chlorhydrin, are produced in some materials, particularly if, like the flexible PVC used for catheters, tubing and giving sets, they contain free chloride ions. As the amount of free chloride in PVC is increased by exposure to ionizing radiations, it is undesirable to use ethylene oxide for resterilizing previously irradiated PVC articles.

Conclusions

Ethylene oxide sterilization is less reliable and more expensive than steam sterilization and should never be used when the latter is practicable. To increase its reliability, microbial contamination of articles to be sterilized should be minimized.

Formaldehyde

Like ethylene oxide this is an alkylating agent but it is generally inferior for use as a sterilizing agent. This is because formaldehyde has poor penetrating power and is readily inactivated by organic matter. Furthermore, high concentrations are difficult to maintain in the atmosphere because it tends to deposit in the form of solid polymers on contact with cool surfaces. Nowadays the chief application of formaldehyde is the fumigation of empty air-flow cabinets and rooms to eliminate microbiological contamination from solid surfaces.

Pure formaldehyde cannot be kept at ordinary temperatures and so it is used either as Formaldehyde Solution (Formalin) BP, which is an approximately 37% w/w solution containing stabilizers to prevent deposition of solid polymers, or as tablets of paraformaldehyde. The gas is vaporized from these sources by heating devices or, in the case of formalin for fumigation, by the addition of potassium permanganate which produces heat by oxidation.

STERILIZATION BY RADIATIONS

Radiations can be divided into two groups which are known as electromagnetic waves and streams of particulate matter. In the former group are infrared radiation, ultraviolet light, X-rays and gamma rays. In the latter group are alpha and beta radiations.

Infrared radiation, ultraviolet light, gamma radiation and high-velocity electrons (a type of beta radiation) are used for sterilization.

Ultraviolet light, with a wavelength in the nanometer (nm) range, and gamma rays with a wavelength in the range $1-10^{-4}$ nm can both directly damage molecules vital to living cells. High-velocity electrons have a similar effect. As they pass through matter, both types of waves and the high-speed particles are each able to excite the planetary electrons surrounding the atomic nuclei. If the electrons acquire sufficient energy they escape from the atoms and ionization results. Both gamma rays and high-velocity electrons have high energy values, over 1.3 million electron-volts (1.3 MeV) and 4 MeV respectively. Both produce ionization and are therefore called ionizing radiations. Ionizing radiations are very effective sterilizing agents. Although ultraviolet light has relatively low energy (5 eV) and rarely causes ionization it does cause excitation of the atomic electrons. Excitation is not as potent a lethal effect as ionization but it nevertheless causes the death of micro-organisms.

Ultraviolet light

Only a narrow range of wavelength (220–280 nm) is effective in killing micro-organisms, and wavelengths close to 265 nm are the most effective. This is because wavelengths of 265 nm and adjacent wavelengths are strongly absorbed by nucleoproteins.

The main method of generating ultraviolet light for sterilization is by passing a low current at high voltage through mercury vapour in an evacuated tube made of borosilicate-type glass.

The intensity of ultraviolet radiation is expressed as the energy received by a specified area, usually in microwatts/mm^2. Intensities of from 10 to 60 μW/mm^2, depending on the type of bacterium, will reduce populations of vegetative cells by 90% in a short period of time. However, the most serious disadvantage of ultraviolet light as a sterilizing agent is its poor penetrating power. This is the result of strong absorption by many substances. Applications are therefore limited to the treatment of clean air and water in thin layers and of hard impermeable surfaces in situations where people are not subjected to direct or high-intensity reflected radiation. This latter precaution is necessary because bactericidal ultraviolet light causes eye problems and erythema of the skin.

Thus, in general, ultraviolet light should not be relied on for sterilization.

Ionizing radiations

Ionizing radiation suitable for commercial sterilization processes must have good penetrating power, high sterilizing efficiency, little or no damaging effect on irradiated materials and be capable of being produced efficiently. The radiations that best fulfill these four criteria are high-speed electrons from machines and gamma rays from radioactive isotopes.

High-speed electrons

This type of sterilizing radiation is most widely used in Denmark and the USA. In a machine known as a van de Graaff accelerator electrons are generated from a suitable source and then accelerated along a highly evacuated tube by a tremendous potential difference between the ends. The particles in the emergent beam are travelling at near to the speed of light and, depending on the accelerating voltage, have energies of from 5 MeV to 10 MeV. The beam, which is narrow and intense, is used to irradiate articles on a conveyor belt.

In England, the travelling wave linear accelerator, in which a different method of acceleration is used, has been developed.

Gamma rays

Most gamma-ray sterilization in this country is carried out at specialized irradiation plants. Radiation from the radioactive isotope of cobalt, ^{60}Co, is used as a source of gamma emission. Most of the disintegrating atoms of this isotope emit two gamma rays in succession (in cascade) which have energies of 1.33 MeV and 1.17 MeV. Therefore irradiated products are treated with gamma radiation having a mean energy of 1.25 MeV.

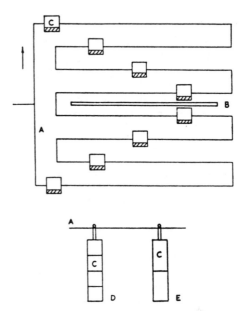

Fig. 21.1 Monorail system for sterilization by gamma radiation. A, Monorail; B, source plaque; C, packages (shown at only a few positions on the rail) — one side is shaded to illustrate exposure of opposite faces on two sides of the source; D, E, tiers of 4 and 2 packages respectively

^{60}Co has a half-life of 5.25 years. It is possible that eventually ^{60}Co will be replaced by the radioactive isotope of caesium, ^{137}Cs, which has a half-life of 30 years. This isotope is a major constituent of spent fuel rods from nuclear reactors. It could be utilized for commercial sterilization rather than being regarded as a waste disposal problem. It emits a gamma ray having an energy of 0.66 MeV. At present ^{137}Cs plus other disintegration products are used at Harwell for some commercial sterilization.

Articles for sterilization by radiation are packed in boxes of standard size which are suspended from a monorail and sterilized by slow passages around the gamma ray source (Fig. 21.1).

Mode of action

Ionizing radiations can cause excitations, ionizations and where water is present free radical formation. Free radicals are powerful oxidizing (OH, HO$_2$) and reducing (H) agents which are capable of damaging essential molecules in living cells. Thus all three processes cause disintegration of essential cell constituents such as enzymes and the DNA of the nuclear apparatus. This results in cell death.

Sterilizing dose

The dose is measured in kGy. The gray (Gy) is the SI equivalent to 100 rads. In the UK and the USA the recognized sterilizing dose is 25 kGy. The choice was based on experiments in which test pieces (e.g. paper discs or strips of plastic or foil, heavily contaminated with different types of organisms including vegetative bacteria, spores, pathogens and non-pathogens) were exposed to various doses of radiation. Absence of survivors after treatment with 25 kGy and the high margin of safety of the dose led to its selection. In fact, in North America a sterilizing dose of 18–22 kGy is sometimes used. This is based on a sterility assurance of not more than one item contaminated in one million.

As the inactivation of bacteria by radiation is exponential the probability of survivors after a particular dose can be calculated. With radiation, the D_{10} value (the decimal reduction dose) is the dose in Gy that reduces the number of viable organisms by a factor of 10. The D_{10} value for *Bacillus pumilis* spores irradiated in air is 1.7 kGy and, therefore, the inactivation factor for the recognized sterilizing dose is $10^{25/1.7} = 10^{15}$ (in the absence of air the factor falls to 10^7). *Bacillus pumilis* spores have been extensively used for investigating radiation sterilization because they are less susceptible to ionizing radiations than most other commonly occurring microbial cells.

Some non-pathogens show exceptionally high resistance to ionizing radiations. For example *Micrococcus radiodurans* has an inactivation factor of only 10^3 when exposed in meat to 25 kGy but, because it is harmless and of rare occurrence an increase of the recognized radiation dose is not considered necessary.

It should be noted, however, that in Denmark a sterilization dose of 45 kGy, is recommended. Apparently the evidence for such a high dose was obtained under artificial and not naturally occurring conditions or in practice conditions. For this reason other countries have kept the 25 kGy sterilization dose.

Sterilization time

The intense beam or pulses of electrons from accelerators can deliver a sterilization dose in a fraction of a second to a few seconds, depending on the size and density of the material or article being irradiated. With isotope sources, because of the diffuse and penetrating nature of their emissions, the dose rate is much less and therefore the sterilizing dose has to be accumulated over several days (e.g. 3 to $3\frac{1}{2}$). However, as partial compensation for this, the volume of material that can be exposed at the same time is much larger than with accelerators.

Control of the process

The actual radiation dose is checked by including dosimeters in packages. The most common type is a Perspex strip or disc containing a radiation-sensitive red dye. Irradiation causes changes in optical density which can be measured in a spectrophotometer and converted to dosage by reference to a calibration curve prepared with a standard source.

It is generally accepted that there is no purpose served in routinely using a biological indicator which is known to be killed by 25 kGy because this dose is accurately checked by the dosimeter.

Undesirable effects

Radiation sterilization appears an attractive method for thermolabile medicaments and equipment because the rise in temperature caused by a sterilizing dose is very small — about 4°C. However, the Association of British Pharmaceutical Industries (ABPI) investigation on the effects of radiation on pharmaceutical products (ABPI Report 1960) led to the conclusion that in many instances 25 kGy produces changes that may make the preparation unacceptable for administration or presentation.

Undesirable effects include chemical decomposition, immediately or after storage, and alterations in colour, texture and solubility. Potency changes range from almost nil or nil (e.g. certain antibiotics and steroid hormones) to serious loss (e.g. insulin, posterior pituitary hormones and cyanocobalamin). Alterations in colour are common and, although sometimes there is no associated loss in activity, the preparation is less acceptable for sale. Because of the indirect effect of radiation, destruction is often greater when substances are irradiated in solution (e.g. heparin).

Ordinary types of clear glass become brown. Special glasses that are unaffected have been developed but are expensive. Silicone rubber is very resistant but butyl and chlorinated rubbers are degraded.

It is inadvisable to resterilize irradiated articles without careful investigation of possible adverse effects. For example, repeated irradiation of certain dressings and plastics causes degradation, as does autoclaving of cellulosic materials that have been subjected to gamma radiation previously. In addition, some radiation-sterilized products become toxic if exposed to ethylene oxide gas.

Applications of radiation sterilization

Articles regularly sterilized on a commercial scale include plastic syringes and catheters, hypodermic needles and scalpel blades, adhesive dressings, single-application capsules of eye ointment and catgut. Containers made of polythene and packaging materials using aluminium foil and plastic films.

A service for hospitals is provided, for example, by the irradiation plant at Wantage. It is for special items that are difficult to sterilize by other methods and not for bulk articles that are readily available from commercial sources.

Radiation sterilization of medicaments is developing slowly because of the adverse effects already described.

Advantages

1. The temperature rise is insignificant.

2. The processes can be continuous because exposure is so short (machine generation) or a large amount of material can be treated at once (isotope generation).

3. There is no aseptic handling since sterilization can be performed *after* packing in the final containers.

4. The methods are reliable and can be very accurately controlled.

5. Dry, moist and, with electrons, frozen materials can be treated.

6. Some bacterial and viral vaccines can be sterilized without loss of antigenicity.

Disadvantages

1. Capital and replacement costs are high. Preferably isotopes should be used 24 hours a day because the radiation takes place continuously.

2. Elaborate and expensive precautions must be taken to protect operators from the harmful effects of ionizing radiations.

For isotopes, the radiation chamber is surrounded by concrete several metres thick; the door is stepped to prevent escape of radiation through the surrounding cracks; and automatic controls are installed, e.g. to prevent raising of the source while the door is open and vice versa. When not in use the source is lowered into a deep (not less than 7 m) water-filled pond in a concrete pit.

The problems are smaller with generating machines because they can be switched off when not in use and the electrons are less penetrating than gamma rays. However, a penetrating form of X-ray known as *bremsstrahlung* is produced by the stopping of electrons by matter and since this escapes in all directions considerable shielding must be provided.

3. Deletrious changes are produced in many medicaments, fats and foods. Nevertheless, at the dose levels normally used there is no danger of residual radioactivity in irradiated products.

BIBLIOGRAPHY

ABPI Report 1960 Report of a working party established by the Association of British Pharmaceutical Industry and others on the use of gamma radiation sources for the sterilisation of pharmaceutical products. Association of British Pharmaceutical Industry, London

Aulton M E (ed) 1988 Pharmaceutics: the science of dosage form design. Churchill Livingstone, Edinburgh

BP 1988 HMSO, London

British Standard 1752 1963 Laboratory sintered or fritted filters. British Standards Institution, London

Burnard L G 1961 Design and production of irradiation plants. In: Symposium on the sterilisation of surgical dressings. Pharmaceutical Press, London, pp 34–35

Christensen E A, Holm N W, Juul F A 1967 Radiosterilisation of medical devices and supplies. In: Radiosterilization of medical products. HMSO, London, pp 265–283

Darmady E M, Hughes K E A, Burt M M, Freeman B M, Powell D B 1961 Radiation sterilisation. Journal of Clinical Pathology 14: 55–58

Dow J 1961 Sterilisation of adhesive dressings. In: Symposium on the sterilisation of surgical dressings. Pharmaceutical Press, London, pp 29–31

Ernst R R, Doyle J E 1968 Sterilisation of ethylene oxide. A review of chemical and physical factors. Biotechnology and Bioengineering 10: 1–31

Ernst R R, Shull J J 1962 Ethylene oxide gaseous sterilisation. II. Influence of method of humidification. Applied Microbiology 10: 342–344

Fraenkel-Conrat H 1961 Chemical modification of viral nucleic acid. I. Alkylating agents. Biochimica et Biophysica 49: 169–172

Gaughran E R L, Goudie A J (eds) 1974 Sterilization by ionizing radiation, vol. 1. Multiscience Publications, Montreal

Gaughran E R L, Goudie A J (eds) 1978 Editors. Sterilization by ionizing radiation, vol. 2. Multiscience Publications, Montreal

Hollaender A (ed) 1954 Radiation biology, vol. 1. High energy radiations. McGraw-Hill, New York

Horne T 1956 Sterilisation by radiation. Pharmaceutical Journal 176: 27–29

IAEA 1967 In: Radiosterilization of Medical Products (Proceedings of a Symposium held by the International Atomic Energy Agency). HMSO, London

Kaye S, Phillips C R 1949 The sterilizing action of gaseous ethylene oxide. IV. The effect of moisture. American Journal of Hygiene 50: 296–300

Ley F J, Winsley B, Harbord P, Keall A, Summers T 1972 Radiation sterilization: microbiological findings from subprocess dose treatment of disposable plastic syringes. Journal of Applied Bacteriology 35: 53–61

Mayr G 1961 Equipment for ethylene oxide sterilisation. In: Symposium on the sterilisation of surgical materials. Pharmaceutical Press, London, pp 90–97

Perkins J J, Lloyd R S 1961 Applications and equipment for ethylene oxide sterilisation. In: Symposium on the sterilisation of surgical materials. Pharmaceutical Press, London, pp 76–90

Phillips C R 1949 The sterilising action of gaseous ethylene oxide. II. Sterilization of contaminated objects with ethylene oxide and related compounds. Time, concentration and temperature relationships. American Journal of Hygiene 50: 280–288

Phillips C R 1961 The sterilizing properties of ethylene oxide. In: Symposium on the sterilisation of surgical materials. Pharmaceutical Press, London, pp 59–75

Powell D B 1961 Application of radiation sterilisation to surgical materials. In: Symposium on the sterilisation of surgical materials. Pharmaceutical Press, London, pp 9–16

USP 1985 United States Pharmacopeial Convention Inc, Rockville, MD,

Royce A, Bowler C 1961 Ethylene oxide sterilisation — some experiences and some practical limitations. Journal of Pharmacy and Pharmacology 13: 87T–94T

Summer W 1952 Cold sterilisation. Manufacturing Chemist 23: 451–455

Tallentire A, Dyer J, Levy F J 1971 Microbiological quality control of sterilized products: evaluation of a model relating frequency of contaminated items with increasing radiation treatment. Journal of Applied Bacteriology 34: 521–534

Trump J G 1961 High energy electrons for the sterilisation of surgical materials. In: Symposium on the sterilisation of surgical materials. Pharmaceutical Press, London, pp 16–28

Wilkinson G R 1960 Sterilisation of medical products. 2. Gas sterilisation. Manufacturing Chemist 31: 479–483

Winar F G, Stumbo C R 1971 Effect of water activity on sterilisation with gaseous ethylene oxide. Journal of Food Science 36: 892–898

22. Aseptic technique

R. M. E. Richards

Aseptic techniques are used to prevent the access of viable microbial and particulate contamination into products used for ophthalmic and parenteral products not intended to be sterilized in the final container, for products sterilized by filtration and for sterility testing of all 'sterile products'.

The applications of aseptic technique include the preparation of intravenous additives (see Ch. 25), the dispensing of cytotoxic agents (see Ch. 26), the compounding of total parenteral nutrition (see Ch. 27) and the production of radiopharmaceuticals (see Ch. 31). The requirements necessary to achieve strict asepsis include:

— Sterile starting materials.
— Sterile equipment.
— Controlled environment.
— Sterile containers.
— Suitable technique by trained personnel.

The methods for sterilizing materials, equipment and containers have been described in Chapters 20 and 21. The design, operation and monitoring of clean rooms and areas suitable for aseptic work are described in Chapter 23. This chapter is concerned with good aseptic technique by the operator in the preparation of sterile products.

Laminar air flow stations

Filtered laminar air flow (LAF), properly utilized, is a great asset in providing suitable conditions. Vertical or horizontal laminar air flow (VLAF and HLAF, respectively) can be used to sweep a working area virtually free from micro-organisms (see Ch. 23) and to provide a suitable working environment for aseptic procedures.

Protective clothing

Within the clean room environment, most airborne contamination results from the personnel using the facility. Jansen et al (1974) estimated that in a 24-hour period each person sheds the outermost layer of their epithelial cells and MacIntosh et al (1978) indicated that this is about 10^9 cells per day. Microbes are often associated with whole skin cells or fragments of these cells. The average size of these bacteria-carrying particles is thought to be about 14 μm (Noble et al 1963) and they will settle in still air under gravitational forces at a rate of about 0.37 m/min (Whyte, 1981). Whyte et al (1976) have estimated that male workers can disperse 1000 bacteria-carrying particles per minute. Therefore it is necessary to prevent contamination of a working area by enclosing each person in that area as effectively as possible within appropriately designed sterile impervious clothing, including gloves, footwear and headgear (see Ch. 23).

Personnel

The numbers of personnel working in a clean area should be as few as possible and the staff involved in aseptic procedures must demonstrate high standards of both integrity and motivation. All personnel should have both formal instruction and suitably validated practical training in the full range of procedures to be undertaken in the work place. It is important that staff of all levels including maintenance staff from outside the pharmacy understand the importance and the significance of the strict controls imposed. Compliance with procedures is likely to be increased if the reason for their imposition is understood.

Clean room personnel should be encouraged to report any minor infections or skin disorders which may render them temporarily unsuitable for aseptic work and regular medical checks should be made.

Operator technique

Basic rules for effective aseptic processing are:

1. Use a 'no touch' technique whenever possible.

Handle small articles with sterile forceps and, when sterile apparatus must be touched, handle as distant as possible from the part which will come into contact with a sterile liquid or solid. For example, the plunger of a syringe must not be touched because it will subsequently come into contact with the inner surface of the barrel and hence a sterile liquid. This rule applies even though sterile gloves may be worn.

2. Reduce air disturbances to a minimum

Standard procedures should be designed to minimize movement of personnel within the clean room. Objects should be positioned within reach under the laminar air flow cabinet. Only the hands and arms should be placed into the cabinet area and operators should not position their hands between the source of air and the objects being manipulated. Sharp and sudden movements should be avoided. Poor aseptic technique can easily negate the benefits of the LAF cabinet.

3. Consider the arrangement of objects under the LAF

Clean air should not flow over dirty articles to contaminate sterile articles. The cabinet should not be loaded with unnecessary equipment. Materials required should be carefully selected and arranged before beginning the procedure. For example, placement of large objects in the airstream of a LAF cabinet will create downstream turbulence in proportion to the size of the object. If a sufficiently large object is located near the front of a horizontal LAF cabinet, contaminants from the room or from the operator can be drawn into the work area behind the obstruction.

4. Refuse to be distracted

No interruption should be allowed until a set procedure has been completed.

Use of the laminar air flow cabinet

The air flow should be switched on and left for 15 minutes before use.

The inner faces of the cabinet should be swabbed with a suitable antimicrobial agent, e.g. 70% IMS.

An appropriate swabbing sequence is:

Horizontal LAF — top, sides, work surface.
Vertical LAF — back, sides, front, work surface.

All equipment and articles should also be swabbed with 70% IMS before placement in the cabinet. The outer wrapping should be removed from wrapped items.

Operator tests

Regular tests to ensure the adequacy of the technique of each operator should be carried out. These usually involve serial transfer of a sterile nutrient medium which is subsequently incubated and examined for the presence of turbidity indicating microbial growth. The test should involve both general transfer techniques and specific operations which form part of the daily routine of the operator. An example of an operator test is provided in Example 23.2.

STERILIZATION BY FILTRATION

Sterilization by filtration is a method permitted by the BP for solutions or liquids that are not sufficiently stable to withstand the process of heating in an autoclave as described in Chapter 20. Passage through a filter of appropriate pore size can remove bacteria and moulds although smaller micro-organisms such as viruses and mycoplasms may not be retained. After filtration the liquid is aseptically distributed into previously sterilized containers which are then sealed. This method has a number of disadvantages and should be used only for those products where sterilization by alternative means is not available.

Filter media

A sterile filter of nominal pore size 22 μm or less is required (DHSS 1983, BP 1988). Filters containing asbestos or any other medium likely to shed fibres or particles may not be used.

Membrane filters

These are usually the preferred type of filter for sterilization. Membrane filters are made from cellulose derivatives or other polymers and there are no loose fibres or particles. The retention of particles larger than the pore size occurs on the filter surface which also makes this type of filter particularly useful for the detection of bacteria (see Ch. 30).

Advantages of membrane filters include:

1. Rigid structure — unaffected by bubbles or pressure surges.
2. High flow rates — 80% of filter surface consists of pores.
3. Non-fibre shedding.
4. Minimal absorption — concentration unaffected.
5. Minimal wastage — little retention of solution.
6. Testable prior to and after filtration

Although re-useable membrane filters are available, the disposable types are generally preferred.

The use of a pre-filter

Membrane filters are generally blocked by particles close in size to the pore size of the filter. Pre-filtration reduces the risk of blockage of the final filter. Since the filtration method of sterilization carries a potentially greater risk of failure than other methods, a second filtration through a sterilized membrane filter provides an additional safeguard.

Sintered glass filters

Sintered glass filters made from borosilicate glass with an appropriate pore size may be used to sterilize solutions. These have the disadvantages of slowness of filtration, fragility and difficulty of cleaning.

Other filters

Filter media that have been used in the past as bacteria proof filters include asbestos pads, ceramic filters and kieselguhr candles.

Testing of filters

The BP requires that the integrity of an assembled sterilizing filter be verified before use and confirmed after use by means of a suitable test.

Bacteriological tests

The filter may be challenged by the passage of a diluted 24–48-hour broth culture of *Serratia marcescens*. A sample of the filtrate is collected aseptically and incubated at 25°C for 5 days. This organism is chosen because it has a small cell size (0.3–0.4 μm across). It grows vigorously in aerobic conditions and produces a readily detected red pigment.

Bubble point test

The bubble point of a test filter is the pressure at which the largest pore of a wetted filter is able to pass air. The pressure varies with the surface tension of the liquid with which the filter is wetted. Details of bubble pressure testing are given in the relevant British Standard (BS 1752:1963). Sterile membrane filters can be tested before use by a bubble pressure method, usually described in the manufacturer's literature.

Sterility testing

In-process controls are not generally available for methods of sterilization by filtration. It is therefore advisable to withold the issue of products sterilized by this method until sterility data is available (see Ch. 30).

BIBLIOGRAPHY

Aulton M E (ed) 1988 Pharmaceutics: the science of dosage form design. Churchill Livingstone, Edinburgh
British Pharmacopoeia 1988 HMSO, London
British Standard 1752 1983 Laboratory sintered or fritted filters including porosity grading. British Standards Institution, London
British Standard 3928 1969 Method for sodium flame test for air filters. British Standards Institution, London
British Standard 5295 1976 Environmental cleanliness in enclosed spaces. British Standards Institution, London
Burton W R, Marshall I W, Midcalf B, Taylor R 1981 Cleaning and disinfection of clean room garments. Pharmaceutical Journal 226: 30–31
Diamond J A 1972 Contamination control in the pharmaceutical industry. Journal of the Society of Environmental Engineers, Issue 55
DHSS 1983 Guide to good pharmaceutical manufacturing practice. HMSO, London
FDA 1985 Draft guidelines on sterile drug products produced by aseptic processing. Division of Drug Quality Compliance, FDA
Jansen L H, Hojyo-Tomako M J, Kligman A M 1974

Improved fluorescence staining techniques for estimating turnover of the human stratum corneum. British Journal of Dermatology 90: 9–12
MacIntosh C A, Lidwell, O M, Towers A G, Marples R R 1978 The dimensions of skin fragment dispersal into the air during activity. Journal of Hygiene 81: 471–476
Noble W C, Lidwell O M, Kingston D 1963 The size distribution of airborne particles carrying micro-organisms. Journal of Hygiene 66: 385–392
Wallhäusser K H 1982 Germ removal filtration. In: Bean H S, Beckett A N, Carless J E (eds) Advances in pharmaceutical sciences. Academic, London, pp 1–116
Whyte W 1981 Settling and impaction of particles into containers in manufacturing pharmacies. Journal of Parenteral Science and Technology 35: 255–261
Whyte W, Bailey P V 1985 Reduction of microbial dispersion by clothing. Journal of Parenteral Science and Technology 39: 51–60
Whyte W, Vesley D, Hodgson R 1976 Bacterial dispersion in relation to operating room clothing. Journal of Hygiene 76: 367–372

23. Design and operation of clean rooms

A. Broad

The resources that are required to achieve good pharmaceutical practice in the compounding of 'non-sterile' pharmaceutical products are described in Part 1 of this book. The areas in which such compounding takes place may be described as 'socially clean'.

The preparation of sterile pharmaceutical products requires special facilities designed to eliminate microbial and particulate contamination at all stages of manufacture. Products to be subjected to a terminal sterilization process should be prepared in a 'clean room' environment. Preparation of products not to be subjected to a terminal sterilization process in the final container should take place under 'aseptic' conditions. Basic environmental standards for clean preparation areas and for aseptic areas are defined in the 'Guide to good pharmaceutical manufacturing practice' (DHSS 1983) and are described in this chapter.

The design and operation of industrial scale clean rooms is described in Chapter 42 of the companion volume (Aulton 1988).

PREMISES

The premises in which the manufacture of sterile products takes place should provide sufficient space to allow an efficient flow of work through all the necessary operations and should include the following facilities:

Storage. Space is required for raw materials, empty containers, labels, etc., some of which may be 'bonded' pending release by quality control (see Ch. 29)

Weighing area. The main use of this area is to measure raw materials used for the product. Some powders may produce a dust hazard.

Bottle washing areas. All bottles should be washed prior to entry into clean rooms. Clean wash areas are sometimes within the clean room areas for washing of ampoules and various components just prior to use.

Laundry/changing areas. Access to clean room areas is only via a changing area. The operative must exchange their outdoor clothing for clean room clothing (see later).

Preparation. Clean room area for collection of water, preparation of solutions, mixing and final bulk product prepared.

Filling areas. The most critical areas. The product is filled into the final container via a suitably sized filter, then sealed and sent out of the clean room area.

Sterilization area. If the product is not aseptically prepared it has to be sterilized. The various equipment is installed here.

Inspection and labelling. Once the product has been sterilized the contents are inspected for particulates. The container is inspected for defects and then labelled.

Bonded area and release. Locable area where the product is kept until it passes all the requirements of the quality control. It is then released for use.

The 'Guide to good manufacturing practice' (DHSS 1983) states that the following principles should be applied to premises where manufacturing takes place.

Buildings should be located, designed, constructed, adapted and maintained to suit the operations carried out in them. The size of the premises should provide sufficient space to allow efficient flow of work and permit effective communication and supervision. The construction, and equipment layout, should ensure protection of the product from contamination, permit efficient cleaning and avoid the accumulation of dust and dirt. Premises should be designed and laid-out in such a way that the risk of mix-up or contamination of one product or material by another is minimised.

Design and construction

The preparation of sterile medicinal products should take place in specially designed departments in which different types of activities are confined to separate rooms, e.g. component preparation, solution preparation,

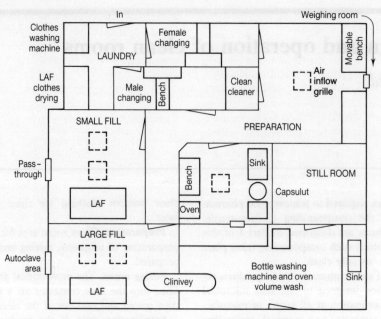

Fig. 23.1   Typical layout of a sterile manufacturing unit

filling and sealing, etc. Figure 23.1 shows a typical layout of a sterile manufacturing unit. The sizes of the rooms should be kept to a practical minimum (maximum 12 m × 14 m × 3 m) to assist cleaning, especially after contamination, and to comply with fire and safety regulations.

Access

Normal (non-emergency) access to and egress from the clean room should be through air locks for both material and personnel. Air locks may be used as anterooms. A low physical barrier (boot barrier) across an anteroom serves to remind personnel of the change from one class of environment to another.

Construction should be such as to prevent leakage of air either into or out of the clean room. Appropriately sited control pressure relief grilles or flaps should be provided in cases when it is needed to ensure that over-pressure is bled to atmosphere (if necessary through adjacent change rooms and outer-rooms). The number of openings should be kept to a minimum and pairs of airlock doors, through-the-wall autoclave and dry sterilizer doors should be interlocked to prevent both being opened simultaneously. Doors should be self-closing and of adequate size to permit the unimpeded entry and exit of specified material and personnel.

Hatchways and airlocks for the passage of materials, equipment and other goods into clean and aseptic areas should be arranged so that only one side may be opened

at any one time. Because of difficulties in cleaning the sliding gear, sliding doors should be avoided. Conveyor belts should not pass through walls enclosing aseptic areas. They should end at the wall, products passing onwards across a stationary surface. Special precautions are necessary to avoid contamination of aseptic areas when articles are passed through airlocks or hatchways. Access to clean and aseptic areas should be restricted to authorized persons, who enter only through changing rooms where normal clothing is exchanged for special protective garments.

Windows

Windows should be non-opening, flush fitting and sealed to prevent ingress of contamination. Good use of windows can aid communication, help supervision and make training easier. Windows on outside walls should be avoided wherever possible in order to reduce heat loss, condensation and noise problems. They should be double glazed and sealed to minimize heat transfer and to aid sound proofing. When blinds are fitted they should be hung between the double glazing to avoid dust traps.

Surfacing materials

The surfaces of walls, floors and ceilings should be smooth, impervious and unbroken in order to minimize the shedding or accumulation of particulate matter, and to permit the repeated application of cleaning agents and disinfectants where used.

Floors in processing areas should be made of impervious materials, laid to an even surface. They should be free from cracks and open joints and should allow prompt and efficient removal of any spillages. Walls should be sound and finished with a smooth, impervious and washable surface. Ceilings should be constructed and finished so that they can be maintained in a clean condition.

Except in vertical flow, unidirectional air flow clean rooms, where the floor forms the exhaust grills, the floor covering should be continuous; where sheet materials are used the joints should be welded and dressed flush or otherwise similarly joined to avoid dirt traps. Coving should be used where walls meet floors and ceilings in aseptic areas (and preferably in other clean areas as well). Care should be taken to ensure that the coving is installed so as not to create additional dust-accumulating ridges.

Services

Piped liquids and gases (e.g. water, compressed air) should be filtered before entering the clean room to ensure that the liquid or gas at the work position will be as clean as, or cleaner than, the air circulating at that point. Non-ferrous or stainless steel piping and pipe fittings should be used wherever possible and blanking covers provided and fitted whenever a service is out of use. All pipes, fittings, etc. should conform to the relevant British Standards. Thought should be given to the type and quantity of piped gases into the clean rooms, e.g. nitrogen, compressed air, vacuum, natural gas, oxygen, propane, etc. All other fittings such as fuse boxes, switch panels, isolators, valves, etc. should be located outside the clean rooms.

Drains should be avoided wherever possible, and excluded from aseptic areas unless essential. They should be of adequate size, and should have trapped gullies and proper ventilation. Open channels should be avoided where possible, but if they are necessary they should be shallow to facilitate cleaning and disinfection. Where installed they should be fitted with effective, easily cleanable traps and with air breaks to prevent back-flow. The traps may contain electrically operated heating devices or other means for disinfection. Any floor channels should be open, shallow and easily cleanable and be connected to drains outside the area in a manner which prevents ingress of microbial contaminants.

Sinks should be excluded from aseptic areas. Any sinks installed in other clean areas should be of stainless steel, without overflow, and be supplied with water of at least potable quality. All water supplied to clean rooms should preferably be taken from the rising mains and not from storage tanks. Drain heaters offer a quick and convenient way of sanitizing the U-bend of any sinks, etc.

Furniture

Furniture, test equipment and lighting should be installed in a manner such that the production of dust particles or other contamination is kept to a minimum. Equipment, such as laminar air flow cabinets, can be built into the walls of the clean rooms to give a flush finish with the minimum number of ledges. Alternatively the cabinets can be mounted on wheels with the advantage that they can be moved throughout the clean rooms if required. This makes servicing of the cabinet easier but has the disadvantage that additional ledges and dust traps are created. The same arguments (fitted or mobile?) can be made for the installation of benches within the clean rooms. If fitted benches are chosen then care must be taken in their construction to ensure that no stress cracks appear in the clean room walls after long-term use. False ceilings should be adequately sealed to prevent contamination from the space above them.

ENVIRONMENTAL CONTROL

A clean room is a room with total environmental control, i.e. control of temperature, humidity, of particulate contamination and, where appropriate atmospheric pressure.

The possible sources of particulate and microbial contamination are the air supply of the room, infiltration of outside air and generation of contaminations within the room. Each of these possible sources can be minimized as described below.

The air supply of the room

The air supply of a clean room can be provided in several ways.

Unidirectional

The air enters the room through a bank of filters which comprises one complete wall (horizontal flow) or ceiling (vertical flow) and leaves through ducts forming part of the opposite wall or floor (Fig. 23.2(a),(b)).

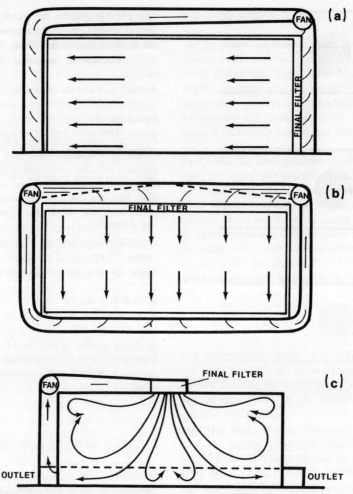

Fig. 23.2 Air movements in laminar air flow (LAF) rooms. (**a**) Horizontal laminar flow (unidirectional); (**b**) vertical laminar flow (unidirectional); (**c**) conventional flow (multidirectional)

Conventional flow

The air enters the rooms through a bank of filters situated either in the ceiling or high up in a wall, and leaves through outlet ducts fitted low down on the wall or in the floor at points remote from the inlet (Fig. 23.2(**c**)). The air flow should be such that the number of air changes should not be less than 20 per hour. This should be the worst case, i.e. at the end of the filters' life, therefore on commissioning the air change rate should be considerably higher.

The air flow should not produce excessive turbulence. The air can be recirculated to save energy (because the air is already heated and cleaned). In which case a proportion of fresh air should be added. Care should be taken that fumes from cleaning solvents are not recirculated to clean rooms and build up.

Laminar air flow theory

Liquid or gas flows in turbulent or streamline (laminar) motion, or in a state intermediate between these two (Fig. 23.3). If air is moving very slowly it will move as a block or mass so that motion is parallel throughout. This is said to be laminar flow. If an object is placed in the airflow, streamlines will form around it so that the lamellae part upstream of the object and reform downstream. There is little movement of material suspended in the air from one streamline to the next (except possibly in a downwards due to gravity direc-

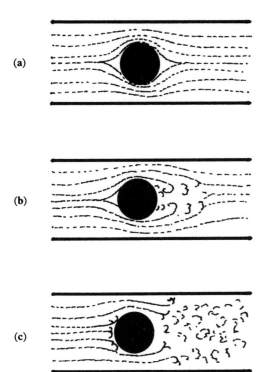

(a)

(b)

(c)

Fig. 23.3 The flow of fluid past an object, illustrating the difference between laminar flow and turbulent flow.
(a) Streamline flow; (b) transitional region; (c) turbulent flow

tion) (Fig. 23.3(a)). As the velocity is increased, eddy currents begin to form downstream of the object so that there are small localized areas where the movement of the air is actually in the opposite direction of the main movement. Once again, however, the streamlines will eventually reform downstream of the object

(Fig. 23.3(b)). If the velocity is increased further a point arises where there is complete turbulent mixing of streamlines around the object. (Figure 23.3(c)).

The concept of laminar air flow rooms and cabinets therefore visualizes all the work being continually bathed in a stream of sterile, particle-free air, any contamination generated by the work itself, or by the worker, being carried away downstream away from the work space. This gives greater freedom to the operators in the sense that there are fewer restrictions on their movement under these conditions, although as will be pointed out later, care is still required when using a laminar air flow cabinet.

Air filtration

The final high-efficiency particulate air (HEPA) filter should be positioned ideally at the inlet to the clean room or as close as possible to it. Pre-filters may be fitted upstream of the HEPA filters to prolong the life of the final filter.

To maintain the integrity of the clean rooms, systems can be designed with a large HEPA filter additionally installed in the main duct before it branches to the various clean areas. Therefore the HEPA filters within the room are rarely being challenged with large quantities of particles and the life-expectancy is greatly extended. The disadvantage is that a large fan system is required to push the air through the additional resistance of a HEPA filter. The fans selected should provide a constant air flow as the pressure drop across the filter increases. Gauges should be fitted upstream and downstream of all banks of filters in order to indicate any restriction in the air flow due to a blocked filter. The gauges may be connected to an automatic alarm

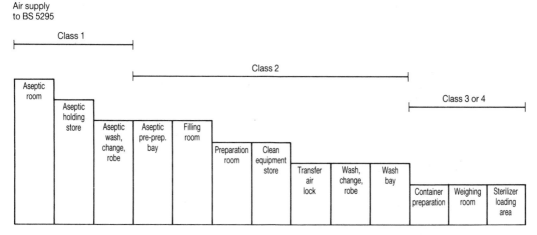

Fig. 23.4 Sterile manufacturing: mechanical ventilation pressure gradient

device. Ducting should be manufactured from materials with corrosion-resistant and non-flaking properties or should be given suitable surface treatment to prevent the introduction of contaminants from the duct.

Ingress of outside air

This is prevented by maintaining the air pressure of the clean room at all times above that of the surrounding areas. The rooms requiring the highest degree of environmental control (aseptic areas) are maintained at the highest pressure and the gradients between successive pressure areas are not less than 15 Pa (Fig. 23.4). The various grades or classes of environmental cleanliness are defined in British Standard 5295 (1976) and summarized in Appendix 1 of the 'Guide to good pharmaceutical manufacturing practice' (DHSS 1983).

Laminar air flow cabinets (contained work stations)

LAF work stations are cabinets that provide a local Class I environment. The cabinets can be bought in various sizes (generally from 300 mm to 2 m in length) depending on the use to which they are put. They are available in two main configurations as far as direction of air flow is concerned — horizontal and vertical (Fig. 23.5). The cabinet may be made from any suitable

material which is sufficiently durable to withstand normal working stresses. If organic materials are used, all surfaces should be covered with a plastic laminate or other material resistant to particle shedding and abrasive action. Inorganic materials should be coated with suitable primers and finish paints so as to produce smooth, durable surfaces, except those surfaces finished with stainless steel, which should be polished to remove burrs and any loose particulate matter resulting from fabrication operations, etc.

Side panels or dust covers, when supplied, should be made of transparent thick plastics or toughened glass with any projecting or unmasked edges rounded off. Consideration should be given to fire risks when organic or other combustible materials are used in the construction. Levelling devices should be fitted.

Enclosed work stations

The techniques employed in the manipulation of radiopharmaceutics and cytotoxics can produce aerosols which can be readily inhaled by personnel and inadvertently distributed to the surrounding environment. Therefore additional requirements for the processing of radiopharmaceuticals and cytotoxics are required not only to protect the product but also the user (see Chs 26, 31). Similar cabinets are also employed for the

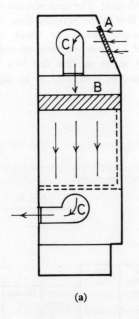

(a)

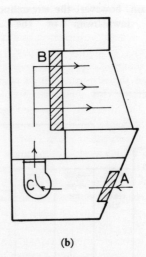

(b)

Fig. 23.5   Laminar air flow cabinet. (**a**) Vertical laminar air flow unit, (**b**) Horizontal laminar air flow unit: A, pre-filter; B, HEPA filter; **c**, fan

manipulation of microbiological organisms. There are three classes of safety cabinet; Class II cabinets are usually used in the hospital pharmaceutical environment (BS 5726 Class II).

They are designed to:

1. Protect personnel from aerosol particles or vapours from products which are known mutagens and are suspected of being carcinogens and teratogens.
2. Protect the pharmaceutical product from micro-organisms and particulates.
3. Protect maintenance personnel.

Part of the cabinet is open-fronted where an inward flow of air through the working aperture creates an air curtain between the operator and the work area. This prevents any aerosol produced from toxic substances being pushed out of the cabinet onto the operator. The air exhausts through a grated work surface often with the aid of a second fan. The incoming air blends with laminar flow air which is then totally exhausted via a suitable duct or a proportion recirculated through the HEPA filter. The units are usually self-balancing and alarmed against fan failure. In normal operating mode the amount of barrier air entering the cabinet from the clean room environment is equal to the volume of air being exhausted through the exhaust filter.

Totally enclosed work stations

As can be seen from the information given on the design of clean rooms and the type of clothing required, the cost of building and equipping clean rooms can be considerable. This has led to the introduction of self-contained units that provide a suitable environment for processing the complete range of pharmaceuticals. The cabinets consist of a glove box system for the sterile and particle-free handling of normal or highly toxic powders and materials. A suitably designed cupboard section is linked to a filtration unit on the rear panel fitted with both fume and particle filters. This allows for flexibility in use, as the cabinet does not need to be connected to laboratory ducting, so avoiding building costs, and allowing movement from site-to-site.

The cabinet offers a high degree of chemical resistance, and the internal design has carefully eliminated dust traps, which make cleaning and sterilizing the interior of the cabinet a relatively simple operation.

In use, air passes into the cabinet through an inlet HEPA filter (to BS 3928) to ensure a Class I particle-free atmosphere. Air leaves the cabinet through an outlet HEPA filter to remove particles, then through a main filter of either activated carbon or chemisorbant material to remove fumes or water vapour, before returning to the cabinet via a centrifugal fan and the inlet HEPA filter.

A valve-operated air inlet and exhaust system allows the pressure in the cabinet to be adjusted either positively or negatively with respect to the outside. For those applications requiring the highest sterility (e.g. preparing parenteral nutrition solutions) the cabinet may be operated at positive pressure. For other applications requiring maximum environmental protection (e.g. handling highly toxic powders) the cabinet may be operated at negative pressure. All air entering or leaving the system passes through two protective HEPA filters. Entry and exit ports are located on the side panels, these are fitted with a double door system and may be optionally flushed with HEPA-filtered air to avoid contamination of the cabinet. Four glove ports are located in the front panel. Electrical switches, a differential pressure gauge to measure cabinet pressure, and lights are located in the top section of the cupboard, isolated from the fumes by a translucent diffuser.

An optional formaldehyde sterilization unit, which includes leak test equipment, is available. A main filter saturation alarm and cabinet airflow indicator may also be supplied.

The *advantages* of this type of cabinet over conventional clean rooms are as follows:

1. The operator works through gloved port holes, therefore alleviating the need to wear and process clean room clothing.
2. The interior of the cabinets can be quickly and safely sterilized.
3. The cabinets are mobile and can be moved from site-to-site.
4. No special rooms are required to house the cabinets.

The cabinets are thus ideal for handling cytotoxics and for total parenteral nutrition (TPN) dispensing operations.

Generation of contaminants within the room

This may be minimized by applying a rigorous cleaning programme, by working within strict procedural guidelines and by the use of effective protective clothing for the personnel.

Cleaning programmes

It has been shown that there is a close parallel between airborne particulate contamination and airborne microbical contamination. Horizontal surfaces are more likely to be contaminated than are vertical faces because of settling due to gravity. Air flow patterns, touching by personnel, static surface charges, etc. will result in some areas becoming more contaminated than others.

Wherever possible the areas of greatest contamination should be identified and subjected to regular effective decontamination.

Methods of cleaning

There are two main cleaning methods, vacuuming to remove gross particulate contamination (size $> 100 \ \mu$m) and wiping with a damp cloth to remove the remaining particles.

Cleaning agents should preferably be:

— Effective decontaminants.
— Non-toxic to personnel.
— Non-flammable.
— Fast drying.
— Harmless to surfaces.
— Cost-effective.

Cleaning agents are used to:

— Remove contamination, e.g. surfactants and soaps.
— Kill micro-organisms, e.g. disinfectants and bactericides.
— Control electrostatic charges.

Wiping materials should be sterilized before and after use and should not shed particles.

A rigorous cleaning protocol should be designed and implemented with daily, weekly and possible monthly routines defined. Rotation of disinfectants may be used to limit the emergence of resistance to a particular agent. Periodic gaseous sterilization (fumigation) may be required (see Ch. 21). Measurable levels of 'cleanliness' for surface and air contamination should be monitored regularly.

Clean room operations (procedural guidelines)

When not under continuous operation, ventilation equipment should be switched on at least 30 minutes before the entry of personnel and switched off not less than 30 minutes after vacation of the clean room.

Any operation likely to result in gross contamination in the clean room should be prohibited.

Procedural guidelines should ensure that the movement and handling of materials by personnel is minimal.

Personnel should be fully trained and motivated to work within a strict protocol.

Protective clothing

The major sources (approximately 80%) of particulate and microbial contamination in any clean room are the personnel. Protective clothing is therefore designed to protect the environment from the operator by acting as a filter and must be made of finely woven material which does not itself shed particles and lint. The material should be antistatic, comfortable to wear, non-flammable and easily washed. In addition, resistance to repeated washing and for aseptic work, to repeated sterilization is also desirable.

Suitable fabrics are closely woven from monofilament yarns of polyamide (nylon) or polyester (terylene) fibres. These are less comfortable to wear than fabrics woven from more conventional multifilament yarns but offer more effective environmental protection. Special processes may be applied to the fabric to reduce the interstices or small gaps between the warp and the weft (see Fig. 33.2). A suitable fabric so produced is called 'ceramic terylene' because it was developed originally to protect workers in the ceramic industry from china clay dust.

A full set of garments should comprise the following. A *surgical mask* to cover the nose and mouth. Suitable *headgear* to cover and enclose the hair and, where beards are worn, special masks or full face headgear. A *smock* which fits closely at the neck and wrists worn with trousers close fitting to the smock and at the shoes or alternatively a *one-piece overall suit* close fitting at the neck, wrists and ankles: these garments should be without pockets. *Particle-free gloves*, as necessary. *Shoes or overshoes*, which should be a close fit at the join with the trousers.

Outdoor shoes should always be removed before proceeding to clean rooms and replaced by antistatic pumps, clogs or clean room slippers. Then depending upon the type of production being carried out, a disposable (for short periods only) or reusable overshoe or overboot should be used. Overboots should consist of a non-porous sole of nylon or vinyl rubber thick enough to offer some protection from broken glass, e.g. ampoules. In addition, the soles should preferably be slip proof in wet conditions. The top should be of a similar material to the other garments, nylon, terylene or ceramic terylene. The leg of the coverall should go down inside the boot cover so that any matter inside the coverall will fall into the boot cover rather than into the atmosphere.

Since it is impossible to sterilize the operators' hands by scrubbing and the use of antiseptics, any object that is handled will always present a cross-contamination risk. Consequently a glove should be choosen to fill the following criteria. It should be particle free, sufficiently strong to prevent puncture during use, provide an impenetrable barrier to hand oils, bacteria and other contaminants, provide a good seal around the wrists of the cleanroom suit and have high tactile qualities for product manipulation and if necessary should be sterile.

Note that there are on average 5 million talc/starch particles per cm^2 on most gloves which are impossible to remove completely by washing with sterile solutions before use. A number of alternatives are available, none of which meet all the requirements. These are: sterile latex surgeons' gloves (which are powder free), p.v.c. gloves, and biogel gloves (which, because a gelatin formulation is used as a lubricant for mould release, are comfortable to wear).

Laundering of clothing

Clean protective clothing should be used for each entry into a clean or aseptic area. The garments should be subjected to rigorous laundering either by 'wet washing' or 'dry cleaning' and inspection should precede packaging for further issue.

Sterilization of clothing

Sterilization is needed to destroy all living organisms. The three methods available are:

1. Autoclaving.
2. Ethylene oxide.
3. Gamma Irradiation.

Autoclaving (see Ch. 20) is clearly effective and if an autoclave is installed at the unit it is both cheap and easy to use. It is unfortunate that as far as synthetic fibre cleanroom clothing is concerned it is by far the worst method to be used. The heat will create considerable shrinkage, so that when fitting new garments it must be remembered to install garments two sizes too large. The fibres are likely to be damaged in a short time and the garment life can be expected to be 50% shorter than non-heat methods of sterilization due to breakdown of the fibres. Autoclaving, quite apart from the hardening of the fabric and thus increasing wearer discomfort, is not very satisfactory as a cleanroom garment process.

It is unfortunate that *ethylene oxide* (see Ch. 21) is increasingly unacceptable as a means of sterilization due to the toxic and explosive nature of the gas. In cleanroom clothing terms it is outstanding in doing the job without any known deterioration of the fibres. The fabric retains its full characteristics and its life-expectancy is extended by a factor of two or three over autoclaving.

As far as cleanroom clothing is concerned *gamma irradiation* (see Ch. 21) is probably the best compromise solution as at the DHSS-approved dose of 25 kGy (2.5 Mrads) there is not only an effective kill of viable organisms but the fabric has reasonable resistance to the cumulative degradation that is inevitable with ^{60}Co

source irradiation. Sterilization is achieved by passing the product to be treated before the ^{60}Co source on a conveyor. The product is treated evenly by virtue of the conveyor passing to both sides of the source (Isotron).

The dose level is a function of the time the product spends exposed to the source. Products to be irradiated are separated physically, from those already treated and administrative controls and records on dosages given are stringently enforced.

Monitoring of clothing

Whatever method of washing, drying and sterilizing is chosen it should be performed using well-documentated procedures. The garments and procedures should be checked regularly.

There are two main testing methods that can be applied to cleanroom garments in order to judge their freedom from particulate contamination.

1. Before commencing work the operators wearing the garments in the clean room can be scanned with an air particle counter; the garments should be assessed at commissioning and when room or laminar flow cabinets are checked.

2. The garments may be tested according to the method of the American Society for Testing Materials (ASTMS designation FS1-68). This method counts the number of particles and fibres actually on the material.

Ideally, cleanroom clothing for hospital manufacturing use should conform with Class B standards, a standard found to be achievable with standard wet-wash and tumble-drying equipment in non-HEPA filtered air supply areas over considerable periods.

Changing procedure

All staff using the clean rooms should be aware of the garment changing procedure and a copy should be displayed in each changing area. The details of the procedure will depend on the type of product being prepared. A typical protocol is illustrated in Example 23.1.

Example 23.1

Changing room procedure for cleanroom clothing

Changing procedure — on entering clean rooms
1. Before entering clean rooms wash hands and remove heavy make-up.
2. Collect jumpsuit, hood and boots (ensure that they do not touch the outer floor), hook hood over hanger and tie boots by string to hook of hanger. Close clear cover of laminar air flow cabinet.

3. Take into changing room hang on bar. Check press-studs on arms and legs are open. Check press-studs on hood are set at required fitting.
4. Remove any jewellery and place in container supplied.
5. Obtain face-mask and gloves from locker.
6. Remove street clothing down to underwear.
7. Remove cleanroom shoes from bench and place on clean side.
8. Step over bench into cleanroom shoes.
9. Hang up cleanroom clothing.
10. Put on face-mask.
11. Put on hood and ensure no hair is protruding (using mirror provided). Adjust hood for snug fit.
12. Put on jumpsuit and ensure hood is tucked into suit. Adjust press-studs on both arms and legs to give a snug fit. Pull up zip then press studs to cover zip.
13. Put on overboots and tie straps.
14. Open gloves and spread package on bench so the gloves are ready to put on.
15. Wash and dry hands thoroughly with the wall unit.
16. Put on gloves and ensure the elasticated end of the gloves covers the sleeves of the jumpsuit.
17. Enter clean rooms by using your backside to open door, do not touch doors with gloves.

Changing procedure on leaving clean room
1. Remove gloves and place on bench.
2. Remove overboots and place on bench
3. Remove cleanroom shoes and place on bench — clean side.
4. Step over bench into 'dirty' area.
5. Remove hood.
6. Remove face-mask and put with gloves and any wrapping place in bin provided.
7. Remove jumpsuit, ensure the press-studs are undone and the zip is pull up to the closed position ready for washing.
8. Put on street clothes and jewellery.
9. Remove jumpsuit, hood and boots and place in laundry basket.

ENVIRONMENTAL MONITORING

Commissioning tests

A number of tests and procedures must be applied when clean rooms and aseptic areas are commissioned for use. These are specified in British Standard 5295 and include testing for leaking in construction joints and leaking around air filters. The efficiency of the air filtration and the control of particulate contamination must also be demonstrated. Tests for environmental conditions, light, temperature, humidity and noise, air pressure and air flow between areas of different pressure are also specified.

Monitoring tests

The results of the commissioning tests provide a baseline for regular routine monitoring tests designed to assure the quality of the environment (see Ch. 29).

Microbiological tests

The appropriate freedom from microbial contamination should be established by using swabs, settle plates and process simulation tests.

Settle plates

Settle plating should be carried out in all rooms in which pharmaceutical manufacturing procedures are performed, including the preparation of radiopharmaceuticals, blood labelling and cytotoxic reconstitution. Changing rooms should also be included. A diagram should be made of each room to be tested, and the various test sites should be numbered on the diagram.

Sites for testing should include laminar flow cabinets, pass throughs, work benches, floors, sinks, drains, window ledges and shelves, with particular attention being paid to the working area (Fig 23.6).

Settle plates should be 90 mm in diameter, and pairs of plates should be laid at each site, one plate containing nutrient agar (test for bacteria) and the other Sabouraud dextrose agar (test for fungi). Alternatively a single blood agar plate may be used for both types of organism, provided that it has been demonstrated that plates from the particular source employed will give results comparable to the nutrient agar/Sabouraud dextrose agar combination.

Plates should be pre-incubated before use in order to detect any contaminated plates

Settle plates should be swabbed before being placed in position, and care must be taken not to contaminate them, either by direct contact or by breathing upon them. Plates should be exposed for a standard length of time, which should be at least 30 minutes. Longer periods may be employed, provided that the testing does not become invalid, for example by drying out of the plates. After exposure, the plates should be covered and incubated at 30°C to 32°C for nutrient agar or 22°C to 25°C for Sabouraud dextrose agar. Counting of colonies should be carried out 5–7 days after exposure of the plates. Blood agar plates should be incubated for 1 day at 37°C before counting.

Settle plates should be set out routinely in aseptic rooms and LAF cabinets during all aseptic manufacture, the plates in the LAF cabinet being as close as is practical to the manufacturing operation that is being/will be carried out. Settle plating of other locations, including rooms used for aseptic dispensing and radiopharmacy units, should be carried out weekly. A routine procedure should be established which should allow for testing to be carried out at different times of the day and on different days of the week, to obtain an overall picture of contamination levels. The nature of any activity being

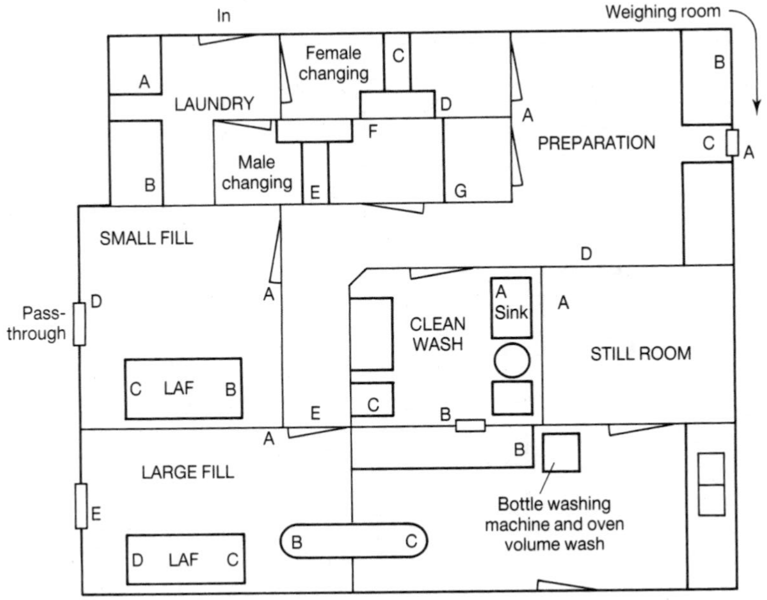

Fig. 23.6 Sterile fluids manufacturing units: routine settle plate map

SETTLE PLATES

Settle plate map (refer to Fig. 23.1 for detail of room use)

Laundry and changing rooms:
A On bench over washing machine
B Under LAF air curtain
C On female change boot barrier
D On clean side female change
E On male change boot barrier
F On clean side male change
G Under PVR in cleaner's cupboard

Preparation room:
A Near female change/cleaner's door
B On large work bench
C Near pass-through hatch
D Under still room outlets
E Under small fill PRV

Clean wash:
A On sink draining board
B Near pass-through hatch (on floor)
C On top of oven

Small fill:
A Behind door
B LAF cabinet bench
C LAF cabinet bench
D Near pass-through hatch (on floor)

Large fill:
A Behind door
B Under clinivey
C LAF cabinet bench
D LAF cabinet bench
E Near pass-through hatch (on floor)

Stills/volume wash:
A Under window of preparation room
B On bench near pass-through hatch
C On top of clinivey

Weighing room:
A On balance bench

Total 28 pairs of plates

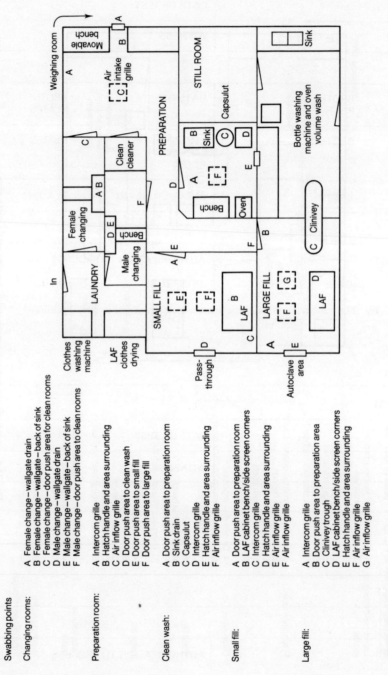

SWABS

Swabbing points

Changing rooms:
A Female change – wallgate drain
B Female change – wallgate – back of sink
C Female change – door push area for clean rooms
D Male change – wallgate drain
E Male change – wallgate – back of sink
F Male change – door push area to clean rooms

Preparation room:
A Intercom grille
B Hatch handle and area surrounding
C Air inflow grille
D Door push area to clean wash
E Door push area to small fill
F Door push area to large fill

Clean wash:
A Door push area to preparation room
B Sink drain
C Capsulut
D Intercom grille
E Hatch handle and area surrounding
F Air inflow grille

Small fill:
A Door push area to preparation room
B LAF cabinet bench/side screen corners
C Intercom grille
D Hatch handle and area surrounding
E Air inflow grille
F Air inflow grille

Large fill:
A Intercom grille
B Door push area to preparation area
C Clinivey trough
D LAF cabinet bench/side screen corners
E Hatch handle and area surrounding
F Air inflow grille
G Air inflow grille

Total = 31 swabs

Fig. 23.7 Sterile fluids manufacturing unit: routine swabbing points

---

RESULT/RECORD FORM   BROTH TRANSFER TEST

HOSPITAL	DATE OF TEST
OPERATOR	WITNESS

COMMENTS

DATE ON	BROTH PLATES	DATE OFF	BROTH PLATES
RESULTS	BROTH	RESULTS LAF ROOM	PLATES
SUBCULTURE / ID	BROTH	SUBCULTURE / ID	PLATES

COMMENTS

RESULTS OF TEST (QC) PASS / FAIL SIGNATURE DATE	AUTHORIZATION TO PROCESS SIGNATURE DATE

Fig. 23.8   Report form for operator test to assess quality of aseptic dispensing.

RESULT/RECORD FORM   AEROSOL TEST

HOSPITAL	DATE OF TEST
OPERATOR	WITNESS

COMMENTS

WIPE RESULT

BAG APPEARANCE

SYRINGE APPEARANCE

COMMENTS

RESULTS OF TEST (QC) PASS / FAIL SIGNATURE DATE	AUTHORIZATION TO PROCESS SIGNATURE DATE

Fig. 23.9   Report form for operator test to assess aerosol formation during liquid manipulations

carried out in the unit during settle plating should be recorded. From the results obtained, it may be possible to reduce contamination levels in consultation with staff, by improved working practices, or changes in cleaning and disinfection procedures.

The results of testing should be tabulated on cumulative cards, showing date and location, so that any trends or unusual results are readily apparent.

Contact plates or swabs

Contact plates or swabs are used to test for surface, rather than airborne, contamination and thus provide a check on cleaning and disinfection procedures. Testing of work surfaces and sinks should be carried out monthly, preferably at the same time as settle plating. Action levels should be set locally, from a consideration of the accumulated testing results in the unit concerned. The action to be taken in the event of unsatisfactory testing results should be defined (Abdou 1980) (Fig. 23.7).

Centrifugal or slit samplers

Air sampling in clean rooms using a centrifugal or slit sample should be carried out on a monthly basis. Remote control accessories are available to enable counts to be made in the unmanned state. Limits are set in Appendix 1 of the 'Guide to good pharmaceutical manufacturing practice' (DHSS 1983) for the maximum permitted number of viable organisms per cubic metre in the unmanned state.

Sampling or laminar flow systems

Laminar air flow units should be periodically checked to ensure efficiency of the filters. The sampler should be mounted at the distal limit of the laminar flow to avoid turbulence inside the unit. The operating time for this application is 4–5 minutes.

Monitoring of the operator

Operator technique is of paramount importance in the preparation of the product. These techniques should be routinely checked by a series of tests which can then be used to monitor the operator's performance. The frequency of the testing would be dependent on each individual operator. Operators who are in the clean rooms on limited occasions would require more frequent testing than those in the clean rooms at all times. An example of a transference is given below (Example 23.2).

Example 23.2

Operator test — aseptic dispensing

The kit contains:

1 × 100 ml clear DIN bottle containing 25 ml of concentrated broth.
4 × 20 ml ampoules of Water for Injections BP.
5 × 30 ml sterile empty vials.
Report form.
Instruction leaflet.
In addition you will require Luer-Lock syringes, needles and settle plates.

The aim of the test is to examine the operator's technique in the manipulation of containers normally associated with aseptic dispensing.

All vials are provided with flip-tops which when removed will expose the rubber inserts.

All precautions should be taken to ensure the test is conducted in the same environment normally used for aseptic dispensing.

Full settle plate monitoring should be carried out at the same time.

Method
1. Add 75 ml of water for injections from the 4 × 20 ml ampoules to the bottle.
2. Shake the 100 ml DIN bottle gently until the media is well mixed.
3. Remove the diluted medium from the 100 ml bottle and add 20 ml portions to each of the five sterile vials.
4. Label the 5 × 20 ml vials with the date and operator's name or code.
5. Send the vials for incubation at 30–37°C for 7 days.
6. The report form (Fig. 23.8) should be completed and returned to the pharmacist in charge of aseptic dispensing.

A further example of technique can be assessed by testing the operator to ensure that no aerosol formation occurs (especially with cytotoxics and radiopharmaceutics) when adding to or extracting from injection containers (Example 23.3).

Example 23.3

Operation test — aerosol formation.

The kit contains:

1 × 30 ml vial containing 5 ml sterile proflavine 1:1000 solution.
1 × 20 ml ampoule of Water for injections BP.
Large clean room wipe.
Report form.
Instruction leaflet.
In addition you will require Luer-Lock syringes, needles, mini-bag and blind hubs.

The aim of the test is to ascertain whether the correct method is being used to fill and remove solutions from vials *without* the production of aerosol sprays.

Method
1. Lay the large cleanroom wipe on the bench. All operations should take place over or on the wipe.
2. Add 20 ml of water for injections to the vial containing the proflavine 1:1000 solution.
3. Remove 10 ml of the proflavine solution and add to the mini-bag.
4. Remove a further 10 ml of proflavine solution from the vial and add a blind hub to the syringe.
5. Remove the mini-bag, syringe and cleanroom wipe for examination by the pharmacist in charge.
6. A report form (Fig. 23.9) is available if required.

Documentation

All procedures which take place within clean and aseptic areas should be fully documented. Product and

manufacturing parameters should be clearly defined and the protocols, processes and procedures necessary to achieve the required parameters derived. It is essential that all personnel are fully trained and motivated to achieve the high standards required.

All procedures should be fully recorded by means which do not impair the cleanroom environment and the principles of quality assurance (see Ch. 29) must be maintained.

REFERENCES

Aulton M E (ed) 1988 Pharmaceutics: the science of dosage form design. Churchill Livingstone, Edinburgh

B S 5295 Environmental cleanliness in enclosed spaces, British Standards Institution, London

Department of Health and Social Security 1983 Guide to good pharmaceutical manufacturing practice. HMSO, London

Smail G A, Marshall I 1982 Intravenous additives. In: Lawson D H Richards R M E (eds) Clinical pharmacy and hospital drug management. Chapman & Hall, London

24. Parenteral products

A. Broad

Parenteral products are dosage forms intended for administration by injection, infusion or implantation via routes that breach one or more biological membranes. Body mechanisms concerned with preventing the access of micro-organisms and other harmful materials are thus circumvented and therefore special care in the formulation, preparation and administration of parenteral dosage forms is required.

The major routes of parenteral administration are discussed in the companion volume (Ch. 21, Aulton 1988) and are listed briefly below.

Intradermal injections are made into the skin between the dermis and the epidermis (Fig. 24.1). Small volumes (0.1–0.2 ml) are injected mainly for diagnosis of allergy and immunity.

Subcutaneous injections are made into the tissues immediately under the dermis (Fig. 24.1). Bolus injections of 1 ml or less are given but the route may be used for slow infusion, e.g. of opiates for relief of chronic pain.

Intramuscular injections are small volumes (maximum 5 ml) injected into a block of skeletal muscle, usually the deltoid in the shoulder or the gluteal muscle in the buttock (Fig. 24.1). Suspensions and oily solutions as well as aqueous injections can be given by this route.

Intravenous injections are made directly into a convenient superficial vein (most often on the back of the hand or in the internal flexure of the elbow). The volumes administered may vary from 1 ml to 500 ml or more. Small volume injections may be given intravenously to produce a rapid effect, e.g. induction of anaesthesia or muscle relaxation for endotracheal intubation procedures. Large volume infusions, administered slowly, are used when the oral route is unavailable for replacement of fluid, electrolytes and nutrients and for the administration of some drugs.

Intra-arterial injections administered directly into an artery are used mainly in diagnostic procedures, e.g. X-ray contrast and to administer drugs to neonates.

Intraspinal injections may be used to administer spinal anaesthetics and occasionally for the administration of antibiotics. Injections are made into the subarachnoid space (intrathecal), into the peridural space (peridural) or into the cisterna magna (intracisternal). Formulation of spinal injections is critical if irreversible damage to delicate tissues is to be avoided.

Intra-articular injections made into the synovial fluid of a joint may be used for the localized administration of corticosteroid anti-inflammatory agents.

Other parenteral routes include ophthalmic and intracardiac injections.

Implants are small non-disintegrating tablets intended for depot medications and are prepared by heavy compression or by fusion. They are implanted subcutaneously or intramuscularly.

FORMULATION OF PARENTERAL PRODUCTS

Injections as drug delivery systems are described in detail in Chapter 21 of the companion volume (Aulton 1988). Some practical aspects of the formulation of in-

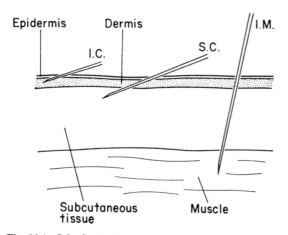

Fig. 24.1 Injection routes

jections are discussed in this chapter.

These aspects include:

— Volume of the injection.
— The vehicle in which the drug is dissolved or dispersed.
— Disperse systems for injection.
— Adjustment to isotonicity.
— Concentration units.
— Adjustment of specific gravity.
— Adjustment of pH.
— Stabilizers.
— Preservatives.

The volume of the injection

The major factors are the required route of administration which may impose a limit on dosage volume and the solubility of the drug in the chosen vehicle.

The vehicle

Water is the preferred injection vehicle since aqueous preparations are well tolerated by the body and easy to administer.

Water

Water is used to clean containers and equipment, and is the main constituent in the majority of pharmaceuticals. Water has a large solvent capacity for a wide range of materials, but it is difficult to purify and difficult to keep clean. Mains water arriving in the pharmacy has only been purified to the extent that it is safe to drink and is compatible with good health. It often contains a wide variety of contaminants such as electrolytes and organic substances, micro-organisms, particulate matter, dissolved gases such as carbon dioxide, ammonia and chlorine. The diverse nature of these contaminants poses a problem for anyone attempting to purify water to a level suitable for pharmaceutical use.

Pure water is a poor conductor of electricity. It has a conductivity of 0.055 μS/cm (microsiemens) at the standard measuring temperature of 25°C. Even low concentrations of dissolved solids will cause a substantial change in conductivity, so conductivity measurement represents a useful means of checking the degree of impurity in a sample of water. This figure can be converted to give a value for the level of total dissolved solids (t.d.s.) by using the formula:

conductivity (μS/cm) $\times$ 0.7 = t.d.s. (p.p.m.)

Conductivity is temperature dependent, changing by about 2% per degree Celsius, and must therefore be corrected to 25°C. As the water approaches absolute purity this temperature variation rises to almost 6% per degree Celsius. Many water purification systems have integral conductivity meters which automatically make the correction for temperature but this correction can be calculated from standard graphs.

There are three general methods of purifying water, by distillation, deionization or reverse osmosis (Cross 1985).

Deionization

Deionization, or ion exchange, removes all inorganic ions and some weak organic ions from the water by exchanging them with hydrogen or hydroxide ions, depending on the charge on the contaminant. The process uses two types of polymeric bead, one bearing anionic reactive groups and the other cationic reactive groups. The resins are known respectively as cation and anion exchange resins:

1. R–H + NaCl $\rightleftharpoons$ R–Na + HCl
2. R–OH + HCl $\rightleftharpoons$ R–Cl + H$_2$O

In stage 1 above an ionic impurity sodium chloride interacts with the resin to produce the salt of the acidic resin and free hydrochloric acid. In step 2 the acid reacts with the basic resin to produce the chloride salt of the basic resin and water. The net result of passing through both resins is therefore the exchange of a molecule of ionic impurity with an equivalent molecule of water. Two kinds of anion exchange resin are commonly used; weakly and strongly basic. Weakly basic resins are economical in use and can yield a product with a conductivity better than 50 μS/cm. Strongly basic resins, such as that shown in the above example, remove chlorides and sulphates as well as weakly ionized species such as silica, carbon dioxide and organic contaminants. They yield a product with a conductivity of 1 μS/cm or less but cost more to run.

Ultra-pure water with a conductivity below 0.1 μS/cm can be produced using mixed-bed systems and these are the type found in most laboratories.

Reverse osmosis

Reverse osmosis is a technique in which pure water and feedwater are separated from one another by a semipermeable membrane, and pressure is applied to the feedwater sufficient to overcome the osmotic pressure exerted by its contaminants. As a result, water is forced from the feedwater side of the membrane to the pure water side leaving the bulk of the contaminant load behind. It is distinct from filtration because 90–95% of ions are removed, as are all contaminants with a molecular weight above about 250.

Reverse osmosis units have low running costs virtually independent of the level of contamination in the feedwater. Membranes are reasonably long lived if handled properly and most small systems can operate simply using mains feedwater pressure. The method can be used with badly contaminated feedwater, although its efficiency falls as the contamination level increases, and it generally produces water with a conductivity in the range 20–80 μS/cm. Under ideal conditions conductivities down to 10 μS/cm can be achieved.

Distillation

Distillation is by far the oldest method and can produce water with a conductivity varying from 0.1 μS/cm to 5 μS/cm depending on the type of still used. The advantages of distillation are that it can be used successfully with water of any level of impurity, and the purity of the distillate and the cost of producing it is independent of that.

The majority of stills consist of an evaporating vessel where boiling water produces steam which is then condensed back to water. Various systems are used to prevent water droplets carrying pyrogens, foreign matter and gases over from the evaporator to the condensor in the water vapour.

Water supplies to the stills should have a high purity to reduce the build up of scale. Scale reduces the transfer of heat and therefore the efficacy of the still is reduced (see the companion volume, Ch. 30, Aulton 1988).

Closed circuit cooling systems can be provided to reduce the water consumption of the still to only that which is required to be converted to distillate. This is particularly suited when water supplies are erratic or inadequate. The cooling water is recirculated via a fan-assisted, air-cooled heat exchanger.

Conductivity meters are used to measure the quantity of ionizable material in the distillate and are installed at the outlet of the stills. A conductivity of 1 μS/cm is accepted as the usual standard for water of injectable quality. Above this level a valve system sends the distillate to waste and triggers an alarm. This measurement of conductivity alone can be misleading since pyrogens, dissolved organic matter and particulate matter may not affect the conductivity. The temperature of the distillate is controlled via valves which pass it through a water-cooled condenser. The distillate is therefore cooled and the feedwater is pre-warmed.

The treated water should be monitored regularly for chemical, microbial and pyrogenic contamination as relevant. Records should be kept of the results of monitoring and of any remedial action.

For a discussion on the types of still suitable for preparing water of the quality appropriate for parenteral products, see Allwood & Fell (1980).

Water for injections

The only process for producing water for injections acceptable to the British and European Pharmacopoeias is distillation, although the USP also allows the method of reverse osmosis.

'Water for Injections' is sterile distilled water, free from pyrogens and prepared in a still fitted with a baffle system to prevent entrainment of water droplets that carry pyrogenic substances. Water for Injections is sterilized by autoclaving in sealed containers immediately (within 4–6 hours of collection) to prevent the development of bacteria from which pyrogens are derived.

For some preparations (e.g. aminophylline injections) the water must be free from dissolved carbon dioxide and for some preparations (e.g. apomorphine injections) the water must be free from dissolved air. This is achieved by boiling freshly prepared apyrogenic water for 10 minutes to dispell dissolved gases and then immediately sealing into its final container for sterilization.

Unsterilized, freshly prepared apyrogenic water may be used in the preparation of injections, provided that the final solution or preparation is then immediately sterilized. It is usual to interpret immediately as 'within 4–6 hours of collection'.

Pyrogens

The injection of distilled water may cause a rise in body temperature; water producing this reaction is said to be *pyrogenic* (meaning 'producing fever') and water free from this effect is described as *apyrogenic*.

Types of pyrogens. There appear to be several different pyrogens with closely related chemical structures. They are produced chiefly by Gram-negative bacteria and may form part of the endotoxin of these organisms. In smooth bacterial forms the endotoxin consists of a complex of a pyrogenic lipopolysaccharide, a protein and an inert lipid. The lipid part of the lipopolysaccharide is the main pyrogenic agent but combination with the polysaccharide increases its activity, probably by making it more soluble. In rough bacteria the active lipid is associated with the protein instead of the polysaccharide and in this form is less active.

Some lipopolysaccharides have been highly purified and found to have a molecular weight of about one million, i.e. they are about the size of a very small virus. Unlike the complete endotoxin, the lipopolysaccharide fraction is water soluble and, consequently, is found in the medium in which the organism is grown. The pyrogens which occur in intravenous fluids are very active because relatively few contaminating bacteria are required to produce a solution which has a pyrogenic effect.

The presence of pyrogens in an injection is most serious when the volume is large. There are three reasons for this: (a) a large volume injection will contain a correspondingly large amount of pyrogens (b) large volume injections (such as infusion fluids) are usually given intravenously and, consequently, the pyrogen will have a more rapid effect and (c) patients receiving infusion fluids are often dangerously ill and the effect of the rise in temperature could be disastrous. Therefore, it is of the utmost importance to eliminate pyrogens from injections, especially those given in large volumes intravenously.

The *sources* of pyrogens in injections may be the solvent, the medicament, the apparatus and the method of storage between preparation and sterilization. Possibly the most important is the solvent.

Pyrogens are difficult to destroy once produced in a product for the following reasons:

1. *Thermostable* — to destroy some types, temperatures much lighter than those used in the official sterilization processes are necessary (250°C for 30 minutes or 200°C for 1 hour).
2. *Water-soluble* — therefore, they are not removed by the usual types of bacteria-proof filters.
3. *Unaffected by the common bactericides.* Consequently none of the methods used to sterilize the injections of the British Pharmacopoeia can be relied upon to eliminate pyrogens. However, they are also:
4. *Non-volatile.* This provides a way of removing them from water. As already stated the still must be of a design that prevents the carry over of water spray from the boiler.

British Pharmacopoeia test for pyrogens. When the volume to be injected into a patient in a single dose is 15 ml or more the preparation must comply with the test for pyrogens in the BP Appendix XIV K as outlined below.

The test consists of measuring the rise in body temperature evoked in healthy rabbits by the intravenous injection of a sterile solution of the substance under test. Details of the selection of animals, the housing of the animals and the equipment to be used are specified in the Pharmacopoeial Appendix. The '*main test*' is preceded by a '*preliminary test*' using sterile

pyrogen-free saline solution and is designed to exclude any animal showing an unusual response to the trauma of injection. The method of carrying out the main test and the interpretation of the results are described in the Pharmacopoeia.

Limulus amoebocyte lysis (LAL) assay

The LAL assay is a specific test method for bacterial endotoxin, the only pyrogen of significance to most manufacturers of pharmaceuticals and medical devices. The test is based on the primitive blood-clotting mechanism of the American horseshoe crab (*Limulus polyphemus*). Several enzymes located with the crab's amoebocyte blood cells are triggered by endotoxin to initiate an enzymic coagulation cascade that concludes with the production of a proteinaceous gel.

The gel that results from the interaction of endotoxin with the LAL reagent can be evaluated by several methods. The most commonly used today are the gel clot endpoint test, the turbidometric assay, the colorimetric (Lowry protein) assay and the chromogenic substrate test. The gel clot endpoint test is the simplest and most widely used assay.

The test should be carried out in a manner that avoids microbial contamination. Before carrying out the test it is necessary to verify that there are no interferring factors in the preparation, the equipment does not adsorb endotoxins (as with some plastics) and the sensitivity of the lysate is known.

LAL test reagent is prepared by lyophilizing lysed *Limulus* amoebocyte cells. An equal volume of LAL reagent and test solution (typically 0.1 ml of each) are mixed in a depyrogenated glass test-tube. The tube is incubated at 37°C for 1 hour, after which the test is read. The tube is removed from the incubator and inverted. A gel clot that remains solid through inversion is evidence of a positive test. When used in this manner, the gel clot endpoint assay is primarily a pass-fail test, limited only by the sensitivity of the LAL reagent employed.

The LAL test is cheaper, quicker and more accurate than other tests. Additionally it can be performed in the pharmaceutical laboratory. The test is specific for endotoxins of Gram-negative origin whereas the rabbit pyrogen test is sensitive for all pyrogens (exotoxins and endotoxins from sources other than Gram-negative bacteria).

The LAL test is particularly useful for the following:

1. Radiopharmaceuticals and cytotoxic agents.
2. Products with marked pharmacological or toxicological activity in the rabbit (e.g. insulin).

3. Blood products which sometimes give misleading results in the rabbit.

4. Water for injection where the LAL test is potentially more stringent and readily applied.

Other water-miscible vehicles for injections

Ethanol

Ethanol is rarely chosen as a vehicle for parenteral products because of its pharmacological activity and capacity for producing pain and tissue damage on injection. It is sometimes included as a cosolvent (see Ch. 11).

Propylene glycol

Propylene glycol may be used as a vehicle or cosolvent. It may cause pain and irritation at the site of injection and formulations designed for administration via intramuscular or subcutaneous routes should include a local anaesthetic, such as benzyl alcohol.

Water-immiscible vehicles

Oily vehicles may be chosen for drugs with poor aqueous solubility, particularly if a sustained-effect, slow-release preparation is required. Oily injections may only be administered by the intramuscular route and should be so labelled. They are generally viscous especially when cold and therefore require a wide-bore injection needle. Injections are often painful.

Fixed oils

A 'suitable' fixed oil may be used for several of the 'official' oily injections. Oils that have been used for injectable products include almond, arachis, cottonseed, maize and sesame oil. Deterioration of fixed oils leading to rancidity and production of free fatty acids must be avoided in injectable products and fixed oils for parenteral use must not contain any mineral oil or paraffins which cannot be metabolized by the body.

Fatty acid esters

A 'suitable' ester may be used as an alternative vehicle for several 'official' oily injections. Low-viscosity esters such as ethyl oleate or isopropyl myristate may be used alone or in combination with an oil. Peroxide-free grades are preferred to minimize the risk of oxidation of any drug and autoxidation of the oil and/or ester. These esters give products which are less viscous and therefore easier to inject, particularly in cold weather, but are less effective as slow-release dosage forms.

Alcohols

Benzyl alcohol or ethanol may be included in the formulation of oily injections containing fixed oils and/or esters to improve the overall solubility of the medicament.

Benzyl benzoate

Benzyl benzoate is included with arachis oil in Dimercaprol Injection BP.

Disperse systems for injection

Suspensions for injection

It is sometimes advantageous to inject a suspension of a drug, particularly as a depot for slow release. Suspensions must not be administered by intravenous injection. The factors which must be considered in designing a suspension for parenteral administration are discussed in the companion volume (Ch. 21, Aulton 1988). The suspension must remain sufficiently stable to allow a dose to be withdrawn from the container and any sediment of the suspended drug must be readily re-dispersible.

Emulsions for injection

The intravenous administration of an oil may be made possible by the formulation of a very stable oil in water emulsion in which the size of the oil droplets should not exceed 3 μm at any time during the product life. (See Ch. 13 for general principles of emulsion formulation.) For parenteral use the chosen emulsifiers and stabilizers must be free from any toxic effects.

Suitable substances include lecithin, polysorbate 80, serum albumin and gelatin.

Other additives for parenteral products

Adjustment to isotonicity

Aqueous solutions which exert the same osmotic pressure as blood plasma are said to be isotonic with plasma. Solutions which exert a different osmotic pressure are said to be paratonic. Those exerting a lower osmotic pressure are hypotonic and those exerting a higher osmotic pressure are hypertonic.

Aqueous solutions for injection should preferably be made isotonic with plasma in order to minimize any possible adverse effects.

Hypotonic solutions injected into the circulation may cause haemolysis, particularly if the solution is very hypotonic and/or of large volume. Hypertonic solutions cause little problem when injected intravenously provided that the chosen vein has a fast blood flow in order to avoid irritation to the vein (phlebitis) and possible thrombosis. Leakage from the injection site to the surrounding tissues should also be avoided when the injected fluid is potentially irritant.

Injections for spinal use must always be adjusted to isotonicity to avoid serious adverse effects.

The substances used to adjust the osmotic pressure of parenteral solutions to that of plasma must be inert and non-toxic. Sodium chloride is the most usual substance used, although dextrose may also be used for intravenous infusions.

Various methods may be used to estimate the amounts of adjusting substance required to render a particular solution isotonic with plasma. Calculations may be based on freezing-point depression, on sodium chloride equivalents, on molar concentration or on serum osmolarity. Full details of the methods of calculation may be found in the Pharmaceutical Handbook (1980) together with comprehensive tables of sodium chloride equivalents and freezing-point depressions.

Units of concentration

The concentrations of the ingredients in parenteral products may be expressed in a number of different ways:

Weight per unit volume

For example, atropine sulphate injection 600 μg/ml; prednisolone injection 25 mg/ml.

Percentage weight/volume

For example, sodium chloride intravenous infusion 0.9%; glucose intravenous infusion 5%; lignocaine injection 0.5%.

Millimoles per unit volume

For example, potassium chloride solution, strong (sterile) 2 mmol each of K^+ and Cl^-/ml; sodium bicarbonate intravenous infusion (usual strength) 150 mmol each of Na^+ and HCl/litre. This is explained further below.

A mole (mol) is the amount of substance containing as many elementary units (atoms, molecules, ions, etc.) as there are atoms in 12 g of the carbon isotope, ^{12}C. The millimole (mmol, i.e. 1/1000 of a mole) is more often used.

The number of atoms in 12 g of carbon-12 is 6.023 $\times 10^{23}$ (Avogadro's number): hence, this is the number of units in a mole. Since 12 is the gram atomic weight of carbon-12 it follows that a mole of atoms of any other element is the same as its gram atomic weight.

However, in the formulation of infusion fluids, the units of interest are the molecules of non-electrolytes, such as dextrose, and the ions of electrolytes.

For molecules, a mole is the same as the gram molecular weight and, therefore, 1 mmol of a non-electrolyte is the molecular weight in milligrams. For example, the molecular weight of anhydrous dextrose is 180.2 and, hence, 180.2 mg is 1 mmol.

Ions. By analogy with atoms and molecules, a mole of an ion is its ionic weight in grams but the number of moles of each of the ions of a salt in solution depends on the number of each ion in the molecule of the salt. For example:

a. Sodium chloride has one sodium and one chloride ion. Hence, 1 mole of sodium chloride provides 1 mole of sodium ions, and 1 mole of chloride ions and the molecular weight of sodium chloride in milligrams provides 1 mmol of sodium ions and 1 mmol of chloride ions.

b. Calcium chloride, however, has one calcium and two chloride ions and, hence, the molecular weight in milligrams provides 1 mmol of calcium ions and 2 mmol of chloride ions.

It follows that the quantity of salt, in milligrams, containing 1 mmol of a particular ion can be found by dividing the molecular weight of the salt by the number of that ion contained in the salt. For example:

Salt	Ion	Quantity of salt (in mg) containing 1 mmol
NaCl	Na^+	mol.wt/1 = 58.5
	Cl^-	mol.wt/1 = 58.5
$CaCl_2$	Ca^{2+}	mol.wt/1 = 147
	Cl^-	mol.wt/2 = 73.5
Na_2HPO_4	Na^+	mol.wt/2 = 179
	HPO_4^{2-}	mol.wt/1 = 258
NaH_2PO_4	Na^+	mol.wt/1 = 156
	H_2PO_4	mol.wt/1 = 156

Weights of salts to provide 1 mmol of commonly used ions are listed in Table 24.1.

Conversion equations

To convert quantities expressed in mmol per litre into weighable amounts, the following formulae may be used:

mg per litre = $W \times M$
g per litre = $(W \times M)/1000$
% w/v = $(W \times M)/10\,000$

where W is the number of mg of salt containing 1 mmol of the required ion and M is the number of mmol per litre.

Table 24.1 Weight of salts required to provide 1 mmol of various ions

Ion	mg of ion equivalent to 1 mmol	Salt	mg of salt containing 1 mmol of specified ion
Na^+	23.0	Sodium acetate $CH_3COONa \cdot 3H_2O$	136
		Sodium acid phosphate $NaH_2PO_4 \cdot 2H_2O$	156
		Sodium bicarbonate	84
		Sodium chloride	58.5
		Sodium phosphate $Na_2HPO_4 \cdot 12H_2O$	179
K^+	39.1	Potassium chloride	74.5
Ca^{2+}	40.0	Calcium chloride $CaCl_2 \cdot 2H_2O$	147
Mg^{2+}	24.3	Magnesium chloride $MgCl_2 \cdot 6H_2O$	203
Cl^-	35.5	Sodium chloride	58.5
		Potassium chloride	74.5
		Calcium chloride $CaCl_2 \cdot 2H_2O$	73.5
		Magnesium chloride $MgCl_2 \cdot 6H_2O$	101.5
CH_3COO^-	59.0	Sodium acetate $CH_3COONa \cdot 3H_2O$	136
KCO_3	61.0	Sodium bicarbonate	84
H_2PO_4	97.0	Sodium acid phosphate $NaH_2PO_4 \cdot 2H_2O$	156
HPO_4^{2-}	96.0	Sodium phosphate $NaHPO_4 \cdot 12K_2O$	358

Example 24.1

Calculate the quantities of salts required for the following electrolyte solution:

Sodium	60 mmol
Potassium	5 mmol
Magnesium	4 mmol
Calcium	4 mmol
Chloride	81 mmol
Water for injections	to 1 litre

From Table 24.1, 5 mmol of potassium ion is provided by 5 × 74.5 mg of potassium chloride which also provides 5 mmol of chloride ion. 4 mmol of magnesium ion is provided by 4 × 203 mg of magnesium chloride which also provides 2 × 4 = 8 mmol of chloride ion, since there are two chloride ions in the molecule. 4 mmol of calcium ion is provided by 4 × 147 mg of calcium chloride which, like magnesium chloride, also provides 8 mmol of chloride ion, 60 mmol of sodium ion is provided by 60 × 58.5 of sodium chloride which provides a further 60 mmol of chloride. The formula becomes:

Although there appears to be inequality between the anions and cations, the charges are equally balanced.

Example 24.2

Calculate the number of millimoles of (a) dextrose and (b) sodium ions in 1 litre of sodium chloride and dextrose injection containing 4.3% w/v of anhydrous dextrose and 0.18% w/v of sodium chloride.
Use the conversion equation — % w/v = $W \times M/10\,000$

$$M = \frac{\% \ w/v \times 10\,000}{W}$$

a. For dextrose
Since dextrose is a non-electrolyte, W = mol.wt

Hence, $M = \dfrac{4.3 \times 10\,000}{180.2} = 239$ mmol

			K^+	Mg^{2+}	mmol Ca^{2+}	Na^+	Cl^-
Potassium chloride	5 × 74.5	= 0.373 g	5				5
Magnesium chloride	4 × 203	= 0.812 g		4			8
Calcium chloride	4 × 147	= 0.588 g			4		8
Sodium chloride	60 × 58.5	= 3.510 g				60	60
Water for injections		to 1 litre					60
					73		81

b. For sodium chloride

$$M = \frac{0.18 \times 10\,000}{58.5} = 31 \text{ mmol}$$

Since 1 mmol of sodium chloride provides 1 mmol of sodium ions and 1 mmol of chloride ions, 1 litre of the solution will contain 31 mmol of sodium ions (and 31 mmol of chloride ions).

Example 24.3

Calculate the number of millimoles of calcium and chloride ions in a litre of a 0.29% solution of calcium chloride

$$M = \frac{0.029 \times 10\,000}{147} = 2 \text{ mmol}$$

But, each mole of calcium chloride provides 1 mole of calcium ions and 2 moles of chloride ions. Therefore, 1 litre of solution contains 2 mmol of calcium ions and 4 mmol of chloride ions.

Adjustment of specific gravity

This is of particular importance in spinal anaesthesia when the position of the patient and the specific gravity of the solution determine the region of anaesthesia. Hypobaric (lower density) solutions tend to rise and hyperbaric (higher density) solutions to sink relative to the cerebrospinal fluid.

Adjustment of pH

It is often desirable to adjust the pH of a parenteral product using an appropriate non-toxic buffer system. Very acid or alkaline solutions injected by the subcutaneous or intramuscular routes may cause pain and tissue damage. Although injection into a fast-flowing stream of blood by intravenous injection results in rapid dilution, leakage from the needle at the injection site may cause phlebitis and possible thrombosis. It may be necessary to adjust the pH in order to increase the stability of the preparation or to enhance therapeutic activity and it may be possible, by buffering the product to a particular pH, to minimize chemical and/or microbial deterioration.

Buffers should not be included in injections intended for intracardiac or intra-ocular injection or which will gain access to the cerebrospinal fluid.

Stabilizers

The common causes of degradation of aqueous pharmaceuticals are hydrolysis, oxidation or photolytic reactions, and a number of procedures may be used to limit these processes. Stabilizers, such as antioxidants, reducing agents and chelating agents may be included in the formulation providing that no toxicity arises from their use.

Suitable antioxidants and reducing agents include:

For aqueous injections: sodium metabisulphite, sodium sulphite, sodium thiosulphate, ascorbic acid and dextrose.

For oily injections: propyl gallate, butylated hydroxyanisole, butylated hydroxytoluene and alpha tocopherol.

Suitable chelating agents include: disodium edetate, calcium edetate, citric acid and tartaric acid.

Methods of removing gaseous oxygen include: use of Water for Injections free from dissolved gases, replacement of the air in the final container with an inert gas such as nitrogen or carbon dioxide.

Other methods of stabilization include: use of buffers to optimum pH, suitable storage conditions (cool, dark, etc.).

Antimicrobial preservatives

Bactericidal substances which will destroy vegetative bacterial cells may be included in parenteral products in which the risk of contamination by microbes is significant. These are products prepared using aseptic precautions, including sterilization by filtration and for which a terminal sterilization process in the final container is not possible. Products packed in multi-dose containers may become contaminated as successive doses are withdrawn. The BP states that aqueous preparations supplied in multi-dose containers should contain a suitable antimicrobial preservative in appropriate concentration except when the preparation itself has adequate antimicrobial properties.

Preparations in which antimicrobial preservatives are not permitted must be presented in single-dose containers and clearly labelled with an instruction to discard any unused material. Preparations intended for administration by the intra-ocular or intracardiac route or into the cerebrospinal fluid should not contain a preservative. Because of the possible toxicity associated with the injection of large quantities of bactericidal substances, injections with a dose volume in excess of 15 ml should also be unpreserved and packed in single-dose containers.

Examples of suitable antimicrobial preservatives for aqueous injections include:

Phenol	0.5%
Chlorocresol	0.1%
o-Cresol	0.3%
Benzyl alcohol	1%
Phenylmercuric salts	0.002%

For oily injections the risk of growth of vegetative organisms is much less, although phenol, o-cresol or chlorocresol may be included at the same concentrations as above if necessary.

The chosen bactericide must be compatible with the medicaments and any other adjuncts in the formulation. As with all preservative systems the response to an appropriate challenge test should be determined on order to demonstrate the efficacy of the selected bactericide. Some bactericides may interfere with the assay for the medicament, particularly those involving light absorption methods. The presence of a bactericide will also modify the approach to testing for sterility of the final product (see Ch. 30).

PREPARATION OF PARENTERAL PRODUCTS

COMPOUNDING

The basic techniques for preparing solutions, suspensions and emulsions for parenteral use are as described for 'non-sterile' preparations in Part 2 of this book. The conditions under which the compounding is carried out and the materials used must be appropriate to the product and designed to minimize particulate and microbial contamination (see Ch. 22, 23 of this book and Ch. 24 of the companion volume (Aulton 1988)). For products sterilized by filtration and other preparations not subjected to a terminal sterilization process in the final container, full aseptic precautions must be observed (see Chs 22, 23).

CLARIFICATION

Solutions for parenteral use should be free from particles, and injections with a volume of 100 ml or more must

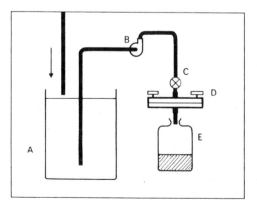

Fig. 24.2 In-line fitration unit: A, Mixing tank; B, pump; C, valve; D, in-line holder containing microporous membrane; E, receiver. (Courtesy of Millipere (UK) Ltd)

comply with the BP test for the absence of particulate matter. Suitable filtration media are sintered glass filters or membrane filters with a pore size of 0.45–1.2 μm.

Usually filters are made part of a unit consisting of a container for the unfiltered solution, the filter and a receiver for the filtrate (Fig. 24.2) The application of positive pressure above, or of negative pressure below the filter increases the rate of filtration. Prolonged filtration times are undesirable because of the risk of the growth of pyrogen-producing bacteria during the filtration process. For a further description of filtration media for clarification and sterilization see Chapter 22.

STERILIZATION

Methods used for terminal sterilization of parenteral products are described in Chapters 20 and 21.

CONTAINERS AND CLOSURES FOR PARENTERAL PRODUCTS

Containers

Containers for parenteral products are produced from one of three types of glass or from one of a variety of plastic materials (see also the companion volume Ch. 12, Aulton 1988).

Types of glass

Type I. Commonly known as neutral glass this material has a high resistance to hydrolysis and withstands autoclaving, weathering and solutions of pH up to about 8.

Type II (sulphated glass). Containers may be treated with moist sulphur dioxide at high temperature to create a neutral surface film with high hydrolytic resistance. Resistance to autoclaving may be less than for Type I.

Type III (soda glass). This offers very little resistance to hydrolysis and should be used only for non-aqueous preparations and powders for reconstitution immediately prior to administration.

Containers made from Type II or III glass should be used once only for parenteral preparations.

Standards for glass containers for parenteral products are given in the BP.

Types of plastic

Materials based on a number of polymers are used to manufacture containers for parenteral products. These include polyethylene, polyvinyl chloride and polypropylene. Desirable characteristics for plastic containers for injectables include some rigidity combined with flexibility, impermeability to air and water vapour, light resistance, resistance to autoclaving, etc. In order to produce plastics of appropriate quality a number of additives may be added to the basic polymer. It is essential that none of the constituents of the plastic are leached out into any fluid in the container, particularly if such constituents could cause deterioration of the product or toxicity in the patient. It is also important that the plastic does not sorb any of the constituents of injection, e.g. drug, stabilizer, preservative, etc. The composition of the plastic should be obtained from the supplier before selection of a plastic container and exhaustive tests under the proposed conditions of use should be made prior to and at regular intervals during full production.

Standards for plastic containers for parenteral products are given in the BP.

Types of container for parenteral products

Parenteral products are supplied in a type and size of container appropriate to the use of the product. The most usual types of container are described below.

Glass ampoules. These are the most common single-dose containers. They are made entirely of glass in a range of sizes from 1 to 50 ml. For aqueous solutions neutral glass is used. The powder ampoule is for sterile solids that are unstable in solution and, since the injection is prepared immediately before use, neutral glass is not essential. Because, after filling, ampoules are sealed by fusion of glass there is no danger of entry of micro-organisms and all the problems associated with the use of rubber are avoided. Good ampoule glass should melt and seal easily and not splinter excessively when the container is opened. Excessive splintering might contaminate the solution with glass spicules.

Amber ampoules are obtainable for protection against light although it is now more usual to rely solely on packaging in a light-tight box.

Ampoules can be used only once and, consequently, they need not be very strong; their walls can be thin with the advantage of lightness, greater resistance to thermal shock and more rapid heat conduction to the contents during sterilization (Fig. 24.3).

A British Standard (BS 795:1983) specifies the materials, dimensions and performance requirements of the types of glass ampoule and specifies a sampling procedure for ampoules that are normally manufactured and sold in bulk. Pre-scored ampoules are not covered in the standard because of the inherent risk of perforation at the score and the possibility of cracks propagating from the score line.

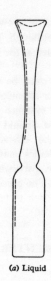

(a) Liquid

Fig. 24.3   Glass ampoule for parenterals

The following performance requirements are specified in the standard:

— Light transmission of amber ampoules.
— Residual stress.
— Freedom from internal impurities.
— Freedom from cracks.
— Eccentricity.
— Verticality.
— Hydrolytic resistance.
— Break force for easy-open ampoules.

The British Standard classifies the various types of ampoules by a reference letter. A type Q ampoule has a flat bottom, narrow stem, is a cut ampoule (for draw-off sealing) and contains a constriction.

The majority of ampoules specified in the standard are designed for draw-off sealing. Tip sealing may produce an inferior closure. Ampoules should be sealed at the gauging point. The objective should be to achieve a minimum wall thickness at the seal of not less than 50% of the ampoule stem wall thickness. An ideal finished seal should be hemispherical in shape, free from spikes, capillaries and cracks.

Closed-neck ampoules. For large-scale production closed-neck ampoules may be preferred since this removes the need for pre-washing.

The closed-neck ampoules are blown from glass tubing and sealed by fusion. The temperature used in the process kills all micro-organisms and any contaminants present in or on the tubing are burnt off to produce a sterile particle-free ampoule. The sterile closed ampoules are usually opened on semi-automatic or automatic machinery. The ampoules are fed from a hopper or by hand into a transport wheel. The wheel delivers the still sealed ampoule to the opening station. The top of the ampoule is heated using an oxygen/gas or oxygen/propane mixture which ensures a hot flame. A small hole is produced in the top of the ampoule which is then enlarged at the next station when the ampoule is spun as a further flame enlarges the opening. The tip of the open ampoule is then seized by a centring system during filling which ensures the neck of the ampoule is centred with regard to the filling needle. In case no ampoule is inserted, no filling takes place.

Advantages of sealed ampoules:
1. Clean and particle free.
2. Sterile.
3. Machine operation gives consistent seals.
4. Quick with the minimum of handling.

Cartridges (Fig. 24.4). These are cylindrical glass which are closed at one end with a rubber stopper or diaphragm (the latter held in position with a metal overseal) and at the other by a rubber plunger. They are used in a special all-metal syringe of which the needle mount is detachable and has a short piercer needle pointing into the barrel. The mount is attached, the syringe plunger is drawn back against a spring and the

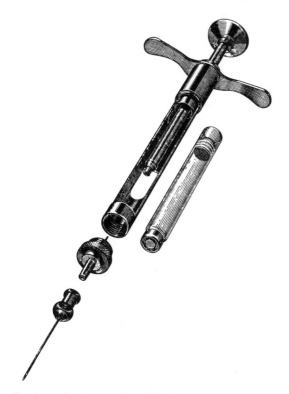

Fig. 24.4 Cartridge and special syringe

cartridge is introduced into the hollow barrel and pushed against the piercer needle to penetrate the rubber diaphragm. Then the cartridge is fully inserted and the plunger released to hold it firmly. A thread on the syringe plunger screws into a corresponding thread in the rubber plunger of the cartridge, which allows steady pressure on the injection and, if required, slight withdrawal of the plunger to discover if the needle is in a blood vessel.

They are still much used by dentists but rarely in general use compared to the ampoule and disposable syringe. Compared with ampoules:

1. They are quicker and easier to use; ampoules have to be opened and their contents carefully measured into a syringe.
2. They are safer; the risk of contaminating the injection during administration is much less and their is no possibility of injecting glass spicules.

Disadvantages are the use of rubber (care: more particulates!), the need for a special syringe and the sterilization of the needle mount (because this is the part touched by the injection).

Prefilled syringes. Prefilled syringes are becoming popular. Their capacities vary from 1 ml to 2 ml in conventional syringes to the larger (50 ml) assembled syringes.

Packaging of parenterals in the USA in disposable units is a common practice in hospitals, where a unit dose drug distribution system is used (Patel et al 1972). The American Society of Hospital Pharmacists published the first general guidelines of single unit packages in February 1967 and a revision in February 1971. The construction of the syringe is an important factor to consider in respect to convenience in routine use at the bedside, in emergency situations wherein speed and accuracy are necessary and in the manual packaging operation in the pharmacy. There are various kinds of syringes available on the market and each has its advantages and disadvantages. Because the disposable single unit package may have to be stored for extended periods of time in disposable plastic syringes, any drug–plastic interactions should be assessed before packing.

Most disposable syringes have rubber-type plunger tips made of various type of materials. Therefore each drug packaged in a single unit syringe should be monitored for compatibility with the components and stability on storage. The majority of drugs may be satisfactorily packaged in syringes with rubber-tip caps. Two exceptions are aminophylline and adrenaline. These solutions are not suitable for packaging in commercially available empty syringes for prolonged periods of time, primarily because the absorption by the rubber of the stabilizers and antioxidants, like disodium edetate and sodium metabisulphite used in the formulation, enhances degradation of the active ingredients.

Contamination of prefilled syringes may occur during or after filling or upon storage. During the filling operation particulate and bacterial contamination may result from (1) personnel, (2) the environment, (3) particulate matter in the contents of the commercially prepared multidose vials, and (4) the syringe itself. Points 1–3 have been covered elsewhere in this book and in the companion volume (Ch. 27, Aulton 1988).

Contamination from the syringe. Dirty (but sterile) syringes themselves, may be a major source of contamination. The syringe can contaminate the solution either from particulate matter adhering to the inside of the barrel and plunger or from lubricant used for the plunger. An improperly processed rubber tip on the plunger may shed particulate matter. Miller et al (1969) showed that up to 2.8 mg of silicone fluid can be found on the rubber tip of a plunger. Silicone fluid is not miscible with the aqueous medium used for most parenteral products and mechanical flushing may deliver up to 10–11 μg of liquid silicone from a 10 ml size disposable plastic syringe. Excess silicone on the rubber-tip plungers is often visible if observed against light.

The whole operation of packing the syringes should take place in a Class I room environment. If necessary, after reconstitution, the product is thoroughly mixed in the original container. The product is drawn aseptically into a 50 ml syringe and a sterile three-way mixing stopcock is placed at the tip of the filled syringe. The desired volume of the product is drawn up into the sterile syringe blanks after attaching them to the other end of the mixing valve. A sterile rubber tip is placed on the hub tip of the syringe. After the filling operation is complete, all the syringes should be inspected visually for particulate matter. Labels with all necessary information are then attached to each syringe. During packaging, provision for solution loss in the hub tip and needle must be calculated and the overfill determined. Overfill usually averages from 0.2 ml to 0.3 ml.

Glass vials. These are glass containers sealed by a rubber closure which permits the penetration of a syringe needle to allow the withdrawal of a dose of the injection. The rubber closure is usually held in place by an aluminium sealing ring which may incorporate a detachable protective cover (Fig. 24.5). Vials may be used to contain single doses for use on one occasion only or may act as multi-dose containers from which successive doses may be withdrawn.

Large volume bottles. These may be used for intravenous infusions and contain volumes of up to 1 litre.

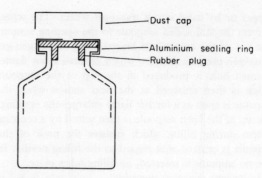

Fig. 24.5   Glass vial

They are also sealed with a rubber closure which permits access to a piercing needle connected to an intravenous administration ('giving') set. Glass containers for intravenous fluids have been largely superseded by the plastic containers described below.

The *disadvantages* of glass infusion bottles include: fragility; expense; weight; air inlet required (risk of air embolism); risk of microbial contamination through air inlet.

Flexible plastic containers (Fig. 24.6). These are the most commonly used containers for intravenous infusions since they offer a number of *advantages* over the older type of glass container. These include unbreakable; disposable; lightweight; no air inlet required; occupy less storage space; less likely to shed particles. *Disadvantages* of plastic containers include: less transparent; more difficult to mix additives; less easy to estimate residue; more difficult to label unless pre-printed; require special autoclave; vulnerable to puncture; risk of leaching/sorption of contents.

Closures

These must provide protection against the access of micro-organisms and other contaminants but allow for the contents to be withdrawn without removing the closure from the container. The term 'elastomer' refers to the complex mixture of ingredients that are used to produce a closure which may be of natural or synthetic origin. The elastomers used must be sufficiently firm and elastic to allow penetration by a needle with minimal shedding of particles. For multiple-dose containers it is important that the hole made by the needle should re-seal immediately and effectively when the needle is withdrawn.

Characteristics of an ideal elastomer:

1. Satisfactory hardness and elasticity.
2. Impermeable to air and water.

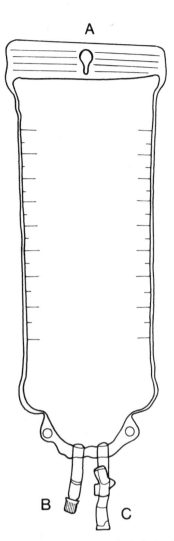

Fig. 24.6 Flexible plastic container for infusion fluid. A, Suspension eye; B, rubber cap for injecting supplementary medication; C, point at which giving set is inserted. (Viaflex, Travenol Laboratories)

3. Resistant to sterilization conditions.
4. Negligible release of constituents.
5. Negligible sorption of ingredients.
6. Good ageing qualities.

To minimize extraction by the closure of the bactericide from multi-dose containers the closures should be equilibrated with a concentration of the bactericide in excess of that in the product. This is achieved by placing the closures in a solution of at least double the concentration in the injection and subjecting to an autoclaving process followed by storage in the same solution. Full details are given in the BP.

Pharmacopoeial requirements for a container and closure

Those detailed are:

1. Sufficient transparency to allow visual inspection of the contents.
2. No adverse effect on the product.
3. Prevent diffusion in or across the walls.
4. Do not yield foreign substances to the product.

Single-dose vs multi-dose containers

Disadvantages of ampoules:

1. Less convenient for variable doses.
2. More difficult to handle.
3. Require some aseptic technique.
4. Danger of glass spicules in injection.
5. Danger of cut fingers (less with 'easy open' type).

Disadvantages of multi-dose containers:

1. Less effective seal than fused glass.
2. Risk of contamination in use.
3. Risk of leaching and/or sorption from solution.
4. May be wasteful in materials.

Methods of filling the containers

Because of the stringent requirements for quality assurance and the high production costs the preparation of parenteral products tends to be limited to commercial manufacturers and to specialized centres within the NHS hospital service. Within such organizations production methods may be streamlined and full use made of mechanization in order to reduce costs and to improve efficiency. On a small scale, products may be produced for a small number of named patients providing that adequate facilities are available.

The following method for filling ampoules is suitable for small-scale production as exemplified by the teaching laboratory.

Washing

Ampoules are supplied clean but can collect dust during packaging, transportation and subsequent storing. Washing before use is essential to remove this dust and any glass fragments generated from broken ampoules.

The most effective washing machines employ ultrasonic agitation as an aid to loosening particles from the inner surface of the ampoule. Ampoules are positioned over needles which inject water inside while at the same time the ampoules may be passed through an ultrasonic bath. The washing water is expelled from the ampoule by injecting filtered compressed air through the needles.

A simple unit often used in small hospital pharmacies is shown in Figure 24.7. The ampoule is inverted over the needle and pressed down so that its neck makes a good seal with the rubber tubing. A vacuum causes a stream of water from the needle to wash the ampoule thoroughly and quickly.

The inverted ampoules are dried in a beaker in a drying oven. If they were used wet the strength of the injection could be significantly lowered. Also, when a wet ampoule is filled the medicament often diffuses quickly up to the neck through the moisture film on the inside and then charring occurs on sealing. This is particularly noticeable with dextrose and citrates. Complete drying of the ampoule requires the use of hot air but care must be taken that the ampoule is not contaminated by any particulate matter and as soon as they are dry they should be stored under laminar air flow until required.

On a larger scale, washers are available that can wash up to 50 ampoules at a time. Several different washes can be given to the ampoule via a system of valves but each ampoule still has to be dried.

If a special washing unit is not available a syringe can be used. The ampoule is held inverted over a sink and

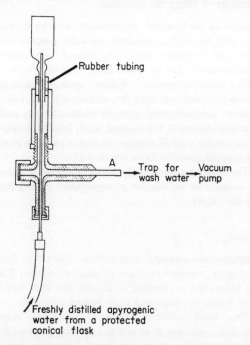

Fig. 24.7 The Manning ampoule washer. Section, slightly diagrammatic

Rubber tubing

A

Trap for wash water

Vacuum pump

Freshly distilled apyrogenic water from a protected conical flask

a syringeful of freshly distilled apyrogenic water is forcibly injected into it, making sure that the jet hits the base. The residual water is shaken out and the process repeated. Then the ampoule is inverted in a small beaker to drain.

As can be seen from the above methods, the washing and drying of ampoules is a very time-consuming occupation. In addition, all washing should take place in a cleanroom area to prevent the recontamination of the ampoule by particulates. This then requires bigger cleanroom areas and a greater chance of growth of bacteria in these 'wet' areas.

Filling of the ampoules

When filling ampoules the main aims must be to measure the volumes accurately and to keep the neck free from liquid. Many medicaments are organic chemicals that char on heating and if there is solution at the point of sealing, an ugly black ring is produced from which pieces may separate and contaminate the injection during sterilization. These ampoules would therefore be rejected on inspection.

A method of filling small quantities of ampoules using a syringe and needle is outlined below:

1. Carefully draw into the syringe a little more than the volume required of the solution. Do this gently to avoid large numbers of air bubbles in the liquid.
2. Invert the syringe to allow the air to rise towards the needle and push up the plunger to expel the bubble and leave exactly the quantity required in the barrel.
3. Wipe the needle on a non-particle-shedding wipe; this will not leave fibres on the needle.
4. Invert the ampoule over the needle, which must be long enough to reach well into the ampoule body. Since the surface of the latter is dry, no liquid will be put on the ampoule neck. If, however, the ampoule is held upright and the syringe is reverted for filling, the weight from the plunger often forces a drop of solution from the tip of the needle, and contamination of the neck is hard to avoid. Expel the liquid, gently and slowly to prevent splashing into the neck.
5. Finally, touch the needle tip against the constriction at the bottom of the neck to dislodge the last drop of liquid and then sharply withdraw the needle without touching the neck.

Filling each individual ampoule by syringe can be a time-consuming occupation. The time factor can be greatly reduced by using equipment that will deliver the required volume quickly and with the minimum of time required for setting up and manipulation of the equipment.

A peristaltic pump is ideal for this sort of operation. Peristaltic pumps are used for four major reasons:

1. The fluid is not contaminated by its passage through the pump.
2. The pump is not contaminated by the fluid.
3. The peristaltic pumping action is particularly gentle.
4. Peristaltic pumps are self-priming.

Instead of stripping and cleaning, the peristaltic pump tube can be discarded and a new tube fitted in minutes or even seconds. A sterile tube creates a sterile pump.

Hand sealing of ampoules

Use a twin-jet burner (Fig. 24.8). Set the platform at a satisfactory height and adjust the flames to a suitable intensity.

The composition of ampoule glass varies and some batches melt more easily than others. Check the behaviour of the type being used by trying an empty, but open, ampoule before sealing the batch. The following instructions are for right-handed operators.

With the left hand, position the ampoule between the flames. Grip the end of the neck with blunt-nosed forceps, held in the right hand, and, when the glass is soft enough, pull off the tops vertically and gently. Leave the tip in the flame a second or two longer, and then remove. The tip should be smoothly and evenly rounded with a small flat blob of glass in the centre (Fig. 24.9(a)).

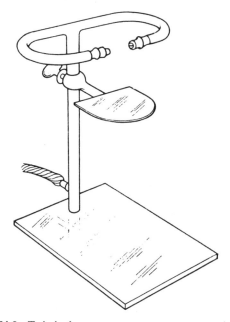

Fig. 24.8 Twin-jet burner

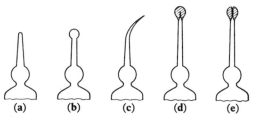

Fig. 24.9 Good and bad ampoule seals

The two most common faults are: (i) leaving the tip in the flame too long after sealing, when expansion of the air inside causes the glass to balloon (Figure 24.9(b)), and (ii) pulling off the top too vigorously; this draws the tip into a fine sharp point that is easily broken and can give a painful prick when the ampoule is handled (Fig. 24.9(c)).

Automatic sealing of ampoules

Draw sealing is recommended in preference to tip sealing and incorrect flame settings for the draw-sealing operation may lead to unacceptable levels of stress in the glass of the stem of the ampoule. The flame settings, particularly of the pre-heat flame, will largely decide the thickness of the final ampoule seal. Thin seals are more susceptible to becoming 'blown'. The correct setting of the filling/sealing machine will avoid weak or damaged seals due to the presence of liquid in the ampoule neck caused, for example, by needle touch or drips from the needle. The seal may be adversely affected if the liquid contents tend to froth easily or are very volatile or if the space between the top of the liquid and the seal is unduly small. With automatic machinery where the contact between hot glass and cold metal machine parts may lead to the formation of stress, care should be taken in the location of guides, supports, etc. It is important at all stages of handling ampoules to avoid glass against glass abrasion.

For draw-sealed ampoules a correctly formed seal will be thickest at the tip, where the glass is pulled and twisted together, and thinnest just around the centre 'pip'. At its thinnest point the seal should be not less than 50% of the original stem thickness.

Sterilization of ampoules

For methods of sterilization see Chapters 20 and 21.

Causes of leaks in ampoules

The fusion of glass in an ampoule seal can result in problems. There are two basic types of ampoule leaks: cracks and faulty seals.

Cracks in the glass arise from two sources:

1. Thermal cracks caused by rapid temperature change.
2. Mechanical cracks caused by impact or abrasion.

Stress can be introduced into glass by rapid cooling from elevated temperatures, e.g. by contact of hot glass with cold metal machine parts. The cracks may not be apparent to the naked eye but may develop later, e.g. during autoclaving. Thermal stress can be also be introduced by ceramic printing and solution dripping on the hot ampoules at the filling/sealing stage. Mechanical cracks are generally caused by ampoules rubbing or colliding together during handling operations.

Tests for leaking ampoules

The test used should ideally detect leaks regardless of their location in the ampoule. All ampoules produced should be tested. For sound ampoules the test must necessarily be non-destructive to both the ampoule and its contents and have no effect on the physical, chemical or biological properties of the contents.

The design of the leak test procedure must take into account the nature of the product and its container. For example, different test procedures may be needed for fluids of different viscosity, aqueous or non-aqueous fluids and powder-filled or lyophilized products. Highly coloured products and products in coloured ampoules could also present difficulties with the dye challenge tests. Ideally the test should be carried out after any operations liable to cause damage to the ampoule. All leak tests have one thing in common; whilst they may show the presence of leaking ampoules they cannot guarantee their absence. Hence an ampoule leak test may be defined as:

A test which gives an indication of the probability that each ampoule within a test load is perfectly sealed.

Since the test is not capable of guaranteeing that all leaking ampoules are detected, it is important that the number of faulty ampoules produced be kept to a minimum. This will reduce the overall probability that a leaking ampoule be accepted.

INSPECTION — GENERAL

It follows that the final stage of manufacture is an inspection stage to satisfy the producer that this product has reached a pre-determined standard. The container can be checked for cracks, chips and any damage to the closure system (Amini 1981) such as a split teat in a eye-drop bottle, but checking the contents of the container is far more difficult. There are at present few, if any, objective standards. Unlike a chemical assay the inspection is hardly objective; indeed it could be argued that the question of approval or rejection depends largely on the attitude of the inspector towards his or her responsibility. Consequently, different inspectors, and even the same inspector at different times, may not examine uniformly (Baldwin et al 1981). It is concluded in general however, that uniformity is achieved. A further complication is the inability of the human eye to detect particles smaller than about 50 μm. The degree of inspection will be dependent on the type of product, minimal for disinfectants but far greater for injectables.

Inspection of plastics

Visual inspection of fluids in PVC containers is feasible provided that the PVC film is of good clarity (Uotila and Santasolo 1981). Polyethylene is rather more difficult but it is claimed that experienced personnel can detect small particles. All containers should be examined for seal failure, preferably by the application of a standard pressure to the walls of the container for a few seconds (Wikner 1973). Following this inspection, it is normal procedure to overwrap with a water-impermeable plastic, such as polyethylene or polypropylene. This material should not obscure the print of the container. It should be remembered that the inside surfaces of this film will not be sterile unless applied before sterilization. This procedure is essential for PVC, moisture loss can be reduced from approximately 10% per annum to 2%. Overwrapping also helps to protect the pack from damage during handling.

Inspection of injectables

It is accepted that injection solutions should be free from foreign particles of varying types but preparing injectable medicinal products which conform to a test for clarity is one of the biggest problems faced when preparing injectables. Despite meticulous care at every stage of manufacture, the ampoules will often contain foreign matter.

There are four basic sources of particles during the preparation of the product:

1. *Introduction of particles into the solution during filtration*. Particles may pass through the filter, be shed from the filter, or introduced into the filtrate from the environment.

2. *Introduction of particles from the container and closure surfaces.* These may be present as debris before and during filling, or they may be generated physicochemically by contact with the contents during or after autoclaving.

3. *Introduction of particles after filling* (flakes of carbon may be produced when an ampoule is heat sealed). Particles may enter around the closure during spray cooling, or for the purpose of testing may enter when the closure is penetrated or removed (breaking of glass ampoules).

4. *Formation of particles (including air bubbles) during storage.* These may be produced by agglomeration, polymerization, precipitation or nucleation. Since there is such a low level of nuclei on which air bubbles can form, air dissolved during autoclaving may take a long time to come out. Users have reported a high count after 1 or 2 weeks from physiological saline that passed specification before, and 2 days after, autoclaving and that again passed specification after 1 month's storage.

Particulate matter can be defined as follows: 'Particulate matter consists of extraneous, mobile, undissolved substances, other than gas bubbles, unintentionally present in parenteral solutions.'

The BP 1980 recommends that injections which are solutions, when examined under suitable conditions of visibility, are clear and practically free from particles. Additionally, where stated in individual monographs, solutions to be injected and which are supplied in containers with a normal content of 100 ml or more comply with the limit test for particulate matter, Appendix XIII.

Visual inspection

In industry the majority of inspection is performed by sophisticated machinery. Hospital pharmacies generally use trained operators for spotting defective products. The container and closure system are examined for obvious defects such as cracked bottles, split eye-drop teats, broken ampoule seals, etc. The contents of the containers are examined using simple light sources with or without polarized light. The container is held horizontally and rotated immediately under an illuminated background. Polarized light helps identification in clear bottles but can cause problems when viewing amber glass depending on the degree of coloration (Groves 1973, Davis et al 1970). The container should then be inverted once or twice to find heavy particles, such as glass. Movement must not be sufficiently vigorous to fill the solution with confusing air bubbles.

The success rate of finding defective containers is totally dependent on the operator. Particulates in solutions can be examined using mechanical methods (Knapp 1981) and is the basis for the BP limit test on particulate matter.

LABELLING

Methods

It was once usual to label containers of injections by means of orthodox paper labels, but for ampoules this method has now largely been superseded by direct printing on the glass. One reason for this is that paper labels are capable of being heavily contaminated with bacteria. These could, perhaps, gain access to the contents when the ampoules are opened, or could contaminate the operator's hands or hypodermic needles. Secondly, in operating theatres ampoules are often stored immersed in antiseptic solutions in order to ensure that their external surfaces are quite sterile; paper labels would not survive this treatment. To overcome this, ampoules which are sterile on the outside are now often provided for certain procedures in operating theatres (epidural injections). They are overwrapped in single- or double-wrapped packages.

For many purposes printing with air-dried inks is satisfactory. This method has the advantage of being carried out on the filled ampoule. However, like paper labels, such inks do not withstand immersion in some of the antiseptic fluids used, so it is often preferable to use ceramic inks applied by an offset method or by silk screening. The inks are subsequently subjected to temperatures approaching the melting point of glass in an electric muffle furnace, or by the direct application of a gas flame. This process can, of course, only be used on empty ampoules but the effect is permanent because the pigment is baked into the glass.

Whatever printing process is used the lettering should be as large as space will allow in order to achieve maximum legibility, and should run parallel to the long axis to facilitate reading.

Labelling requirements

The information included on the label of a parenteral product must conform to the requirements of the Medicines Act (1968) and subsequent regulations and the Misuse of Drugs Act (1971) and Regulations (1985). These general labelling requirements for medicines are described in Chapter 10 and Appendix 1 of the book.

Special labelling requirements for parenteral products are given in the British Pharmacopoeia and include:

— The strength expressed in terms of the amount of active ingredient in a suitable dose volume.

— The name of any added substance.

— An indication that a single-dose preparation should be discarded after first use.

There are also special labelling requirements for particular types of product, e.g. powders for reconstitution, and concentrated solutions requiring dilution.

PRODUCT RECALL

Finally after formulating, filling, sterilizing, inspecting and quality controlling the product, problems can occur. The problem could be a wrongly labelled product, a stability problem or a multitude of other problems and a method must be employed to recall the affected product. The 'Guide to good pharmaceutical manufacturing practice' (DHSS 1983) states:

A complaint, or otherwise reported product-defect, may lead to the need for a recall. Any action taken to recall a product suspected or known to be defective or hazardous, should be prompt in accordance with a pre-determined plan. The procedures to be followed should be specified in writing and made known to all who may be concerned.

The cause of the problem should be investigated and rectified as quickly as possible. The incidence of recall should be minimal as the whole philosophy of dispensing and manufacture is to try and anticipate the problem BEFORE it happens.

BIBLIOGRAPHY

Aulton M E (ed) 1988 Pharmaceutics: the science of dosage form design. Churchill Livingstone, Edinburgh

Baldwin H J, Howard S A, Leelarasamee N Visual ampoule inspection by experienced and non-experienced inspectors. Journal of Parenteral Science and Technology 35 (4): 148–151

British Standard 795. 1983 British Standard specification for ampoules

Cross J 1985 Water ways. Laboratory Practice 1: 11–15

Davis N M, Turco S 1971 A study of particulate matter in I.V. infusion fluids — Phase 2. American Journal of Hospital Pharmacy 28: 620–623

Davis N M, Turco S, Sively E 1970 A study of particulate matter in I.V. infusions. American Journal of Hospital Pharmacy 27: 822–826

Department of Health and Social Security 1983 Guide to good pharmaceutical manufacturing practice. HMSO, London

Groves M J 1973 Parenteral products. William Heinemann Medical Books Ltd

Knapp J Z, Kushner M K, Abramson L R 1981 Particle inspection of parenteral products: an assessment. Journal of Parenteral Science and Technology 35(4): 176–185

Patel J A, Curtis E G, Phillips G L 1972 Single unit packaging of parenterals in the hospital pharmacy. American Journal of Hospital Pharmacy 29(11): 947–951

Smail G A, Marshall I 1982 Intravenous additives in Clinical Pharmacy and Hospital Drug Management. Lawson D H, Richards R M E (eds), Chapman and Hall, London

Trueman G 1973 Journal of Hospital Pharmacy 31: 239

Uotila and Santasol 1981 New concepts in the manufacturing and sterilisation of LVP in plastic bottles. Journal of Parenteral Science and Technology 35(4): 170–175

Wikner M 1973 Svensk Farmaceutisk Tidskrift 77: 773

25. Intravenous additives

A. Auld

Introduction

Intravenous injections are usually aqueous solutions injected into a prominent vein. The dose volume of an intravenous injection may vary from a fraction of a millilitre given as a bolus injection to 500 ml or more given as a slow injection and termed an 'intravenous infusion'. Intravenous injections should be pyrogen free if greater than 10 ml and preservative free if greater than 15 ml in volume.

Large-volume intravenous infusions are used to replace fluid losses in patients unable to take adequate oral fluid and also to administer electrolytes to restore any imbalance and to correct any deficit. Solutions infused into a peripheral vein should be isotonic with plasma. The administration of more concentrated solutions should be made into a central vein.

It may be necessary or convenient to administer one or more drugs via an intravenous infusion, either by adding the drug to the infusion fluid or by injecting into the giving set or intravenous cannula. Some of the limitations and precautions associated with this method of administration are described in this chapter.

METHODS OF ADMINISTRATION OF INTRAVENOUS INFUSIONS

Administration sets

Administration sets, or giving sets, are used to carry the infusion fluid from the infusion container to the patient and to control the rate of administration of the infusion fluid. They are made of plastic. Control of infusion rate can be achieved by various methods — from the simple 'V'-track controller and drip chamber to the more sophisticated devices described below.

The use of plastic in the manufacture of giving sets can pose problems. Most sets are made of PVC which can absorb drugs from solution.

Light transparency is a problem when a drug is significantly degraded by light, e.g. sodium nitroprusside,

vitamin A (Kirk 1985) and frusemide (Yahya et al 1986). Giving sets are available which filter out harmful light.

Adsorption of drugs onto PVC has been demonstrated with nitroglycerin, chlormethiazole, isosorbide dinitrate and diazepam.

Giving sets made of polybutadiene and methacrylate butadiene styrene have been shown not to adsorb isosorbide dinitrate, nitroglycerin or diazepam (Lee 1986).

Infusion control devices

Infusion pumps are electromechanical devices which are designed to automatically control intravenous infusion ensuring greater precision and therefore safety when compared to the traditional gravity flow infusion. They are used to infuse parenteral nutrition solutions and drugs which require careful control, e.g. dopamine. There are four basic types available: gravity feed controllers, drip-rate pumps, volumetric pumps and syringe drivers.

Gravity feed controllers

The infusion pressure is supplied by gravity and control of the infusion is via drip rate. They are cheap, use conventional infusion sets and carry a low risk of extravasation since they do not pump the intravenous injection into the vein. Once set up they require little attention and will sound an alarm should the pre-set rate not be maintained or when the infusion container is empty. They do have several disadvantages however. As in gravity infusion, pressure is limited by the height of the container and is unable to cope with changes in infusion resistance such as a rise in venous pressure or a change in the patient's position. The maximum infusion rate is limited by solution viscosity and the bore of the cannula. Their greatest drawback is reliance on the counting of drops to fix the flow rate. Drop size varies with the viscosity and surface tension of the drug solution and so gravity feed controllers are unable to accurately control volume flow rate.

Drip-rate pumps

In this case infusion pressure is supplied by the peristaltic action of rollers (rotary peristaltic) or of mechanical fingers (linear peristaltic), on deformable tubing. This may be part of the standard giving set or a special giving set with an insert of softer tubing. The infusion rate is controlled by drip rate. As with drip-rate controllers, volumetric accuracy is poor due to drop-size variability. Factors which vary drop size are the giving set used, the rate of infusion, and the temperature, viscosity and surface tension of the fluid. These pumps are able to produce high pressures which carry the risks of extravasation and pressure build up when there is a blockage. Pressure-limiting devices are often fitted to prevent the patient receiving a bolus injection when the blockage is relieved. A further problem with pressurized systems is the risk of injecting air. Air detectors and bubble traps can reduce the risk but correct priming and the use of the correct giving set are essential. The advantages of these pumps are that they often use low-cost giving sets and that high flow rates can be achieved even with viscous fluids through small bore cannulae.

Volumetric pumps

Volumetric pumps avoid the problems of drop-size variability by using a piston-type pump or special insert into a peristaltic pump of known capacity. These pumps are able to accurately control infusion volume, they are not affected by changes in resistance to the infusion and have a variety of alarms to prevent injection of air and warn of faults with the pump. The disadvantages of volumetric pumps are the possibility of extravasation (i.e. leakage of drug outside the vein), they have an oscillatory flow pattern, air bubbles in the volumetric part of the giving set can lead to overestimation of the volume infused due to reduction of stroke volume. They are also the most expensive to buy, and, because of their dedicated infusion sets, to run.

Syringe drivers

Syringe drivers are used for the continuous infusion of small volumes of drug solutions. A standard syringe loaded with the drug in a suitable vehicle is fitted onto the device which then compresses the plunger at a pre-set rate. They may be clockwork or electromechanical. These devices do not rely on drop counting and are therefore not affected by properties of the drug solution.

The electromechanical devices have alarms to warn of malfunction. Drugs often administered in this way are heparin, insulin and diamorphine. For instance, diamorphine is sometimes given as a 24-hour subcutaneous infusion for the control of chronic pain.

In-line filtration

Removal of pyrogen-producing bacteria

The manufacturing processes for the production of intravenous infusion exclude pyrogens from the final product. During use the product can become contaminated with micro-organisms from the environment. These can be filtered out by in-line filters with a pore size of 0.2 μm (Holmes et al 1980). When in-line filters are used for longer than 24 hours, however, their ability to retain pyrogens released from the trapped bacteria becomes important. Filters made from cellulose ester polyacrylate, polypropylene and polyethylene allow pyrogen to pass, whereas filters made from posidyne nylon 66 retain pyrogen for up to 96 hours (Baumgartner et al 1986).

Removal of particles

It is inevitable that intravenous fluids contain particles. These particles originate from the packaging and the environment during manufacture and after opening. The number of particles due to the packaging and the environment has been reduced by improvements in the manufacturing techniques (Davis et al 1970, Davis & Turco 1971, Turco & Davis 1973a), but the risk of introduction afterwards, by opening ampoules or inserting needles through vial bungs, still remains.

Infusion of particles is associated with phlebitis which is the most common side-effect of intravenous therapy. Other associated factors include the size of the vein, the site of the infusion, the fluid being infused, the cannula used, the duration of the infusion and the rate of flow through the cannula (Lewis & Hecker 1985).

It would therefore be logical to reduce the infusion of particles by terminal filtration. This can be achieved by using an in-line filter which is fitted between the end of the giving set and the intravenous cannula.

The incidence of phlebitis during infusion of large volumes (Rusho & Bain 1979) and antibiotic infusions (Maddox et al 1977, Bivens et al 1979) has been reduced by in-line filtration with pore sizes varying between 0.2 and 0.5 μm. However, the systemic effects of infused particles are not clear. Granulomas in rabbit lung after intravenous infusion have been described (Garvan & Gunner 1964). In humans, lesions in lung, kidney, liver, spleen and brain have been linked with infused particles but the clinical importance is unknown (Turco & Davis 1973b). Pulmonary capillaries have a diameter of 10–12 μm and glass particles with diameters over 20 μm which have been found in opened glass ampoules (Shaw & Lyall 1985) may lodge in them.

In-line filters do have disadvantages: they cost more; they decrease the flow rate of colloidal solutions and lipid suspensions; they add an extra site for disconnection and some drugs are absorbed by the filters, notably vincristine and insulin (Butler et al 1980).

INFUSION ADDITIVES

In critically ill patients, it is often necessary to infuse more than one drug at the same time. This can be achieved by adding a drug to an infusion fluid or by infusing drugs along the same line. This procedure is not without hazard, quite apart from the risk of microbial and particulate contamination there is the danger of producing and administering unstable or incompatible mixtures.

In the UK, concern about the problems of adding drugs to infusion fluids led to the establishment of a working party by the Department of Health and Social Security. The Report of the Working Party on the Addition of Drugs to Intravenous Infusion Fluids (Breckenridge Working Party Report 1976) includes guidance for pharmacists, doctors and nurses when drugs are administered by intravenous infusion. Their main recommendation was that ways in which pharmacy staff could prepare the necessary drug infusion admixture be examined and that such mixtures should be supplied by the pharmacy. Where such a service was not feasible the pharmacist should advise on the training of doctors and nurses on intravenous infusion therapy and should provide advice and reference data for medical and nursing staff concerned with intravenous drug prescribing, preparation and administration.

The report defines the responsibilities of the pharmacist to include, in addition to the above, (i) monitoring of prescriptions for drugs to be added to i.v. infusions with special reference to stability and compatibility and (ii) provision of pharmaceutical advice and information to medical staff.

Stability and compatibility

Definitions

Drug — a single drug chemical.

Drug preparation — a drug formulated with additional substances to form a product for a specified route of administration. The additional substances can include antioxidants, buffers and preservatives. The exact formulation can vary depending on the manufacturer, hence it is important to discriminate between manufacturers.

Instability

Instability is considered to have occurred when an intravenous fluid admixture loses greater than 10% of its labelled potency from the time of preparation to the time of completion of the infusion.

Incompatibility

Incompatibility occurs when by physicochemical means an intravenous admixture is produced that is unsuitable for administration.

Causes of instability and incompatibility

Addition of a drug preparation to a sterile intravenous infusion fluid carries the risk of microbial and particulate contamination and the preparation of an unstable or incompatible mixture. This unstable or incompatible mixture can be caused by one or more of the following factors as described by Smail and Marshall (1982): inadequate mixing; the ability of the drug or drug preparation to interact with or degrade the infusion fluid; the effect of the infusion fluid on the stability of the drug; and other aspects such as light and air on the stability of the admixture.

The effect of inadequate mixing

Drugs are added to infusion fluids as solutions in appropriate solvents. These solutions may have a specific gravity which is significantly different from the infusion fluid resulting in layering. As a result of inadequate mixing, the patient can receive a bolus of the drug which in the case of potassium chloride could be life threatening (Petrick et al 1977).

The ability of the drug to interact with or degrade the infusion fluid

The addition of drugs to intravenous lipid emulsions can result in aggregation and increases in drop size without macroscopic change. Should such an admixture be infused, embolization of the small blood vessels could occur. Intravenous infusions of mannitol are prone to crystallization when drugs are added. These and other effects were recognized in the Breckenridge Report which recommended that drugs should not be added to blood, plasma or lipid preparations, or infusions of mannitol or sodium bicarbonate.

The effect of the infusion fluid on the stability of the drug

The addition of a drug to an intravenous infusion fluid can result in chemical or physical changes deleterious to the drug and in addition expose the drug to light, air and altered temperature. The outcome may be an altered therapeutic response, an inactivated drug or harmful byproducts.

Inactivation of a drug in an infusion fluid can occur due to various chemical mechanisms including hydrolysis, oxidation, polymerization and photolysis. The effect of temperature on these reactions can be described by the Arrhenius equation:

$$k = Ae^{\frac{-E_a}{RT}} \qquad (25.1)$$

where k is the observed first-order rate constant for the reaction, A is a constant, E_a is the observed energy of activation, R is the gas constant and T is the absolute temperature. Deviation from Arrhenius behaviour is uncommon, except for extremes of temperature and with biologicals and, in general terms, increase in temperature increases the rate of degradation. For instance, the degradation of a 1% sodium ampicillin solution in 0.9% sodium chloride solution over a 4-hour period at 0°C is 0.4%, at 5°C, 1% and at 27°C, 1.8%. Decreases in temperature below freezing generally further reduce the rate of degradation but there are exceptions, such as sodium ampicillin. At −20°C the same ampicillin solution as described above loses 1.2% of its activity after 4 hours (Savello & Shangraw 1971).

Many drugs for parenteral administration are water-soluble salts of sparingly soluble weak acids or bases. The solubility of a weak acid can be predicted from the Henderson–Hasslebalch equation (see the companion volume, Aulton 1988, for more details).

$$pH = pK_a + \log [salt]/[acid] \qquad (25.2)$$

Weak acids and bases are often formulated in buffered or pH-adjusted solution which is at the optimum for the solubility and stability of the drug. When this formulation is added to an infusion fluid the resultant pH may vary from the optimum.

Poorly water-soluble salts may be maintained in solution with water-miscible cosolvents such as ethanol and propylene glycol. The solubility of drugs in cosolvent — water mixtures is not a linear function of the cosolvent concentration.

Phenytoin combines these two solubility problems. Phenytoin is a weak acid ($pK_a = 8.3$) which is poorly water soluble. The commercial formulation contains 10% ethanol, 40% propylene glycol with the pH adjusted to 12 with sodium hydroxide (Stella 1986). Should this formulation be diluted to aid intravenous administration the pH of the solution is lowered and the cosolvents are diluted so that they are no longer able to maintain the phenytoin acid in solution (Cloyd et al 1978).

METHODS OF ADMINISTRATION OF INTRAVENOUS ADDITIVES

There are three methods of administration of drugs added to an infusion: continuous infusion, intermittent infusion and addition to the drip tubing. The two former methods have the advantage that the drug may be added to sterile infusion fluid away from the bedside and using full aseptic precautions if available.

Continuous infusion

This method is suitable for very stable drugs required to be given very slowly to avoid irritant or toxic effects or where a sustained therapeutic effect is required. The drug is added to a large volume container of infusion fluid and infused over a long period.

Intermittent infusion

This may be achieved by replacing a large-volume infusion container with a small-volume container of the same fluid into which the drug has been mixed. This is administered over a relatively short period after which the large volume infusion container is replaced. Alternatively a 'piggy-back' technique may be employed in which the drug is added to a small secondary container of infusion fluid which is then administered through a Y-connection with the primary infusion. The secondary solution is usually administered within 30 minutes.

Addition via the drip tubing

In this method a solution of the drug is drawn into a syringe and injected through the tubing of the giving set using aseptic precautions. Administration time is comparatively short and compares with a bolus injection into an uncannulated vein.

Choice of a method

The factors outlined above must be taken into consideration when deciding on the most appropriate method of administration for a particular drug. A comprehensive table of guidelines for commonly used drugs and infusion fluids is provided in Appendix 2 of the BNF. For drugs not included, or for further information, the product data sheet and/or the product manufacturer should be consulted. The intravenous route is the least favoured route of administration and the addition of drugs to infusion fluids should be made only when there is no suitable alternative method and when the proposed combination of drug and fluid has been thoroughly researched.

BIBLIOGRAPHY

Allwood M C, Fell J T 1980 Textbook of hospital pharmacy. Blackwell, Oxford

Aulton M E (ed) 1988 Pharmaceutics: the science of dosage form design. Churchill Livingstone, Edinburgh

Baumgartner T G, Schmidt G L, Thakker K M et al 1986 Bacterial endotoxin retention by in-line intravenous filters. American Journal of Hospital Pharmacy 43: 681–684

Bivins B A, Rapp R P, DeLuca P P et al 1979 Final in-line filtration: a means of decreasing the incidence of infusion phlebitis. Surgery 85: 388–394

Breckenridge Working Party Report 1976 Report of the working party on addition of drugs to intravenous infusion fluids, HC(76)9, Department of Health and Social Security. HMSO, London

British National Formulary 1988 16th edn. British Medical Association and Royal Pharmaceutical Society of Great Britain, London (updated twice yearly)

Butler L D, Munson J M, DeLuca P P 1980 Effect of in-line filtration on the potency of low dose drugs. American Journal of Hospital Pharmacy 37: 935–941

Cloyd J C, Bosch D E, Sawchuck R J 1978 Concentration–time profile of phenytoin after admixture with small volumes of intravenous fluids. American Journal of Hospital Pharmacy 35: 45–48

Davis N M, Turco S 1971 A study of particulate matter in i.v. infusion fluids – phase 2. American Journal of Hospital Pharmacy 28: 620–623

Davis N M, Turco S, Sively E 1970 A study of particulate matter in i.v. infusions. American Journal of Hospital Pharmacy 27: 822–826

Fachuk K H, Peterson L, McNeil B J 1985 Micro-particulate-induced phlebitis: its prevention by in-line filtration. New England Journal of Medicine 312: 78–82

Garvan J M, Gunner 1964 The harmful effects of particles in intravenous fluids. Medical Journal of Australia ii: 1–6

Holmes C J, Kemdsin R B, Ausman R K et al 1980 Potential hazards associated with microbial contamination of in-line filters during intravenous therapy. Journal of Clinical Microbiology 12: 725–731

Kirk B 1985 The evaluation of a new light protective giving set. British Journal of Parenteral Therapy 6: 146–151

Lee G M 1986 Sorption of four drugs to polyvinyl chloride and polybutadiene intravenous administration sets. American Journal of Hospital Pharmacy 43: 1945–1950

Lewis G B H, Hecker J F 1985 Infusion phlebitis. British Journal of Anaesthesia 57: 220–233

Maddox R R, Rush D R, Rapp R F 1977 Double-blind study to investigate methods to prevent cephalothin-induced phlebitis. American Journal of Hospital Pharmacy 34: 29–34

Nipride Data Sheet 1986 Roche Products Ltd. Welwyn Garden City, Herts

Petrick R J, Loucas S P, Cohl J K, Mehl B 1977 Review of current knowledge of plastic intravenous fluid containers. American Journal of Hospital Pharmacy 34: 357–362

Savello D R, Shangraw R F 1971 Stability of sodium ampicillin solutions in the frozen and liquid states. American Journal of Hospital Pharmacy 28: 754–759

Shaw N J, Lyall E G H 1985 Hazards of glass ampoules. British Medical Journal 291: 1390

Smail G A, Marshall I 1982 Intravenous additives. In: Lawson D H, Richards R M E (eds) Clinical pharmacy and hospital drug management. Chapman and Hall, London, pp 239–260

Stella V J 1986 Fundamentals of drug stability and compatibility. In: Trissell L A (ed) Handbook on injectable drugs. American Society of Hospital Pharmacists, pp XI–XXII

Turco S, Davis N M 1973a Particulate matter in intravenous infusion fluids — phase 3. American Journal of Hospital Pharmacy 30: 611–613

Turco S, Davis N M 1973 Clinical significance of particulate matter: a review of the literature. Hospital Pharmacy 8: 137–140

Yahya A M, McElnay J C, D'Arcy P F 1986 Burette administration sets. International Journal of Pharmaceutics 31: 65–68

26. Dispensing of cytotoxic agents

C. Hirsch

Cytotoxic agents have been used for some years in the treatment of cancer. Some of the agents used have been associated with carcinogenicity when used in therapeutic doses to treat certain types of malignant disease. In 1979 a letter in *The Lancet* by Falck et al raised concern for the staff who handled the cytotoxic agents when administering them to patients. His studies showed possible absorption of cytotoxics in nurses who mixed the drugs. Since then many studies and guidelines for working procedures with cytotoxic agents have been published. Much of the work done however is speculative but the following information should provide insight into the basics for new developments.

What is a cytotoxic chemotherapeutic agent?

By definition anything which is *cytotoxic* is capable of killing cells. It is for this reason that cytotoxics are employed in the treatment of cancer, to destroy tumour cells. So far, however, these agents have been non-selective and destroy some healthy tissue as well.

The drugs act in various ways to prevent replication of DNA or RNA within the cells and so stop tumour growth. They are often classified according to their different modes of action (Table 26.1). Some of the drugs may be administered orally but many are given parenterally.

POTENTIAL HAZARDS TO OPERATORS HANDLING CYTOTOXICS

Many injectable cytotoxics are powdered preparations which need reconstituting before use, although there is a trend towards producing formulations in solution. As cytotoxic agents can damage living tissue, it follows that personnel handling the drugs may be at risk if sensible precautions are not taken.

Mustine hydrochloride (mechlorethamine) was one of the first cancer chemotherapeutic agents used therapeutically. Mustine is extremely irritant to mucous membranes, eyes and skin. Anecdotal evidence is available of nurses who have experienced lightheadedness, dizziness, nausea, headache and allergic reactions after preparing drugs without proper protection in poorly ventilated areas (Crundi 1980, Reynolds et al 1982). There is evidence that secondary malignancies were induced in those patients who received chemotherapy for cancers in the 1940s and 1950s. Some patients seemed to have a higher incidence of leukaemias. This may have been due to drug-induced chromosome damage (Sieber 1975). Antineoplastics have been implicated in teratogenesis and infertility in patients who had received them. Fetal loss has been reported among nurses in Finnish hospitals, thought to be associated with handling cytotoxics. Liver damage has been reported amongst nurses working on an oncology ward thought to be re-

Table 26.1 Modes of action of cytotoxic agents

Alkylating agents	Antimetabolites	Vinca alkaloids	Antitumour/antibiotic	Miscellaneous
Mustine	Methorexate	Vincristine	Actinomycin	Cisplatin
Cyclophosphamide	5- Fluorouracil	Vindesine	Mithramycin	Carboplatin
Chlorambucil	6-Thioguanine	Vinblastine	Doxorubicin	Procarbazine
Melphalan	6-Mercaptopurine		Daunorubicin	Mitozantrone
Ifosfamide	Cytosine arabinoside		Epirubicin	Dacarbazine
Busulphan			Bleomycin	Etoposide
Thiotepa			Mitomycin C	
Carmustine				

lated to their exposure to antineoplastic agents. However, it should be noted that few if any safe handling procedures were observed in these reports.

Methods of monitoring exposure of personnel

Unfortunately, there are still no reliable tests to 'measure' exposure to cytotoxics or the degree of hazard that personnel might experience while preparing these drugs.

The Ames test for mutagenicity

The Ames test uses the organism *Salmonella typhimurium*, a histidine auxotrophic strain, which is susceptible to reversion back to prototrophy in the presence of a variety of mutagens, i.e. a substance capable of causing mutation. Varying quantities of the substance to be tested are added to the bacteria grown on an agar plate. A trace of histidine is added to the agar to allow background growth of bacteria but not permit full formation of colonies. If the agent added to the plates is mutagenic, the plate will become granular in appearance. The number of bacteria reverting to prototrophy is measured by counting the number of colonies present after incubation for 48 hours. Several studies have been carried out using the Ames test. Staliano et al (1981) tested the urine of eight subjects handling cytotoxic agents who were controlled for smoking, medication, alcohol and diet. Some mutagenicity was apparent in the urine of workers who had not taken safety precautions or had worked with a horizontal laminar flow cabinet. This indicated that they must have absorbed some of the cytotoxics. Those working with cytotoxics using a vertical laminar flow cabinet and wearing gloves, etc. showed no mutagenicity, i.e. no sign of absorption of cytotoxics (Anderson 1982). There are, however, many environmental factors which could confound mutagenicity results. Urine of cigarette smokers for instance was found to be mutagenic (Anderson 1982, Bos 1983). Baker et al (1982) detected mutagenic activity in human tissue after meals of fried pork or bacon. A further problem is that although the Ames test gave negative mutagenic results when pharmacists were tested after handling cytotoxic agents safely in a vertical laminar flow cabinet, the test may not be sensitive enough to detect very low levels of chronic exposure. For these reasons it has been decided that the Ames mutagenicity test is not a reliable indicator of cytotoxic hazard.

Sister chromatid exchange

The term 'clastogen' is used to describe a substance which causes chromosome damage. Gaps or breaks in the chromosome may be seen under a microscope at mitosis. New techniques now exist to measure sister chromatid exchange (SCE), i.e. the rearrangement of genetic material in a chromosome. The tissue is incubated with the substance suspected of causing chromosome damage for two cycles of DNA replication in the presence of 5-bromodeoxyuridine. The material is then stained and viewed under a microscope. This method is very sensitive and gives results at very low clastogen levels. However, very low clastogen levels may not cause significant damage to human tissue as it has an efficient DNA repair mechanism. Positive results have occurred with a range of substances, including cytotoxics, caffeine, ethanol and oral contraceptives. Drugs such as phenytoin also cause SCE. This technique may prove a useful addition to existing methods of monitoring operator exposure.

Measurement of a urinary platinium marker

Venitt et al (1984) studied a group of pharmacists and nurses exposed to cytotoxic drugs using a mutagenic test and found that the control group of workers, unexposed to cytotoxics, also showed positive urinary mutagenicity. He looked therefore for an alternative method of monitoring. Platinum-containing cytotoxic drugs were used as markers of absorption by hospital personnel, as platinum would not normally be encountered during a working day unless by handling these types of agent. Urine from patients treated with cisplatin was also tested. Platinum levels in the urine of the 'exposed' group were found to be no higher than unexposed controls. However, the urine of patients treated with cisplatin was found to contain 7000 times more platinum. Disposal of patients' urine would, therefore, pose a hazard to nursing staff.

The paper concluded that direct chemical analysis of the urine of workers handling cytotoxics along with an environmental monitoring system would be a more reliable guide to drug absorption than the use of urinary mutagenicity assays.

Recommendations for safe handling

Studies have shown that measurable exposure may be minimized by instituting safe handling practices. If procedures are followed, areas of possible direct exposure such as skin contact, inhalation of aerosolized drug or ingestion can be eliminated.

Preparation areas

In many large oncology centres, responsibility for reconstitution and dispensing of intravenous cytotoxics has been accepted by the pharmacy department. If the workload is large a special vertical laminar air flow cytotoxic cabinet may be used, providing a Class I (BS 5295) environment. The cabinets vary in design but provide two basic functions. The first, product protection, requires that air entering the cabinet is free of contaminated particles — cabinets must conform to BS 5295. The second, operator protection, is achieved by the downward laminar air flow. This contains any cytotoxic contamination within the cabinet. The air is then circulated within the cabinet · and filtered before being recirculated into the room or vented outside. Cabinets should conform to BS 5276 for operator protection. All cabinets should be fitted with gauges to show pressure differentials and audible alarms which should activate if optimum velocities of air flow are not achieved, indicating a failure in cabinet safety. The cytotoxic cabinet should be reserved solely for preparation of cytotoxic agents. Cabinets may be placed in a clean area, for example, a pharmacy aseptic suite. Alternatively it may be decided to site the cabinet in a side room in a normal environment, here, however, the filters may need changing more often. Cabinets should be regularly serviced by qualified personnel. Where the number of cytotoxic agents being used is small the cost of such a work station may be prohibitive. It must also be noted that if few cytotoxics are prepared the handling risk will be less. If pharmacists are not able to provide a reconstitution service during 24 hours a day, it may be necessary for medical staff to perform reconstitutions. In this situation a side room or area away from the general traffic of the ward or clinic should be designated for cytotoxic preparation. Ventilation should be adequate, but doors and windows should be closed to exclude draughts. The working surface should be non-porous to substances being handled an be easily cleaned. A supply of running water should also be close at hand.

Eating, drinking, smoking and the application of cosmetics should be prohibited in the area. Equipment and stocks of cytotoxic drugs should be arranged in a safe and orderly manner to avoid accidents. Neutralizing solutions to cope with spills should also be close to hand. If a side room has to be used or cytotoxics have to be made up in the community (e.g. district nurses), consideration should be given to provision of special packs containing protective clothing and disposal facilities.

Horizontal laminar flow cabinets should never be used to reconstitute cytotoxics as particles and aerosols could be blown towards the operator.

Techniques and precautions

When dispensing a cytotoxic agent for intravenous administration the drug must be reconstituted and dispensed into a suitable dosage form whilst maintaining sterility of the product and also ensuring the maximum degree of safety to the operator.

Three main ways that personnel exposure may occur are from skin contact, inhalation or ingestion of the cytotoxic agents.

Prohibiting eating, smoking, drinking and application of cosmetics in the work area should prevent ingestion. Skin contact may be prevented by wearing suitable protective clothing and gloves. If reconstitution is being carried out in an aseptic environment in the pharmacy, cleanroom clothing should be worn. In a non-sterile area normal clothes should be protected either with a special gown (which may be sterile and preferably non-fibre shedding) or a plastic apron. Gloves made of latex should be worn unless directed otherwise by specific instructions from the manufacturer. PVC gloves were recommended in Guidance Note MS21 from the Health and Safety Executive as they seem to be impervious to most cytotoxic agents. PVC gloves were shown to be less permeable than latex gloves to mustine and carmustine. However, new research seems to indicate that surgical latex gloves are less permeable to many cytotoxics than PVC. New guidelines were published in the *Pharmaceutical Journal* (Working Party Report) to support this.

Surgical face-masks will not completely prevent inhalation of aerosols but they may help. American recommendations state that an efficient respirator should be used if a vertical laminar air flow cabinet is not available. Goggles to protect the eyes should be worn conforming to BS 2092 and should be washed in water after use.

If protective clothing and gloves do not totally cover the skin, protective lint-free armlets should be used to cover exposed skin.

When working with cytotoxics good aseptic technique is essential in order to protect both the product from bacterial contamination and the operator from contamination with the product.

Reconstitution should be carried out on a solid surface that can be cleaned easily. A broad-edged tray may be suitable if a vertical laminar air flow cabinet lacks a continuous solid surface (i.e. the working area is perforated). Plastic-backed paper may also be used as a work surface as long as it does not compromise a stable working surface.

Prevention of aerosol formation from cytotoxic vials

Aerosolization of cytotoxic agents should always be prevented. Aerosolization may occur when pressure differentials occur between the inside and outside of a vial.

This can be prevented by equalizing pressure between syringe and vial, i.e. by replacing the volume of fluid drawn out of the vial with an equal volume of air from the syringe. Always ensure, however, that negative pressure is maintained within the vial. This can be achieved practically by withdrawing the syringe driver to withdraw solution then allowing the syringe driver to find its own equilibrium. A volume of air or fluid should never be pushed directly into the vial but added in small volumes, allowing equalization of pressure. An alternative method is to vent the vial, this may be done using a needle connected to a hydrophobic filter. This allows air in and out of the vial but prevents fluid and particles being expelled. Many devices are marketed to provide a safe venting function. Diluents should always be introduced slowly into the vial. Powder should be thoroughly wet before agitation.

Aerosols may also be produced when opening ampoules. To prevent this, any material in the top of the ampoule should be tapped down gently. A sterile wipe should be wrapped around the neck of the vial to prevent cuts. The neck of the vial may be scored with a file if necessary. The ampoule neck should be snapped in a direction away from the operator. Diluent should be slowly introduced down the wall of the ampoule.

If air bubbles have to be expelled from the syringe these may be vented back into the container if an air vent is used, or into the needle sheath of the syringe with non-fibrous gauze wrapped around. 'Luer-Lock' fittings on syringes and apparatus should always be used when handling cytotoxics to prevent the needle and syringe becoming detached. Wide-bore needles are also useful to prevent pressure build up in the syringe. However, some experienced personnel believe that wide-bore syringes are more likely to drip.

Training procedures and methods

It is essential that all personnel involved in the use of cytotoxic drugs receive training in the relevant techniques and procedures involved in their safe handling. Detailed written policies and procedures should be prepared locally.

Staff directly involved in reconstituting and drawing up cytotoxic drugs for intravenous administration should be taught aseptic technique. This should be assessed before the operator is allowed to handle cytotoxics. Training may be done initially using a process of transferring water for injection from ampoules to empty vials. Out-of-date vials of medication are sometimes useful for training. Assessment may be carried out by direct observation of the operator at work

and also by a broth transfer test (see Ch. 23) which involves the transfer of a concentrated broth solution into vials which are then incubated to detect any microbial contamination. A positive result (i.e. growth in the broth) will indicate failure of the test and further training will be required. This tests aseptic technique. In order to handle cytotoxics safely, aerosolization should be prevented at all times. A solution of quinine may be used in the transfer which will fluoresce under ultraviolet light and may be used to detect clumsy technique. Staff performance should be regularly evaluated and 'refresher' courses in technique provided if necessary.

All training procedures should be written down along with safe procedures for individual manipulative techniques, general handling and checking. In addition, local policies should be drawn up preferably by a multidisciplinary committee which covers practice both in hospitals and the community. These policies should include advice on the storge and administration of the cytotoxic agents. Staff involved in receiving delivery of cytotoxics and those engaged in transport should be aware of the potential hazard if spillage should occur and be trained in the appropriate course of action.

Coping with spills and waste disposal

It is essential the procedures are written down and distributed to all staff handling cytotoxic agents, detailing action to be taken if spillage should occur. A general procedure should be available to ensure prompt first-line action. Spills and breakages should be cleaned up immediately or as soon as a procedure can be safely interrupted. Protective clothing should be worn including gloves (PVC or latex as recommended), surgical face-mask, protective goggles or glasses and a disposable apron.

The spillage should be wiped up with a damp cloth — this ensures that if powder has been split it will be dampened and thus prevent dust being inhaled. Contaminated waste should be sealed in a plastic bag and disposed of in a high-risk waste-disposal bag. Contaminated surfaces should be washed with copious amounts of water. If spillage on the skin occurs soap and copious quantities of cold water should be used. If the eyes are contaminated, immediate irrigation with a saline eye wash should be carried out and medical help sought. Should skin puncture occur from needles attached to syringes containing cytotoxic material, the area should be washed well with soap and water. The employee should then receive a medical examination. Occasionally chemicals may be used as a second line to deal with spillage of certain cytotoxics as recommended

Table 26.2 Procedures in case of accidental contact

Drug	Manufacturer's recommended action on contamination
Actinomycin D.	Rinse off immediately with water for 10 min; finally rinse with buffered phosphate solution
Melphalan	Sodium carbonate 3% w/v solution
Methotrexate	For skin stinging — aqueous cream. For systemic absorption of large amounts use calcium leucovorin
Mustine	Use water plus sodium carbonate 3% w/v or isotonic sodium thiosulphate 2.98%
Vinblastine Vincristine Vindesine	Large quantities of water; heparin (Hirudoid) cream if accidental injection
Doxorubicin	Hypochlorite with 1% available chlorine

by the manufacturer. Those for which more detailed information is available are shown in Table 26.2. All accidents and spillages should be documented.

Disposal

Equipment used to prepare cytotoxics, intravenous administration sets, and other contaminated materials should be placed in high-risk waste-disposal bags. Disposal of sharp objects, e.g. syringes and needles, empty vials and ampoules, should be placed in suitable rigid containers and labelled with a hazard warning seal. Persons collecting waste should be aware of the hazard and that the waste should be incinerated. The temperature of incineration of particular drugs may be obtained from the manufacturers. Some drugs may be degraded using chemical methods. Some commonly used chemical and thermal methods are listed in Table 26.3.

Cytotoxic drugs and their metabolites are excreted in urine, faeces and other body fluids. Nurses should be made aware of this and take appropriate precautions. It may be felt that patients and relatives should also be informed of the potential hazard.

STABILITIES AND COMPATIBILITIES OF CYTOTOXIC AGENTS

Many cytotoxic drugs for intravenous use are presented as dry powders as they have limited stability in solution.

1. Stability may be affected by the diluent or infusion fluid used, e.g. manufacturers state that cisplatin is most stable in 0.9% sodium chloride.

Table 26.3 Commonly used cytotoxics and methods of disposal

Drug	Chemical	Temperature
Actinomycin	Large volumes of sodium phosphate	
Azathioprine	10% sodium bicarbonate for 24–48 h then flush to drain	
Bleomycin	Chromic acid	
Busulphan	10% sodium thiosulphate for 20 h	
Carmustine	Chromic acid	
Cisplatin		1000°C
Cyclophosphamide	0.2 mol/l potassium hydroxide in methanol; copius amounts of water; 5% sodium hyperchlorite for 24 h	
Cytarabine	1 mol/l hydrochloric acid then flush down drain	
Dacarbazine	10% sulphuric acid for 24 h	
Daunorubicin	Sodium hypochlorite for 24 h	700°C
Doxorubicin	Sodium hypochlorite for 24 h	700°C
Ethoglucid	Conc. hydrochloric acid (acid: Epodyl 1 : 3) for 0.5 h in a fume cupboard. Add 10% sodium hydroxide to pH 6–8 then flush down drain	
Etoposide	Chromic acid	
5-Flurouracil	Conc. sodium hydroxide 700°C	
Ifosfamide	As cyclophosphamide	
Methotrexate	Chromic acid	
Mithramycin	10% trisodium phosphate	700°C
Mitomycin	Dilute sodium hydroxide for 3–4 h	
Mitozantrone	5.5 parts of calcium hydroxide	

2. Agents may be light sensitive, e.g. dacarbazine which must be protected with special light resistant infusion sets when infusion is prolonged.

3. Stability may be affected by the concentration of the drug in solution. Etoposide is less stable in more concentrated solution.

4. pH may affect stability of drugs.

5. Some drugs including vincristine and actinomycin are adsorbed onto certain types of filters which may be used in drug preparation.

6. A rise in temperature may accelerate drug degradation but conversely some agents precipitate if cooled. Examples are cisplatin, 5-fluorouracil and etoposide.

7. Requests may be made by medical staff to mix certain antineoplastic agents either together or with antiemetics or other agents. Stability work should be carried out (both in hospitals and industry) to establish stabilities of admixtures. If there is doubt concerning stability of mixtures, agents should be administered separately.

8. As more studies are carried out on cytotoxic agents it seems that many drugs are reasonably stable from a chemical point of view but contain no preservatives. If these agents are made up in the normal environment and kept at room temperature they should be discarded after 8 hours. If however, they are reconstituted aseptically and refrigerated immediately it may be possible to extend their shelf-life. Work is also currently on-going in the stability of drugs which have been deep frozen and then thawed in a microwave oven.

METHODS OF ADMINISTRATION

Procedures should be drawn up for the administration of cytotoxics, usually carried out by experienced medical or nursing staff. They must take care to handle the cytotoxic agent without exposing themselves or the patient to any hazard but at the same time without causing alarm to the patient. The injection of cytotoxics can be traumatic for the patients who will be anxious and apprehensive. This very often leads to constriction of the veins which makes injection more difficult. Intravenous infusion sets and containers should be assembled carefully to avoid leakage. The patient's eyes, skin and mucous membranes should be protected from contact with the drug.

If direct bolus injection is carried out, needles used during drug preparation should be changed before injection and then discarded so that drugs are not in contact with tissue. Extravasation of cytotoxics (i.e. leakage of drug outside the vein) can cause extensive irreversible tissue necrosis. It is therefore essential that the administrator is trained in injection technique.

The presentation of the cytotoxics can assist the administrator if dispensing is carried out in the pharmacy. The drug may be requested in a syringe which can be capped with a 'Luer-lock' cap. This may be given as a slow bolus injection into a butterfly cannula or into the side arm of a fast-running infusion. Syringes may also be placed in syringe drivers for slow infusion. It is possible for home chemotherapy to take place in this manner by use of a portable battery-operated syringe driver. Alternatively, the drug may be added to an appropriate infusion fluid — large volumes up to 3 litres for slow infusion and smaller volumes, 50–100 ml, for short infusions. If the pharmacy department have dispensed a cytotoxic in one of these forms care must be taken with labelling. Checking must always be an integral part of the procedure.

Labels should state:

1. That there is a cytotoxic substance in the preparation.

2. The total amount of drug and the total volume of the preparation.

3. The time and date after which it should not be used.

4. Storage recommendation.

Local procedures should also be developed for the safe transport of cytotoxics. Specially designed containers may be used. Provision should also be made for infusions to be protected from light during administration if necessary.

PHARMACY INVOLVEMENT IN COMPOUNDING INTRAVENOUS CYTOTOXICS

Pharmacists are well placed to provide a cytotoxic reconstitution service. They have extensive knowledge in areas of pharmaceutics, pharmacology, pharmaceutical chemistry and pharmacokinetics, all of which are basic to the understanding of the action of cytotoxics in the body and their stability in solution. Pharmacists and technicians are well trained in aseptic technique, recording and checking procedures to ensure that the patient receives an appropriate dose of the correct drug which often has a small therapeutic range.

The pharmacy can serve as an information centre for medical and nursing staff, and also for the patient.

As trends move towards the use of more complicated cytotoxic regimens and home chemotherapy, it will be essential for the pharmacist to utilize his pharmaceutical knowledge to the full to provide a safe and efficient service for the dispensing of cytotoxic drugs.

BIBLIOGRAPHY

Anderson R W, Puckett W H, Dana W J, Neuyen T V, Theiss J C, Matney T S 1982 Risk of Handling Injectable Antineoplastic Agents. American Journal of Hospital Pharmacy 1982: 39: 1881–7

Baker R S U, Arlauskas A, Bonin A M, Angus D S 1982 Detection of mutagenic activity in human urine following fried pork or bacon meals. Cancer Lett 16: 81–89

Bos R P 1983 Mutgenicity of urine from nurses handling cytostatic drugs, influence of smoking. Int Archives Occupational Environmental Health. 50: 359–69

Connor T H et al 1984 Permeability of latex and PVC gloves to carmustine. American Journal Hospital Pharm 41: 676–679

Crundi C B 1980 A compounding dilemma. I've kept the drug sterile but have I contaminated myself? National Intravenous. Therapy Journal 77–80

Drug induced Chromosome Damage 1874 Adverse Drug Reaction Bulletin, April

Falck F, Gröhn P, Sorsam, Vanio H, Heinone E, Holsti L R 1979 Mutagenicity in urine of nurses handling cytostatic drugs. Lancet 1: 1250–1251

Dodds L 1985 Handling of Waste from Patients receiving cytotoxics. Pharm J 235: 289–291

Laidlaw J L, Connor T H, Theiss J C, Anderson R W, Matney T S 1985 Permeability of four protective clothes materials to seven antineoplastic drugs. American Journal Hospital Pharmacy 42: 2449–2454

OSHA work-practice guidelines for personnel dealing with cytotoxic (antineoplastic) drugs 1986 American Journal Hospital Pharmacy 43: 1193–1204

Selevan S, Hemminki K, Lindbohm M L 1985 A study of occupational exposure to antineoplastic drugs and fetal loss in nurses. New England Journal Medicine 313: 1173

Sieber S M 1975 Cancer Chemotherapeutic agents and Caranogenesis, Cancer Chemotherapy Rep. 59: 915–918

Sotaniemi E A , Sutinen S, Arranto A J, Sontaniemi K A, Lehtola J, Pelkonen R D 1983 Liver damage in nurses handling cytostatic agents. Acta Medica Scandinavica 214: 181–189

Staliano N, Gallelli J F, Adamson R H, Thorgeirsson S S 1981 Lack of mutagenic activity in urine from Hospital Pharmacists admixing antitumour drugs. Lancet 1: 615–616

Venitt S, Baker R, Liber H, Zeiger E 1984 Monitoring exposure of nursing and pharmacy personnel to cytotoxic drugs urinary mutation assays and urinary platinium a markers of absorption. Lancet 1: 74–77

Working Party Report Guidelines for the Handling of cytotoxic Drugs. Pharmaceutical Journal 1983: 230: 1

Working Party Report. Guidelines for the handling of Cytotoxic drugs: Amendment. Pharmaceutical Journal 1987: 238: 414

27. Total parenteral nutrition

C. E. Bude

Introduction

The provision of adequate and appropriate nutrition is a necessary part of total care for any patient. The enteral (gastric) route is preferred whenever possible and, for patients unable to swallow a normal diet, feeding via a nasogastric tube is the method of choice.

For patients unable to tolerate any form of enteral feeding, the administration of fluid and nutrients via a parenteral route is necessary. In the short term (e.g. immediately postoperative) administration of fluid and dextrose may be adequate, but for long-term care a balanced diet containing all the essential nutrients, including vitamins and trace elements, must be provided.

It has been shown (Johnston 1978) that an undernourished patient whose gastrointestinal tract is temporarily or permanently unusable can increase lean body tissue and also lay down fat if fed a suitable combination of nutrients intravenously. This form of therapy is known as *total parenteral nutrition* (TPN) and was pioneered by workers such as Dudrick et al (1967).

This chapter gives an overview of TPN therapy with emphasis on the role of the pharmacist.

CLINICAL ASPECTS

With an understanding of the clinical aspects of TPN, pharmacists can recommend regimens to fulfil the needs of the patient as diagnosed by the physician. Possible interactions with concomitant medication may be identified and advice given on suitable administration systems.

Indications

The main indications for TPN are as follows:

Adults

Pre- and postoperative support
Malignancy
Inflammatory bowel disease
Gastrointestinal fistulae
Pancreatitis
Severe trauma
Burns
Sepsis
Hepatic failure
Renal failure

The intravenous route for nutrition should only be used where the oral or nasogastric routes are not readily available.

Children (see Harries 1978)

Protracted infantile diarrhoea
Major alimentary tract surgery in newborns
Prematurity

In comparison with the adult, the paediatric patient has very little reserve of fat and protein to call upon during periods of malnourishment (Harries 1978).

The data in Table 27.1 is adapted from Harries (1978). The table lists the expected duration of survival of children and adults during starvation and shows that the effect of nutritional deprivation is thus quite dramatic in the neonate as compared to the adult.

As with adults, where a child requires nutritional support, the enteral or nasogastric route must be used wherever possible. Where this is infeasible, intravenous feeding should be instituted rapidly.

Table 27.1 Duration of survival during starvation

Age group	Duration of survival (days)
Small premature (1 kg)	4
Large premature (2 kg)	12
Full-term infant (3.5 kg)	32
One-year-old	44
Adult	90

Administration

Powell-Tuck et al reported in 1978 a technique for administration of the total daily requirement for TPN via one single container. This was a significant advance over the multiple-bottle method of administration.

Three-litre bag therapy, however, is not ideal for all patients. In an intensive care unit, for example, requirements for fluids and electrolytes may change rapidly throughout the day and require the careful titration that can only be obtained with smaller volume fluids and injections.

Choice of entry sites

Many of the individual solutions required for TPN, such as high-strength glucose, together with mixed 3-litre regimens are generally hypertonic. For short-term therapy rotation of peripheral entry sites may provide a simple means of administering TPN without the complications of initiating central vein access. However, for longer-term therapy a catheter placed into the superior vena cava is reported as being the safest method of entry providing rapid dilution of the hypertonic solution (Silk 1983).

Flow control

Adult TPN patients generally receive 2–3 litres of fluids per day. Rapid, uncontrolled infusion of this amount of fluid would cause renal overload and would be of no benefit to the patient. It is thus vital that some form of flow control device is employed. This may range from simple clamps through to electronic drip controllers (see Ch. 5).

Patient assessment and monitoring

Once TPN has been initiated on a patient it is essential that routine monitoring is carried out. The clinical pharmacist should have an understanding of the relevance of these routine tests (particularly those such as 24-hour urine analysis which is the main determinant of nitrogen requirements) in order to make adjustment to the TPN formulation.

Home TPN

Patients with severe Crohn's disease, excessive bowel resection, etc., who may require long-term, if not permanent, TPN therapy may be ideal candidates for home TPN provided that their home environment is suitable.

The majority of patients use the 3-litre bag system administered overnight via an alarmed pump system.

The patient requires a period of training whilst hospitalized which encompasses aseptic technique, product storage and handling, reporting of side-effects or complications, use of ancillary items and pumps, before they are capable of treating themselves at home.

FORMULATION OF TPN

The proportions and mix of components of solutions used for intravenous nutrition can vary considerably depending upon the patient's nutritional status and underlying medical or surgical condition. The components available for TPN are detailed below.

Nitrogen

The main objective of parenteral nutrition is to supply the undernourished patient with sufficient utilizable nitrogen to re-establish nitrogen balance, i.e. where the amount of nitrogen administered is approximately equal to that excreted (mainly as urea).

Choice of amino acid

The body's relative requirements of the individual amino acids is expected as follows:

Essential, i.e. which cannot be synthesized by man. All the commercially available solutions contain the eight essential amino acids in varying proportions.

Non-essential, i.e. those amino acids which can normally be synthesized by the body. These amino acids are used to increase the amount of nitrogen available from the solutions and the optimum ratio of essential to non-essential amino acids has yet to be agreed between workers.

Semi-essential, i.e. those amino acids which although they can in theory be synthesized by the body, may occasionally need to be provided in the TPN solution due to the patient's age or disease state.

Non-nitrogen energy

The malnourished patient requires, in order to utilize administered nitrogen in the form of amino acids, an independent energy source. There are many such individual sources available which have been utilized historically although many have now fallen out of favour due to undesirable side-effects. Examples of these are fructose, sorbitol, xylitol and ethanol. The use of combinations of mixed calorie sources for parenteral nutrition have been reported but these appear to have no major benefits over and above the use of glucose alone.

Glucose

From the literature it would appear that glucose is the carbohydrate of choice in nutrition, however, it is not without metabolic complications. Woolfson (1979) suggested that glucose handling in the sick patient becomes complicated due mainly to an imbalance in the normally well regulated hormonal systems which are in existence. This can lead to hyperglycaemia, hypoglycaemia, hypophosphataemia etc. Careful design of TPN regimens plus the use of lipid as a complementary calorie source can minimise such effects.

Lipid

Intravenous lipid emulsions are utilized clinically both as a calorie source and as a source of essential fatty acids. Their administration, whilst providing some benefits to the patient, is not without clinical difficulties such as interference with diagnostic tests and deposition in tissues such as the lung.

Administration of lipid emulsion on a daily, twice or three times weekly basis appears to provide a balanced mixture of nutrients for the patient requiring long-term feeding.

Electrolytes

This section explains the requirement for the electrolytes sodium, potassium, calcium, magnesium and phosphate. Table 27.2 shows some of the small volume electrolyte additive solutions available.

Sodium

Sodium is of critical importance in the fluid balance of both healthy and sick subjects. Sodium losses and gains are generally accompanied by similar shifts in chloride ions and a consequent movement in water. Severe losses may lead to hypovolaemia, circulatory failure and shock. Generally a serum concentration of 135–145 mEq/litre is thought to be normal (Normal Laboratory Values 1980).

Potassium

Potassium is essential for the normal operation of the cell and is an important determinant of cell membrane resting potential. Thus abnormally high or low levels can result in poor nerve impulse conduction, fluctuations in heart rhythm and even death due to heart failure. It also plays a vital role in distribution of body water.

Table 27.2 Electrolyte content of some small volume additive solutions

| | Content per ml | | | | | | | | | | | | |
| | mmol | | | | | | μmol | | | | | | |
	Na^+	K^+	Mg^{2+}	Ca^{2+}	Phos	Cl^-	Zn^{2+}	Mn^{2+}	Cu^{2+}	Cr^{3+}	$Fe^{2+/3+}$	F^-	I^-
Sodium Chloride BP 30%	5.1					5.1							
Potassium Chloride BP 15%		2.0				2.0							
Magnesium Sulphate BP 50%			2.0										
Calcium Chloride EUR.P. 5 mmol Ca^{2+} in 10 ml				0.5		1.0							
Potassium Acid Phosphate BPC 1949 10 mmol K^+ in 10 ml		1.0			1.0								
Sodium Acetate BP 20 mmol Na^+ in 10 ml	2.0												
Calcium Gluconate BP 20%				0.45									
Addamel (Kabi Vitrum)			0.15	0.5		1.3	2.0	4.0	0.5		5.0	5.0	0.1
Ped-el (Kabi Vitrum)			0.025	0.15	0.075	0.35	0.15	0.25	0.075		0.5	0.75	0.01
MTE-4 (Lyphomed)							15.3	1.8	6.3	0.077			
Addiphos (Kabi Vitrum)	1.5	1.5			2.0								

Calcium

Absence of calcium from TPN in the long term may produce symptoms of hypocalcaemia such as muscle spasms and numbness. The effect of lack of calcium on the growing child on TPN could understandably have a dramatic effect on growth and development of bones and teeth. Abnormalities involving both high and low levels of calcium may be responsible for a wide variety of clinical conditions.

Magnesium

Magnesium has many physiological actions. The most clinically significant effects of magnesium imbalance are associated with changes in neuromuscular or cardiovascular function.

Phosphate

By virtue of its buffering action phosphate helps maintain body acid–base balance. If phosphate is not provided in the TPN solution hypophosphataemia may develop which can give rise to impaired red blood cell function and poor function of many organs. Hypophosphataemia may also be induced as a result of infusion of high glucose loads (Knochel 1977).

Trace elements

Table 27.3 summarizes the primary use of the individual trace elements which are considered to be clinically significant.

Vitamins

Patients on long-term TPN therapy will generally require some vitamin supplementation. Table 27.4 shows the commercial preparations of vitamins available along with recommended daily requirements which seem to vary according to the current available recommendations.

Fluid

In the human body, water is the predominant chemical entity, generally accounting for more than half of the total body weight. Total body water content varies with age, sex and obesity. Table 27.5 shows the relative proportions of body water for an average male, female and infant. An inverse relationship exists between the amount of body fat and the amount of body water present in an individual.

Table 27.3 Trace elements in TPN

Trace elements	Uses etc.
Zinc	Participates in wound healing and normal immune function (Kay et al 1976). Diarrhoea, crusting dermatitis, alopecia, etc., noted as signs of zinc deficiency (Karper & Peden 1972). Onset of varying duration. Skin conditions can be corrected rapidly, sometimes within 48 h, alopecia reversal takes longer (Kay et al 1976)
Copper	Deficiency observed primarily as bone abnormalities such as osteoporosis, soft-tissue calcification etc., mainly in infants (Lowry et al 1979). This is due to reduced activity of copper-containing enzyme lysyl oxidase, necessary for cross-links in collagen and elastin (Kay et al 1976). Clinical signs appear slowly. Neutropenia and refractory hypochromic anaemia also noted (Shenkin et al 1976)
Selenium	Clinical deficiency symptoms rare (Kay et al 1976). Prolonged i.v. feeding commonly shows biochemical signs of depletion. Two clinical syndromes have been identified; cardiomyopathy and skeletal muscle myopathy
Chromium	Rare reports of chromium deficiency during TPN, possibly due to chromium contamination of commercial preparations of amino acids and glucose (Shenkin 1987). Deficiency may have impact on glucose metabolism in the form of hyperglycaemia and glycosuria
Iron	Difficulty in assessing iron status as injury, infection, etc., may alter serum transferrin levels, independently of the iron status. Although need for iron is well established, give only basal levels by the i.v. route (Kay et al 1976)
Manganese	Again, may be a contaminant of TPN preparations. Manganese is a co-factor for many enzymes in human tissue although little clinical evidence of deficiency states available (Kay et al 1976)
Cobalt	Deficiency not reported during TPN. Adequate tissue levels can be achieved by administration of vitamin B12 in suitable amounts (Kay et al 1976)
Molybdenum	Only one report of presumed deficiency noted (Kay et al 1976). Intolerance to amino acid infusions was observed which was reversed by administration of ammonium molybdate i.v.

Table 27.4 Commercially available vitamin preparations

Vitamin		Recommended daily Intake i.v. Adult		Solivito	Vitlipid Adult	Vitlipid Infant	Multi-bionta	Select-a-jet Mult. vit.	Parent-rovite
		(American Medical Association 1979)	(Review 1980)	10 ml	10 ml	10 ml	10 ml	sol. 10 ml	1 VHP 1 + 2
A	Retinol (IU)	3300	700		2500	333	10 000	10 000	
B1	Thiamine (mg)	3	1.4	1.2			44.6	4.5	223
B2	Riboflavine (mg)	3.6	2.1	1.8			7.3	10	4
B6	Pyridoxine (mg)	4	2.1	2			12.43	12.3	41.1
B12	Cyanocobalamin (μg)	5	2.0	2					
B	Nicotinamide (mg)	40	14	10			100	100	160
B	Biotin (mg)	0.06	0.35	0.3					
B	Pantothenic acid/dexpanthenol (mg)	15	14	10			25	25	
B	Folic acid (mg)	0.4	2	0.2					
C	Ascorbic acid (mg)	100	35	30			500	500	500
D	Calciferol (IU)	200	100		120	100		1000	
E	Tocopherol acetate (IU)	10	30				5	50	
K	Phytomenadione (μg)	285–570	140		150	50			

n.b. Constituent levels adjusted for consistency, e.g. thiamine base calculated where thiamine hydrochloride quoted in data sheet

Table 27.5 Total body water as a percentage of body weight

Constituent	Adult male	Adult female	Infant
Body water	60%	50%	77%
Fats and fat-free solids	40%	50%	23%

From Fundamentals of Body Water and Electrolytes (1981), Travenol Laboratories, Deerfield, Illinois, USA

Body water control mechanisms

Total water gains and losses in the healthy adult fall within the range of 1500–3000 ml daily. Thus, where the patient requires TPN, the volume administered will fall into this range and may need to be supplemented by additional fluids in the special cases of burns, etc. Careful patient monitoring is required to ensure that they do not become dehydrated.

Requirements for neonates and infants

Neonates and growing children may have special requirements for amino acids, fluid, calcium, etc. Harries (1978) provides useful further reading.

Requirements and regimens

Figure 27.1 from Elia (1982) shows nomograms used to determine patient requirements at Addenbrookes

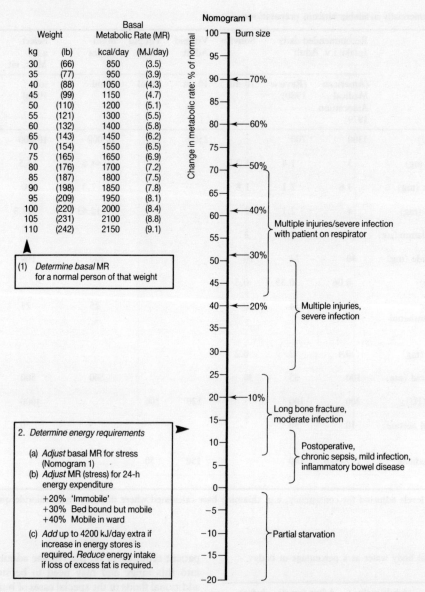

Fig. 27.1 Estimation of energy and nitrogen requirements. Reproduced by kind permission of M. Elia, Department of Gastroenterology, Addenbrookes Hospital, Cambridge

Hospital, Cambridge. Patient nitrogen and calorie requirements are determined using this system and then compared to the constituents of commercially available solutions in order to develop a regimen which both closely fits these requirements and is practical to administer.

For example, if a patient required 14.3 g nitrogen, a solution providing 14 g per litre of nitrogen would generally be acceptable. The degree of accuracy

required would be dictated by the patient type and medical preference, i.e. neonates will require finer 'tuning' of quantities than will the average adult patient.

Whereas some clinicians will favour use of a different mixture for each patient, recent work (Oxford Parenteral Nutrition Team 1983) has shown that in a major centre, standardized regimens fulfilled the requirements of 70% of TPN patients.

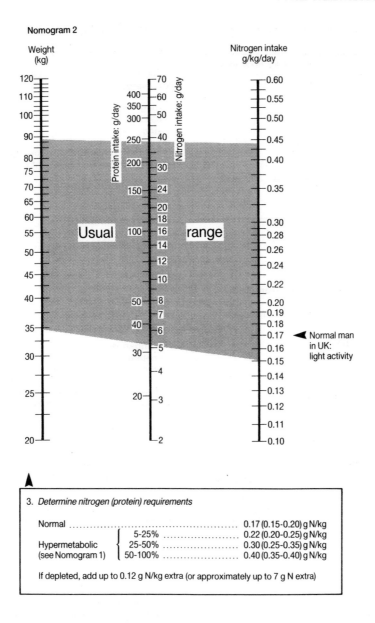

Nomogram 2

3. *Determine nitrogen (protein) requirements*

Normal		0.17 (0.15-0.20) g N/kg
	5-25%	0.22 (0.20-0.25) g N/kg
Hypermetabolic	25-50%	0.30 (0.25-0.35) g N/kg
(see Nomogram 1)	50-100%	0.40 (0.35-0.40) g N/kg

If depleted, add up to 0.12 g N/kg extra (or approximately up to 7 g N extra)

Fig. 27.1 (contd)

Formula build-up

The build-up of a formula generally starts with either the nitrogen or calorie requirement of a patient. Once these have been determined, the next stages are to identify requirements for electrolytes, lipid, vitamins, etc., taking into account any constraints on volume.

Where the 3-litre bag presentation of TPN is required, the pharmacist must review the proposed mixture in terms of stability (see later in this chapter), particularly where lipid is present.

Sample regimens

Clark (1980) suggests adult daily requirements for the major components of TPN. These are listed in Table 27.6.

Table 27.6 Adult daily requirements for major components of TPN

Component	Amount/kg body weight
Water (ml)	30–40
Sodium (mmol)	1.0–1.5
Potassium (mmol)	0.7–1.0
Energy (kcal)	
Medical patient	23–30
Postoperative patient	30–45
Hypercatabolic patient	45–75
Nitrogen (g)	
Medical patient	0.11–0.20
Postoperative patient	0.20–0.31
Hypercatabolic patient	0.25–0.74

Example 27.1

Using these figures we can work out an example as follows.

First let us consider the requirements for nitrogen, energy and water.

For a 65 kg postoperative patient
Nitrogen requirement @ 0.20–0.31 g/kg
$$= 65 \times (0.20–0.31)$$
Range = 13–20 g

Energy requirement @ 30–45 kcal/kg
$$= 65 \times (30–45)$$
Range = 1950–2925 kcal

Water requirement @ 30–40 ml/kg
$$= 65 \times (30–40)$$
Range = 1950–2600 ml

The following mixture would meet these requirements:

Synthamin 14 (Baxter)	1000 ml
glucose 50%	1000 ml
glucose 10%	500 ml

This will provide:

nitrogen	14 g
energy	2200 kcal
water	2500 ml

Further calculations

The above regimen already contains electrolytes intrinsic to the amino acid solutions. Patient electrolyte requirements will be determined from results of blood tests combined with any local policy or standard regimen procedures.

Using the calculation method from Example 27.1 above we can apply Clark's (1980) theory to calculate sodium and potassium requirements.

Sodium requirement @ 1.0–1.5 mmol/kg
$$= 65 \times (1.0–1.5)$$
Range = 65–97.5 mmol

Potassium requirement @ 0.7–1.0 mmol/kg
$$= 65 \times (0.7–1.0)$$
Range = 45.5–65 mmol

Let us assume that this patient also requires the following:

magnesium	10–15 mmol
calcium	6–8 mmol
zinc	50 μmol

With reference to the following tables a suitable mixture for our 65-kg patient may now be:

Synthamin 14 (Baxter)	1000 ml
glucose 50%	500 ml
glucose 40%	500 ml
Nutracel 400 (Baxter)	500 ml

This provides:

nitrogen	14 g
glucose	2200 kcal
sodium	70 mmol
potassium	60 mmol
magnesium	14 mmol
calcium	7.5 mmol
zinc	40 μmol
manganese	40 μmol
acetate	130 mmol
chloride	103 mmol

However, this still does not provide enough zinc. Thus a small volume additive is also required:

Zinc

We are short of 10 μmol of zinc. This could be achieved using zinc sulphate (Lyphomed) — 1 mg zinc per ml (15.3 μmol).

Content = 15.3 μmol of Zinc per ml
Therefore volume required = (10 ÷ 15.3) ml = 0.65 ml

The final formulation would now be:

Synthamin 14 (Baxter)	1000 ml
glucose 50%	500 ml
glucose 40%	500 ml
Nutracel 400 (Baxter)	500 ml
zinc sulphate (1 mg zinc/ml) (Lyphomed)	0.65 ml

This will provide:

nitrogen	14 g
glucose	2200 kcal
sodium	70 mmol
potassium	60 mmol
magnesium	14 mmol
calcium	7.5 mmol
zinc	50 μmol
acetate	130 mmol
chloride	103 mmol

Thus a 3-litre bag containing the base solutions plus the additives identified will meet the stated requirements of our patient.

Note: stability data should be checked.

These calculations are somewhat simplistic and the picture can become more complex once we include lipid, vitamins, volume restrictions, etc.

ASPECTS OF STABILITY AND COMPATIBILITY

Combining all the constituents of a daily TPN feed into one container can result in the production of very complex pharmaceutical systems, particularly where lipid is present.

With so many chemical entities present there is much opportunity for interactions and incompatibilities which may affect the therapeutic value of the preparation or increase its toxicity.

Basic principles of chemistry indicate that changes in temperature, pH, light, oxygen levels, etc., can have an impact on the potential for interactions to take place. This potential continues even after all product mixing within the pharmacy aseptic suite has been completed. Adverse temperature conditions, during storage or within the ward environment, e.g. administering product in direct sunlight, may lead to a disturbance of product stability.

Pharmacists involved in TPN should have a thorough understanding of the potential stability issues in these mixtures and be able to advise physicians accordingly.

Maillard reaction

Amino acids and glucose can participate in a number of chemical reactions. The interaction between amino acids and glucose (Maillard reaction; Fry & Steglink 1982) may not only reduce the therapeutic effect of the components but also present a risk of toxicity to the patient.

Calcium and other electrolytes

Calcium appears to be the electrolyte with the most potential to challenge mixed TPN systems, particularly where lipid is employed as a calorie source.

The requirement for concomitant administration of both calcium and phosphate in the same solution introduces the potential for the precipitation of calcium phosphate. This can be influenced by many parameters (Niemiec & Vanderveen 1984), of which pH is by far the most significant since it influences the equilibrium of phosphate ions.

Modification of pH in TPN mixtures is somewhat difficult due to the buffering capacity of amino acids. Amino acids also have the ability under suitable conditions to combine with calcium and phosphate to form soluble complexes.

Other electrolytes and trace elements

Monovalent cations in therapeutic quantities do not appear to give problems with stability, even with lipid-containing mixed TPN systems.

As trace elements are added to TPN solutions in very small amounts, there is generally not a great potential for interaction. Available literature should be consulted for specific issues, e.g. the effect of copper on vitamin C degradation (Allwood 1984).

Vitamins

Niemiec & Vanderveen (1984) highlight that vitamin stability in TPN systems may be affected by solution pH, presence of electrolytes, trace elements and other vitamins, environmental temperature, light and storage time.

Thus, vitamins, if required, should be added to TPN mixtures immediately prior to administration and should not be stored in excess of 24 hours from the time of mixing.

Lipid

In order to minimize risks of instability, attention must be paid to the following points during formulation and manufacture of TPN mixtures containing lipid:

1. Level of cations, particularly di- and trivalent.
2. pH of resultant mixture.
3. Order of mixing of constituents.
4. Choice of plastic container.
5. Conditions of storage and administration.
6. Manufacturer's recommendations.

Instability of lipid emulsion systems progresses through 'creaming' to 'cracking' or separation of the oil and water phase (see Ch. 16, 16 of the companion volume, Aulton 1988). Administration of such unstable mixtures can give rise to fatty deposits in the lung and other tissues. Thus comprehensive testing should be carried out on potential mixtures to ascertain their suitability for administration to the patient. This should include direct microscopic examination as well as particle size measurements. Davis (1983) is useful further reading.

Drugs and miscellaneous additives

Due to the complex nature of TPN mixtures in single containers, further additions of drugs, etc., should be avoided. Where this is necessary, i.e. where patient's vein access is limited, the addition should be carried out aseptically in the hospital pharmacy if possible and then only if manufacturers or literature have been consulted. Table 27.7 summarizes current recommendations (at date of preparation of this chapter).

Microbiological considerations

Allwood (1984) reviews papers which have examined growth of specific organisms in TPN mixtures and

Table 27.7 Issues of stability for drugs added to TPN mixtures

Drug	Stability issues
Heparin	Visual compatibility reported in concentrations up to 20 000 u/litre (Kobayashi & King 1977, Athanikar et al 1979). Does not appear to bind to glass, plastic or tubing (Niemiec & Vanderveen 1984)
Aminophylline	Stability reported by Kirk & Sprake (1982). 100% recovery of aminophylline reported after 24 h in three TPN formulae by Neimiec et al (1983). In combinations with low amino acid level and high calcium and phosphate levels, calcium phosphate precipitation noted following addition of aminophylline.
Insulin	Insulin will bind to PVC, polyethylene and glass. Bolton (1982) reports 40% loss after addition to TPN bag. Extent of adsorption depends on (Niemiec & Vanderveen 1984) length of administration set, temperature, electrolytes, etc.
Cimetidine	Moore et al (1981) report no apparent adverse effects of mixing cimetidine with TPN solutions. Rosenberg et al (1980) note no loss of cimetidine 7 days after mixing. Tsallas & Allen (1982) show compatibility with TPN mixtures containing Synthamin
Antibiotics	The review article by Niemiec & Vanderveen (1984) gives compatibility data on 15 different antibiotics

recommends storage at between 2 and 6°C in order to minimize effects.

ASEPTIC PRODUCTION

This section looks at the parameters of control for aseptic TPN compounding.

Facility and environment

As with all aseptic processes, the environment used for manufacturing can contribute considerably to product quality and must thus be designed, cleaned, maintained and monitored to the highest achievable standard as described in Chapters 22 and 23.

Personnel and training

Aseptic preparation of TPN solutions should only be carried out by personnel who have undergone a suitable documented training programme. This should cover not only aseptic technique and validation but also theoretical aspects such as patient requirements and use of products.

Documentation

A work sheet should be generated for each TPN-dispensing activity to be carried out for recording materials, patient name, label details, etc. The format for such a work sheet should be agreed between the production and quality control departments of the hospital in accordance with local policy.

This is by no means the only documentation which is required to control the overall aseptic process. Raw material testing, environmental monitoring records, cleaning records, operator training records, patient records should all form part of the documentation packages which are developed and retained to best fit the requirements of the hospital or industrial environment and the standards laid down in BS 5295 and recommended in the 'Guide to good pharmaceutical manufacturing practice' (DHSS 1983).

Manufacturing procedures

Manufacturing procedures or guidelines should be drawn up jointly by production and quality control staff depending upon the manufacturing environment. These should be adhered to by all personnel involved in the process, updated regularly and audited periodically to ensure conformance. This is essential to the quality assurance of the operation.

These procedures should cover all the activities in the department down to specific tasks, such as use of syringes, etc.

METHODS AND EQUIPMENT

The steps in the dispensing of TPN solutions in the hospital facility are detailed below.

Receipt of prescription

The documents used for the prescribing of TPN solutions at ward level may vary from adaptation of a basic fluids chart to a custom-made TPN chart often developed jointly by pharmacy and medical staff.

On receipt of the request for TPN the pharmacist should check that the requested combination is feasible, stable and within normal clinical limits. Information can then be transferred to the dispensing worksheet.

Collection of materials and preparation

Once the documentation for a bag or number of bags has been generated and checked the manufacturing process proper may commence.

The first stage in this process will be the identification and collection together of all materials required to be taken into the aseptic suite.

A typical 'shopping list' for the dispensing of one patient-specific TPN bag is listed in Tables 27.8 and 27.9.

Table 27.8 Source components for one TPN bag

1 × 1000 ml amino acid solution
1 × 500 ml glucose solution
1 × 500 ml electrolyte solution
1 × 500 ml i.v. lipid
2 × 10 ml additive ampoules (Na, K, etc.)
1 × 10 ml trace element solution
1 × 10 ml water-soluble vitamins
1 × 10 ml fat-soluble vitamins

Table 27.9 Equipment (sterile) required to prepare one TPN bag

1 × empty 3-litre bag
5 × 10 ml syringes
5 × 21 g needles
2 × quill
5 × individual filter (5 μm, 0.22 μm)
Swabs, cloths, etc.

The components assembled are then checked against the work sheet by the pharmacist who should initial the sheet. At this stage either the work sheet or label containing a copy of the formulation should be passed through with the ingredients, utilizing a transparent pocket which can be swabbed (see Ch. 22).

Entry into preparation area

This is best effected using a controlled pass-through hatch or chamber with interlocking doors in order to prevent the ingress of dirty air from the surrounding environment. Specially designed trays, trolleys or plastic containers may be utilized for this purpose provided that they are sanitizable and effect bag or batch control and segregation during handling and transit throughout the manufacturing process.

First-stage preparation

In order to minimize the microbiological bioburden on the final aseptic process all excess packaging should be removed and discarded at this stage and all surfaces should be cleaned.

The cleaning process is normally effected using a 70% alcoholic solution (e.g. industrial methylated spirit or isopropyl alcohol) together with sterile lint-free swabs or cloths utilizing a systematic and thorough wiping routine.

Where more than one bag is being processed in the preparation room, care should be taken to avoid cross-contamination of source materials, labels, etc., and another reconciliation should be carried out prior to the passage of materials into the aseptic (Class I) room.

Second-stage preparation

Entry of materials into the Class I area should again be effected by means of a pass-through system with interlocking doors.

Following a defined and thorough decontamination of the laminar air flow cabinet (see Chs 22, 23), materials passed into the area from the Class II room should then be subjected to a repeat of the surface cleaning process before being passed directly into the laminar air flow cabinet.

As with all aseptic operations, materials should be placed well within the laminar air flow cabinet making use of all the available space and organized in a manner which will facilitate the pre-defined systematic steps in the dispensing process and cause minimum disruption of air flow.

The container (empty bag)

Original silicone-based bags (Solassol & Joyeux 1973) were superseded by polyvinyl chloride (PVC) and eventually ethylvinyl acetate (EVA) which permitted the inclusion of intravenous fat emulsions into TPN mixtures — a process which had previously been avoided due to concerns regarding the potential leaching of diethylhexylphthalate (DEHP) plasticizer from PVC into fat.

Hardy (1987) summarizes the standards and testing required for i.v. containers in his review of TPN therapy developments since 1977. He highlights other container-related issues such as retention of dust particles by the plastic caused by the residual eletrostatic charge left after certain steps in the manufacturing process. Developments in the extrusion process may help to reduce this. Rubber stoppers in the ports of the bag may give rise to electrolytes, antioxidants, etc. as contaminants to the filled solution.

Development work continues in order to produce the optimum design for empty TPN containers.

Additives and connections

Operational procedures should define these activities in order to ensure consistency of approach between individuals. This is necessary not only from the microbiological standpoint but also from a compatibility perspective as the addition of say calcium salts directly into lipid can have an adverse effect on the stability of the resultant mixture, as can the order in which the bulk components are mixed.

It is not recommended to use the additive port on the 3-litre bag itself for small volume additions as this should be reserved for any last minute additions at ward level, if this is permissible. Thus, one of the following techniques should be employed:

Method 1 (addition to flexible PVC source containers)

The measured contents of the syringe of additive solution should be fully discharged into the additive port of the PVC source container, e.g. sodium chloride 0.9% Viaflex. The additive port is then firmly squeezed to dispense residual quantities of small volume solution into the bulk fluid. The PVC container should then be agitated thoroughly to ensure even mixing of the additive solution with the vehicle.

Should a second or third additive be required, the process may be repeated, paying special attention to any potential chemical compatibility issues if the same source PVC container is to be used. Where possible, additives should be spread between several source containers.

Method 2 (addition to bottles)

The rubber cap of the bottle will indicate where the needle is to be inserted to make an addition.

Such source container bottles, e.g. amino acid solutions, electrolyte solutions, will generally contain a vacuum above the level of the fluid which can be utilized to suck in the contents of the additive syringe.

Method 3 (via the in-line additive port)

Where the empty TPN bag contains an in-line additive port additions may be made sequentially at this point using the gravity or assisted flow of bulk fluids to effect immediate dilution. However, once the bag is filled, it should still be well agitated to encourage thorough mixing of all components. This is necessary to ensure that patients get a regular, even flow of nutrients and no high doses of, for example, undiluted potassium chloride.

Filling process options

Gravity filling

Where a small number of bags need to be dispensed in a hospital pharmacy the method of choice for filling may be to utilize gravity.

Spiked source containers are suspended from a suitable rack or retort stand under the laminar air flow cabinet and allowed to drain into the empty TPN bag. This may take in the order of 20 minutes depending upon the viscosity of the source components, however, this time may be well utilized in making the required small volume additions as described in the previous section.

Negative pressure

In order to speed up the filling process one of the assisted systems available is negative pressure filling. Commercial companies, e.g. Miramed, Baxter, Pfrimmer, have developed chambers made from reinforced plastics into which the empty TPN containers are placed once they have been connected to source components. A lid with a suitable gasket then covers the chamber allowing only the filling tube of the empty bag to pass through it.

Source containers are suspended from a suitable rack or stand and a pre-defined level of vacuum is applied to the chamber. Filling can be effected in 3–4 minutes.

Positive pressure

Several methods now exist for positive-pressure bag filling. Some pharmacists may chose to utilize the standard pumps used for a variety of hospital manufacturing activities, however, specialist systems for TPN do exist (Automix (Baxter), Fillmat 2000 (Miramed)), which may also be combined with volumetric measuring systems providing a useful means of dispensing paediatric TPN solutions.

Inspection and labelling

Inspection

The completed nutrition bag should be inspected to check for integrity of all ports, leaks, splits and particulates for which TPN solutions should conform to the BP 1988 criteria together with the limit test for particulate matter.

Labelling

In general the following information will be required on the label:

Patient name/number
Ward
Product constituents
Batch (dispensing number)
Expiry date/time
Storage conditions

Other instructions such as guidance on administration rate or technique, limitations on further additions etc., may also be required. Example 27.2 shows an example of label format which takes these factors into account.

Dispensing

Once the product has been filled and labelled a pharmacist should perform a final check against the prescription prior to sending the product to the ward.

This check should include the patient's name, ward, etc. and should once again compare the constituents requested against the final label. Details of further additions, storage conditions, expiry date, etc. should also be confirmed and the batch number or other reference allocated should be checked to facilitate traceability in the event of any difficulties arising subsequent to dispensing, e.g. precipitation, discoloration, etc.

The hospital pharmacist may be involved in development of nursing care guidelines with particular reference to further additions, storage, etc. It may also be useful for the ward pharmacist to check that TPN is being cor-

Example 27.2

Labelling example (after Allwood 1984)

Parenteral Nutrition Mixture		
Total energy supplied in 24 hours is . . . . kcal is . . . . ml.		
Contents:	Nitrogen	g
	Carbohydrate	kcals
	Sodium	mmol
	Potassium	mmol
	Phosphate	mmol
	Calcium	mmol
	Magnesium	mmol
	Trace elements	
	Cu: Zn: Cr: Mn: F: I: Fe.	
	Vitamins	
	A: B Co: C: E: Folate: Biotin.	
	Final volume	ml
	Patient	Ward
	Expiry date	
Date:	Prepared by:	Batch no:
Warning:	Protect from light. Contains approx. 20% w/v dextrose, do not infuse too rapidly. Refrigerate until ready for use.	
	Do not make any further additions to this container.	

rectly administered to the patient, i.e. with correct flow control device, away from direct sunlight, etc.

Storage and packaging

Storage

Allwood (1984) recommends that compounded TPN solutions should be stored at 2–6°C in light of both microbiological and chemical considerations (see 'Aspects of stability and compatibility' earlier in this chapter).

The pharmacy/ward/home patient — refrigerators should be calibrated to ensure that they are able to maintain this level of temperature, as bags, particularly those containing lipid, should not be allowed to freeze and should not be stored at room temperature for periods in excess of the 12–24 hours required for administration.

Packaging

Where supplies of compounded product are to be made to hospitals or home patients away from the site of manufacture, the quality of the packaging system to maintain product temperature during transit should be validated to the satisfaction of local quality control standards. Insulated polystyrene containers may be useful for this purpose.

Costs

Providing a TPN compounding service within a hospital may be a costly venture for the pharmacy department. Amino acid and lipid presentations are, by their specialist nature, expensive items to purchase. The materials cost of compounding is easy to identify, however, dispensing into a 3-litre bag requires other, sometimes not so apparent, costs such as labour input, overheads, consumables, etc.

All these factors must be considered when developing true service costs and deciding whether to produce in-house or obtain product from a regional hospital or commercial source.

BIBLIOGRAPHY

Abbott W M 1976 Indications for Parenteral Nutrition. In: Fischer J E (ed) Total parenteral nutrition, 1. Little Brown, Boston

Allwood M C 1984 Compatibility and stability of TPN mixtures in big bags. Journal of Clinical and Hospital Pharmacy 9: 181–198

Allwood M C, McHutchinson D, Elia M Ongoing A guide to the operation of a TPN service. Addenbrookes Hospital/Baxter Laboratories, Cambridge, UK

American Medical Association 1979 Multivitamin preparations for parenteral use. Journal of Parenteral and Enteral Nutrition 3: 258–262

Athanikar N, Boyer B, Deamer R et al 1979 Visual compatibility of 30 additives with parenteral nutrient solution. American Journal of Hospital Pharmacy 36: 511–513

Aulton M E (ed) 1988 Pharmaceutics: the science of dosage form design. Churchill Livingstone, Edinburgh

Black C D, Popovich N G 1981 A study of intravenous emulsion. Compatibility effects of dextrose, amino acids and selected electrolytes. Drug Intelligence and Clinical Pharmacy 15: 184

Bolton D 1982 Insulin adsorption during total parenteral nutrition. Proceedings of the Guild 14: 45–46

Clark R 1980 Nutritional requirements in different nutritional states. British Journal of Pharmaceutical Practice (Symposium Suppl: Complete parenteral nutrition in perspective)

Davis S S 1983 The stability of fat emulsions for intravenous administration. In: Johnston IDA (ed) Advances in clinical nutrition. MTP Press, Lancaster

Dawes W H, Groves M J 1978 The effect of electrolytes on phospholipid-stabilised soybean oil emulsions. International Journal of Pharmacy 37: 673–674

Dudrick S J, Wilmore D W, Vars H M 1967 Long term parenteral nutrition and growth in puppies and positive nitrogen balance. Surgical Forum 18: 356

Elia M 1982 The effects of nitrogen and energy intake on the metabolism of normal depleted and injured man. Considerations for practical nutritional support. Clinical Nutrition 1: 173–192

Farwell J A 1980 Pharmaceutical factors in long-term parenteral nutrition. Proceedings of the Guide of Hospital Pharmacists 8: 3–40

Fielding L P, Humfress A, Mouchizadeh J, Dudley H, Gilmour M 1981 Parenteral Nutrition: experience with three-litre bags. Pharmaceutical Journal 226: 590–592

Fry L K, Stegink L D 1982 Formation of Maillard reaction products in parenteral alimentation solutions. Journal of Nutrition 112: 1631–1637

Guidelines for the Nursing Care of Patients Receiving Parenteral Nutrition. British Intravenous Therapy Association. (B.I.T.A.) Guide. Baxter Laboratories, Thetford

Hardy G 1987 Ten years of TPN with 3-litre bags. Pharmaceutical Journal 239: 26–28

Harries J T 1978 Aspects of intravenous feeding in childhood. In: Johnston I D A (ed) Advances in parenteral nutrition. MTP Press, Lancaster, pp 267–280

Hirsch J, Bradley D 1983 Clinical applications of 20% fat emulsions. In: Johnston I D A (ed) Advances in clinical nutrition. MTP Press, Lancaster, pp 189–192

Irving M 1983 Intestinal failure and its treatment by home parenteral nutrition. In: Johnston I D A (ed) Advances in clinical nutrition. MTP Press, Lancaster pp 269–388

Johnston I D A 1978 Metabolic foundations of intravenous nutrition. In: Johnston I D A (ed) Advances in parenteral nutrition. MTP Press, Lancaster, pp 3–20

Karpet J T, Peden V H 1972 Copper deficiency in long-term parenteral nutrition. Journal of Pediatrics 80: 32–36

Karran S J, Alberti K G M M 1980 Carbohydrates in parenteral nutrition. In: Karran S J, Alberti K G M M (eds) Practical nutritional support. Pitman Medical, London

Kay R G, Tasman-Jones C, Pybus J, Whitney R, Black H 1976 A syndrome of acute zinc deficiency during total parenteral alimentation in man. Annals of Surgery 183: 331–340

Kirk B, Sprake J M 1982 Stability of aminophylline. British Journal of Intravenous Therapy 3: November 4–8

Knochel J P 1977 The pathophysiology and clinical characteristics of severe hypophosphataemia. Archives of Internal Medicine 137: 203–220

Kobayashi N H, King J C 1977 Compatibility of common additives in protein hydrolysate/dextrose solutions. American Journal of Hospital Pharmacy 34: 589–594

Lowry S F, Goodgame J T, Maher M M, Brennan M 1979 Abnormalities of zinc copper during total parenteral nutrition. Annals of Surgery 189: 120–128

Moore R A, Feldman S, Treuting J et al 1981 Cimetidine and parenteral nutrition. Journal of Parenteral and Enteral Nutrition 5: 61–63

Niemiec P W Jr, Vanderveen T W 1984 Compatibility considerations in parenteral solutions. American Journal of Hospital Pharmacy 41: 893–911

Niemiec P W Jr, Vanderveen T W 1984 Compatibility considerations in parenteral nutrient solutions. American Journal of Hospital Pharmacy 41: 893–911

Niemiec P W, Vanderveen T W, Hohenwarter M W et al 1983 Stability of aminophylline injection in three parenteral nutrient solutions. American Journal of Hospital Pharmacy 40: 428–432

Normal Laboratory Values 1980 New England Journal of Medicine 302: 37–48

Nunn A J 1980 Aspects of pharmacy involvement. British Journal of Pharmaceutical Practice 2: (Symposium Suppl)

O'Kane M, Knott C 1982 New parenteral nutrition facility. Pharmaceutical Journal 228: 599–601

Oxford Parenteral Nutrition Team 1983 Total parenteral nutrition: value of a standard feeding regimen. British Medical Journal 286: 1323–1327

Powell-Tuck J, Farwell J A, Nielsen T, Lennard-Jones J E 1978 Team approach to long-term intravenous feeding in patients with gastrointestinal disorders. Lancet 2: 825–828

Review 1980 Adult parenteral nutrition: which preparation? Drug and Therapeutics Bulletin 18: 85

Rosenberg H A, Doughtety J T, Mayron D et al 1980 Cimetidine hydrochloride compatibility I. Chemical aspects and room temperature stability in intravenous infusion fluids. American Journal of Hospital Pharmacy 37: 390–392

Shenkin A 1987 Essential trace elements during intravenous nutrition. Intensive Therapy and Clinical Monitoring 8: March/April 38–47

Shenkin A, Fell G S, Halls D J, Dunbar P M, Halbrook I B, Irving M H 1986 Essential trace element provision to patients receiving home IVN in the United Kingdom. Clinical Nutrition 5: 91–97

Silk D B A 1983 Nutritional support in hospital practice. Blackwell Scientific, Oxford

Solassol C, Joyeux H 1974 Nouvelles techniques pour nutrition parenteral chronique. Annals de l'Anesthesiologie Francaise 2: (Special), 75

Tsallas G, Allen L C 1982 Stability of cimetidine hydrochloride in parenteral nutrition solutions. American Journal of Hospital Pharmacy 39: 484–485

Woolfson A M J 1979 Metabolic considerations in nutritional support. Research Clinics Forums 1: 35

28. Ophthalmic products

L. Titcomb

Introduction

Ophthalmic products include:

Eye drops. Sterile solutions or suspensions of one or more drugs in an aqueous or oily vehicle intended for instillation into the conjunctival sac.

Eye ointments. Sterile, semi-solid preparations of homogeneous appearance containing one or more drugs intended for application to the conjunctival sac or eyelid margin.

Eye lotions. Sterile aqueous solutions used undiluted for washing or bathing the eyes.

Contact lens products. Sterile, aqueous solutions used for the cleaning, disinfection, storage and wetting of contact lenses.

EYE DROPS

Eye drops are used both for diagnostic and therapeutic purposes and contain drugs which act on the anterior segment of the eye: the cornea, conjunctiva and anterior uvea. Drugs acting on the eye which are formulated as eye drops include antimicrobial agents (antibacterials, antifungals and antivirals), artificial tears, corticosteroids and non-steroidal anti-inflammatory agents, cycloplegics, diagnostic stains, drugs used in the treatment of glaucoma, local anaesthetics, miotics and mydriatics.

The eye is normally protected against infection by a variety of mechanisms. The eyelashes help to prevent small particles of dust entering the eye, the blink reflex is initiated when objects are perceived to be travelling towards the eye and the eye is continually washed by the tear fluid which contains lysozyme, an antibacterial enzyme. However, when the eye is infected, inflamed or damaged by accidental injury or surgery, the most important defence mechanism, the integrity of the outer layers of the eye, is lost and the opportunist pathogen is given access to deeper tissue. As this tissue is non-vascular, its resistance to infection is low and ulceration and even penetration can occur. Since eye drops are frequently administered when the eye's defence mechanisms are compromised, it is imperative that they are sterile.

The outer tissues of the eye, the cornea and conjunctiva, are well supplied with nerve endings and their sensitivity is increased when the tissue is inflamed. Irritation, apart from being unpleasant, stimulates tear production and therefore results in a reduction in the time that the drug is in contact with the eye. In order to achieve maximum comfort and therapeutic effect, possible causes of irritation in eye drops must be minimized.

Certain drugs such as idoxuridine and rose bengal are inherently irritant. This effect is unrelated to other causes of irritancy such as pH or tonicity of the eye drop formulation.

FORMULATION OF EYE DROPS

Vehicle

Most drugs used in the form of eye drops are formulated as aqueous solutions or suspensions. However, certain drugs are unstable in aqueous solution and are formulated as oily eye drops. For example, tetracycline hydrochloride is formulated as an oily suspension of the drug in sesame oil.

Ecothiopate iodide eye drops are unstable at room temperature. The commercially available preparation is presented as a sterile, freeze-dried powder together with a sterile, aqueous diluent containing the preservative and stabilizers, intended to be mixed immediately before issue to the patient. The reconstituted solution has a shelf-life of 1 month, the recommended period over which eye drops may be used in the domiciliary situation.

Particulate matter

To avoid irritation in the form of a foreign body sensation it is important that eye drops in the form of solutions do not contain particles and that the particle size of eye drop suspensions is limited. The British Pharmacopoeia specifies that eye drop solutions are practically free from particles and lays down stringent limits on particle size for eye drops which are suspensions. These standards may be achieved by the clarification of solutions by filtration and the use of medicaments in the form of ultra-fine powders for the preparation of suspensions.

Adjuvants used in eye drops

Eye drops may contain added substances to maintain the sterility of the preparation, to adjust the tonicity or viscosity, to adjust or stabilize the pH, to increase the solubility of the medicaments or to stabilize the preparation.

Any substance used in this way should be:

1. Physically, chemically and therapeutically compatible with the active ingredient(s) and any other adjuvants included in the formulation.
2. Compatible with the container in which the formulation is housed.
3. Unaffected by the method of sterilization to be employed.
4. Non-toxic and non-irritant to the ocular tissue.
5. Effective over the period that the product is intended to be used at the concentration at which it is employed and the conditions under which the product is to be stored.

Antimicrobial agents

If an eye drop is to be used on more than one occasion, it must contain an agent which will prevent the growth of organisms which are inadvertently introduced during use. Thus eye drops intended for multiple use must contain antimicrobial preservatives.

In addition to the ideal mentioned above the preservative should be active against a wide range of organisms (bacteria and fungi), be capable of withstanding the test for efficacy of antimicrobial preservatives in pharmaceutical products as described in the British Pharmacopoeia, and its activity should not be affected by the pH of the solution into which it is introduced.

A substance fulfilling all these ideals is yet to be found but the preservatives in use today possess many of these characteristics.

Note that eye drops supplied for use during intraocular surgery should not contain preservatives as there is a chance that the preservative will enter the anterior chamber of the eye and damage the corneal endothelium.

The antimicrobial substances commonly included in eye drops are described below.

A list of suitable preservatives useable in a range of eye drops is provided in Table 28.1.

Benzalkonium chloride. This is a quaternary ammonium compound, a cationic surfactant, and is used at a concentration of 0.01% w/v. This is often expressed as 0.02% v/v Benzalkonium Chloride Solution BP, a formulation of the preservative containing 50% w/v.

Benzalkonium chloride is bactericidal against a wide range of Gram-positive and some Gram-negative organisms. Its antimicrobial activity, which is greatest at pH 8 and reduced in acidic pH, is due to an increase in the permeability of bacterial cell membranes. The activity of benzalkonium chloride is decreased in the presence

Table 28.1 Suggested preservatives for eye drops

BAC,
  Carbachol
  Cyclopentolate
  Hypromellose
  Phenylephrine
  Physostigmine
  Physostigmine and Pilocarpine
  Pilocarpine
  Prednisolone

CHA
  Cocaine and Homatropine

BAC or CHA
  Homatropine
  Hyoscine

PMA or PMN
  Amethocaine
  Chloramphenicol
  Fluorescein
  Hydrocortisone and neomycin
  Lachesine
  Neomycin
  Zinc sulphate
  Zinc sulphate and adrenaline

PMA, PMN or BAC
  Atropine sulphate

PMA, PMN or CHA
  Cocaine

PMA, PMN or TM
  Sulphacetamide

BAC, Benzalkonium chloride solution BP 0.02% w/v; CHA, Chlorhexidine acetate 0.01% w/v; PMA, Phenylmercuric acetate 0.002% w/v; PMN, Phenylmercuric nitrate 0.002% w/v; TM, Thiomersal 0.01% w/v.

of hypromellose, magnesium, calcium and potassium ions, but enhanced by benzyl and phenethyl alcohols, disodium edetate and phenylpropanol.

Benzalkonium chloride is incompatible with citrates, iodides, nitrates, salicylates, some sulphonamides and zinc sulphate. It is inactivated by fluorescein and forms a precipitate when it comes into contact with rubber lubricated with microcrystalline polyethylene or stearates. It is significantly adsorbed onto rubber.

It is very soluble in water, solutions are stable when stored in airtight containers, protected from light and may be sterilized by autoclaving.

Solutions containing 0.02% w/v benzalkonium chloride are well tolerated by the eye but concentrations above 0.1% w/v are irritant.

The surface activity of this preservative is used therapeutically to enhance the transcorneal penetration of non lipid-soluble drugs such as carbachol. However, this property of benzalkonium chloride can result in solubilization of the protective oily layer of the tears resulting in instability of the tear film. This effect precludes the use of this preservative in combination with local anaesthetics. Such a combination will abolish the blink reflex and prevent the reformation of the tear film.

Patients who wear soft contact lenses are often warned against using eye drops containing benzalkonium chloride but although this type of lens will absorb and concentrate the preservative when stored in a solution containing benzalkonium chloride, intermittent use of one drop of an eye drop containing the preservative does not normally lead to irritation or damage. Certain patients show allergic sensitivity to benzalkonium chloride and must be treated with preparations containing an alternative preservative.

Chlorhexidine acetate. Chlorhexidine is a cationic disinfectant employed at a concentration of 0.01% w/v. It is effective against many Gram-positive and some Gram-negative bacteria, acting by attacking and rupturing the cell membrane. It is ineffective against acid-fast bacteria, bacterial spores, most fungi and viruses.

It is most active at neutral or slightly alkaline pH. Its activity is reduced in the presence of organic matter and insoluble magnesium, zinc and calcium compounds, and enhanced by benzyl and phenethyl alcohols, phenylpropanol and disodium edetate. Chlorhexidine acetate is soluble in water and aqueous solutions may be sterilized by autoclaving although there is some decomposition to 4-chloroaniline. Considerably less breakdown occurs when solutions of chlorhexidine are held at 100°C for 30 minutes. It is more stable in acidic than alkaline solutions, the rate of decomposition being least at pH 5–6.

At the concentrations employed in eye drop formulations (0.01% w/v) it is compatible with most anions used in these products, other than sulphates.

Chlorhexidine acetate is generally well tolerated by the eye although allergic reactions do occur.

Chlorbutol. This compound, often known as chlorbutanol or chlorobutanol, is a chlorinated alcohol used at a concentration of 0.5% w/v.

Chlorbutol is a very effective preservative, being active against Gram-positive and Gram-negative bacteria and fungi, and is bactericidal when exposure is prolonged. It is compatible with most compounds used in ophthalmic preparations but is inactivated by fluorescein.

It is soluble 1 in 130 of water, therefore at the concentration at which it is normally employed it is close to its saturation point at low temperatures and crystallization may occur. Lower concentrations of chlorbutol have been used in preparations of drugs with intrinsic antibacterial activity such as amethocaine.

It is volatile and easily lost from solution and will diffuse through polyethylene containers. It is stable in acid but not in neutral or alkaline solutions in which it hydrolyses to form hydrochloric acid with a resultant decrease in the pH of the solution. The increased rate of this hydrolysis at high temperatures means that there is appreciable decomposition on autoclaving or steaming. Solution containing chlorbutol should be protected from light.

Chlorbutol is well tolerated by the eye.

Phenylmercuric salts. Phenylmercuric acetate and nitrate are organic mercurials employed at a concentration of 0.002% w/v. The former is often preferred because of its greater solubility, but both compounds are only slightly soluble in water.

Phenylmercuric salts are active against bacteria and fungi over a wide pH range, although their activity is bacteriostatic rather than bactericidal and is reduced in the presence of body fluids. They are ineffective against bacterial spores. Their activity is increased in the presence of phenethylalcohol and in the presence of sodium metabisulphite at acid pH but decreased in the presence of this compound at alkaline pH. Their activity is also decreased by the addition of disodium edetate, sodium thiosulphate and anionic emulsifying and suspending agents.

These preservatives are incompatible with halides, aluminium and other metals, ammonia and ammonium salts and with some sulphur compounds such as those found in rubber. There is a significant amount of absorption onto the rubber components of containers in which their solutions are stored.

Phenylmercuric salts are non-irritant at the concentrations used in ophthalmic preparations. However, they should not be used in eye drops which are to be administered over long periods of time, such as those containing drugs in the treatment of glaucoma, because their prolonged use can lead to intra-ocular deposition of mercury (mercurialentis) and the development of band keratopathy, a similar deposition in the cornea.

Thiomersal. Thiomersal is an organic mercurial, employed at a concentration of 0.005–0.01% w/v.

It is bacteriostatic and fungistatic, forming covalent bonds with the sulphydryl groups of cellular enzymes. Its activity is reduced in the presence of disodium edetate and sodium thiosulphate.

It is incompatible with benzalkonium chloride, iodine, heavy metal salts and many alkaloids.

Thiomersal is very soluble in water and is more stable at neutral than alkaline pH. In acidic solutions the compound is converted to the corresponding acid which decomposes to form insoluble products. It is stable to autoclaving but decomposes in the presence of light. It is adsorbed onto the rubber components of containers in which it is housed.

Thiomersal does not disrupt the lipid layer of the tear film but allergy to this preservative is common. It has been implicated in the development of band keratopathy but is less likely to cause mercurialentis than the phenylmercuric salts.

Other compounds. Other compounds such as hydroxybenzoates, phenethyl and benzyl alcohols, cetrimide and sodium pentachlorophenate are used as preservatives in eye drops but are not used as the sole agent unless the drug itself is an antimicrobial. A complete list of the preservatives used in branded eye drops may be found in the 'Monthly Index of Medical Specialities' (MIMS).

Benzalkonium chloride, chlorhexidine acetate, the phenylmercuric salts and thiomersal are the preservatives which were approved by the British Pharmacopoeia (1980) to be employed in that method of sterilizing eye drops known as 'heating with a bactericide' (see Ch. 20).

Tonicity modifiers

Although in the past it was common practice to adjust the tonicity of eye drops, so that the solution was isotonic with tears (approximately equivalent to a 0.9% w/v sodium chloride solution), it is now known that the eye can tolerate solutions having an isotonicity range equivalent to 0.6–2.0% w/v sodium chloride. However, as very hypotonic solutions can cause temporary oedema of the cornea which will result in impaired vision, and grossly hypertonic solutions can produce discomfort due to the inability of the tears to adequately or rapidly dilute the solution, it is wise to adjust the tonicity of hypotonic eye drops by the addition of sodium chloride to bring the solution into the range tolerated by the eye and to avoid non-essential increases in the tonicity of hypertonic solutions. If the tear film is deficient, the patient's tolerance of eye drops which are not isotonic is decreased. Therefore eye drops such as Hypromellose Eye Drops BPC 1973 ('artificial tears') used in these conditions are made isotonic.

Phenylephrine Eye Drops 10% w/v BPC 1973 and Sulphacetamide Eye Drops 10–30% w/v BP 1988 give rise to stinging on instillation due to their unavoidable hypertonicity.

Sodium chloride may be added to hypotonic eye drop formulations to bring the tonicity within the range tolerated by the eye. Methods for calculating the amount of sodium chloride required are given in the 'Pharmaceutical Handbook' (1980) and the 'Pharmaceutical Codex' (1979).

Viscosity modifiers

Aqueous solutions of drugs do not remain in contact with the eye for long periods. The instillation of 50 μl (1 drop) of a fluid into the conjunctival sac (the normal capacity of which is 7–10 μl and the maximum capacity 25 μl) results in immediate overflow onto the lids and into the naso-lacrimal drainage system. Most of the drug will have disappeared from the conjunctival sac within 30 seconds and the total amount instilled will have disappeared within 10–20 minutes.

Increasing the viscosity of instilled liquid to 15 mPa s (15 cP) causes a marked decrease in tear drainage, thus the ocular contact time and the bioavailability of the drug can be increased by the incorporation of a viscolizing agent.

Viscolizing agents used in ophthalmic preparations include substituted cellulose ethers (methylcellulose and its derivatives) and polyvinyl alcohol.

Substituted cellulose ethers. The use of methylcellulose in ophthalmic preparations was first described in 1945. Since then many derivatives of this compound including hydroxyethylcellulose, hydroxypropylcellulose, carboxymethylcellulose and hydroxypropyl methylcellulose have been employed.

Methylcellulose is slowly soluble in cold water but, being insoluble in hot water, separates out on autoclaving, re-dissolving on cooling. Solutions of methylcellulose are neutral, odourless, tasteless and stable in the pH range tolerated by the eye. Solutions of the pure compound do not support bacterial or fungal growth and are unaffected by light or ageing.

The refractive index of a solution of the 4000 grade of methylcellulose, which is normally employed in ophthalmic preparations, is similar to that of distilled water, therefore its use does not distort the vision. It is used at a concentration of 0.5–2.0% w/v in eye drop formulations. More concentrated solutions form gels which are best administered from ointment tubes.

Methycellulose is almost inert chemically but the viscosity of its solutions is increased by the presence of large amounts of electrolytes. Highly surface active agents such as amethocaine are adsorbed by the colloid so that their penetration of tissue is retarded.

Hypromellose, the hydroxypropyl derivative of methylcellulose, is now more commonly employed than the parent compound. Hypromellose has better solubility characteristics, its mucilages have greater clarity and contain fewer undispersed fibres, and its aqueous solutions are tolerant to salts.

Polyvinyl alcohol. This compound, usually employed at a concentration of 1.4% w/v, is gaining popularity as a viscolizing and wetting agent. Like the substituted cellulose ethers, it is soluble in water, its solutions are transparent and colourless and may be sterilized by autoclaving.

Its great advantage is that it has excellent contact time on the eye despite the low viscosity of its solutions, which, unlike those of methylcellulose can easily be passed through a 0.22 μm filter, allowing sterilization by filtration.

Solutions of polyvinyl alcohol may be thickened or gelled by certain agents including sodium bicarbonate, sodium borate and inorganic sulphates but generally it is compatible with ophthalmic drugs and preservatives.

Other compounds used as viscolizing agents include polyethylene glycol, polyvinylpyrrolidone and dextran.

pH buffers

There is usually a particular pH or pH range at or within which a drug in solution is most stable. Adjustment of the pH of the solution to this value by the use of appropriate buffers is desirable to achieve maximum stability of the product. Unfortunately, maximum stability cannot always be achieved at a pH at which it is comfortable for the patient to use the drops, and a compromise must be sought.

Tears have a great capacity to buffer solutions instilled into the conjunctival sac to their normal pH of 7.4, therefore solutions varying in pH from 3.5 to 10.5 may be instilled without discomfort. However, solutions buffered to an acidic or alkaline pH, or very acidic solutions such as those of adrenaline acid tartrate or pilocarpine hydrochloride, will cause stinging on instil-

lation. Eye drop formulations for these drugs contain adjuvants to bring the pH into the range which will be tolerated by the eye.

Single compounds such as sodium bicarbonate and boric acid may be added to eye drop formulations to adjust the pH. Buffers may be used to maintain the pH of the eye drops at an optimum to minimize chemical degradation, but may also be included to increase comfort for the user and enhance therapeutic effect.

Examples of buffers used in eye drop formulations are:

Borate buffer (boric acid/borax) — pH range 6.8–9.1. This buffer system is incorporated into Chloramphenicol Eye Drops BP 1988 to maintain the pH at 7.5 and into Hypromellose Eye Drops BPC 1973 to maintain it at 8.4.

Phosphate buffer (sodium acid phosphate/sodium phosphate) — pH range 4.5–8.5. This buffer system is incorporated into Neomycin Eye Drops BPC 1973 and Prednisolone Sodium Phosphate Eye Drops BPC 1973 to maintain the pH of these preparations at 6.5 and 6.6 respectively.

Citrate buffer (citric acid/sodium citrate) — pH range 2.5–6.5. This buffer is incorporated into benzylpenicillin and idoxuridine eye drops to maintain the pH at approximately 6.

The components of all these buffer systems are stable to autoclaving and non-toxic to the eye in the concentrations used.

Borate and phosphate buffers are incompatible with many alkaloidal salts and inorganic compounds including the salts of zinc. Borate buffers form chelates with polyols including glycerol, catecholamines and polyvinyl alcohol.

Stabilizers

Several drugs used in the form of eye drops oxidize on exposure to air with loss of potency. The stability of adrenaline, proxymetacaine and sulphacetamide eye drops is improved if the air in the bottle is replaced by an inert gas such as nitrogen. Inclusion of an antioxidant is recommended for eye drops containing these drugs and for those containing amethocaine, phenylephrine and physostigmine. Autoxidations are often catalysed by light and trace metals, therefore the inclusion of a chelating agent and protection from light will increase the stability of solutions.

Antioxidants employed in eye drop formulations are reducing agents which are preferentially oxidized to maintain the drug in its active, reduced form.

Sodium metabisulphite is employed in acid preparations while sodium sulphite is preferred for alkaline formulations. Both compounds are soluble in water and stable in solution if protected from light. Sodium metabisulphite also has antimicrobial properties at the concentration usually employed in eye drops (0.1% w/v). At acid pH it is effective against most bacteria, fungi and yeasts, its antimicrobial action being due to the presence of sulphur dioxide and sulphurous acid liberated by the reaction between the metabisulphite and the acid. Sodium metabisulphite is incompatible with prednisolone phosphate, adrenaline, chloramphenicol and phenylephrine, forming sulphonic acids with little or no activity. The presence of sodium metabisulphite affects the activity of phenylmercuric nitrate.

Chelating agents. Chelating agents may be included in eye drop formulations to remove traces of heavy metals where the presence of such impurities catalyses breakdown of the drug. These agents are often used in conjunction with an antioxidant as oxidation processes are frequently catalysed by heavy metals.

Certain chelating agents enhance the activity of preservatives and are included in formulations containing lower concentrations of preservatives than are normally used. For example, the concentration of benzalkonium chloride may be safely reduced to 0.004% w/v if disodium edetate at a concentration of 0.02% w/v is included.

Disodium edetate, which is soluble in water and stable to autoclaving, is the most commonly employed chelating agent in eye drops.

Factors affecting bioavailability

The site of action of many drugs applied to the eye in the form of eye drops is the anterior uvea (the iris and ciliary body). The drug must reach this area in a suitable concentration to exert its therapeutic effect. Factors affecting the bioavailability of a drug administered as an eye drop include its degree of ionization, its water/lipid solubility coefficient and the ocular contact time.

Degree of ionization. For a topically applied drug to cross the cornea, which has been described as 'a fat-water-fat sandwich', its molecules must exist in forms which are soluble in both layers. Weak acids and weak bases, which exist as equilibrium mixtures of ionized (hydrophilic) and unionized (lipophilic) forms at physiological pH, penetrate the cornea readily. Drugs which exist in solution only in the ionized form, such as fluorescein sodium, do not penetrate the corneal epithelium.

Atropine sulphate and pilocarpine nitrate are weak bases which exist as the ionized, water-soluble salts at acidic values of pH, but form lipid-soluble alkaloidal bases as the pH rises. Thus, these drugs will cross the cornea if the tears are able to buffer the solution to pH 7.4 but will not be available for corneal penetration if buffered in the eye drop solution to an acidic pH.

As these drugs are most stable at acidic pH, a compromise between drug stability, bioavailability and patient tolerance must be made.

Water/lipid solubility coefficient. Forms or derivatives of a drug which are more lipophilic than the parent drug cross the cornea better and are, therefore, more potent. Thus, dipivalyladrenaline, a pro-drug of adrenaline, which is more lipophilic than the parent compound, has been found to produce an effect equal to that of 2% w/v adrenaline when applied to the eye at a concentration of 0.1% w/v.

Storage and shelf-life

A drug presented in the form of an eye drop must retain its potency over the intended period of use. Chemical degradation products may not only be inactive but irritant or even toxic to the eye. To minimize such degradation the nature of the vehicle, the storage temperature, the pH and the effects of oxygen, light and trace metals must be considered during formulation.

The stability of solutions of several drugs used as eye drops is improved by refrigerated storage. Idoxuridine, proxymetacaine and thymoxamine eye drops should be stored between 2°C and 8°C. Chloramphenicol Eye Drops BP 1988 may be expected to retain their potency for 18 months from the date of preparation when stored in a refrigerator but the shelf-life is reduced to 4 months if stored at room temperature.

Containers for eye drops

A container for an eye drop must protect the contents from the ingress of moisture, air and microbial contamination and must not adversely affect the product by removing substances from or leaching substances into the product. The container must be free from particles and if the product is to be sterilized in the container, all parts of the container must withstand the sterilization process.

Eye drops are supplied in single- or multiple-dose containers which are made of plastic or glass.

Single-dose containers

The most widely used type of single-dose eye drop preparation in Great Britain is the 'Minims' range manufactured by Smith and Nephew Pharmaceuticals Ltd.

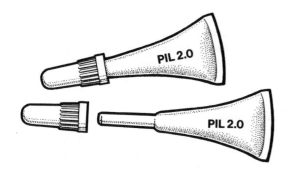

Fig. 28.1 Minims single-use eye drop unit. (Reproduced with permission from Smith & Nephew Ltd)

The stabilized, preservative-free eye drop solution is contained in an injection-moulded polypropylene container which is heat sealed at one end and has a nozzle section closed with a cap at the other end (Fig. 28.1).

The unit is enclosed in a heat-sealed pouch with peel-off paper backing. The eye drop is sterilized in this form by autoclaving.

Plastic bottles

Commercially prepared eye drops are normally supplied in plastic bottles with integral droppers (Fig. 28.2). These bottles are usually made of polyethylene or polypropylene and are sterilized by ionizing radiation and then filled aseptically with the sterilized solution or suspension.

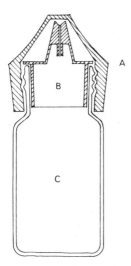

Fig. 28.2 Plastic eye drop bottle. A, Rigid plastic cap; B, polythene friction plug containing baffle that produces uniform drops; C, polythene bottle

Glass bottles

Eye drops dispensed extemporaneously are generally supplied in glass bottles, a complete specification for which is given in British Standard 1679: Part 5: 1973 (Amended 1974).

The eye dropper bottle consists of a bottle of 10 ml capacity fitted with a cap, teat and dropper tube as shown in Figure 28.3.

The bottle should be made of either amber neutral glass or amber soda glass which has been surface treated during manufacture by a process that reduces the amount of alkali released from the interior surface when it is in contact with aqueous liquids. Only the former type may be autoclaved more than once as repeated autoclaving of soda glass may lead to alkali release. The bottle may be ribbed vertically so that it may be distinguished by touch as containing a liquid for external use, but an adequate plain surface should be available for labelling.

The dropper tube should be of clear, colourless neutral glass annealed after manufacture. It consists of a glass tube with a flanged rim at one end with a ball-ended delivery hole at the other. It may be straight or angled and of such a length that when the complete eye dropper bottle is assembled, the dropper tube is approximately 5 mm from the base of the bottle.

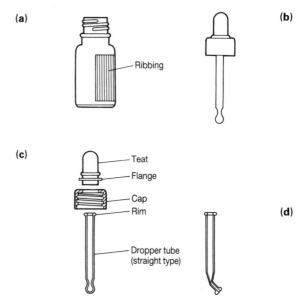

Fig. 28.3 Eye dropper bottle to BS 1679: Part 5: 1974. (a) Bottle; (b) assembled closure; (c) components of closure; (d) dropper tube (angled type). (Reproduced with permission from the British Standards Institution (complete copies can be obtained from BSI at Linford Wood, Milton Keynes, MK14 6LE))

The flanged teat should be made of good-quality rubber, either natural or synthetic. Natural rubber teats will withstand autoclaving at 115°C for 30 minutes but will not withstand dry heat sterilization. Silicone rubber teats will withstand dry heat sterilization and are therefore suitable for use with oily eye drops but are slightly permeable to water vapour. For this reason the shelf-life of eye drops closed with a closure including a silicone rubber teat must be limited to 3 months. If eye drops for which a silicone teat is appropriate are to be stored for more than 3 months, the complete dropper assembly should be supplied separately as a wrapped sterilized unit.

The screw cap which is perforated to hold the teat should be made of a phenolic plastics material such as 'Bakelite' which will withstand heat sterilization at a temperature of up to 115°C for 30 minutes without distortion.

Teats and caps should not be used more than once.

As the final product must be practically free from particles, all components of the eye drop container should be clean and free from extraneous matter. This may be achieved by thorough washing, rinsing in filtered, distilled or de-ionized water, drying in an oven and storing in a clean area until required.

Rubber teats tend to adsorb preservatives from eye drop formulations during autoclaving and storage. To prevent this, teats should be impregnated with the preservative, and antioxidant if present, as described in the sterilization section of the Pharmaceutical Codex, and stored in the impregnating solution until required for use.

Immediately before filling, the eye drop container should be assembled taking care not to contaminate those parts of the container which will come into contact with the preparation.

PREPARATION OF EYE DROPS

The extemporaneous preparation of an eye drop consists of three main parts:

1. Preparation of the solution.
2. Clarification of the solution.
3. Filling and sterilization.

Preparation of the solution

The vehicle for the solution should be prepared before the active drug is added. This allows for dissolution of relatively insoluble preservatives such as the phenylmercuric salts and ensures that the active ingredient is introduced into a vehicle formulated to preserve the stability of that drug in solution by the inclusion of antioxidants and buffers. The pH of unbuffered solutions may be adjusted after addition of the active ingredient immediately before the product is made up to its final volume.

Clarification

To meet the stringent standards of the British Pharmacopoeia on the absence of particulate matter, eye drop solutions will normally require clarification by filtration before filling and sterilization. As filter paper tends to yield fibres into the filtrate, sintered glass filters or membrane filters of pore size 0.45–1.2 μm are generally employed. The clarified solution should be expressed directly into the final container unless the solution is to be sterilized by filtration, when it should be housed in a container which has been cleaned, dried and stored in such a way that it is practically free from particles. If the eye drop is a suspension, the vehicle should be clarified before the active ingredient is suspended in it.

Filling and sterilization

The British Pharmacopoeia specifies several methods suitable for the sterilization of eye drops. The most commonly employed methods are described below.

Heating in an autoclave

The aqueous product is transferred to the final containers which are then closed to exclude microorganisms and exposed to saturated steam for a sufficient time to ensure that the whole of the contents of each container is maintained for an effective combination of time and temperature to ensure sterility (see Ch. 20).

This method should be used whenever possible. The following combinations of temperature and time are appropriate for sterilization of eye drops by heating in an autoclave: 115°C for 30 minutes and 121°C for 15 minutes.

Combinations involving higher temperatures cannot be employed for eye drop bottles as pressures above 2 bar (15 p.s.i.g) achieved at 121°C cause the rubber teats and/or the bottles to explode.

Heating with a bactericide

The aqueous product containing one of the prescribed antimicrobial substances is transferred to the final containers which are then closed to exclude micro-organisms and heated for a sufficient time to ensure that the whole of the contents of each container is maintained at 98–100°C for 30 minutes.

Five preservatives at specified concentrations are listed in the BP 1980 as 'prescribed antimicrobial substances'. These are: benzalkonium chloride at 0.01% w/v, chlorhexidine acetate at 0.01% w/v, phenylmercuric acetate or nitrate at 0.002% w/v and thiomersal at 0.01% w/v.

The specialized apparatus employed for sterilization by this method is called a steamer but sterilization by this method can be performed using simpler apparatus as long as the water used is kept at boiling point.

The BP 1988 no longer recognises 'heating with a bactericide' as an 'official' method of sterilization.

Filtration

The aqueous solution is sterilized by filtration and transferred, by means of an aseptic technique, to sterile containers which are then closed to exclude micro-organisms (Chs. 22, 23).

Strict aseptic technique must be employed throughout the filling of eye drops sterilized by this method. Filling should be undertaken under Class I laminar air flow conditions.

The recommended pore size for a bacterial filter is 0.22 μm. This type of filter may be placed in a separable Swinnex-type filter holder (Fig. 28.4) and the filter assembly autoclaved before filling or be employed as a Millex disposable filter (Fig. 28.5).

If the active ingredient is unstable in the presence of

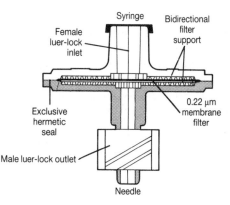

Fig. 28.5 Millex bacterial filter unit. (Reproduced with permission from Millipore (UK) Ltd)

air and the air in the bottle is to be replaced by gas during the filling of a product sterilized by this method, the gas must be sterilized by passing it through a hydrophobic, bacterial gas filter.

Other methods (see also Chs 20, 21)

Dry heat sterilization must be employed for non-aqueous preparations such as liquid paraffin eye drops, although it must be remembered that natural rubber teats will not withstand the temperature required for this type of sterilization (160°C) and silicone rubber teats must be used.

Exposure to ionizing radiation is the only suitable method for sterilizing heat-labile drugs formulated as an oily suspension.

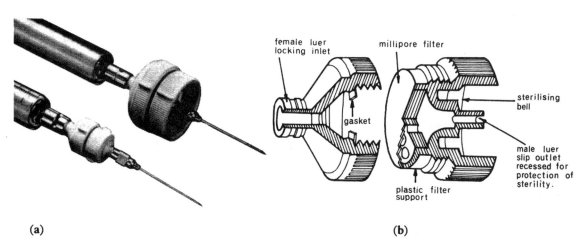

(a)   **(b)**

Fig. 28.4 Swinnex holders for bacterial filters. (a) 13 mm and 25 mm types filled to syringes. (b) Cutaway view of 25 mm type. (Reproduced with Permission from Millipore (UK) Ltd)

The method chosen for the sterilization of a particular eye drop can only be made after the consideration of a number of factors:

1. The stability to heat of the active ingredient(s) and preservative(s), e.g. drugs such as chloramphenicol and prednisolone and the preservative chlorocresol will not withstand the temperature attained during the autoclaving process.
2. The presence and type of an antimicrobial agent. The second method mentioned above, 'heating with a bactericide', cannot be employed unless one of the prescribed antimicrobial substances at the concentration specified above is included in the formulation.
3. The form of the preparation. Filtration of a suspension would result in a sterile vehicle with the active ingredient deposited on the filter!

Following sterilization the closure of the eye drop should be covered with a readily breakable seal, such as a viskring, to distinguish between opened and unopened containers.

Labelling of container

The label on an eye drop should:

1. Fully identify the product — the title should either include the name and concentration of active ingredients or refer to an official monograph in which these details are specified. If the monograph allows for variation in the concentration of the active ingredient, the concentration of that ingredient must be stated, e.g.:

Adrenaline Eye-drops, Neutral BPC 1973
Atropine Eye Drops BP 1% w/v
Zinc Sulphate and Adrenaline Eye Drops BP 1980
2. Specify the conditions of storage, e.g.

> Store in a cool place

or

> Protect from light

3. State a date after which the product should not be used (expiry date).
4. Include the warning

> Not to be taken

5. Specify the volume of the preparation.

6. Ensure correct use, e.g.

> Shake the bottle

for an eye drop suspension.

Additional information to be included on an eye drop label is dependent on the form of the product and the intended user.

Eye drops supplied as a dry powder and vehicle

Eye drops supplied in this form must be labelled as follows:

1. The label on the container states

> Powder for eye drops

2. The label on the container or package states the directions for the preparation of the eye drops.

Guidance on the correct use of eye drops in various environments is given in a Department of Health and Social Security health service circular issued in 1975 (HSC(IS)122).

Hospital use

In addition to the details listed above, eye drop labels for hospital use should include the concentration of active ingredient, i.e. reference to an official monograph is insufficient, the name and concentration of any added antimicrobial substance, the words

> Sterile until opened

the date of issue and the batch number.

Use on hospital wards

The recipients of eye drops used on hospital wards are generally more prone to infection than patients in the domiciliary situation, therefore certain additional measures to avoid contamination of such drops are followed.

Patients on hospital wards must be issued with individual bottles, i.e. a 'stock' bottle must not be used, and separate bottles should be issued for each eye if both eyes are to be treated. Bottles of eye drops on hospital wards must be discarded 7 days after first opening the container. Therefore, in addition to the labelling requirements already mentioned, an eye drop for use on a hospital ward must include the patient's name, the eye to be treated with that bottle and the date of opening and/or the date on which the eye drops must be discarded.

Use in operating theatres

Eye drops issued to operating theatres should not contain preservatives because of the damage which could ensue if the preparation entered the anterior chamber of the eye. Preservative-free eye drops should be used once only and any remaining solution discarded. A warning to this effect must therefore appear on the label of eye drops used in operating theatres.

Single-application presentations (Fig. 28.1) are preferable as the outside as well as the contents of the unit can be sterile. As the container of this type of presentation is too small to include all the labelling information, the eye drop tube is identified with an approved drug code (see BP 1988 Appendix XIX) and the strength of the active ingredient. A greater amount of detail is given on the backing paper of the overwrap.

Use in outpatient clinics and accident and emergency departments

As there is a risk of cross-infection in these situations, unit dose eye drops are the preparations of choice in these areas.

If a single-dose preparation is not available, a multi-dose container may be used for 1 day only in an outpatient department, although any patient requiring outpatient surgery must be treated from a previously unopened container. However, in external eye disease clinics and ophthalmological accident and emergency departments, every container which is used, whether single- or multi-dose, should be discarded after being used once. Appropriate warnings to this effect must appear on the labels of eye drops issued to these areas.

Note: In all areas of the hospital, fluorescein eye drops and other diagnostic dyes must be used only from single-application packs.

Domiciliary use

When a patient is issued with a bottle of eye drops to use in the home, that patient will be extracting multiple doses of the preparation from the bottle. As some preservatives included in eye drop formulations are bacteriostatic rather than bactericidal, and bactericidal preservatives do not have an unlimited capacity, the warnings

> Avoid contamination during use

and

> Discard one month after first opening

should be included on the label and the patient instructed on maintaining the cleanliness of the preparation.

The label should include instructions for use of the eye drop. Details of dose (i.e. ONE drop, as even this quantity is in excess of the capacity of the conjunctival sac), the eye to be treated (right, left or both), frequency of instillation and, if the preparation is not for continual use, the period of treatment.

As with all dispensed medicines, eye drops issued for use in the home should include the patient's name, the date of dispensing and the warning

> Keep out of the reach of children

EYE OINTMENTS

Eye ointments are used for therapeutic and diagnostic purposes and contain drugs such as antimicrobial agents (antibacterials and antivirals), corticosteroids and non-steroidal anti-inflammatory agents and mydriatics. Eye ointment bases such as Simple Eye Ointment BP 1988 may be used for their soothing and lubricating effect. Eye ointments may be considered a logical extension of viscolized eye drops and are employed where a prolonged contact time is required.

Eye ointments should be sterile and practically free from particulate contamination and precautions should be taken to preserve the stability of the preparation throughout its shelf-life and its sterility during use.

FORMULATION OF EYE OINTMENTS

Bases for eye ointments

The basis for eye ointments normally consists of liquid paraffin, wool fat and yellow soft paraffin in the proportions 1:1:8, the wool fat being present to facilitate the incorporation of water. However, the proportion of the paraffins may be varied or hard paraffin incorporated when the product is to be used in tropical or subtropical climates where the high temperatures make the basis too soft for convenience. Aliphatic alcohols, for example cetyl and stearyl alcohols, and compounds such as cholesterol and beeswax may be included in the basis, in addition to or instead of the wool fat, to facilitate incorporation of water to produce water-in-oil emulsions (see Ch. 13). A limit for particle size in eye ointments containing dispersed solid particles is given in the British Pharmacopoeia. This standard may be met by reducing all suspended solids to extremely fine powder (<25 μm) before incorporation.

Adjuvants used in eye ointments

Although medicaments formulated in an eye ointment base are less prone to chemical and microbial degradation than in an aqueous eye drops, suitable antimicrobial agents, antioxidants and stabilizing agents may be included in an eye ointment formulation.

Antimicrobial agents

Eye ointments are less likely than eye drops to become contaminated during use for a number of reasons:

1. The aqueous vehicle of most eye drops is a more favourable environment for microbial growth than the paraffins used in eye ointment bases.
2. As eye ointments are packed in tubes with very small apertures and the ointment is delivered to the eye directly from the tube or via a glass rod which does not enter the product, contamination is less likely to be introduced into an eye ointment than into an eye drop, especially one supplied in an eye dropper bottle where the medication is delivered by a pipette.
3. The use of collapsible tubes for eye ointments ensures that there is no air space in this type of container and the risk associated with the ingress of contaminated air is obviated. This advantage is lost with the use of plastic tubes.

However, antimicrobial agents may be incorporated into the eye ointment base. This is desirable when bases containing water are used and is required by law in the USA. Chlorbutol, methyl- and propyl-hydroxybenzoates and phenethyl alcohol are examples of preservatives incorporated into eye ointments (see Ch. 14).

pH buffers

Irritation may occur if the pH of the aqueous phase of the ointment is outside the limits tolerated by the eye.

The pH of the aqueous phase of Sulphacetamide Eye Ointment BP 1988, for example, is adjusted before incorporation into the oily phase as concentrated solutions of sulphacetamide sodium are very alkaline.

Containers for eye ointments

Eye ointments must be supplied in collapsible tubes made of metal or a suitable plastic. The tube, of which the capacity should not exceed 5 g, must be fitted with a nozzle of a suitable shape to facilitate application of the ointment without contamination. Eye ointment tubes must be as free as possible from contaminants and, unless the product is to be sterilized by ionizing radiation, must be sterilized before use.

Metal tubes

A complete specification for metal tubes is given in BS 4230: 1967. This standard specifies that the tube must be made of aluminium, tin or a tin alloy and gives dimensions for a range of capacities of eye ointment tubes.

Eye ointment tubes must be supplied fitted with caps made of a suitable thermoplastic or thermosetting material, the latter necessitating the inclusion of suitably faced wads.

The British Standard and United States Pharmacopiea set limits for the number and size of metal particles in eye ointment tubes.

Preparation of eye ointments

Although eye ointments may be sterilized by ionizing radiation, they are normally prepared using aseptic techniques by incorporating the finely powdered medicament or a sterilized concentrated aqueous solution of the medicament into the sterile eye ointment basis.

The apparatus used in the preparation of eye ointments must be thoroughly cleansed and sterilized.

Preparation, clarification and sterilization of eye ointment basis

The wool fat, yellow soft paraffin and liquid paraffin are heated together and filtered while hot through a coarse filter paper in a heated funnel into a container which will withstand dry heat sterilization. The container is closed to exclude micro-organisms and the basis is sterilized by maintaining the whole of the contents of the container for an effective combination of time and temperature to provide adequate assurance of sterility (see BP 1988, Appendix XVIII).

Incorporation of medicament

If the medicament is readily soluble in water, forming a stable solution, it is dissolved in the minimum quantity of Water for Injections BP. The solution is then sterilized by autoclaving or filtration and incorporated gradually in the melted sterile basis, the mixture being stirred continuously until it is cold.

If it is not readily soluble in water or if the aqueous solution is unstable, the medicament is finely powdered, thoroughly mixed with a small quantity of the melted sterile basis, and then incorporated with the remainder of the sterile basis.

Immediately after preparation, the eye ointment is transferred to the final sterile container, which is then closed so as to exclude micro-organisms.

The screw cap should be covered with a readily breakable seal or, alternatively, the whole tube should be enclosed in a sealed package from which the tube cannot be removed without breaking the seal: suitable outer packages include paperboard cartons with sealed flaps and sealed pouches of paper, plastic, or cellulose film.

Labelling

In addition to the general labelling requirements the label on the container or on the sealed outer package enclosing an eye ointment should indicate that the contents are sterile provided that the container has not been opened.

EYE LOTIONS

Eye lotions are used to irrigate the eye to aid the removal of conjunctival discharge, foreign bodies and chemicals.

A solution of normal saline is used for simple irrigation while solutions of buffers and chelating agents are sometimes used in the treatment of chemical burns.

Formulation

As the volume of eye lotion applied to the eye greatly exceeds that of the tears (cf. eye drops), eye lotions should be isotonic with tears and of a neutral pH to avoid discomfort to the user.

Containers and labelling

Eye lotions should be housed in containers which are sealed to exclude micro-organisms and labelled with the words

> Sterile until opened

and

> Not to be taken

and the expiry date. Although it is recommend that eye lotions should be supplied in coloured, fluted bottles, for convenience for first-aid use, commercial plastic packs are often used.

These preparations are generally intended for use on one occasion only and do not contain any antimicrobial agent. Such eye lotions should be labelled with a warning to use once and discard any remaining solution.

Preserved eye lotions should be labelled with the warnings

> Avoid contamination during use

and

> Any remaining solution should be discarded 7 days after first opening

CONTACT LENS PRODUCTS

Products used in the care of contact lenses include: a) cleaning, disinfecting, soaking and wetting solutions for hard and gas-permeable lenses, (i.e. those made of the hydrophobic polymers polymethylmethacrylate, cellulose acetate butyrate and silicone methylmethacrylate) and b) cleaning, disinfecting and soaking solutions for soft or hydrogel lenses, (i.e. those made of polyhydroxyethylmethacrylate).

In 1976, following the publication of reports which gave cause for concern about the efficiency of contact lens fluids withstanding microbial contamination, the Department of Health and Social Security brought contact lens fluids under the control of the Medicines Act. Since January 1980 no new product may be marketed without a product licence and the manufacturers of products already on the market were given 3 years to provide data on safety, quality and efficacy of the products in order to obtain such a licence. The supply of contact lens solutions is restricted to pharmacists and opticians only.

Cleaning solutions

All contact lenses are liable to become contaminated with organic materials from the tear film and corneal epithelium, insoluble salts, cosmetics and atmospheric pollutants. These contaminants must be regularly removed to ensure maximum comfort, efficacy and life of the lens.

Daily cleaning with a solution containing a non-ionic surfactant such as polysorbate 80 is suitable for cleaning hard lenses. Deposits on soft lenses tend to be more tenacious and so for this type of lens a regular immersion in a proteolytic/mucolytic enzyme solution is necessary in addition to the daily cleaning. As enzymes used to clean contact lenses are not stable in solution they are supplied in the form of tablets for dissolution in sterile water immediately before use.

Cleaning solutions may be isotonic or hypertonic. The latter is often preferred as concentrated solutions of sodium chloride have mucolytic properties and cleanse soft lenses by a hydraulic effect. Use of hypotonic solutions should be avoided.

Disinfecting solutions

The insertion of a lens contaminated with micro-organisms into the eye could have very serious consequences. Contact lenses must, therefore, be effectively disinfected before insertion.

An overnight soak in an antimicrobial solution is suitable for hard lenses while soft lenses may be disinfected by cold chemical or thermal methods.

Hard lenses are soaked in a solution containing one of the antimicrobial agents used as preservatives in eye drops. Benzalkonium chloride, thiomersal, chlorhexidine and chlorbutol are all used for the disinfection of this type of lens.

Soft lenses may be disinfected using this method, but as benzalkonium chloride and chlorbutol are concentrated in this type of lens during soaking, and would lead to irritation and damage to the corneal epithelium on insertion of the lens, these compounds are not used in disinfecting solutions for this type of lens. Chlorhexidine and thiomersal are the most commonly used antimicrobials for the disinfection of soft lenses but as these compounds are common causes of allergy, alternative cold disinfection methods using hydrogen peroxide have been developed.

Boiling soft lenses in unpreserved saline is an inexpensive method of disinfection which avoids the use of potentially irritant chemicals. The limitations of thermal disinfection are that the method is time consuming, spores are not killed and any protein deposited on the lens will coagulate on heating leading to opacities in the lens.

Soaking and storing solutions

Although there has been some controversy over the best way to store hard lenses after removal, it is now generally agreed that wet storage is preferred over dry storage. Soft lenses must be stored wet to prevent dehydration.

Soaking solutions designed to maintain the correct degree of hydration of the lens must be isotonic with lachrymal secretions and of physiological pH.

Soaking solutions contain antimicrobial preservatives to protect the solution from contamination. Solutions designed to be used with soft lenses do not contain benzalkonium chloride or chlorbutol.

If disinfection of the lens is by a cold chemical method, the disinfection and storage requirements of the lens may be met by the use of a combined soaking/disinfecting solution.

Wetting solutions

The insertion of a hydrophobic hard or gas-permeable lens is facilitated and made more comfortable by the use of a solution containing an agent such as polysorbate 80 which coats the surface of the lens making it hydrophilic.

Wetting solutions also contain hydrophilic polymers such as polyvinylpyrrolidone, hydroxyethylcellulose and polyvinyl alcohol to make the preparation slightly viscous so that it will cushion the lens on the eye.

As wetting solutions can remain in contact with the eye for some time, they are made isotonic, are of neutral pH or weakly buffered and contain low levels of preservatives to avoid irritation by these chemicals or reversion to a hydrophobic state, as can occur with the use of a cationic surfactant such as benzalkonium chloride at a concentration of 0.01% w/v. Disodium edetate is used in combination with benzalkonium chloride and chlorhexidine to allow lower concentrations of these preservatives to be used.

Containers

Contact lens solutions are packaged in containers designed to minimize the chance of accidental microbial contamination of the product. Many multi-dose preparations are housed in plastic containers with in-built droppers which prevent the return of used or excess solutions to the container. Preservative-free solutions are supplied in single-dose sachets or vials which cannot be reclosed or aerosols in which the one-way valve prevents ingress of microbial contamination.

As very low levels of preservatives are included in contact lens solutions, it is imperative that the concentration of preservatives in these products is maintained throughout their shelf-life and not reduced by adsorption onto or interaction with the container.

Information to be included in information sheets on contact lens products

The type of information about contact lens products which must be included in information sheets and data sheets for these products was defined in The Medicines (Contact lens fluids and other substances) (Advertising and Miscellaneous amendments) regulations 1979 (SI 1979 No. 1760).

BIBLIOGRAPHY

Bartlett J D, Jaanus S D 1984 Clinical ocular pharmacology. Butterworth, Guildford

Bloomfield S F 1986 Control of microbial contamination. British Journal of Pharmaceutical Practice 8: 72–79

British Pharmacopoeia 1980 HMSO, London

British Pharmacopoeia 1988 HMSO, London

British Standard 1679: 1973 Specification for containers for pharmaceutical dispensing Part 5. Eye dropper bottles (amended 1974). British Standards Institution, London

British Standard 4230: 1967 Specification for metal collapsible tubes for eye ointment. British Standards Institution, London

Department of Health Memorandum 1975 (H.S.C. (IS)122). HMSO, London

Deim K, Lerner C (eds) 1970 Documenta Geigy scientific tables, 7th edn. Geigy

Grant W M 1974 Toxicology of the eye, 2nd edn. Thomas, Springfield, IL

Havener W H 1983 Ocular pharmacology, 5th edn. C.V. Mosby, St Louis

Healey J N C 1982 A guide to contact lens care. Pharmaceutical Journal 229: 650–655

Higuchi T, Schroeter L C 1959 Reactivity of bisulfite with a number of pharmaceuticals. Journal of the American Pharmaceutical Association Scientific Edition 48: 535–540

Krishna N, Brow F 1964 Polyvinyl alcohol as an ophthalmic vehicle. American Journal of Ophthalmology 57: 99–106

Leer S E 1986 Contact lenses and their care. Pharmaceutical Update 2: 14–20

Li Wan Po A 1982 Non-prescription drugs. Blackwell Scientific, Oxford

Lowbury E J L, Geddes A M, Williams J D (eds) 1975 Control of hospital infection. Chapman & Hall, London

Mandell A I, Podos S M 1977 Dipivalyl epinephrinee (DPE): a new prodrug in the treatment of glaucoma. In: Leopold I H, Burns R P (eds) Symposium on ocular therapy, vol 10. Wiley, New York, pp 109–117

Martindale, see Reynolds J E F

The Medicines (Contact lens fluids and other substances) (Advertising and Miscellaneous amendments) regulations 1979 (S.I. 1979 No. 1760)

Minims 1984 The comprehensive range of sterile, single-use, disposable eye drops. Smith & Nephew Pharmaceuticals Ltd, Romford, Essex

Monthly Index of Medical Specialities (MIMS). Medical Publications, London

Mullen W et al 1973 Ophthalmic preservatives and vehicles. Survey of Ophthalmology 17: 469–483

Norton D A, Davies D J G, Richardson N E, Meakin B J, Keall A 1974 The antimicrobial efficiences of contact lens solutions. Journal of Pharmacy and Pharmacology 26: 841–846

O'Brien C S, Swan K C 1942 Carbaminoylchloine chloride in the treatment of glaucoma simplex. Archives of Ophthalmology 27: 253–263

Pharmaceutical Codex 1979 11th edn. The Pharmaceutical Press, London

Reynolds J E F (ed) 1989 Martindale: The Extra Pharmacopoeia, 29th edn. The Pharmaceutical Press, London

Richards R M E, Fell A E, Butchart J M E 1972 Interaction between sodium metabisulphite and PMN. Journal of Pharmacy and Pharmacology 24: 999–1000

Richardson N E, Davies D J G, Meakin B J, Norton D A 1979 Containers, preservatives and contact lens solutions. Pharmaceutical Journal 223: 462–464

Smail G A, Marshall I 1982 Intravenous additives. In: Lawson D H, Richards R M E (eds) Clinical pharmacy and hospital drug management. Chapman and Hall, London

Swan K C 1945 Use of methylcellulose in ophthalmology. Archives of Ophthalmology 33: 378–380

United States Pharmacopeia 1985 21st edn.

Wade A (ed) 1980 Pharmaceutical handbook, 19th edn. The Pharmaceutical Press, London

29. Principles of quality assurance

R. Lund

Introduction

This section is intended to provide an introduction to the 'quality control' aspects of 'quality assurance' and to the duties of the 'quality control' personnel in this context.

What is quality assurance?

Quality assurance is a concept embracing a wide variety of activities. These start with product design and follow through all stages of manufacture, to and beyond the final release of the product for use.

The aim of quality assurance is to ensure that each batch of a medicinal product complies with its specification and is fit for its intended use in terms of safety, efficacy and acceptability (Martin 1982). The philosophy underlying this aim is that quality must be built into a product, it cannot be assured by merely testing the finished product.

Two useful definitions are:

Quality assurance — is the sum total of the organized arrangements made with the object of ensuring that products will be of the quality required by their intended use.

Quality control — is that part of 'Good pharmaceutical manufacturing practice' (DHSS 1983) which is concerned with sampling, specification and testing, and with the organization, documentation and release procedures which ensure that the relevant tests are, in fact, carried out and the materials are not released for use, nor products released for sale or supply, until their quality has been judged to be satisfactory (DHSS 1983).

Who is responsible for quality assurance?

In the setting of industrial manufacture, the overall responsibility lies with the quality controller who must be a 'Qualified Person' (Medicines Act Leaflet (MAL) 45, 1982). In the NHS within the UK, responsibility is usually delegated jointly to the production and quality control managers of the unit concerned, with overall responsibility falling to the Regional Pharmaceutical Officer or Regional Quality Control Pharmacist as appropriate.

DOCUMENTATION

The documenting of processes involved in pharmaceutical manufacture is a key feature of quality assurance. It includes both procedural documentation intended to ensure that processes are correctly carried out and batch production records which state the formula and indicate the method of manufacture. Documentation specifically for manufacturing has been adequately covered elsewhere (see Chs 5, 24) and need not be considered here.

Quality control documentation is somewhat similar, and may conveniently be organized as follows:

1. Procedural

— A set of standard operating procedures (SOPs) for instruments and equipment.
— A set of 'analytical procedures' (APs) to cover frequently used methods.
— A set of specifications for testing starting materials and packaging components.
— A set of specifications for testing finished products.

2. Work records

Cumulative records (trend sheets) for each product to enable ready access to results and detection of trends.

Individual records of batches tested. These may be in a laboratory note-book or on individually generated sheets. They should include records of all tests, instrument readings, calculations and comments which may be of assistance should problems arise in the future.

Clearly, other schemes which adequately perform these functions are acceptable.

Well-designed documentation is crucial to its effective use and so the entire scheme requires careful thought. It seems sensible that a minimum of documentation without unnecessary duplication is most readily managed and used. Thus, specifications should cross-refer to SOPs and APs wherever necessary, and be written in clear, concise steps.

Records of batch manufacture and testing of both ingredients and finished products must be retained for 5 years. Copies of any superseded documents should be identified as 'obsolete' and retained for the same period. Reference samples constitute a part of the production records and sufficient sample to allow repetition of all tests must be retained for the following periods: ingredient samples — a minimum of 2 years; finished products — at least until their expiry date Guide to good pharmaceutical manufacturing practice (GMP) (DHSS 1983).

ENVIRONMENTS AND MONITORING

The design and use of controlled environments is discussed in Chapter 23. The responsibility for commissioning and monitoring of the performance of these areas however falls to the quality controller. These activities may be divided into two groups;

1. Monitoring of physical parameters

This is necessary to ensure that the air-handling plant and other equipment continues to meet design and performance criteria. This involves monitoring of the air inflow to rooms and laminar air flow (LAF) work stations for particulate contamination and velocity (to provide the required number of air changes per hour). Measurement of differential pressures between rooms and across high-efficiency particulate air (HEPA) filter banks is used to confirm that air flows are from 'clean' to 'dirty' areas and to give an indication of filter condition (the pressure differential across filters increases as they become blocked with debris and may decrease if they are punctured).

At commissioning, and if problems arise, 'smoke pencils' can be useful to demonstrate the directions of air flows.

Temperature, humidity, light intensity and noise levels should be monitored periodically as they directly affect operator comfort, and thus performance.

2. Microbiological monitoring of 'clean' areas

This is necessary to ensure that the air handling and other plant provides an environment of the required standard, that procedures to minimize the introduction of contamination (e.g. clothing) are effective and that cleaning procedures continue to be effective.

The routine exposure of 'settle plates' is the most fundamental activity, it is easy and relatively inexpensive, and can usefully highlight potential problems. Settle plates do however have one major shortcoming — they demonstrate only the ability of micro-organisms to settle and survive and are at best semi-quantitative. A more rigorous method is to sample known volumes of air onto agar impinger strips or plates (see the 'Guide to good pharmaceutical manufacturing practice', Appendix 1 (DHSS 1983)). This is rather more expensive than settle plating, but does allow quantification of the number of viable organisms in air and, if the sampler is carefully selected, it can sample large volumes giving more accurate results. Their major drawbacks are that sampling whilst work is in progress can cause congestion in clean areas and may hamper operations, and that care is necessary to prevent drying of the agar to the point where it is unable to support microbial growth.

Surface contamination can be measured by swabbing and plating of areas difficult to clean, e.g. door handles, drains and sharp angles on LAF work stations. These again are only semi-quantitative and if a more rigorous approach is required, contact plates giving a count of viable organisms over a known surface area may be used. Contact plates may leave traces of culture medium on surfaces and care must be taken to remove these, otherwise microbial growth may be encouraged at these points.

All aspects of physical and microbiological monitoring must be rigorously undertaken at commissioning and at regular intervals thereafter. Results of such monitoring are best recorded on cumulative charts so that trends may be detected readily.

Typical schemes for environmental monitoring together with acceptable ranges of results are set out in Table 29.1. The necessary equipment is described later in this chapter.

INGREDIENTS

An important aspect of quality assurance is the use of the appropriate quality of ingredients. It is of course useful to build up confidence with reputable suppliers and in the hospital setting this is facilitated by regional and, in some cases, national discussion.

Within the NHS in the UK, manufacturing and quality control are organized on a regional basis. Within regions, practices for testing of ingredients are generally uniform, and only small variations exist between regions. These generally involve agreed levels of testing, acceptance of results from other laboratories within the

Table 29.1 Summary of environmental monitoring activities

Parameter		Class 1A	Class 1B	Class 2	Class 3	Class 4	Suggested test frequency	Comments
Particles in air per m^3 Sizes in μm	> 0.5	3 000	3 000	300 000	3500 000	—	Quarterly	Required class of air to be attained at filters and room air inlets and throughout the room unmanned. A short clean-up period should be allowed after personnel have left. DOP smoke test should be performed bi-annually on Class I or II system where the air supply does not present a challenge sufficient for particle counting alone to be adequate
	> 5	0	0	2 000	20 000	200 000		
	>10	0	0	30	4 000	40 000		
	>25	0	0	—	300	4 000		
Viable micro-organisms in air per m^3		<1	5	100	500	—	Monthly	Use a slit sampler or plate/strip type impinger
Air inflow velocity or equivalent room changes per hour		HLAF velocity 0.35–0.55 ms^{-1} VLAF velocity* 0.25–0.35 ms^{-1}	Room changes per hour 20	20	20	10	Monthly	Use a vane anemometer 100 mm from the filter face. Care is required to ensure a true average, especially where baffle plates are fitted
Settle plates (suggested average number of viable organisms for plate)†		Not more than 1 per work station	1	2	5	10	Weekly	If action levels exceeded, investigate. Expose full set of plates for each aseptic batch and for filling of terminally sterilized solutions as necessary
Surface swabs and plates		Set acceptable levels based on past results					Monthly	Use a sterile moistened swab to sample known or suspected problem areas and transfer to plates
Differential pressure		Not less than 1.5 mm water gauge between successive clean/dirty areas					Daily	Use inclined manometer water gauge. Check zero monthly
Application		Unidirectional work station	Room for aseptic filling (within LAF work station)	Filling of solutions for terminal sterilization (within LAF work station)	Solution preparation	Non-sterile manufacturing		

LAF, laminar air flow; HLAF, horizontal laminar air flow; VLAF, vertical laminar air flow.
* The special case of VLAF work stations for handling cytotoxics or radiopharmaceuticals should be considered separately.
† The total number of colonies divided by the total number of plates for a given area.

region and acceptance of agreed features of certificates of analysis from certain 'approved' suppliers (see 'Guide to good pharmaceutical manufacturing practice', Appendix 3 (DHSS 1983)).

The quality standards most often applied to ingredients are those of the various pharmacopoeias and many materials are sold as complying with these standards. Occasionally, it is necessary to purchase 'reagent' materials — these only become, say, 'BP' quality when all the monograph tests have been satisfactorily completed. In general terms, when reagents must be purchased, it is preferable to opt for a good 'analytical grade' which is intended to comply with a written standard rather than a 'laboratory grade' material. The latter should be used only when there is no alternative. Alternatively, for industrial manufacture where ingredients may be synthesized in-house or where there is no relevant pharmaceutical standard, an in-house standard must be drawn up. This is a somewhat complex process and involves consideration of synthetic routes to determine likely contaminants and the nature of the material to determine physical properties and acceptable purity.

Appendix 4 of the 'Guide to good pharmaceutical manufacturing practice' (DHSS 1983) recommends that discretion should be exercized with respect to the sampling and testing of ingredients, based largely upon experience with the supplier. A typical scheme, frequently adopted by NHS quality control laboratories, is as follows:

1. All containers of ingredients should be examined physically for adequacy and integrity of packaging and labelling and the contents for appearance. Simple tests to confirm identity should be performed on the contents of each container.

2. Each batch of ingredient should be subjected to assay for content of active material, together with any associated limits such as loss on drying. Discretion should be exercized with regard to the issue of retest dates or expiry dates when a second delivery of a batch of ingredient is received some time after the first.

3. Each batch of ingredient should be subjected to a programme of limit testing for known impurities, the precise nature of the testing being determined by the intended use of the ingredient.

The quality of parenteral products is critical and every batch of ingredient received for use in injectables should be subjected to the full range of tests. Ophthalmics, oral and certain topical preparations are less critical and a portion of the limit tests are performed such that the complete range is covered over a small number of batches. The remaining topical preparations and non-medicinal disinfectants require only a small proportion of limit tests to be performed on each batch received. The entire range of tests is normally performed on perhaps five batches.

Exceptions to the above include materials known to be unstable, e.g. aspirin where a salicylic acid limit test should be performed on each delivery, and instances where certificates of analysis or analytical data from other laboratories are accepted.

A number of ingredients are of natural origin and susceptible to microbial contamination, e.g. tragacanth, acacia, celluloses and starch. Total viable count limits of 1000 organisms per millilitre or gram should be applied. All ingredients for sterile production should be subject to a programme of examination for total viable count, the frequency depending upon the likelihood of contamination; a limit of 100 organisms per millilitre or gram is suggested. Certain official monographs require that the absence of particular organisms be demonstrated, these tests should be performed in addition to any total viable counts.

Expiry or retest dates are assigned to approved ingredients based on consideration of their physical and chemical stability. These typically range from 6 to 24 months from the date of testing. Materials should not be retested more than once and a useful rule of thumb is to give retested materials an expiry date equivalent to half the initial retest period.

Official monographs for a small number of materials require that biological safety tests are performed to detect abnormal toxicity or pyrogenicity. These are best undertaken by a specialist contractor with the necessary facilities.

Purified water for manufacturing must be considered as an ingredient, the supply and control of purified water from stills is considered elsewhere (see Ch. 24). In addition to the routine continuous measurement of conductivity, it is necessary to perform the full set of compendial tests at regular intervals, the frequency of testing being dictated by circumstance and the use to which the water is put.

Total viable counts should be performed on distilled water, sampled from the point of use at regular intervals. Where water is to be used in sterile production, samples should be counted at least weekly. If, however, the water is used exclusively for non-sterile production the frequency may be reduced. It is important to consider the past performance of the water when deciding on levels of monitoring.

Suggested limits for microbial contamination of water are that one or more organisms per millilitre should be investigated to determine the source, whilst a level of ten or more organisms per millilitre should cause the water to fail. The reasons for failure should be investigated, faults rectified and satisfactory results obtained before the water is approved for use.

Storage conditions for stocks of ingredients should be controlled such that they do not adversely affect the materials (e.g. humidity and temperature are important) and should allow adequate rotation of stocks.

PACKAGING SYSTEMS

Containers

The packaging system is an integral part of any pharmaceutical product and as such deserves careful attention. The product and its packaging are in intimate contact and can clearly exert marked effects upon each other. It is vital then that the product and its container be mutually compatible, both chemically and physically, that the packaging be well designed for ease of manufacture and acceptable to the user. For more general information on packs and packaging, see Ch. 12, 44 of the companion volume (Aulton 1988).

Once the packaging system for a product has been designed or selected, quality considerations fall into two groups:

1. The packaging must meet design criteria intended to minimize physical product damage. Examples include hydrolytic resistance of glass containers (citrates can produce a 'snowstorm' of glass particles when autoclaved in containers of inferior glass) and the resistance of eye dropper teats to leach preservatives from the product.

2. The packaging must meet design criteria intended to prevent 'environmental product damage'. Examples here include effective container sealing (vital for sterile products), light transmission and permeability to water vapour.

A large number of 'official' standards apply to packaging components, notable are those of the pharmacopoeias, especially the BP and EP for glass type and composition, the British Standards Institution — ampoules (BS 795: 1983), eye dropper bottles (BS 1679: Part 5: 1973) — and German DIN standards — the 'DIN' bottle/closure system for sterile fluids (DIN 58363). Such official standards tend to be rather complex and a number of the tests require special equipment. As with ingredients it is important to build up a relationship with reputable suppliers who are able and competent to certify compliance with relevant standards. In-house testing may then be reduced along the following lines:

— Visual checks for serious defects, markings and excessive aesthetic defects.

— Checks on the hydrolytic resistance of the glass used.
— Checks of critical dimensions, e.g. neck diameter and depth, stopper diameter and cap depth.
— Checks on resistance to preservative leaching.
— Checks on complete packaging systems for adequate sealing, especially where these are built up from different supplier's components.

If serious defects do become apparent, it is important to assess the problem accurately. This can be complicated since the problem may be confined to bottles from a single mould or affect the entire batch. Any one consignment will contain containers from many different moulds and batch identification is difficult. Sampling and examination should be conducted in accordance with BS 6000 and 6001 or the equivalent Federal Standard. Some guidance on acceptable quality levels (AQLs) may be obtained from the DHSS specification for DIN bottles.

Where plastic containers are purchased for use, broadly similar considerations to those described above will apply. If the containers are produced on-site, a system of testing and approval must be designed based on considerations of the processes applied and ingredients used.

Labels

Product labelling is the sole means of communication of product details to the user, it is therefore critical to control the suitability of labels.

The degree of examination applied to the labelling materials depends upon their source. All labels should be checked for completeness and accuracy of information and legibility. Labels obtained from a contract printer should be checked for continuity of rolls and identity either side of any joins.

Label security to avoid mislabelling is vital, particularly where labels are printed with batch numbers, and adequate systems must be implemented to ensure control over label issue.

FINISHED PRODUCTS

The end examination of finished products is most commonly considered to be the role of the quality control section and, whilst in the context of quality assurance, less emphasis is placed upon it, examination of batches of product remains an important activity.

Samples of completed batches (Table 29.2) are tested to and must comply with a written specification (cf. documentation above). This specification may be, or be

Table 29.2 Sampling for quality control examination

1. Sterility testing	The techniques used are discussed elsewhere (Ch. 30). The EP/BP sampling schemes should be used; with samples being taken from any known autoclave cool spots and all 'layers' of containers in the sterilizer, these may include 'visual particle rejects' if appropriate
2. Pyrogen testing	Sufficient containers should be supplied to provide a minimum of 5–6 ml from near the end of the filling run. Water is a special case and requires a sample of at least 100 ml
3. Chemical testing	Depending on container size, at least two containers — 'first and last' filled as these theoretically represent the worst case, and may help to highlight stratification due to poor mixing. It is also useful to examine containers from the middle of the batch to ensure consistency of mixing

based upon an official monograph or be devised in-house.

Examination can conveniently be divided into groups of checks:

Documentation

All sections of the batch manufacturing record must be completed. Numbers of units produced, rejects, quality control samples and labels used must all be reconciled. The labels used must be the correct ones, and batch numbers and expiry date must match throughout. All raw materials and packaging components must have been approved for use. In the case of sterile products, evidence of adequate processing in approved equipment (e.g. bubble point for terminal filtration, chart trace for autoclaves) must be presented.

Packaging

The container system used must be as specified, undamaged and clean.

Appearance

The product is inspected visually for colour, clarity and other characteristics such as viscosity. The odour of the product can be inspected with caution, but tasting is not recommended and should not be performed in the laboratory on grounds of safety.

Identification of active and other ingredients

Where assay methods are not sufficiently specific (in many cases where assay is by u.v. absorbance), a wavelength scan will confirm identity. Otherwise, simple colour reactions or, less commonly, i.r. are employed.

Assay of active ingredients

Assay should be by the most appropriate and specific method available. The limits applied to content of active ingredients are determined by:

1. Capability of the manufacturing process.
2. Formulation and stability of the product.
3. Capability of the assay method.
4. The intended use of the product.

As a general rule, ± 5% of the intended content is adequate, with ± 10% acceptable in certain circumstances, e.g. some ophthalmics and topicals. With impurities are known or expected to be a problem, e.g. degradation products or processing contaminants, they should be tested for and acceptable levels identified.

If the methods are well designed, a technique such as h.p.l.c. can perform identity, assay and limits of impurities in a single operation. It is thus a potentially powerful tool in analysis of this kind.

Physical characteristics

These should be checked where appropriate. pH control is important in buffer systems and those products with a known pH/stability relationship. For the majority of products pH is not critical but the build up of a 'trend' gives added product assurance. Viscosity should be measured where it is important, e.g. certain topical semi-solids and eye drops, limits should be assigned. Weight per millilitre can give a guide to the content of ingredients such as alcohol; limits should be assigned. For solid dose forms (tablets, capsules, etc.) the dissolution/disintegration rate should be measured, along with uniformity of weight (preferably 'on-line' if possible), breaking strength, friability and melting point as appropriate.

Microbiological tests

All sterile products should be subjected to a sterility test using the sample sizes and techniques described in the pharmacopoeias (see Table 29.2 and Ch. 30). In addition to routine settle-plating, settle plates should be exposed under the laminar airflow work station during filling of terminally sterilized products and a complete set exposed during manufacture of aseptic batches. Non-sterile products containing a preservative should be challenged with micro-organisms to demonstrate preservative efficiency.

Particulate contamination

The 1988 BP requires that parenteral preparations in containers of 100 ml or greater be subjected to measurement of subvisual particulate contamination. Visual 'passes' should be counted using a suitable instrument. A standard dealing with acceptable limits of particulate contamination in small volume parenterals has recently been introduced to the USP, it seems likely that other pharmacopoeias will add similar standards.

Pyrogen testing

The official pharmacopoeial test should be performed where required, and on any other products in which pyrogens may be a problem. This test is based on the summed temperature rise of a group of rabbits following injection of the sample. Where the rabbit test is not required or is impractical (e.g. cytotoxics or radiopharmaceuticals), the limulus amoebocyte lysate (LAL) pyrogen test may be valuable (Weary 1986). This test is based upon the clotting system of the limulus (horseshoe) crab and is performed entirely in vitro. Its major limitation is that only Gram-negative pyrogens can be detected.

In-process controls

In-process controls are being applied increasingly to manufacture and may provide useful information in addition to a valuable contribution to, the overall assurance of product quality. They fall into two major sections;

1. Documentation scrutiny and rapid 'chemical' tests for appearance, identity and content of active ingredients and pH as appropriate. These are to ensure that the product is likely to meet specification thus avoiding undue waste of packaging materials and time. In certain instances, these determinations may not be repeated on the finished product.

2. Microbiological testing of sterile products includes total viable counts of washed containers, water (as an ingredient), the bulk solution before filtration and packing and the packed product before sterilization. These ensure that processes continue to meet required standards, that acceptable biological loads are presented for

sterilization and minimize final product pyrogen load. It is suggested that for product prior to filtration and sterilization, a level of 20 organisms per millilitre should be investigated whilst 100 organisms per millilitre should cause the batch to fail. Limits of contamination of washed containers should be based upon past performance of the equipment used.

For non-sterile products, the efficacy of preservative in the formulation may be assessed by challenge testing.

QUARANTINE

The correct identification of the status of products, ingredients and packaging materials is essential. This is usually achieved by segregation of items awaiting approval, a convenient method is to use a locked quarantine store with restricted access. Thus, ingredients and packing components should be labelled and quarantined such as to permit identification of individual consignments and batches. When testing is satisfactorily completed, the quality controller may approve release of materials for use and transfer into stock.

Following manufacture of products, batches are transferred to the quarantine store to await completion of testing and authorization for release into stock by the quality controller.

RELEASE PROCEDURES

When testing to all aspects of the specification is completed, the product may be evaluated for release by the quality controller (or deputy).

In addition to the documentary, physical, chemical and microbiological tests described above, consideration must be given to current environmental monitoring results (see above), and sterilizer performance tests (see Chs 20, 21) before release. The bulk of the batch should then be inspected for appearance, packaging and labelling acceptability and to ensure product accountability. If all aspects prove satisfactory, the batch may be released for use.

In the case of batches which constitute a 'border-line fail', consideration must be given to the likely effects of using the product, the risk to the patient, the urgency with which the product is required and likely causes of the failure before a final decision is reached. *Note —* this does NOT apply where sterility or apyrogenicity is in question. If the decision is taken to fail the batch, its subsequent fate, destruction or recovery, should be documented such that all materials can be accounted for and the recovered material identified.

OTHER RESPONSIBILITIES OF THE 'QUALITY CONTROL' DEPARTMENT

1. As part of the overall scheme of quality assurance, it is necessary to check the calibration of both production and quality control equipment. Balances, measures, mixing tanks and instruments should all be challenged with known standards. Checks should be repeated at regular intervals and the results documented. If items of equipment do fall outside acceptable performance ranges, they should be withdrawn from use and steps taken to restore performance before retesting and return to use.

2. The quality controller must be satisfied that maintenance and testing of sterilizers is adequately and properly undertaken. This consists of:

— Planned preventative maintenance activities
— Routine testing of sterilizer performance

Plans for these activities are detailed in Health Technical Memorandum 10.

3. Expiry dates and storage conditions for finished products should be assigned on the basis of accumulated results from pilot stability studies accelerated testing and re-testing of batch samples at the end of their shelf-life. The responsibility for testing and assessment of data falls to the quality controller. Study schemes should be carefully set up to generate the required data and the data and results properly documented.

4. The unique blend of expertise found in the quality control department often leads to their involvement in therapeutic drug level monitoring (particularly in the hospital pharmacy). A number of techniques may be involved — g.l.c., h.p.l.c. and immunoassay, some of which are also used in routine analysis. It is important that appropriate measures are taken for the safe handling of biological specimens and the prevention of contamination of pharmaceuticals. Ideally, such activities should take place in a designated area away from the rest of the laboratory.

5. Occasionally, identification of drug materials from a variety of sources may be required. This can be a difficult undertaking involving a number of techniques — t.l.c., u.v., i.r. and chemical colour reactions. However, excellent guidance is available from literature sources (e.g. Stead et al 1982, Clarke 1986) and these should be consulted.

6. It is the responsibility of the hospital quality controller to ensure the quality of purchased products. This may include testing of 'generics' submitted for regional drug contracts, and examination of materials purchased from manufacturers under the 'specials' exemption to the Medicines Act. In either case, guidelines are drawn up regionally to cover testing and the acceptance (or not) of certificates of analysis.

7. Within the NHS in the UK, the quality control pharmacist is almost invariably nominated as the 'suitably qualified person' for the purposes of testing of piped medical gases. The standards applicable to piped medical gas installations are set out in Health Technical Memorandum 22, the most relevant sections deal with the permit to work system and the testing of installations at commissioning and following 'high hazard work'.

Testing may be divided into four parts;

1. Freedom from macroscopic debris: this may be checked by venting the gas through a coarse membrane filter or piece of clean white cloth for a short period.

2. Identification: a number of techniques may be used including thermal conductivity devices, i.r. spectrophotometry and inferred identity from a para-

Table 29.3 Testing of piped medical gases

	Oxygen	Nitrous oxide	Entonox	Air
Particulate matter	all outlets	all outlets	all outlets	all outlets
Identity	all outlets	all outlets	all outlets	all outlets
Oxygen content	>99%	Approx. 0%	50 ± 0.5%	Approx. 21%
Carbon dioxide	<300 p.p.m. v/v	<300 p.p.m. v/v	<300 p.p.m. v/v	<500 p.p.m. v/v
Oil mist	—	—	—	*
Moisture	—	—	—	<1 mg/l*†
Carbon monoxide	—	—	—	<5 p.p.m. v/v*

* Test if the air is supplied from a compressor, but not if it is from a cylinder.
† For accuracy, moisture should be determined by dew point, with a limit of −40°C at atmospheric pressure or −18°C at 727 kPa 7.2 bar (105 psi) which is a pressure usually found in the piped supply.

magnetic oxygen analyser. I.r. spectophotometry is least prone to interferences but sampling can be a problem.

3. Purity is most commonly checked using a paramagnetic oxygen analyser, although purity for gases other than oxygen is by inference. G.l.c. is a rather better method, but again sample transport can be difficult.

4. Freedom from known or suspected contaminants: brazing residues, carbon monoxide and carbon dioxide can be tested by using Draeger tubes or a similar device. Water vapour may be crudely quantitated by Draeger tube or more accurately by measurement of dew point. Gross carry-over of oil mist from compressors may be seen in the test for particulate contamination and accurately quantitated using a Porton-type impactor.

Testing is performed to regionally agreed standards, a typical scheme is shown in Table 29.3.

When testing of an installation is completed to the satisfaction of the *suitably qualified person* and the *authorized person* (usually an engineer), it is their joint responsibility to approve and return the installation to use.

QUALITY CONTROL LABORATORY AND EQUIPMENT

The laboratory can be considered to consist of the building, furniture and services and, in the planning of new laboratories and upgrading of old, much thought should be given to these basics (Sprake et al 1979). It is important when finalizing the layout of the laboratory to ensure adequate work and storage space, allow free movement and, where possible, space for expansion.

Chemical reagents and solutions may be considered as basic equipment and the grades specified in the pharmacopoeias should be obtained as necessary.

A good range of glassware is essential. Volumetric ware should be of 'Class A' wherever possible. General glassware (flasks, beakers, tubes, etc.) plus some reaction/distillation apparatus of the ground glass joint type is required.

A small library consisting of relevant pharmacopoeias, analytical and microbiological texts and reference works is indispensable in the drawing up of standards and resolution of problems.

Once the basic laboratory and equipment has been considered, attention may be given to instruments and larger items. The costs of such equipment are often quite high and the following points may be borne in mind before purchase.

Table 29.4 Equipment care

For instruments to function correctly, it is essential that they be carefully sited and looked after, a number of things contribute to this:

1. A written set of operating instructions should be available for each piece of equipment to enable it to be used properly and effectively
2. Equipment should be maintained regularly by either the manufacturer or other person competent to carry out such work (in many hospitals, the medical physics departments can undertake this)
3. The calibration of instruments should be regularly tested by challenge with known standards. The pharmacopoeias and manufacturers' manuals are helpful here
4. Instruments should be sited away from factors likely to influence their performance, e.g. draughts, temperature fluctuations, mechanical vibrations and electrical interference. Again, manufacturers' manuals are often helpful

1. *Reliability* — information regarding instrument performance is frequently available from colleagues in other laboratories (see also Table 29.4).

2. *Ease of operation* — since a variety of grades of staff may use an instrument, it is essential that it be straightforward to use to obtain reliable results.

3. *Accuracy and suitability* — equipment should be selected to suit the intended purpose and any likely expansion. It is fruitless to invest large sums of money in equipment with capabilities far beyond those which are likely to be required.

4. *Availability of accessories* — pharmaceutical laboratories tend to deal with a wide range of products and so accessories are often required to accommodate this. Instruments should be capable of operation with any such items which may reasonably be needed. It may also be an advantage that instruments be capable of interfacing to a microcomputer where this is useful for data collection or control purposes.

5. *Cost* is often a limiting factor, the cost of the entire installation including accessories should be considered along with other factors when selecting an instrument.

6. *Maintenance and repairs* should be readily available, locally if possible, certainly nationally. In the hospital setting, other departments may be able to assist. Maintenance contracts with manufacturers may be considered.

Basic equipment requirements

1. The analytical balance

An accurate balance is fundamental to the majority of operations, it should be selected and looked after carefully. A four-decimal place (of grams) balance, properly sited on a solid, vibration-free table, is adequate for most purposes, some of the new electronic models are excellent.

2. Top-pan 'rough' balance

A less accurate (to two decimal places of grams) balance is useful for less accurate, rapid weighing.

3. pH meter

This is used for checking sample pH where necessary and for non-aqueous and other titrations where potentiometric end-point determination is required.

4. Spectrophotometry

A spectrophotometer which is sensitive in visible and ultraviolet wavelengths is of great importance in the quantitative analysis of pharmaceuticals and finds other uses in confirmation of identity, and limit measurements. Ideally, a good double-beam scanning instrument with chart recorder should be obtained. Useful accessories include apparatus for derivative spectrophotometry and, in certain instances, flow cells, e.g. for dissolution studies. Ultraviolet/visible light is widely applicable to quantitation of solutions in water or dilute acid and simple colour complexes in solution, but may be applied to gases, turbid liquids and volatile liquids.

Infrared is principally used for the confirmation of identity of starting materials, this usually involves comparison of spectra with known reference spectra. Identity of liquid and semi-solid finished products may also be confirmed by i.r. Sample presentation may be as a KBr disc (sample is incorporated into KBr and the mix fused into a disc using a hydraulic press), a mull in liquid paraffin or hexachlorobutadiene, or as a thin film between sodium chloride windows. Gas cells are available. Quantification is possible, but somewhat involved if conventional means are used.

Fluoresence is applicable to a small number of pharmaceuticals (e.g. quinine, warfarin) and has potential for other materials (such as amines, e.g. adrenaline) at low concentrations. It may also be used in detectors for h.p.l.c. systems. The technique is not generally applicable, but may be of interest to some laboratories.

5. Elemental analysis

Flame emission is most useful for sodium, potassium, lithium and possibly calcium. It is cheap, rapid,

easy to use and relatively safe (cf. atomic absorbtion) but tends to suffer from non-linearity at high concentrations and limited application.

Atomic absorption is a much more sophisticated technique, applicable to a wide variety of metallic elements provided that lamps are available. It is an extremely accurate and sensitive technique but is very expensive and rather more hazardous in use than flame emission (much hotter flame, possibility of production of toxic vapours).

6. Chromatography

Thin layer involves minimal equipment and is useful for a small number of official identification tests and for investigative work. Plates can largely be purchased ready-coated onto plastic film and containing a u.v.-fluorescent medium which is quenched by the 'spots'. There is thus little need for plate-pouring equipment and the plates may be preserved as a part of laboratory records.

Gas–liquid. The first rapid chromatographic technique capable of ready quantitation. It was developed by Martin & Synge in 1941. The major area of application is to volatile materials, e.g. alcohol, and much effort has been given to making volatile derivatives of chemicals to allow analysis by g.l.c. The technique is very sensitive, up to 1 part in 10^9 is possible depending on the detector used.

High-pressure liquid H.p.l.c. has largely superseded g.l.c. in the analysis of pharmaceuticals. It is (generally) an ambient-temperature technique, does not require materials to be volatile and can use aqueous-based mobile phases. It is thus an ideal tool for examination of pharmaceuticals and drugs in body fluids. The initial cost is high and some expertise is required to achieve satisfactory results.

7. Particle counting

For large volume injectable products and for monitoring of cleanroom environments, some form of particle counting and sizing equipment is necessary.

Microscopy is the most basic technique, the air or liquid is sampled through a filter membrane which is dried (if necessary) under ultraclean conditions and examined microscopically. It has the advantages of low cost, large sample size and the possibility of particle characterization, however, it is a time-consuming and somewhat difficult technique.

Light scattering or obscuring techniques e.g. Royco, Hiac) are widely used. A light (or laser) beam is passed through the sample, any particles cause deflection or blocking of the beam which is detected and electronically processed to give a size and count. The technique may be non-destructive to the product, is rapid and simple, not generally volume limited and does not require a polar sample. Disadvantages are high cost, inability to identify particles, the counting of particle aggregates as single particles and interference from flaws in container walls.

Electrical zone-sensing methods (e.g. Coulter) are also widely used. A conducting sample is drawn through an orifice between two electrodes, particles cause changes in the conduction characteristics between the electrodes which allow sizing and counting of the particles. Advantages include accuracy, variable size threshold and relatively low cost. On the other hand, the orifice tube is fragile and expensive, the technique is destructive, lengthy calibration is required (and needs regular checking), identification is not possible, the sample must be conducting or made so, some expertise is required in use, and the instrument must be sited away from draughts, vibrations and electrical noise.

8. Other instruments

Polarimeter for quantitation of dextrose and other sugars and certain other materials. 'Optical-mechanical' instruments are tedious and sometimes difficult to use, the electronic type are much more preferable.

Refractometer for official limit tests and, following calibration, quantitation of certain mixtures, e.g. glycerol/water.

9. Specialized equipment

A number of more specialized items may be required in some laboratories, examples include:

Electronic titration equipment is very useful where a large number of similar titrations are to be performed and for techniques such as Karl Fischer determination of water which are difficult by conventional means.

Dissolution/disintegration apparatus is essential where tablets and capsules are to be manufactured. The 'rig' may be linked to a spectrophotometer and controlled by a microcomputer if desired.

Equipment for measurement of physical characteristics of solid dosage forms is required where these are to be manufactured. This includes measurements of dimensions, friability and breaking strength.

10. Microbiological equipment

Where sterility testing and environmental monitoring are to be performed by the laboratory staff, the equipment described under sterility testing in Chapter 30 will be required, along with basic microbiological equipment — microscope, staining materials and chemical reagents. Whenever possible the sterility testing and microbiological equipment should be located in a separate suite from the chemical test facilities.

Under this broad heading, an air sampler of the slit or impinger type may be included. This device is used for measurement of numbers of viable colonies in a known volume of air and is essential for cleanroom monitoring.

BIBLIOGRAPHY

Aulton M E (ed) 1988 Pharmaceutics: the science of dosage form design. Churchill Livingstone, Edinburgh
Australian Standard. AS 2567: 1982 Laminar flow cytotoxic drug safety cabinets for personnel and product protection
Beckett A J, Stenlake J 1970 Practical pharmaceutical chemistry, parts 1 and 2, 2nd edn. Athlone Press, London
BS 6000: 1972: Guide to the use of BS 6001. British Standards Institution, London
BS 6001: 1972: Specification for sampling procedures and tables for inspection by attributes. British Standards Institution, London
BS 1679: Part 5: 1973: Containers for pharmaceutical dispensing: eye dropper bottles. British Standards Institution, London
BS 5295: 1976: Environmental cleanliness in enclosed spaces. British Standards Institution, London
BS 5726: 1979: Specification for microbiological safety cabinets. British Standards Institution, London
BS 795: 1983: Ampoules. British Standards Institution, London

Clarke (ed) 1986 Clarke's isolation and identification of drugs 2nd edn. Pharmaceutical Press, London
Couper I, Driver N 1980 In: Allwood M C, Fell J T (eds) Textbook of hospital pharmacy. Blackwell, Oxford, pp 199–228
Department of Health and Social Security 1977 Health equipment information no. 67. HMSO, London
Department of Health and Social Security 1981 Medicines Act Leaflet 99. HMSO, London
Department of Health and Social Security 1982 Medicines Act Leaflet 45. HMSO, London, pp 25–33
Department of Health and Social Security 1983 Guide to good manufacturing practice. HMSO, London
Glenn A L 1980 In: Allwood M C, Fell J T (eds) Textbook of hospital pharmacy, Blackwell, Oxford, pp 229–273
Groves M J 1973 Parenteral products. Heinemann, London, Ch 6
Health Technical Memorandum 10 (1980) Sterilisers. HMSO, London
Health Technical Memorandum 22 (1986) Piped medical gases,

medical compressed air and medical vacuum installations. HMSO, London

Li Wan Po A, Irwin W J 1980 Journal of Clinical and Hospital Pharmacy 5: 107–144

Martin I A Quality assurance, Personal communication

Martin A J P, Synge R L M 1941 A new form of chromatogram employing two phases. I. A theory of chromatography. II. Application to the microdetermination of the higher monoamino acid proteins. Biochemical Journal 35: 1358–1368

Safety in Laboratories 1983 Giba–Geigy Horsham

Sprake J M et al 1979 Pharmaceutical Journal 223: 560–561

Stead A H, Gill R, Wright T, Gibbs J P, Moffat A C 1982 Standardised thin-layer chromatographic systems for the identification of drugs and poisons. Analyst 107: 1106–1168

Weary M 1986 Pyrogen testing with the limulus Amebocyte Lysate best Pharmacy International 799–102

Willard L, Merritt L, Dean L 1981 Instrumental methods of analysis, 6th edn. Van Nostrand Reinhold, New York

Williams D H, Fleming I 1980 Spectroscopic methods in organic chemistry, 3rd edn. McGraw Hill, New York

30. Sterility testing

R. M. E. Richards

Sterility testing of pharmaceutical preparations purporting to be sterile is a procedure that has limitations both inherent (technical and biological) and imposed (numerical and economical), which means that it can only provide partial answers to the state of sterility of the product batch under test.

The EP 1980 introduces the section on sterility testing with the following comments.

The test is applied to substances, preparations or articles which, according to the Pharmacopoeia, are required to be sterile. However, a satisfactory result only indicates that no contaminating micro-organism has been found in the sample examined in the conditions of the test. The extension of this result to the whole of a batch of a product requires the assurance that every unit in the batch has been prepared in such a manner that there is a high degree of probability that it would also have passed the test. Clearly this depends on the precautions taken during manufacture. In the case of products sterilised in their final sealed containers, physical proofs, biologically based and automatically documented, showing correct treatment throughout the batch during sterilisation are of greater assurance than the sterility test. The latter, however, is the only analytical method available to the various authorities who have to examine a product for sterility.

Thus it is acknowledged that sterility testing is inadequate as an assurance of sterility for a terminally sterilized product. Nevertheless, the test is still a regulatory test in most countries. However, there appears to be a trend towards exempting from the test manufacturers who provided evidence of good manufacturing practice combined with properly validated and controlled sterilization cycles. On the other hand, sterility testing has valuable application in aseptic processes such as filtration.

Stated very simply, sterility testing attempts to reveal the presence or absence of viable micro-organisms in a sample number of containers taken from a batch of product. Based on the results obtained from testing the sample a decision is made as to the sterility of the batch.

Thus major factors of importance in sterility testing include: the environment in which the test is conducted;

the quality of the culture conditions provided; the test method; the sample size and sampling procedure.

Sterility testing is also discussed in Ch. 28 of the companion volume (Aulton 1988).

Environmental conditions

The basic requirement of the facility used for carrying out sterility testing is that it should be designed to provide conditions which avoid accidental contamination of the product during the test. A suitable environment is a laminar air flow cabinet (Grade 1/A BS 5295) located in a clean room (Grade 1/B BS 5295) (see Ch. 23). Regular microbiological monitoring with contact swabs, settle plates, etc. should be carried out.

Any chemical antimicrobial agents should be used with care. There must be no possibility of such an agent adversely affecting either micro-organisms which may be present in the sample under test or the culture medium subsequently inoculated with the test sample.

Culture conditions

Since sterility testing involves testing for viable micro-organisms which are likely to have been damaged by the sterilization process it follows that appropriate conditions for the growth of any surviving organisms should be provided by the culture media selected. Fundamental aspects of microbiology are discussed in the companion volume (Ch. 24, Aulton 1988). The following account of factors affecting the growth of micro-organisms indicates the importance of selecting the most appropriate culture conditions for sterility testing.

FACTORS AFFECTING GROWTH OF BACTERIA

Nutrition, moisture, air, temperature, pH, light, osmotic pressure and the presence of growth inhibitors are all important factors which affect the growth of bacteria.

Nutrition

All bacteria need mineral salts and sources of carbon and nitrogen. Some, like the denitrifying bacteria, can use very simple materials, e.g. carbon dioxide as the source of carbon and ammonium salts or nitrates as the source of nitrogen. Most, including the pathogens, must be provided with much more elaborate compounds, e.g. carbohydrates or organic acids as carbon sources and proteins or, more often, their degradation products as sources of nitrogen.

The synthesis of bacterial protoplasm is the result of chains of chemical reactions. Certain compounds, known as essential metabolites, form vital links in these chains and therefore growth stops if they are not available. As some bacteria cannot synthesize these substances they must be included in the growth medium and are then known as *growth factors*. Important examples are para-aminobenzoic acid, thiamine hydrochloride (vitamin B_1), cyanocobalamin (vitamin B_{12}) and folic acid.

Thus it can be seen that to produce vigorous growth of bacteria, suitable and adequate sources of carbon, nitrogen, mineral salts and growth factors must be present in the culture medium.

Moisture

Bacteria require moisture in order to utilize the aforementioned food substances. Usually a medium for the growth of bacteria must contain at least 20% of water. In the absence of moisture bacteria cease to multiply but spore-bearing forms may continue to exist in spore form for many years.

Air

Many bacteria will grow in the presence of air and are called 'aerobes', e.g. *Pseudomonas aeruginosa*; others can multiply only in the absence of oxygen and are known as 'anaerobes', e.g. *Clostridium tetani*. A third group, 'facultative anaerobes', are able to grow with or without air, e.g. *Escherichia coli*.

Anaerobic bacteria may be sucessfully cultivated either by providing an oxygen-free atmosphere or by adding reducing substances to the growth media.

The state of oxidation or reduction of a medium can be measured and is known as the oxidation-reduction potential.

Temperature

Most pathogenic bacteria multiply best at normal human body temperature, i.e. approximately 37°C. However,

some common and serious contaminants of wounds, eye drops and injections (e.g. *Pseudomonas* spp.) have an optimum growth temperature of about 30°C and may not be detected at 37°C. The USP, EP and BP all recommend an incubation temperature of 30–35°C.

Some saprophytes have an optimum range of 55–80°C and are known as 'thermophiles'. The spores of some species, e.g. *Bacillus stearothermophilus*, are extremely heat resistant and are used to test the efficiency of heat sterilization processes.

At temperatures approaching 0°C and below most organisms stop multiplying, but they remain alive, and this behaviour is utilized in the preservation of cultures of micro-organisms by freeze-drying.

Temperatures above 50°C are harmful, particularly if moisture is present. All vegetative cells are killed by exposure to dry heat at 100°C for 1.5 hours or moist heat at 80°C for 1 hour. Spores are more resistant.

pH

The optimum pH for growth is about 7.4, although this varies with different organisms. Growth is less rapid as the reaction of the liquid is made more acid or more alkaline. Solutions that are strongly acid or alkaline are bactericidal.

Light

Exposure to sunlight in the presence of air has a harmful action on bacteria and may inhibit growth or destroy the organism. It is for this reason that the incubators used for growing bacteria have no windows. The damage is caused chiefly by light waves from the ultraviolet region and this explains the occasional use of ultraviolet lamps for reducing the contamination of atmospheres and surfaces.

In addition to its action on bacteria, light may also produce changes in the medium in which the bacteria are growing and render the medium unsuitable for supporting growth. Hence it is important to store culture media in a dark place and to use them as soon after preparation as possible.

Osmotic pressure

Bacteria respond rather slowly to changes in osmotic pressure, but they are plasmolysed by strongly hypertonic solutions and they swell and may burst when placed in hypotonic medium. Suspensions of bacteria used for test purposes should be suspended in diluents of optimum osmotic pressure. When used in sterility testing the inhibitory effect of strongly hypertonic solutions must be allowed for.

Growth inhibitors

Many substances can inhibit the growth of bacteria. Substances that prevent the growth of bacteria without destroying them are called 'bacteriostats' while substances that kill bacteria are called 'bactericides'. However, substances can be bacteriostatic at low concentrations and bactericidal at high concentrations and bacteria may die if subjected to prolonged contact with bacteriostatic concentrations.

Bactericides are extensively used in injections as preservatives.

Application to sterility testing

Consideration of the foregoing factors is necessary to establish the most suitable conditions for the growth of bacteria. Thus to produce the rapid and luxuriant growth required in the preparation of bacterial cultures or testing for sterility it is necessary to provide ample nutrients, sufficient water and a suitable hydrogen ion concentration. The temperature will also need to be maintained in the optimum region by using an incubator which will exclude light. For anaerobes precautions must be taken to ensure a low oxidation-reduction potential. In all cases the presence of excessive quantities of substances having bacteriostatic or bactericidal action must be avoided.

Multiplication of organisms may be prevented by maintaining them in complete dryness, by cold storage, by adjustment of the pH to an unsuitable value for growth and/or by adding a suitable bactericide. With solutions to be injected it is not usually possible to control all these factors and the course normally adopted to prevent multiplication of organisms inadvertently introduced during use is the addition of a bactericide. However, it should be borne in mind that the medicament itself may in some cases produce a solution having a hydrogen ion concentration or tonicity unfavourable to the growth of bacteria.

PHASES OF BACTERIAL GROWTH

Four distinct phases of growth are exhibited when bacteria are freshly inoculated into a satisfactory liquid medium and incubated under optimal conditions (Fig. 30.1).

Lag phase

Immediately after inoculation there is an interval of rest during which the bacteria seem to rejuvenate them-

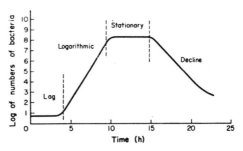

Fig. 30.1 Phases of bacterial growth

selves. This is followed by a period of considerable growth activity in which although there is no cell division the cells increase in size and metabolism is very high. Towards the end of the phase multiplication begins and soon increases in rate.

This phase usually lasts 2–3 hours but its length is affected by a number of factors of which the following are of particular importance in sterility testing.

Inoculum size

The smaller the inoculum the longer the lag. It appears that before an organism can make use of certain nutrients in a culture medium it must convert them into more suitable forms and it does this by liberating enzymes. If the number of cells in the inoculum is very small these enzymes together with the products of their activity may be rapidly dispersed and diluted by diffusion. In these circumstances the bacteria fail to multiply and the lag phase is lengthened and may be indefinitely prolonged. On the other hand, if a large inoculum is transferred the necessary concentration of suitable metabolites is quickly built up. Another factor is that in a large inoculum it is likely that part of the inoculum will consist of medium containing the metabolites and furthermore part of the inoculum will likely consist of dead cells which will break down and release metabolites. Thus the viable cells in the large inoculum start reproducing fairly quickly and the lag phase is short.

Pharmaceutical products are tested for sterility by incubating samples in culture media. Only rarely will these samples be heavily contaminated. Therefore there is a danger that the small numbers of bacteria present may not multiply sufficiently to produce the detectable turbidity used as an indicator of contamination. Consequently the sample of product taken for the test should be as large as other factors allow to ensure that as many organisms as possible are transferred to the culture media.

Sensitivity of medium

Some culture media contain nutrients that are very easily metabolized by bacteria which renders them more sensitive or conducive to promoting the growth of small inocula than others. Such media are essential for sterility testing.

Previous history of organism

Bacteria that are rapidly multiplying under ideal conditions when transferred will have a short lag time, but organisms suffering from the toxic effects of a previous environment will take longer to recover and a prolonged lag will result.

Bacteria in pharmaceutical preparations will most likely have been subjected to adverse conditions such as heat treatment, long contact with a bactericide or a solution of unfavourable pH. Therefore they may show a long lag time even in an optimal medium. For this reason incubation times of at least 7 days are prescribed for sterility tests.

Logarithmic phase

This follows the lag phase and usually lasts for about 6 hours. During this period growth is at its maximum and the number of bacteria increase logarithmically. That is the graph obtained by plotting the logarithm of the number of bacteria per millilitre against the incubation time is a straight line. The number of organisms required to render the medium turbid varies slightly with the size of the organisms but turbidity can usually be detected when about 10 million organisms/ml are present. The time at which detectable turbidity is produced depends upon the size of the original inoculum, the nutritive properties of the medium, the incubation temperature and the rate of multiplication of the cells. Under ideal conditions the rate of multiplication of a given strain of bacteria is reproducible but different species of bacteria have varying rates of multiplication.

Stationary phase

In this phase division is slower and a point is reached where the number of new bacteria formed is approximately balanced by the number dying. The reasons for the decreased reproduction rate include depletion of essential nutrients and in some cases the accumulation of toxic byproducts.

Decline phase

The stationary phase proceeds into one in which the number of organisms dying increasingly outnumbers the newly formed bacteria. Division ultimately ceases.

FACTORS AFFECTING GROWTH OF MOULDS AND YEASTS

Although there is an overlap in the growth requirements of moulds and yeasts with those required by bacteria there are also some differences. The similarities and differences are pointed out in the following comments on the factors affecting the growth of moulds and yeasts.

Nutrition

Moulds and yeasts require the same classes of nutrients as bacteria but the carbohydrate and nitrogen sources are particularly important.

A supplementary source of carbohydrate must be added to most media because a high concentration is essential. Examples are 2% dextrose, 3% sucrose and 4% maltose.

Extracts are used as nitrogen sources and are often obtained from vegetable materials such as malt and potato extracts. However, the pathogenic fungi grow better in media containing extracts from animal sources. Thus the Soyabean casein digest medium used in the fungal sterility test of the USP, EP and BP contains tryptone (a pancreatic digest of casein) as well as the vegetable extract (soya peptone). Peptones are often used to supplement or replace extracts and special mycological grades have been developed that give rapid and luxuriant growth of moulds and yeasts.

Some moulds, like certain bacteria, grow profusely in stored distilled water.

Air

The common saprophytic moulds are very aerobic but yeasts can grow both aerobically and anaerobically. For example, anaerobic growth can occur deep in large containers of unpreserved syrups, or syrupy preparations, producing alcohol and carbon dioxide which may eventually expel the stopper or burst the container. However, special anaerobic media are unnecessary.

Temperature

The optimum temperatures for the growth of most moulds and yeasts lie between 20°C and 25°C. As many moulds grow rather slowly, tests should be incubated for at least 7 days.

Cultures may be freeze-dried but in general mould spores are more sensitive to heat than bacterial spores. Exposure to dry heat at 115°C for 1.5 hours is reported to kill all mould spores and they are rapidly killed by moist heat at 100°C.

pH

Moulds and yeasts prefer a pH well on the acid side of neutrality. Test media are usually adjusted between pH 5 and 6. A pH of less than 5 is avoided when the medium contains agar because this is hydrolysed with consequent loss of gel strength if autoclaved at low pH. If a higher acidity is essential it is obtained by adding sterile acid after sterilization.

Light

Most moulds and yeasts grow equally well in the light and dark. Since incubators are not made with windows it is more convenient to incubate in the dark.

Osmotic pressure

Moulds and yeasts are more tolerant of high osmotic pressure than bacteria and are often found as contaminants of unpreserved syrups, semi-solid creams and ointments. Additional sodium chloride is unnecessary in mould media.

Growth inhibitors

Substances used to prevent the growth of moulds and yeasts are known as 'fungistats' while substances used to kill them are called 'fungicides'. These must be neutralized or 'diluted out' in sterility testing.

CULTURE MEDIA FOR STERILITY TESTING

Culture media suitable for sterility testing must be capable of initiating and maintaining the vigorous growth of a small number of organisms. These organisms may consist of aerobic and anaerobic bacteria and the lower fungi. The former include common saprophytes, pyogenic cocci (*Staphylococcus aureus* and *Streptococcus pyogenes*, Group A) and spore-bearing bacteria pathogenic to man. The lower fungi include yeasts and moulds responsible for spoilage.

The BP 1988 suggest the use of two dual-purpose or joint media. These are Fluid Mercaptoacetate Medium (Fluid Thioglycollate Medium) and Soya-bean Casein Digest Medium. The fluid mercaptoacetate medium is intended primarily for the culture of anaerobic bacteria but will also sustain the growth of aerobic bacteria. The formulation contains a number of ingredients and some have a specific role. For example, reducing conditions are promoted by mercaptoacetic acid and glucose. Resazurin is included as an oxidation-reduction indicator and agar is present to increase the viscosity and thus reduce the inward diffusion of oxygen into the medium.

The nutrients include sodium chloride, glucose and pancreatic digest of casein. Yeast extract is present as a growth factor and the amino-acid L-cystine is included to encourage the growth of certain Clostridia.

The formulation is suitable for the detection of anaerobes if not more than the upper 30% of the medium in a container, such as a 100 ml bottle, has been oxygenated. This is indicated by a pink coloration of the medium. If necessary, reduced conditions can be restored immediately before using by heating the medium in a water-bath until the pink colour disappears and then cooling rapidly. However repeated reheating can give rise to toxic degradation products.

A medium with the top 10% oxygenated is very suitable for use because aerobic growth will be more quickly initiated under such conditions and anaerobic growth will also take place.

Soya-bean casein digest medium

The soya-bean casein digest medium is intended primarily for the growth of aerobic bacteria but also supports the growth of fungi. Due to the inclusion of tryptone (from casein) and soya peptone, this medium is particularly supportive to injured or fastidious aerobic bacteria, that grow slowly in fluid mercaptoacetate medium (especially if trapped in the anaerobic region), because of the low oxidation-reduction potential. In addition, it has given good results in the membrane filtration method of sterility testing (Bowman et al 1971).

Other media may be used provided that they have been demonstrated to support the growth of a wide variety of organisms. The media used must also be shown to comply with certain tests. These tests must be either carried out previous to, or in parallel with, the sterility test on the product being examined. They should be designed to demonstrate the sterility of the medium, its nutritive properties and its effectiveness in the presence and absence of the preparation being examined.

The explanations that follow relate to the tests described in the BP 1988 and the EP 1980. It is important to note the periods of incubation. Where there is a need to establish the absence of micro-organisms a minimum period of 7 days is suggested. Where there is a need to demonstrate the provision of adequate growth conditions then a maximum incubation period to 7 days is recommended. An emphasis on the early detection of growth is also made.

Sterility of the media

Assurance that the media to be used in the sterility test are sterile is necessary in order to eliminate the possibility of false positives arising from contaminated media. This assurance is obtained by incubating portions of the media at appropriate temperatures for not less than 7 days. Media intended for the detection of bacteria are incubated at 30–35°C and media intended for the detection of fungi are incubated at 20–25°C. Sterility is confirmed by the absence of microbial growth.

Nutritive properties of the media — fertility control

Tubes of the chosen media are individually inoculated with 100 viable micro-organisms of one of a selection of culture types. These organisms are representative of the various types of contaminant that the test is seeking to detect. The BP 1988 suggests the use of *Staphylococcus aureus*, NCTC 7447 (an aerobe), *Bacillus subtilis*, NCIB 8054 (a spore-forming aerobe), *Clostridium sporogenes*, NCTC 532 (an anaerobe) and *Candida albicans*, NCYC 854 (a fungus).

Incubation at the appropriate temperature for bacteria and fungi is for not more than 7 days. Early and copious growth of the micro-organism confirms the suitability of that medium.

Effectiveness of media under test conditions — growth control

This test is to demonstrate whether or not culture conditions are satisfactory in the presence of the product being examined or membrane filter, where applicable. This should be repeated for culture media for aerobic bacteria, anaerobic bacteria and fungi. A control set of cultures is included to provide a means of comparing the rate of onset and the density of growth in the presence and absence of the material being examined. The initial inoculations should be carried out in a separate laboratory.

Aerobic bacterial test

An appropriate sample, as used in the test for sterility, of the preparation being examined is added to at least two containers of selected medium. Each container is then inoculated with 0.1 ml of a suspension of a suitable aerobic organism, such as *Staphylococcus aureus*, diluted to contain approximately 1000 viable organisms/ml. It should be noted that if the preparation being examined is an antibiotic then the organism used must be sensitive to that antibiotic.

A control set of containers is prepared without the addition of the product being examined. All containers are incubated at 30–35°C for not more than 7 days.

Anaerobic bacterial test

This is performed in a similar manner to the aerobic bacterial test except that a suitable strain of anaerobic organism (such as *Clostridium sporogenes*) and a suitable medium for anaerobic organisms are used.

Fungal test

The test is carried out similarly to the aerobic bacterial test except that a suitable strain of a fungus (such as *Candida albicans*) and a suitable medium for fungi are used. Incubation is at 20–25°C for not more than 7 days.

If cultures containing the preparation being examined show equivalent growth to the cultures in the absence of the preparation, it indicates that the preparation has no antimicrobial action under the conditions of the test. Therefore the test for sterility of the preparation may be carried out without modification. If weaker growth, delayed growth or no growth occurs in the presence of the preparation compared with the control cultures then the material being examined has antimicrobial action. This must be eliminated before or during the test for sterility of the preparation. Suitable methods may be neutralization, dilution or filtration. Whichever way is chosen it must be demonstrated as being effective by repeating the foregoing test procedure.

TEST METHOD FOR TESTING THE STERILITY OF THE PRODUCT

Two methods are described in the BP 1988 and the EP 1980. The methods are referred to as the membrane filtration method (Method I of the BP) and the direct inoculation method (Method II of the BP). The EP 1980 introduces the two tests as follows.

The test may be carried out using the technique of membrane filtration or by direct inoculation of the culture media with the product to be examined. The technique of membrane filtration described below is to be preferred whenever the nature of the product permits, that is, for filtrable aqueous preparations, for alcoholic or oily preparations and for preparations miscible with or soluble in aqueous or oily solvents which do not have an antimicrobial effect in the conditions of the test.

Membrane filtration

Membrane filters having a nominal pore size of 0.45 μm and having had their effectiveness established in the retention of micro-organisms are recommended for this method. Filters of the appropriate composition for filtering the various solvents are available. For example, cellulose nitrate filters for aqueous, oily or weakly alcoholic solutions and cellulose acetate for strongly alcoholic solutions.

Filter discs commonly used are about 50 mm in diameter and the technique described in the BP 1988 and EP 1980 is based on this size of filter. For filters of different diameter, the volumes of dilutions used may have to be adjusted.

The filtration system and membrane are first sterilized by appropriate means and should be so designed that solutions to be examined are introduced and filtered under aseptic conditions. One of two procedures may then be followed. Either the membrane is removed intact (or divided into two) and aseptically transferred to one (or two) containers of appropriate culture medium. Alternatively, culture medium is passed through the closed system to the membrane which is then incubated in situ in the filtration apparatus. The latter technique may be conveniently performed with one of the commercially available systems. For example, the Sartorius system which consists of a multiple suction filtration device. The system is capable of being sterilized by autoclaving at 121°C for 30 minutes (a deliberate excess) prior to use.

Millipore produce a transparent blister-packed system which has been sterilized by ethylene oxide. The system known as Steritest uses a peristaltic pump to provide pressure filtration. After completion of the test the plastic test system is disposed.

Various fully automatic systems have been developed (Krüger and Herschel 1977).

Aqueous solutions

Each membrane is prepared by moistening with a small quantity of suitable sterile diluent such as 0.1% w/v neutral solution of meat or casein peptone. This renders the membrane less liable to damage and reduces the retention of inhibitors.

The quantity of the preparation to be examined depends on the end-use of the product. Tables 30.1 and 30.2 summarize the BP and EP requirements. The appropriate quantity is transferred from the container or containers to be tested to the membrane or membranes. If necessary dilution is made to about 100 ml with suitable sterile diluent and filtration is carried out immediately. For those solutions being tested that have

Table 30.1 Minimum samples to be used in each culture medium in the test for sterility of parenterals. Based on the BP 1988 and the EP 1980

		<1	1–<4	4–<20	20–100
Liquids	Volume in container (ml)	<1	1–<4	4–<20	20–100
	Sample volume (ml)	All	Half	2	10%
Solids	Weight in container (mg)	<50	50–<200	200 or more	
	Sample weight (mg)	All	Half	100	

Table 30.2 Quantities to be combined and quantities to be used in the test for sterility of ophthalmic and other non-injectable preparations. Based on the BP 1988 and the EP 1980

Type of preparation	Quantity to be combined	Quantity to be used for each culture medium
Solutions	10–100 ml	5–10 ml
Preparations soluble in water or appropriate solvents	1–10 g	0.5–1 g
Insoluble preparations, creams and ointments (suspend or emulsify)	1–10 g	0.5–1 g

antimicrobial properties, the membrane is immediately washed with three successive 100 ml quantities of the chosen diluent. Where necessary a suitable antimicrobial inactivating substance is added to the diluent or to the medium (Table 30.3).

A membrane is transferred to each of the culture media or each medium transferred onto a membrane in the sealed apparatus. The media are incubated for not less than 7 days at 30–35°C for the detection of bacteria and 20–25°C for the detection of fungi.

Alternatively the combined quantity of the material being examined for all media is transferred to the membrane — diluting, filtering and washing as previously described. The membrane is then aseptically cut into the appropriate number of equal parts. One of the parts is transferred to each medium. Incubation is then carried out for not less than 7 days at the appropriate temperatures as just described.

Soluble solids

For each medium the appropriate quantity (indicated in Tables 30.1 and 30.2) is dissolved in a suitable solvent

Table 30.3 Inactivating agents for selected antimicrobials

Antimicrobial	Inactivating agent
Alcohols	None (dilution 1 to 50)
Arsenic compounds	Thioglycollate (<0.5%)
Cephalosporins 　Cephaloridine 　Cephalotin	Cephalosporinase
Hydroxybenzoates	Polysorbate 80 (1%) or (dilution 1 to 50)
Mercury compounds	Cystine (0.1%) or thioglycollate (0.05%) + polysorbate 80 (3%)
Penicillins 　Ampicillin 　Carbenicillin 　Penicillin G 　Penicillin V 　Phenethicillin 　Propicillin	Penicillinase
Phenols, cresols	Polysorbate 80 (1%) or (dilution 1 to 50)
Quaternary ammonium compounds	Polysorbate 80 (3%) + lecithin (0.3%)
Sulphonamides	p-Aminobenzoic acid (25 mg will neutralize up to 5 g sulphanilamide)

such as 0.1% w/v neutral solution of meat or casein peptone. The test is then followed as described for aqueous solutions. If a non-aqueous solvent is used it may be necessary to use membranes made of a material other than cellulose nitrate.

Oils and oily solutions

At least the quantities indicated in Tables 30.1 and 30.2 are used for each medium. Using a dry membrane, oils and oily solutions may be filtered without dilution. Isopropyl myristate, or some other suitable diluent having no antimicrobial activity under the conditions of the test, is used to dilute viscous oils. In fact heat-sterilized isopropyl myristate may be toxic. Therefore a high grade filtration-sterilized isopropyl myristate should be used.

After the oil has been in contact with the membrane and has penetrated the membrane by gravity then filtration should be commenced by applying either pressure or suction gradually. The membrane is then washed at least three times with 100 ml quantities of sterile solution containing a suitable surface-active agent. Neutral meat or casein peptone 0.1% w/v containing either 1% w/v polysobate 80 or 0.1% w/v (4-tert-octylphenoxy) polyethoxyethanol are suitable washing fluids. The

divided membrane or whole membranes are then transferred to the appropriate culture media. Alternatively the culture media are transferred to the membranes as described for the aqueous solutions. Incubation is also as described in the procedure for aqueous solutions.

Ointments and creams

The minimum quantities for each medium are shown in Table 30.2. Again isopropyl myristate forms a suitable diluent and it can be used to dilute ointments in a fatty base or water-in-oil emulsions to 1%. If necessary gentle heat may be used up to a maximum of 40°C, followed immediately by filtration as described under oils and oily solutions. Both the BP 1988 and the EP 1980 permit heating to not more than 45°C in exceptional cases but the test is reaching the limits of credibility under such conditions.

After filtration, washing and incubation procedures are carried out similar to those described for the oils and oily solutions.

Advantages of the filtration method

1. Wide application. It can be used for:
   a. Solutions with or without inhibitory properties.
   b. Soluble solids with or without inhibitory properties.
   c. Insoluble solids without inhibitory properties.
   d. Oils.
   e. Ointments, provided a non-inhibitory solvent or dispersing medium can be found.
   f. Articles, such as syringes, that can be rinsed with a sterile fluid.
2. A large volume can be tested with one filter. Therefore the method is applicable to the testing of poorly soluble solids.
3. A much smaller volume of broth is required than for testing by direct inoculation into culture media.
4. It is applicable to substances for which no satisfactory inactivators are known, e.g. certain antibiotics.
5. Some strongly adsorbed antibacterial agents, such as the mercurials and quaternary ammonium compounds, can be inactivated on the filter by treatment with the appropriate neutralizing solution.
6. Subculturing is often eliminated, e.g. for oils and oily preparations and substances that, like the barbiturates, give precipitates in broth.

Disadvantage of the filtration method

1. An expensive facility, highly trained staff and a consistently high level of operation is required. However, there is no easy alternative.

Direct inoculation method

The quantity of the preparation to be examined (as shown in either Table 30.1 or 30.2) is transferred directly into the appropriate culture medium. Antimicrobial properties are neutralized as previously described in the membrane filtration method (see earlier in this chapter).

To ensure that the sample does not excessively dilute the ingredients and so impair the growth-promoting properties of the medium the volume of culture medium must be at least 10 times the liquid sample volume. For solids it is recommended that the proportion of medium to sample is 100 to 1 in order to negate any effect of the dissolved solid on the nutritive properties of the medium. However, when the volume of sample is large it is difficult for bacteria and yeasts to produce a detectable turbidity in the correspondingly large volume of medium within the incubation period of the test. Therefore in such circumstances it is better to use a concentrated medium which when diluted with sample gives the correct strength of medium. Where appropriate the concentrated medium may be added directly to the preparation in its container.

Oily liquids

When oily liquids are being examined it is necessary to add to the media used an appropriate emulsifying agent which has no antimicrobial activity under the conditions of the test. The two agents described under the membrane filtration test are suitable, i.e. 1% w/v polysorbate 80 or 0.1% w/v (4-tert-octylphenoxy)-polyethoxyethanol.

Ointments and creams

The sample is diluted ten-fold in suitable sterile diluent (0.1% w/v neutral solution of meat or casein peptone) containing the chosen emulsifying agent. The emulsified diluted product is transferred to medium not containing an emulsifying agent.

Incubation for the direct inoculation method is for not less than 14 days at 30–35°C (mainly for the detection of bacteria) and 20–25°C (mainly for the detection of fungi). This longer incubation time, compared with membrane filtration is a disadvantage. The cultures are observed periodically throughout the incubation period, preferably every day. This is because some bacteria produce a detectable turbidity at first which later settles as an insignificant deposit at the bottom of the tube or bottle and leaves clear, apparently uncontaminated medium above. Therefore it is advisable to swirl con-

tainers gently before examination to stir up any sediment. It is also necessary to gently shake media containing oily products daily. However, great care must be taken with the mercaptoacetate medium not to destroy the anaerobic conditions at the base of the medium.

Daily examination of the medium also means that repeat tests (where these are permitted) can be commenced immediately contamination is detected.

Interpretation of the results

The batch passes the test for sterility if there is no sign of growth in any of the test media. When microbial growth is present then the sample fails the test for sterility. In such a situation the media showing growth are kept to one side. If it can be demonstrated that there was a break down in the aseptic technique then the test is declared invalid and the initial test may be repeated. Where there is no evidence that the test was invalid it is possible to proceed to a retest to demonstrate whether or not the growth obtained originated from the product under test. Should the retest have no growth in any of the containers then the batch passes the test for sterility on the evidence of the retest. However, if the retest also results in growth of micro-organisms then tests are undertaken to determine whether or not the micro-organisms which grew in both tests are similar or quite distinct. If in fact the micro-organisms growing as the result of the two tests are readily distinguishable then a second retest is allowed by both the BP and the EP using twice the number of samples. No evidence of microbial growth occuring as the result of the second retest allows the product being examined to pass the test. However, should there be evidence of growth of any micro-organism in the second retest then the preparation being examined fails the test for sterility. The interpretation of the results is set out in Figure 30.2.

It is recognized that there will be a low incidence of accidental contamination or false positives obtained during sterility testing of a sample that is actually sterile. This is especially the case when a number of manipulations are required for testing as in the membrane filtration technique. It will also depend on the testing personnel and the environmental conditions during the the test. Odlaug et al (1984) stated that the rate of false positives was in the range 0.1–2%. Avallone (1985) stated that the incidence of false positives should not exceed 1%. The latter author pointed out that value of reviewing the type of organism which caused the growth. The type of organism, together with an assess-

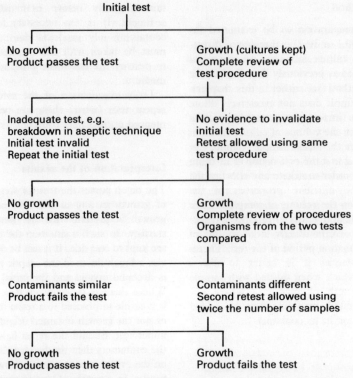

Fig. 30.2 Interpretation of results obtained with the EP 1980 and BP 1988 test for sterility

ment of its ability to survive the manufacturing process to which the product being examined had been subjected, could provide valuable information as to whether it was in fact likely to be a false positive or not. The example is given that *Escherichia coli* would not be expected to be present in a sterility testing environment and thus if growth in the media was due to *Escherichia coli* then it would not be interpreted as a false positive. On the other hand, if the growth was due to *Staphylococcus epidermis* which was also found to be readily killed by the preservative used in the product being examined then it could not be interpreted as originating in the product under test. Rather it would appear to have originated as a skin contaminant from an operator involved in conducting the test for sterility. Therefore there would be justification for classifying the *Staphylococcus epidermis* as a false positive.

Nevertheless the current situation allows different manufacturers to interpret their results obtained from testing for sterility in widely different ways. This is undoubtedly an unsatisfactory aspect of the interpretation of the test. For example, Avallone (1985) reported the case of a manufacturer who, if on the first test found

either 'mold or Gram-negative bacilli', failed the batch on this evidence alone. The opposite extreme was also reported where a manufacturer accepted a batch 'which had an initial contamination of a mold, a Gram-negative bacillus and a Gram-positive cocci'.

Some manufacturers include a product known to be sterile in their testing procedure. This is referred to as a 'negative control'. The negative control may be an ampoule or ampoules of sterile medium or media. On the other hand, the negative control may be samples of the product being tested, e.g. antibiotic powder, which has been terminally sterilized. The negative control is of assistance in interpreting false positives and provides a check on operator technique.

Applications of the test

Guidelines are necessary for those faced with the task of testing for sterility for a wide range of sterile products and materials. The BP 1988 and the EP 1980 contain advice on how to apply the test to injectables, ophthalmic products and other non-injectables and also to surgical dressings, catgut and other surgical sutures.

Injections

With the membrane filtration method it is best to use the whole contents of the container whenever possible, otherwise the quantities indicated in Table 30.1 are used. Where it is necessary to dilute the sample, it is diluted to about 100 ml with a suitable sterile solution (e.g. 0.1% w/v neutral meat or casein peptone).

With the direct inoculation method the quantities shown in Table 30.1 are used.

The tests to detect bacterial and fungal contamination are carried out on the same sample of the product being examined. In the situation where the amount contained in a single container is insufficient to carry out the test then the contents of two or more containers are combined and used to inoculate the different media. In those cases where the contents of the container exceed 100 ml the membrane filtration method is the procedure of choice.

Ophthalmic and other non-injectable preparations

For these products the contents of an appropriate number of containers are combined to provided not less than the minimum and not more than the maximum quantities shown under 'Quantity to be combined' in Table 30.2. Then from the well-mixed sample the amount shown under 'Quantity to be used for each culture medium' in Table 30.2 is used.

Surgical dressings

The procedure for surgical dressings follows a similar pattern to previous tests. That is, the test is carried out in a microbiologically controlled environment. The sealed package is opened using aseptic precautions and appropriate portions are removed from three different parts of the package. For absorbent cotton wool, 1 g portions are used and for woven materials 10 cm^2 portions are considered appropriate. For gauze compresses, whether individually wrapped or not, three complete compresses are taken from different parts of the pack. Portions from each location of the pack, three in all, are used for each culture medium. The quantity of medium used should be sufficient to cover the selected portions of dressing (20–150 ml).

In the membrane filtration method the test portion is shaken for 10 minutes together with at least 50 ml of sterile nutrient broth containing 0.07% w/v lecithin and 0.5% w/v polysorbate 80 as a combined antimicrobial inactivating and washing solution. Then as quickly as possible the washings are filtered through a membrane filter previously moistened with a small amount of cul-

ture medium. Subsequent to filtration the membrane is rinsed with at least three successive 50 ml quantities of the chosen diluent. The membrane is then transferred to the appropriate culture medium or the medium is transferred to the membrane as previously described under 'Aqueous solutions' above.

In the direct inoculation method three test portions are transferred to separate containers of each type of medium.

Catgut and other surgical sutures

The direct inoculation method is used into medium in wide-mouthed containers. The test sample consists of whole strands from freshly opened packages, usually containing one strand per package. Five strands are transferred to a separate container of 20–150 ml of each type of culture medium. If the sutures are present in multistrand packages then the five strands must be taken from five different packages.

The growth control test must be carried out to show that small numbers (about 100) of selected organisms are able to grow satisfactorily in the presence of the sample of product under examination. If the sample inhibits growth then the antimicrobial activity has to be inhibited and the growth control test repeated.

Incubation at the specified temperatures for bacterial and fungal media should be for not less than 14 days. This longer incubation time is necessary for the following reasons. Catgut is made from the intestines of sheep which in the slaughterhouses often become heavily contaminated with the spores of dangerous pathogens such as *Clostridium tetani* and the *Clostridium* spp. responsible for gas gangrene. During manufacture these may be trapped deep inside the threads, and as it is essential to detect any that escape sterilization, the incubation period of the sterility test is lengthened. This gives time for the culture medium to permeate the threads and the organisms to recover and multiply into detectable turbidity.

If it is necessary to carry out a retest or a second retest for any of these surgical dressings, catgut or other surgical sutures, then the same number of test portions are used as in the original test and each must be taken from a separate freshly opened package.

SAMPLING

The selection of samples and the number of samples to be taken from any given batch of sterile product or materials is obviously an important aspect of testing for sterility.

Selection of the samples

Samples must be representative of the whole of the bulk material and each batch of final containers.

For the bulk, the material must be thoroughly mixed before the sample is taken.

For the final containers, the sample must be selected at random, but:

1. When a load from a heat sterilization process is being tested, samples should be taken from every shelf and from any parts of the sterilizer in which less satisfactory conditions are believed to exist.

2. For aseptically processed preparations samples must be taken throughout the filling operation. The USP XXI defines the latter as a period not exceeding 24 consecutive hours during which no interruptions or changes affecting the integrity of the filling assembly have occurred and in which an identical group of containers has been filled with the same product from the same bulk lot.

3. For articles sterilized by a continuous process, such as radiation sterilization, samples are selected from the total number of similar items subjected to uniform sterilization during an appropriate period which the USP XXI suggests should not exceed 24 consecutive hours.

Samples size

There has been much debate on sample size. This has involved statistically based arguments related to the lack of assurance that the test for sterility will detect low levels of contamination. The present situation, however, has changed to where the test is seen as part of a total process aimed at providing assurance of sterility. This has reduced the reasons for criticism of the test. The test is not expected to 'stand alone' as an assurance of the sterility of a product. In fact it may be omitted in some cases. For example, the USP XXI states:

For effectively terminally sterilised products, however, the lower microbial survival probability may direct the use of a less extensive test than the compendial procedure specified under 'Sterility tests', or even preclude the necessity altogether for performing one.

The EP 1980 and the BP 1988 suggest minimal sample sizes for various products. These are summarized in Table 30.4. This is by way of guidance to manufacturers who have to include in their decisions on the size of samples such factors as: the environmental conditions of manufacture, the volume of preparation per container and any other special considerations applying to the preparation concerned. The suggestions summarized in Table 30.4 assume that the preparation has been manufactured under conditions designed to exclude contamination.

Sterility test record

An example of the type of records that need to be kept of each test for sterility that is carried out is given in Figure 30.3.

Table 30.4 Minimum sample size related to batch size. Based on the BP 1988

Product	Batch* size (containers/packages)	Minimum sample size (containers/packages)
Injectables	≯100	10% or 4 whichever is the greater
Single-dose ophthalmics	>100 but <500	10
Single-dose non-injectables	>500	2% or 20
Surgical dressings		whichever is the less
Ophthalmics and other non-injectables	≯200	5% or 2 whichever is the greater
	>200	10
Catgut and non-absorbable surgical sutures	≯1000	2% or 5 whichever is the less
	each additional 1000	Add 2 up to ≯40 strands
Bulk solids	<4	Every one
	4 to ≯50	20% or 4 whichever is the greater
	>50	2% or 10 whichever is the greater

* Batch = homogeneous collection of sealed containers so prepared that the possibility of microbial contamination is uniform.

Sterility test record.
Direct innoculation method

Date test commenced _____   First test _____   Retest _____   Second retest _____
Product _____ Batch no. _____ Method of sterilization _____
Vol/wt in each container _____ Vol/wt of sample _____ No. tested _____
Antimicrobial and conc. _____ Inactivator/diluent _____

Results of incubation. Day number 1, 2, 3, 4, 5, 6, 7, 14

	Mercaptoacetate medium 31°C		Soya-bean casein digest medium 25°C	
Test	Anaerobic	Aerobic	Aerobic	Fungal
Control organisms	*Cl. sporog.*	*S. aureus*	*S. aureus*	*C. albicans*
Density of growth Scale 1–3 — 'Fertility'				
'Growth'				
Controls — 'Negative'				

Conclusion: Sample passed _____   Batch passed _____
              Sample failed _____   Retest allowed _____
              Sample failed _____   Batch failed _____

Signed _____   Date completed _____

Fig. 30.3 Sterility test record: direct inoculation method. 'Fertility control' = media + organism; 'Growth control' = media + organism + product and for the membrane filtration method + membrane; 'Negative control' = sterile media, or terminally sterilized product + media. This latter control is to check the operator technique and should be negative. *Note*: The same sterility test record format can be used for the 'Filter membrane method' noting the difference in the 'Growth control'

USP STERILITY TEST

The USP XXI has a very similar sterility test procedure to that which has been described and which is based on the EP 1980 and the BP 1988. Differences that do occur relate to the following.

The anaerobic bacteria suggested for the test is *Bacteroides vulgaris*, but *Clostridium sporogenes* is suggested as an alternative if a spore-forming organism is desired. *Staphylococcus aureus* is not used but *Bacillus subtilis* is the aerobic test organism suggested with *Micrococcus luteus* as an alternative if a spore-forming organism is not wanted. *Candida albicans* is the recommended fungal test organism.

The inoculum for the 'fertility control' and the 'growth control' is recommended to be within the range 10–100 viable organisms which should result in a slightly lower inoculum than with the EP and BP test.

Two types of thioglycollate media are suggested in the USP. The medium that is different from the EP and BP is called the alternative thioglycollate medium which does not contain agar or resazurin sodium. This medium must be freshly prepared or heated in a steam-bath and allowed to cool just prior to use. It is useful for testing devices which have a narrow lumen into which the more viscous fluid thioglycollate medium will not enter.

The number of representative containers selected to be tested is standardized as 20 for each medium used. This is independent of the batch size and for small batches will represent a larger test sample than that required for the EP and BP test.

When isopropyl myristate is used as a solvent for ointments and oils it is specified that the isopropyl myristate used must have a pH of water extract not less than 6.5. It must be sterilized by filtration through a 0.22 μm membrane filter.

The maximum temperature allowed for melting an ointment or warming a solvent is 44°C.

Interpretation of results is a little different. The USP refers to the initial test for sterility as the 'first stage'. The product tested passes the test for sterility if no growth is observed in the test samples at this stage. If microbial growth is found in the sample of product under examination and it can be shown by review of

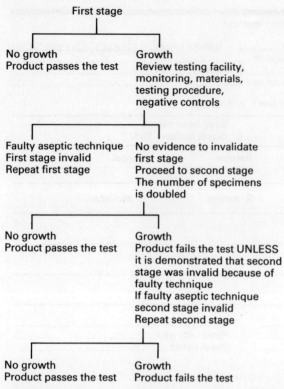

First stage

No growth
Product passes the test

Growth
Review testing facility,
monitoring, materials,
testing procedure,
negative controls

Faulty aseptic technique
First stage invalid
Repeat first stage

No evidence to invalidate
first stage
Proceed to second stage
The number of specimens
is doubled

No growth
Product passes the test

Growth
Product fails the test UNLESS
it is demonstrated that second
stage was invalid because of
faulty technique
If faulty aseptic technique
second stage invalid
Repeat second stage

No growth
Product passes the test

Growth
Product fails the test

Fig. 30.4 Interpretation of results obtained with the USP XXI sterility test

testing facility, monitoring, materials used, testing procedures and negative controls that the test was inadequately performed then the first stage can be repeated (as a first stage test). This is equivalent to the repeat of the initial test in the EP and BP procedure.

The second stage is carried out if a review of procedures gives no ground for invalidating the first stage. For the second stage the minimum specimens of product is doubled. Thus this is different from the retest of the EP and BP which uses the same number of specimens as in the initial test.

If no microbial growth is found at the second stage then the product passes the test for sterility. The presence of growth confirms the failure of the article to pass the test for sterility. However, if it can be demonstrated that the second stage was invalid because the aseptic technique was inadequate then the second stage may be repeated. This is set out in Figure 30.4.

Thus the main difference between the USP test on the one hand and the EP and BP test on the other is in the number of samples selected for testing. That is, the number of samples taken from the batch of product in the first instance and the number of samples required for the second-stage test of the USP differs from the equivalent retest stage of the BP and EP.

The inclusion of samples known to be sterile, as negative controls to evaluate operator technique, provides very useful information to assist with deciding whether a particular test is valid or not.

BIBLIOGRAPHY

Aulton M E (ed) 1988 Pharmaceutics: the science of dosage form design. Churchill Livingstone, Edinburgh

Avallone H L 1985 Control aspects of aseptically produced products. Journal of Parenteral Science and Technology 39: 75–79

Bowman F W, White M, Calhoun M P 1971 Collaborative study of aerobic media for sterility testing by membrane filtration. Journal of Pharmaceutical Sciences 60: 1087–1088

British Pharmacopoeia 1988 HMSO, London

British Standard 5295: 1976 Environmental cleanliness in enclosed spaces. British Standards Institution, London

Brown M R W, Gilbert P 1977 Increasing the probability of sterility of medicinal products. Journal of Pharmacy and Pharmacology 27: 434–491

Department of Health and Social Security 1983 Guide to good pharmaceutical manufacturing practice. HMSO, London

European Pharmacopoeia 1980 2nd edn. Maisonneuve, S.A. Saint Ruffine, France

Krüger D, Herschel J 1977 Die erste Vollautomatisierung der sterlitatsprufung con parenteralen Arzneimitteln im geschlossenen system. Pharmaceutical Industry 39: 60–65

Odlaug T E, Ocwieja D A, Purohit K S, Riley R M, Young W E 1984 Sterility assurance for terminally sterilised products without end product testing. Journal of Parenteral Science and Technology 38: 141–147

United States Pharmacopeia 1985 XXI Mack, Easton, PA

Wallhäusser K H 1982 Germ removal filtration. In: Bean H S, Beckett A N, Carless J E (eds) Advances in pharmaceutical sciences. Academic, London, pp 1–116

PART 4

Radiopharmacy

31. Techniques in radiopharmacy

S. R. Hesselwood

INTRODUCTION

Radiopharmaceuticals are dosage forms which incorporate a radionuclide (radioactive isotope) and hence are radioactive. In addition to the pharmaceutical standards required it is necessary to consider the protection from radiation of the patient and of the personnel preparing the radiopharmaceutical product.

The ionizing radiation emitted from radioactive isotopes may be in the form of electromagnetic radiation (e.g. gamma (γ) rays) or particulate (corpuscular) radiation (e.g. alpha (α) and beta (β) particles).

Particulate radiation

Alpha particles are positively charged and heavy. They have a very short range and are not used in pharmaceutical preparations.

Beta particles have the same mass as an electron and may be negatively charged β^- (electron) or positively charged β^+ (positron). The range of beta particles is a few metres in air or about 10 mm in body tissues. Positron emission takes place if the nucleus is deficient in neutrons. A proton changes to a neutron and a positron is emitted. Positrons have only a brief existence, each combines with an electron to yield two gamma rays in opposite directions (annihilation radiation).

Electromagnetic radiation

Gamma (γ) radiation is energy in the form of very short wavelength radiation which since it has no mass or charge, travels with the speed of light and is very penetrating. High-energy rays can pass through several feet of solid matter. When γ radiation reacts with matter it behaves as if composed of discrete packets or quanta of energy (photons).

Most of the radioactive isotopes that are used in medicine emit either β radiation or β and γ radiation.

Half-life

The rate at which the atoms of a particular radioisotope disintegrate depends on the degree of instability of their nuclei and is a characteristic of the radioisotope. The time taken for half the radioactive nuclei to disintegrate (i.e. for the activity to fall to half of its original value) is known as the *physical half-life* ($t_\frac{1}{2}$). Each radioisotope has a characteristic half-life which may vary from a fraction of a second to many years.

Most of the radioisotopes used in medicine have half-lives in the range of minutes to months. Radiopharmaceuticals with a short half-life must be prepared at or close to the point of use by the pharmacy staff since the rapid rate of physical decay prevents transport over great distances from commercial manufacturers.

Radiopharmaceuticals are administered for therapeutic, or more commonly, diagnostic purposes. The requirements of these situations are quite different, therefore different radionuclides are used.

THERAPEUTIC RADIOPHARMACEUTICALS

The intention with therapeutic radiopharmaceuticals is to use the radiation emitted to damage selectively specific tissues within the body. Examples are treatment of thyrotoxicosis by disrupting thyroxine synthesis in the thyroid gland and treatment of certain tumours in order to kill neoplastic cells. Thus it is important that the radiopharmaceutical localizes in the required part of the body and the radiation emitted achieves the desired result without causing widespread tissue damage. Hence radiopharmaceuticals for therapeutic use normally contain a radionuclide that decays by emitting a β^- particle. The energy of the β^- particles should ideally be within the range 0.5–1.0 MeV to prevent widespread dissemination of radiation from the target. The half-life is normally of the order of several days in order to provide

Table 31.1 Radionuclides used in therapeutic radiopharmaceuticals

Radionuclide	Physical half-life (days)	Energies of β^- particles (MeV)	Energies of principal γ rays (keV)
Iodine-131	8.05	0.61, 0.81	364
Phosphorus-32	14.3	1.71	None

prolonged radiation and achieve a better radiobiological effect.

Radionuclides commonly used in therapeutic radiopharmaceuticals are given in Table 31.1.

DIAGNOSTIC RADIOPHARMACEUTICALS

Diagnostic radiopharmaceuticals are used to obtain information about the patient, for example, the structure or position of an organ within the body or how well it is functioning. In view of the potential harmful effects of radiation it is always essential to ensure that the value of administering a radiopharmaceutical to a patient greatly outweighs its potential danger. An ideal diagnostic radiopharmaceutical therefore contains a radionuclide that decays by the emission of γ rays only. Since rays are electromagnetic radiation, their interaction with tissues of the body is much less than with particulate (e.g. β) emissions. Consequently, the damage caused to the tissue is significantly less. It also means that it is possible to administer a radiopharmaceutical containing a γ emitter to a patient and detect the radiation externally. A system using a scintillation detector, called a *gamma camera*, enables the distribution of the gamma emitting radionuclide within the patient's body to be imagined. By coupling the gamma camera to a computer system, it is possible to perform more sophisticated imaging procedures and functional studies by following changes in distribution of radioactivity with time. For optimal detection efficiency by a gamma camera system, γ energies of between 100 keV and 200 keV are desirable. If the energy is below 100 keV external detection is hampered by attenuation of γ rays by tissue within the body and energies greater than 200 keV decrease the quality of the image formed because of limitations of the detection system.

Another factor to be considered in a diagnostic radiopharmaceutical is the physical half-life of the contained radionuclide, which should be related to duration of the diagnostic procedure since the shorter the half-life the lower is the radiation dose to the patient. The majority of current diagnostic procedures can be com-

Table 31.2 Radionuclides used in diagnostic radiopharmaceuticals

Radionuclide	Physical half-life (h)	Gamma rays emitted (keV)
Technetium-99m	6	140
Iodine-123	13	159
Indium-111	67.2	173, 247
Thallium-201	73.5	140, 170*
Gallium-67	78	93, 189, 296

* These, however, are of such low abundance that they are not used for imaging purposes.

pleted within one working day and it is uncommon for procedures to last more than one week. Consequently radionuclides having a physical half-life of a few hours to a few days are commonly used. Currently, one radionuclide, technetium-99m, predominates because of its desirable physical properties. Characteristics of some radionuclides commonly used in diagnostic radiopharmaceuticals are listed in Table 31.2.

It can be seen that some of the materials used are nuclides of very toxic elements, notably indium and thallium. However, toxicity problems do not arise since the chemical quantity of the element administered to a patient is of the order of micrograms per test and repeated administrations are not often performed.

Positron emitting radionuclides

Positrons are positively charged β particles and immediately after emission they interact with a β^- particle in an annihilation reaction that results in the conversion of both particles into electromagnetic radiation since two γ rays, each having an energy of 511 keV, are produced. The two γ rays are emitted at 180° to each other and by using two detectors and appropriate electronic circuitry it is possible to localize more precisely the point within the body from which the emission emanated.

Another advantage of many positron emitters is that they are nuclides of elements occurring naturally in organic molecules. Thus labelling with the radioactive

Table 31.3 Positron emitting radionuclides

Radionuclide	Physical half-life (min)
Carbon-11	20
Nitrogen-13	10
Oxygen-15	2
Fluorine-18	110

nuclide will produce a radiopharmaceutical whose biological distribution and fate will be identical to a naturally occurring compound.

Table 31.3 lists some positron emitting radionuclides that are used, but because of the cost of their production, the inconveniently short half-lives and the expense of the detection equipment, their use is likely to remain limited.

FACILITIES REQUIRED FOR PREPARATION OF RADIOPHARMACEUTICALS

Radiopharmaceuticals are administered either orally, by inhalation or by injection and the facilities required for their preparation need to take into account both the radioactive nature of the product and the pharmaceutical implications of the route of administration. For radiopharmaceuticals administered orally or by inhalation, the requirements of operator protection predominate. Preparation is usually carried out in a fume cupboard which ensures any released activity is carried away from the operator and discharged to the atmosphere. Suitable shielding may also be placed inside the fume cupboard. However, the majority of radiopharmaceuticals, whether for therapeutic or diagnostic purposes, are administered intravenously. They must, therefore, comply with pharmacopoeial requirements for injectable materials, including sterility. It is important to remember that no radiopharmaceutical is self sterilizing by virtue of the radiation it emits.

Furthermore, the majority of diagnostic investigations are performed with radiopharmaceuticals containing short-lived radionuclides which have to be prepared and used on the same day. Terminal sterilization by autoclaving is not normally performed on such preparations because of constraints of time. Great reliance is therefore placed on aseptic technique and the skill of the operatives is of paramount importance.

It is therefore necessary to give careful consideration to the facilities used and comprehensive guidance is given in 'Guidance notes for hospitals on the premises and environment for the preparation of radiopharmaceuticals' issued by the Department of Health and Social Security (1982).

Laminar flow cabinets

Manipulations are performed within laminar flow cabinets which provide a Class I BS 5295 environment. Vertical as opposed to horizontal flow is used in order to avoid the possibility of radioactivity being blown towards the operators. Greater operator protection is provided by having a cabinet that complies with BS

5726 for containment of particles generated within the cabinet.

An example of such a cabinet is shown in Figure 31.1. It can be seen that air flows through a high efficiency particulate air (HEPA) filter and vertically downwards over the work surface. Air is then drawn through grilles in the work surface and through a second HEPA filter. Approximately 70% of the air is then recirculated within the cabinet whilst the remainder is discharged. In order to compensate for the discharged air, further air is taken into the cabinet via the grilles at the front of the working surface. This net inflow of air prevents any radioactive particles liberated within the cabinet from reaching the operator. In addition, this air does not flow over the materials being prepared until it has been circulated through the HEPA filters.

Maintenance of these air flow patterns and hence operator protection is dependent on careful setting of the fans within the cabinet. It is also important that the working surface inside the cabinet is kept as clear as possible to minimize turbulence. However, it is normal to perform all manipulations on impervious plastic or metal trays placed on the working surface, so that any spillage of radioactive material can be contained.

Operator protection can also be enhanced by the incorporation of local shielding in the cabinet. Cabinets with acrylic lead visors, rather than perspex, are available. In addition, lead shielding can be fitted beneath the work surface without disrupting air flow patterns. Extra shielding in the form of lead bricks or screens may be fitted inside the laminar flow cabinet providing it can be demonstrated that they do not compromise operator protection.

Radiation protection of operators

The handling of syringes and vials containing radioactive solutions means that the hands of the operators inevitably receive a radiation dose. During a working session preparing and dispensing radiopharmaceuticals, it may be necessary to make many transfers of radioactive materials in syringes and it is therefore necessary to reduce the radiation dose to the fingers as much as possible. This can be achieved in the following ways:

1. Maintenance of as large a distance as possible between the fingers and the radioactive source. This is because the radiation dose from a source is inversely proportional to the square of the distance from the source. For example, it has been calculated that for a 2 ml syringe containing 370 MBq of technetium-99m in 0.5 ml, the dose rate over the bolus is 40 times greater than at the end of the syringe barrel. Some departments

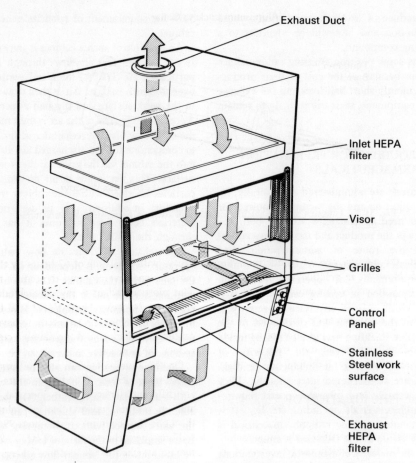

Fig. 31.1 Vertical laminar flow cabinet used for preparation of radiopharmaceuticals. Arrows indicate direction of airflow. (Courtesy of Envair (UK) Ltd)

advocate the use of oversize syringes in order to increase the distance between the fingers and the radioactive solution. Similarly, when vials are removed from their pots for measurement of radioactivity, they should be handled with forceps rather than fingers.

2. Minimize the time spent handling the radioactive material. This obviously depends on the expertise of the personnel and it is worthwhile making new workers practice their manipulative skills with non-radioactive solutions before preparing or dispensing radio-pharmaceuticals.

3. The use of shielding material to reduce the dose rate. Shields are normally made of dense materials such as lead or tungsten which provide efficient attenuation of gamma rays emitted by radiopharmaceuticals. Vials containing radioactivity should be handled in suitable pots and syringe shields can be used when transferring solutions or dispensing patient injections.

A tungsten syringe shield is shown in Figure 31.2. The barrel is an alloy of 90% tungsten and 10% nickel/iron and is 3 mm thick. The nickel/iron is necessary to improve the machining properties of the tungsten. There is a lead glass window in the barrel through which the syringe can be seen. Visualization is enhanced by painting the inside of the barrel white or yellow. The syringe is held in place by means of a rotating aluminium collar at the end of the shield.

The thickness of shielding material necessary is dependent on the γ ray energy source, the higher the energy, the thicker the shield required. Calculations show that attenuation of 50% of the gamma rays of technetium-99m (140 keV) is achieved by 0.3 mm lead or 0.4 mm tungsten. This thickness is usually referred to as the half thickness or half value layer (HVL). A 3 mm tungsten syringe shield is 7.5 HVLs (i.e. 3/0.4)

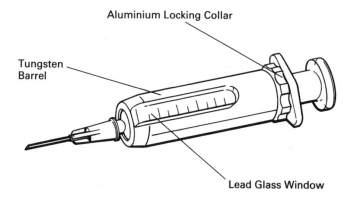

Aluminium Locking Collar

Tungsten Barrel

Lead Glass Window

Fig. 31.2 Tungsten syringe shield. (Courtesy of Medical Equipment Manufacturers (Sheffield) Ltd)

and will attenuate the gamma rays of technetium-99m $2^{7.5}$, i.e. 181-fold. However in practice, the dose to the fingers will not be reduced by this amount, since it is necessary to handle the syringe during withdrawal from the syringe shield for measurement of contained radioactivity. Similarly a 3 mm lead pot is approximately 10 HVLs and will reduce the radiation from a vial of technetium-99m approximately 1000-fold ($2^{10} = 1024$).

PRINCIPLES OF FORMULATION OF RADIOPHARMACEUTICALS

In hospital radiopharmacy departments the radionuclide technetium-99m is the most widely used because of its almost ideal physical properties and in many departments constitutes over 90% of the workload. It is used in the preparation of a wide variety of radiopharmaceuticals which have different biological fates and hence are used for various diagnostic investigations.

Technetium generators

The 6-hour half-life of technetium-99m is suitable for the majority of radiopharmaceutical investigations. However, it is inconveniently short for ordering and transport from a manufacturer. In 24 hours technetium-99m will go through four half-lives which means 94% of the original activity will have decayed in this time period.

Radiopharmacies do not therefore purchase technetium-99m directly, but instead purchase a technetium generator which contains its parent nuclide molybdenum-99. The construction of a typical generator is shown in Figure 31.3. Molybdenum-99 is absorbed in the form of molybdate ions on an alumina column, which acts as an anion exchanger. Molybdenum-99

decays with a half-life of 67 hours by the emission of β^- particles and several γ rays to produce technetium-99m. The most abundant γ ray of molybdenum-99 has an energy of 740 keV. The HVL of lead for this energy is 6.4 mm, therefore it is necessary to have shielding a few centimetres thick round the alumina column in order to reduce the dose rate.

On the alumina column an equilibrium is set up between molybdenum-99 and technetium-99m. Since they are different elements, their chemical properties differ and on passing sodium chloride solution (0.9% w/v) through the column, technetium-99m is eluted as sodium pertechnetate, ($NaTcO_4$). Molybdate ions remain attached to the alumina where they continue to decay to produce technetium-99m. Equilibrium between molybdenum-99 and technetium-99m on the column is re-established approximately 23 hours later. Another elution with sodium chloride solution will then yield further sodium pertechnetate. This process can be repeated on a daily basis until the yield of sodium pertechnetate is inconveniently small because the molybdenum-99 has decayed to low levels. Thus a fresh supply of technetium-99, as a sterile solution of sodium pertechnetate in sodium chloride, is available each day. In practice hospital radiopharmacies purchase technetium generators on a weekly standing order from a commercial manufacturer. The generators are supplied as sterile units and elution is performed automatically by means of a sterile evacuated vial which draws sterile sodium chloride solution from a reservoir through the alumina column. This means that manipulations involving technetium generators are kept to a minimum, which reduces radiation exposure of personnel and minimizes chances of introducing contamination. Between elutions, the delivery needle is covered by a vial containing antiseptic to maintain its sterility.

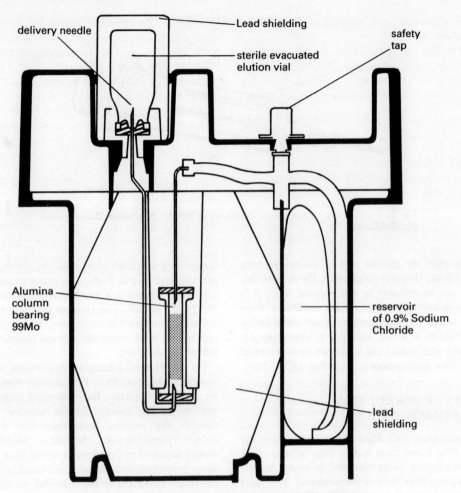

Fig. 31.3 Technetium generator. (Courtesy of CIS (UK) Ltd)

Sodium (^{99m}Tc) pertechnetate has monographs in the European Pharmacopoeia and is used as the starting material for the preparation of the wide range of technetium-99m radiopharmaceuticals.

Preparation of technetium radiopharmaceuticals using kits

Much work has been carried out in order to simplify the preparation of technetium radiopharmaceuticals as far as possible. The simplest and most widely available formulation consists of a single, sterile, freeze-dried, rubber-capped vial which contains all the necessary non-radioactive ingredients to prepare a specific radiopharmaceutical. Such vials, commonly referred to as 'kits', can be obtained commercially and are available

for all technetium-99m radiopharmaceuticals in routine use.

The preparation of the radiopharmaceutical is achieved by the single-step addition of sterile sodium pertechnetate to the kit in accordance with the manufacturers instructions.

Kits offer the following advantages:

1. Most of the formulation work is done with non-radioactive materials and hence there is no radiation exposure during their manufacture.

2. They are stable and quality assurance programmes, including tests for sterility, and pyrogenicity, and radioactive labelling efficiency can be completed by the manufacturer prior to supply of the kits.

3. The single-step addition of the radionuclide mini-

mizes time spent handling radioactive material and hence radiation exposure.

4. The number of manipulations in the radiopharmacy is minimal. This means the chance of introducing foreign matter or micro-organisms into the final radiopharmaceutical is greatly reduced.

Each kit vial normally contains sufficient components to prepare several patient doses.

In addition to the compound being radioactivity labelled, kits contain a stannous salt, which acts as a reducing agent for the sodium pertechnetate, in which technetium is present in the +7 valency state. Reduction to a lower valency state is necessary before the technetium will enter chemical reactions and thus produce radiopharmaceuticals. During these reactions the stannous ion is oxidized to stannic ion. In order to prevent this oxidation occurring spontaneously in the vial prior to the addition of sodium pertechnetate, the air in the vial is normally replaced by nitrogen.

Kits may also contain antioxidants, such as ascorbic acid or para-aminobenzoic acid, which prevent reoxidation of the technetium to a higher valency state after reconstitution of the kit. Materials to control pH and tonicity of the final injection may also be present.

A typical procedure for the preparation of a technetium radiopharmaceutical using a kit is as follows. It is necessary to use aseptic technique throughout to maintain sterility of the final product and to ensure adequate protection of the operator from radiation.

1. Place the kit vial in a suitable shielding container and swab the rubber closure with isopropyl alcohol or other suitable antiseptic.

2. Calculate the activity of sodium pertechnetate injection required. This depends on the number of doses to be obtained from the vial and the activity to be injected into each patient. Manufacturers normally specify the maximum activity that can be added to the vial.

3. Draw the required volume of sodium pertechnetate into a sterile syringe. If necessary, it may be diluted to a convenient volume using Sodium Chloride Injection BP (0.9%). The minimum and maximum volume to be added to a kit is normally specified by the manufacturer.

4. Inject the sodium pertechnetate solution into the shielded vial. Withdraw an equivalent volume of gas from the space above the solution before withdrawing the syringe from the vial. This is necessary to equalize the pressure within the vial and to prevent the ingress of air. A positive pressure left in the vial could be hazardous, both on withdrawing the syringe from the vial and on subsequent occasions when dispensing from the vial.

5. Shake the shielded vial to dissolve the contents. During this time, the sodium pertechnetate is reduced by the stannous ion and the technetium radiopharmaceutical is formed.

6. Measure the radioactivity in the vial and label appropriately. Details required on the label include the name of the radiopharmaceutical, the total volume in the vial and the activity measured at a specified time.

The radiopharmaceutical is then ready for dispensing. The dose required for a patient is calculated and the appropriate volume is dispensed in a sterile syringe. The activity present in the syringe is measured and recorded before it is issued for patient administration.

It is important to remember that because of the decay of technetium-99m, the volume of the radiopharmaceutical required for a given dose of radioactivity will increase during the day. Different volumes inevitably mean that patients receive different quantities of ingredients. In the extreme case, one patient may receive the entire contents of one kit vial and it is therefore essential that toxicity studies have demonstrated that this will not be dangerous to the patient.

The precise chemical structure of technetium-99m radiopharmaceutical is often not known. This is because the chemical quantity of technetium-99m added to the kit is generally less than 1 μg, therefore many analytical techniques are not sufficiently sensitive to permit such determinations. Studies are further hampered by the fact that technetium does not have a stable nuclide, which could be used to elucidate structures.

BIBLIOGRAPHY

British Standard BS 5295: 1976 Parts 1, 2 & 3. Environmental cleanliness in enclosed spaces. British Standards Institution, London

British Standard BS 5726: 1979 Specification for microbiological safety cabinets. British Standards Institution, London

Department of Health and Social Security 1982 Guidance notes for hospitals on the premises and environment for the preparation of radiopharmaceuticals. HMSO, London

European Pharmacopoeia 1981 2nd edn. Radiopharmaceutica, S.A., Maisonneuve, 57 Saint Ruffine, France p 125

Frier M, Hesselwood S R (eds) 1980 Quality control of radiopharmaceuticals. A guide to hospital practice. Chapman & Hall, London

32. Clinical applications of radiopharmaceuticals

S. R. Hesselwood

Introduction

Radionuclide incorporation into various tissues and organs of the body depends on the physiological and biochemical properties of those tissues and organs.

Radiopharmaceutical preparations are designed to utilize the ability of different structures to accumulate different radionuclides in order to aid visualization of the organs of interest or to deliver a dose of radiation to a target site.

RADIOPHARMACEUTICALS USED FOR DIAGNOSTIC PURPOSES

Technetium radiopharmaceuticals in common use

A large number of technetium compounds are used as radiopharmaceuticals, and developments are constantly taking place. In order to image a particular organ of the body, it is necessary for the radiopharmaceutical to localize there after intravenous administration. The major types of radiopharmaceuticals used are described below and are only illustrative of various localization mechanisms employed.

Brain agents

Sodium pertechnetate obtained directly from a technetium generator can be used for brain imaging. In the normal situation, radioactivity is excluded from the brain by the blood–brain barrier, but activity can be visualized in tumours, abscesses or intracerebral bleeds.

Thyroid agents

The pertechnetate ion has a similar size and shape to the iodide ion and is therefore taken up by the thyroid by active transport. In the euthyroid patient approximately 3% of the dose is taken up, which is sufficient to perform thyroid imaging.

Bone agents

Bone-seeking radiopharmaceuticals based on technetium are used for the detection of diseases of the skeleton including metastases from bronchogenic, breast and prostatic carcinomas, and other conditions such as Paget's disease.

Certain phosphate compounds have a high affinity for bone and labelling of such compounds with technetium-99m yields suitable agents. The first compound, monofluorophosphate, was introduced in 1971 but has since been superceded. Methylene diphosphonic acid, also known as medronic acid, was introduced in 1975 and is now the most widely used agent. Three hours after injection at least 30% of the dose has accumulated on the skeleton and images are obtained at this time.

Lung agents

Imaging of the lung is useful in detection of pulmonary emboli and chronic obstructive airways disease. Perfusion of the lung is determined by the intravenous injection of labelled particles of heat-denatured human serum albumin. The particle size is in the range 10–100 μm, with the majority of the order of 50 μm. Particles of this size are immediately retained in the lung by capillary blockade.

Lung kits contain sufficient heat-denatured albumin to produce several million particles per vial and normally a patient will receive half to one million particles. It has been calculated that this number and size of particles will block less than 1% of the total capillary network of the lung and thus their administration is safe. The biological half-life of the particles is only a few hours, as they are rapidly cleared from the lungs by the body's natural defence mechanisms. Imaging is therefore performed immediately after administration of the radiopharmaceutical. When performing lung studies, greater information can be gained by studying both ventilation and perfusion simultaneously. Ventilation studies can be performed by asking the patient to inhale a radioactive gas, such as xenon-127, xenon-133 or krypton-81m. Alternatively, the patient can inhale an aerosol of suitable particles, either liquid or solid, labelled with technetium-99m.

Liver agents

These are used for detection of liver disease such as cirrhosis or metastatic deposits of certain carcinomas. The radiopharmaceutical is formulated as a colloid with a particle size of a few hundred nanometres. After intravenous injection, the particles are removed from the blood by phagocytosis by the cells of the reticulo-endothelial system and within 20 minutes sufficient activity is present within the liver to permit imaging. Several different colloid formulations are commercially available. Some are presented as freeze-dried vials which are reconstituted with sodium pertechnetate in the usual way. The complex formed may be a technetium-tin colloid or a technetium-sulphur colloid. Other liver radiopharmaceuticals consist of a two or more component kit which necessitates formation of the colloid in situ by boiling. An example is the formation of a technetium-sulphur colloid by boiling sodium thiosulphate solution with a dilute acid in the presence of sodium pertechnetate. After boiling, the vial is allowed to cool and a sterile solution of a buffer is added to neutralize the pH of the final colloidal radiopharmaceutical.

Kidney agents

Technetium kidney agents are used to study either the structure or the function of the kidney. Structural studies are performed with dimercaptosuccinic acid (DMSA) which, after labelling with technetium, is accumulated by the renal cortex. It is necessary to allow a minimum of 4 hours accumulation before obtaining images.

Functional studies can be carried out with diethylene-triaminepenta-acetic acid (DTPA). This compound is excreted by glomerular filtration in the kidney. Therefore, by using a gamma camera connected to a suitable computer system, it is possible to see how the activity of technetium-DTPA in the kidney varies with time and construct time — activity curves to assess renal function.

Technetium-DTPA is also used as a brain-imaging agent. Although accumulation in abnormalities is no greater than with sodium pertechnetate, rapid renal excretion means that background radioactivity is lower and hence clearer images can be obtained.

Blood pool agents

Labelling of a patient's own erythrocytes with technetium-99m is readily achieved by treating the cells with stannous ions and then mixing them with sodium pertechnetate. By careful technique, damage to erythrocytes can be minimized and the labelled cells remain within the blood stream. They are used to study functioning of the heart, particularly the left ventricle. With suitable computer equipment and software, it is possible to calculate whether the atria and ventricles are beating in phase and the ejection fraction of the left ventricle.

Radiopharmaceuticals based on iodine-123

Iodine-123 has physical characteristics (half-life 13 hours, γ emission 159 keV) that are suitable for gamma camera imaging. Furthermore, the chemistry of iodine has been well documented so synthesis of a range of compounds can be achieved. The major drawback to iodine-123 is its availability, since there is no generator system available, production costs are high and there is the logistics problem of transport from the manufacturer to the hospital.

Sodium (^{123}I) iodide is used in thyroid imaging and is usually the starting material for synthesis of other iodine-123 radiopharmaceuticals. Kit formulations are available for a small range of radiopharmaceuticals, the most commonly used being sodium (^{123}I) iodohippurate. This agent is excreted via the kidney by both glomerular filtration and tubular secretion and therefore gives an estimate of renal plasma flow.

Radiopharmaceuticals based on indium-111

Indium-111 has a half-life of 67 hours and is commercially available in several formulations. When indium-111 is complexed with a lipophilic carrier, such as oxine (8-hydroxyquinoline), it is used to label a patient's own leucocytes. Upon re-injection, the labelled leucocytes are used to identify areas of infection or inflammation within the body, since they accumulate in such sites. Labelling requires an extremely well-controlled technique to minimize damage of the leucocytes, as this may result in the loss of their function and hence usefulness as a radiopharmaceutical.

Radiopharmaceuticals based on other nuclides

Radionuclides which have half-lives of 2 days or longer can conveniently be formulated by a manufacturer and presented in such a form that is suitable for patient administration. Thus hospital radiopharmacies are involved with dispensing, rather than manufacture, of such materials. A range of radionuclides is used in a variety of radiopharmaceuticals. Only the most commonly used are described here. Their characteristics are described in Table 31.2.

Thallium-201 is used as thallous chloride in the study of myocardial perfusion. The underlying principle of accumulation is that thallium is a monovalent cation analagous to potassium, which is essential to myocardial function. After intravenous injection of thallous chloride, areas of myocardium that are not perfused do not accumulate the radionuclide and such areas can be detected by the gamma camera. Lack of perfusion may be due to infarction of that part of the myocardium or disease in the coronary artery that supplies it.

Thallium-201 is not an ideal radionuclide since although it emits γ rays of suitable energy, their abundance is too low to be of practical value. Myocardial images are therefore obtained on X-rays emitted by a daughter product of thallium-201. The energy of these emissions is below 100 keV and hence significant attenuation problems occur.

Gallium-67 is available as gallium citrate and was initially introduced as a bone-imaging agent but is no longer used as such. Accumulation of gallium-67 occurs in a variety of lesions and mechanisms of uptake appear to be complex. Nevertheless, it is clinically useful in several situations, notably identification of infected hip prostheses and abscess localization. However, after intravenous injection of gallium citrate the radionuclide is excreted by the bowel and thus the identification of abdominal abscesses is less reliable than it is with indium-labelled leucocytes.

Gallium citrate is also accumulated by some soft-tissue tumours, for example lymphomas, and can be used to assess the extent of disease within the body.

Iodine-131 is used in diagnostic radiopharmaceuticals in certain instances, despite the fact that its physical characteristics (see Table 31.1) are not ideal. The fact that it is also used in therapeutic radiopharmaceuticals indicates its unsuitability for most diagnostic procedures. However, it is mainly used as sodium (^{131}I) iodide for thyroid studies or in other formulations where a more satisfactory radiopharmaceutical is not available.

RADIOPHARMACEUTICALS USED FOR THERAPEUTIC PURPOSES

Iodine-131 is the radionuclide most commonly used in therapeutic radiopharmaceuticals. The most frequently used formulation is sodium (^{131}I) iodide which is purchased as a capsule for oral administration in treatment of thyrotoxicosis in patients where therapy with carbimazole cannot be tolerated or is unsuccessful. Higher doses are also used in the treatment of thyroid carcinomas.

Sodium (^{131}I) iodide is also available as an oral solution for patients unable to swallow capsules and as a solution for intravenous injection. Such liquid formulations require greater manipulation during dispensing and thus are less convenient for the operator.

Advances in immunology since 1980 have meant that antibodies specific to certain tumours can now be isolated. If labelled with iodine-131, the antibodies offer the possibility of highly specific radiopharmaceuticals for both diagnosis and treatment, producing maximum radiation dosage at the site of the tumour.

Phosphorus-32 is most frequently used as sodium (^{32}P) phosphate injection in the treatment of polycythaemia rubra vera, a condition characterized by excessive production of erythrocytes. The sodium phosphate accumulates in the bone marrow and the radiation emitted disrupts erythropoiesis.

BIBLIOGRAPHY

British Standard BS 5295: 1976 Parts 1, 2 & 3. Environmental cleanliness in enclosed spaces. British Standards Institution, London
British Standard BS 5726: 1979 Specification for microbiological safety cabinets. British Standards Institution, London
Department of Health and Social Security 1982 Guidance notes for hospitals on the premises and environment for the preparation of radiopharmaceuticals. HMSO, London
European Pharmacopoeia 1981 2nd edn. Radiopharmaceutica, S.A., Maisonneuve, 57 Saint Ruffine, France p 125
Frier M, Hesselwood S R (eds) 1980 Quality control of radiopharmaceuticals. A guide to hospital practice. Chapman & Hall, London

PART 5

Additional pharmaceutical products

INTRODUCTION

In addition to the compounding, dispensing and supply of drugs in a range of dosage forms, the pharmacist is involved, particularly in the community, with the supply of surgical dressings and appliances, invalid aids and a variety of sick room requisites.

The Drug Tariff lists those articles and substances which may be supplied on NHS prescription forms under the general headings of 'appliances', 'chemical reagents' and 'domiciliary oxygen therapy'.

This part of the book describes three major groups of appliances, namely wound management products and surgical dressings (Ch. 33), elastic hosiery (Ch. 34) and stoma care and incontinence appliances (Ch. 35). The reader is referred to the Drug Tariff for details of these and other appliances such as contraceptive devices, hypodermic equipment and trusses.

Chapter 36 describes some aspects of the supply of medical gases, particularly in the domestic situation.

33. Wound management products and surgical dressings

D. M. Collett

INTRODUCTION

Wound management products and surgical dressings include a range of materials and items designed to medicate, absorb secretions from, protect and/or support wounded or damaged areas of the body. The community pharmacist is concerned mainly with the supply of prepacked dressings and wound care products often via the community nurse. The role of the pharmacist is to ensure that dressings of suitable quality are purchased from a reputable source and stored appropriately, i.e. in a cool, dry and well-ventilated place. Many dressings and appliances may not be prescribed on NHS forms and the pharmacist should consult the Drug Tariff and the NPA Guide for current regulations (see Appendix 2). The community pharmacist may also act as an advisor on the purchase of suitable items for first aid treatment and wound care in the home.

In the hospital situation the cost-effectiveness of wound management may be of paramount importance. For example, if the use of a relatively expensive product can be shown to reduce the length of inpatient stay it may be preferred to a cheaper but less effective alternative.

Many surgical dressings and the fibres and fabrics used in their manufacture are the subject of pharmacopoeial monographs (BP 1988). The entry on surgical dressings in the Pharmaceutical Codex (1979) provides a detailed description of a wide range of materials and products. Some of the older types of dressing are the subject of monographs in the BPC 1973.

In this chapter surgical dressings are categorized as wound dressings, surgical absorbents, surgical adhesive tapes and bandages. Some of the terms used to describe fabric surgical dressings are listed in Table 33.1.

WOUND DRESSINGS

Intact skin provides a mechanical, protective barrier against the outside environment. Access of pathogenic

Table 33.1 Terms used to describe fabric surgical dressings

Plain weave	A weave in which the threads pass alternatively over and under the threads running at right angles (Fig. 33.2)
Selvedge	A fabric edge woven so that it is fast and the threads do not become loose (Fig. 33.2)
Threads per unit length	The number of threads per specified length (usually 10 cm) of warp and weft. Indicates whether the fabric has an open or closed texture
Twist	The direction in which the fibres are twisted in spinning the yarn. It may be intensified for special purposes as in crêpe bandage
Warp	The yarn running the long way of the fabric
Weft	The yarn running across the fabric (wight to weft!)
Weight per unit area	Detects an excess of 'fillers' used to 'dress' a fabric to give it a desired appearance
Yarn	The thread spun from the fibres
Yarn count (Tex count)	The weight in grams of 1 km of yarn which gives a measure of the thickness

micro-organisms through broken skin should be prevented. Thus dressings applied to open wounds or raw surfaces should be sterile and should protect against the ingress of pathogens.

Wound healing following damage which causes loss of epidermal and dermal layers of the skin involves the production of fibrous and vascular tissue (granulation), followed by migration of epidermal cells from the edges of the wound to cover the granulation tissue. It is important that this newly forming tissue is not damaged by the application and removal of dressings. A fabric with a pore size of less than 8 μm will ensure that newly developing capillary loops do not penetrate the dressing and hence become damaged when the dressing is changed.

Wound healing is enhanced if an optimum degree of wound hydration is achieved. It is desirable that exudates are absorbed but that the dressing does not stick to the wound causing pain and damage when it is removed.

Traditional materials for dressings include fabric and fibrous compound absorbents made from cotton, cellulose or regenerated cellulose (viscose). These materials may be impregnated with substances designed to minimize adherence, to inhibit the growth of micro-organisms or to aid healing. Newer materials include calcium alginate fibre, non-woven pads and hydrocolloid dressings bonded to PVC or polyurethane support materials.

Wound dressing pads

These are absorbent pads which may or may not be enclosed in a woven or non-woven fabric sleeve. The pads are retained over the wound by means of adhesive tape or a retention bandage. Different types of dressing pads are available for use on different types of wounds, e.g. *highly absorbent* ones for heavily exudative wounds requiring frequent dressing changes, ones with *low absorption* capacity for postoperative and low exudate wounds and *low adherence* for use on ulcerative and other granulating wounds. Dressings incorporating activated charcoal are used to deoderize discharging infected and malodorous wounds and ulcers.

Non-adherent wound contact dressings

These are intended to be placed directly onto the wound to prevent adherence of a dressing pad placed on top.

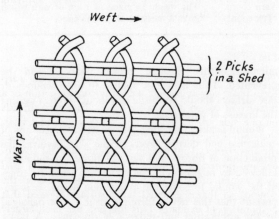

Fig. 33.1 Arrangement of threads in leno weave fabric

A gauze of special weave (leno fabric) designed to remain flat when lifted by a corner forms the basis for tulle dressings (Fig. 33.1). The gauze of tulle is impregnated with yellow or white soft paraffin (Paraffin Gauze Dressing BP) and may also be medicated with antimicrobial substances, e.g. chlorhexidine acetate or framycetin sulphate.

A semipermeable, adhesive, polyurethane foam may be applied directly to a wound, with or without the use of an absorbent pad. These dressings are waterproof but permeable to water vapour and are used for operation sites, stoma care, etc. to provide a protective cover in order to prevent skin breakdown.

Polyurethane foam dressings with low adherence and high absorbence may be applied to burns, open granulating wounds and ulcers. Silicone foam may also be used for dressing of cavity wounds. It has less absorbent capacity but low adherence.

Self-adhesive dressing pads

These consist of an absorbent pad attached directly to an adhesive plaster and may be in the form of single wound dressings with an adhesive margin all round or dressing strips with adhesive margins only at the sides parallel to the warp.

The pad which may be medicated and coloured yellow is faced with a film of perforated net to reduce wound adhesion. The pad has a low absorptive capacity which is a disadvantage. The adhesive backing may be perforated, ventilated and semipermeable (i.e. waterproof but permeable to air and water vapour) or occlusive (i.e. non-permeable waterproof), depending on the purpose for which the dressing is intended.

Other wound dressings

A number of aerosol wound dressings are available. These contain acrylic polymers and can be sprayed onto the skin to leave a flexible porous protective film for surgical wounds and around stomata.

Dressing packs

Sterile dressing packs

These are used mainly for wound cleansing in community nursing and may be supplemented by selected wound dressings.

Standard dressings

These are sterile dressings for first aid treatment packed individually to prevent access of micro-organisms.

Details of these standard dressings can be found in the Pharmaceutical Codex (1979).

ABSORBENTS

Absorbent materials are used in pre-operative skin preparation, during surgery and postoperatively. Absorbents are also used to apply medicaments to the skin for routine skin cleansing, to absorb wound exudate and to absorb large volumes of fluid in incontinence. The fibres used in absorbent products include cotton, viscose and cellulose. Cotton and viscose may be made into fabric or used like cellulose in the fibrous state.

Fibrous absorbents

Absorbent cotton wool

Cotton wool is available in a number of different grades. Pharmacopoeial qualities contain less dust and have a relatively longer staple (fibre length). This quality must be used for wound cleansing and for pre-operative skin care. Hospital quality has a shorter staple length and contains more dust but is suitable as a general purpose absorbent and for routine cleansing of incontinent patients.

Absorbent viscose wadding

Viscose wadding is made from regenerated cellulose (rayon). It has a high absorptive capacity and is a useful substitute for the poorer grades of cotton wool, having the advantages of relative freedom from dust and loose fibres. However, it tends to be slippery in use and is best when mixed with some cotton fibres.

Cellulose wadding

This consists of delignified fibres prepared from bleached wood pulp and compressed into sheets. Like cotton and viscose it is a good absorbent although like viscose tends to collapse when wet. It should not be used directly on wounds but may be combined with other materials in absorbent pads.

Fabric absorbents

Note: Table 33.1 lists some of the terms used to describe fabrics.

Gauze

Absorbent cotton in the form of spun threads either alone or mixed with viscose threads may be woven into

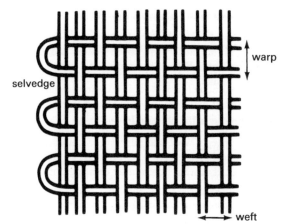

Fig. 33.2 Arrangement of threads in plain weave fabric

a gauze fabric for use as an absorbent. Gauze is a fabric of plain weave (Fig. 33.2, Table 33.1), usually supplied in pieces 900 mm wide and in various lengths folded lengthwise. Various types of gauze are defined by the closeness of the weave (threads per cm) and the weight per unit area. Gauze may also be woven in the form of ribbons of various widths and lengths with a selvedge.

Gauze may be used to prepare swabs, pads, strips, etc. for pre-operative skin preparation, for various purposes during surgery and for postoperative wound care. Some of the products may be colour coded, and for use during surgery swabs with a radiopaque marker may be used to allow radiological detection if accidentally enclosed in a wound.

Muslin

This is a bleached cotton cloth of plain weave, known in commerce as butter muslin. It may be used for applying either wet or dry dressings.

Lint

This consists of a cloth of plain weave in which the warp threads are cotton and the weft may contain cotton or a mixture of cotton and viscose fibres. The warp threads on one side are 'raised' to give a fleecy nap that gives the cloth a thicker and softer appearance and increases the absorbency. Lint is used as a home first-aid absorbent and protective dressing. Traditionally lint was used as a wound dressing (with the plain side next to the wound) so that the linted outer surface allowed that evaporation of exudate. This function has been largely replaced by newer non-adherent dressings.

Fibrous and fabric absorbent products

The gauze fabrics described above may be used to enclose fibrous absorbents as in Gauze and Cellulose Wadding Tissue BP and in Gauze and Cotton Tissue BP (gamgee tissue).

Wool products for chiropody

Fibrous sheep's wool and surgical or chiropodial wool felt are used as protectives in chiropody. Animal wool is particularly useful in retaining dressings on toes.

SURGICAL ADHESIVE TAPES

These are used to retain wound dressings, to secure tubing during parenteral therapy and to immobilize small areas. Adhesive bandages (see below) are used to provide support and to restrict movement for orthopaedic purposes. Surgical adhesive tapes consist of a self-adhesive mass spread on a supporting material that may be permeable, semipermeable or occlusive. The supporting material may be woven or non-woven or a plastic film. This tapes may be extensible, inextensible or elastic. The adhesive masses may vary in adhesiveness, in the residue left after removal and in the frequency of inducing skin irritation.

Permeable surgical adhesive tapes

Fabric-based products include the well-known Zinc Oxide Plaster BP and its counterpart Zinc Oxide Elastic Adhesive Tape BP which stretches in the direction of the warp. The adhesive mass used in these products frequently induces skin reactions and should not be considered for long-term use unless patch testing has been carried out.

As an alternative Permeable Woven or Non-woven Surgical Synthetic Adhesive Tapes BP spread with a polymeric adhesive may be considered.

For dressings in which immersion in water without loss of adhesiveness is an advantage, Permeable Plastic Adhesive Tape BP may be preferred.

Semipermeable surgical adhesive tapes

These are waterproof and therefore protect wounds from the ingress of micro-organisms and the environment from the possible spread of infection from the wound. At the same time the passage of air and water vapour is allowed to minimize overhydration of the site.

Occlusive surgical adhesive tapes

These are used to secure or cover dressings where total exclusion of air and water vapour is required, for example to isolate infected wounds.

BANDAGES

The term 'bandage' includes a number of product types which may be classified in different ways. In terms of function, bandages are used:

— to retain dressings in place;
— to provide support and/or compression for injuries or varicose conditions;
— to apply a medicated paste directly to the skin surface in dermatological conditions.

Bandages may be:

— extensible (elastic) or non-extensible (non-elastic);
— adhesive or non-adhesive;
— woven or knitted;
— flat or tubular.

Retention bandages — non-stretch

Open-wove Bandage BP

These bandages are most frequently used for the retention of absorbent dressings, for securing splints and for providing slight support for minor strains and sprains. Open-wove bandage has a cotton warp and a weft of either cotton, viscose or a combination of the two. It is produced in three types or qualities and many sizes. Since the bandage is generally intended for use on a single occasion the edges are simply cut parallel to the warp threads but must be reasonably free from loose ends.

Triangular Calico Bandage BP

This consists of unbleached calico in the form of a right-angled triangle and may be used as a sling.

Domette Bandage BP

This bandage is of plain weave with either a cotton or a cotton and viscose warp and a woollen weft. It is used to provide support with warmth.

Retention bandages — stretch fabric

Cotton Conforming Bandage BP

This bandage is woven using crimped cotton threads which imparts elasticity to both warp and weft. It is useful to retain dressings over awkward shaped areas, such as joints.

Polyamide and Cellulose Contour Bandage BP

This was previously known as nylon and viscose stretch bandage and may also be used to retain dressings.

Tubular bandages and stockinettes

These consist of knitted fabrics in tubular form manufactured on a circular knitting machine either in plain or ribbed knitting. The fibres may be cotton, viscose, cotton and viscose, or polypropylene. Elasticated tubular bandage is also available. Tubular bandages are used to retain dressings on the limbs, trunk and abdomen and may also be used as protective dressings with tar-based and other non-steroid ointments.

Elastic net surgical tubular stockinette is used for the retention of dressings, particularly on awkward sites, and is designed for long-term re-use.

Support and compression bandages

Non-adhesive woven extensible bandages

These include cotton and rubber elastic bandage and web bandages (used for providing high compression and support over varicose veins) and paste bandages, cotton suspensory bandages (for scrotal support) and crêpe bandages (for light support over strains, sprains and varicose veins). Crêpe Bandage BP is the best known elastic bandage. It is an elastic fabric of plain weave in which the warp threads are of cotton and wool and the weft threads are of cotton. The arrangement of the warp threads is shown in Figure 33.3 and is:

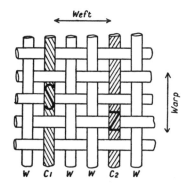

Fig. 33.3 Arrangement of threads in Crêpe Bandage BP. W, Wool thread; C_1, two-fold cotton thread with an S-twist; C_2, two-fold cotton thread with a Z-twist

1 × two-fold thread with an S-twist
2 wool threads
1 × two-fold cotton thread with a Z-twist
2 wool threads

This is repeated to the edges which are fast and secured by two-fold cotton threads.

The opposite twists of the alternate cotton threads give the bandage its considerable elasticity; much of this is lost during use but is largely restored by washing in hot soapy water.

Adhesive woven extensible bandages

Adhesive elastic bandages have the advantages for ambulent patients of providing good support and compression whilst staying in position and not causing undue restriction of movement. The main disadvantage of all adhesive bandages is the tendency to cause damage to the skin on removal. Depilation of the skin prior to application will aid both adherence and subsequent removal. Patch tests should be performed if sensitivity to ingredients of the adhesive is suspected. Organic solvents may be required to remove the sticky residue left on the skin after removal of the bandage.

Elastic self-adhesive bandages

These are woven fabrics, elastic in the warp and spread fully or partially with adhesive mass. They are used for compression of leg ulcers, compression and support for fractured ribs or clavicles, and for swollen and sprained joints.

Extension Plaster BP is a woven fabric extensible in the weft and spread with zinc oxide adhesive mass. This is also used for support of light strains, for joints and limbs recently removed from plaster casts, fractured ribs and for traction bandaging.

Diachylon Elastic Adhesive Bandages BPC 1973

These consist of an elastic cloth spread evenly with diachylon and suitable adhesives. Diachylon is a mixture of lead soaps of higher fatty acids. These bandages may be used for compression in the treatment of leg ulcers and varicose veins especially in patients sensitive to zinc oxide and rubber adhesive bandages. The bandages are occlusive and must be warmed before application in order to ensure adhesion.

Cohesive elastic bandages

These adhere to themselves but not to the patient's skin and may be used to support sprained joints.

Medicated bandages

These consist of a cotton bandage impregnated with a suitable paste or cream. They are used to treat chronic skin conditions and varicose ulcers.

Medicated bandages are retained in position by support or compression bandages. The medicaments used include zinc oxide, coal tar and ichthammol and the dressings may remain in position for several weeks. In the treatment of infantile eczema and other irritating skin disorders hydrocortisone-impregnated bandages may be used.

Plaster of Paris Bandage BP

This is a cotton cloth of leno weave (see Fig. 33.1) impregnated with dried calcium sulphate together with adhesives and setting-time modifiers. It is soaked in water before application and sets within 8 minutes to form a splint. Plaster of Paris Bandage BP is used for the immobilization and splinting of fractures, correction splinting, the construction of body supports, rest splints and similar purposes.

STANDARDS FOR SURGICAL DRESSINGS

For those dressings that are the subject of a pharmacopoeial monograph a number of detailed standards are described (see, for example, BP 1988). Standards for older dressings may be found in the BPC 1973. Non 'official', prescribable dressings may be the subject of specifications described in the Drug Tariff.

Dressings required to be sterilized must also comply with tests for sterility (see Ch. 30) and must be packed and stored so as to preserve the sterile state.

BIBLIOGRAPHY

British National Formulary 1988 16th edn. British Medical Association and Royal Pharmaceutical Society of Great Britain, London (updated twice yearly)
British Pharmacopoeia 1988 HMSO, London
British Pharmaceutical Codex 1973 Pharmaceutical Press, London
Drug Tariff current edition HMSO, London (updated monthly)
Hospital Pharmacists Group 1988 Wound management. Pharmaceutical Journal 241: 666

NPA Guide to the Drug Tariff 1987/88 National Pharmaceutical Associations, St Albans
Pharmaceutical Codex 1979 11th edn (incorporating the British Pharmaceutical Codex). Pharmaceutical Press, London
Thomas S 1988 New Drug Tariff dressings. Pharmaceutical Journal 240: 752–753
Thomas S, Loveless P, Hay N P 1988 Comparative review of the properties of six semipermeable film dressings. Pharmaceutical Journal 240: 785–78

34. Elastic hosiery

D. M. Collett

Elastic hosiery fashioned into a range of garments may be used to provide therapeutic compression for a number of pathological conditions in addition to soft-tissue support and relief of joint sprains and strains.

INDICATIONS FOR COMPRESSION THERAPY

Varicosities

An upright posture induces considerable hydrostatic stress on the veins of the legs. The leg muscles provide adequate support for the deep veins but the superficial veins may become dilated and tortuous. The valves necessary for effective venous return become incompetent and blood stagnates producing the blue blemishes characteristic of varicose veins. In the early stages the patient may seek help for cosmetic reasons, other early symptoms are tiredness, aching and heaviness, particularly at the end of the day. As the condition progresses the symptoms become more serious and include oedema, pigmentation, eczema and skin ulcers which may be very slow to heal. Predisposing factors include a family history associated with fewer vein valves than normal, pregnancy and occupations which involve prolonged standing.

Treatment of varicose veins may involve the surgical removal or stripping of affected veins followed by injection of recurrent varices with a sclerosing solution. External elastic support of varicose veins relieves the symptoms and may delay the progression of the disease.

The degree of compression required to control the symptoms depends on the severity of the varices. Early varices require light or mild support, varices of medium severity require medium or moderate support and gross varices require strong support.

Varicose ulcers

These may be treated with bed rest with elevation of the legs above the heart but for ambulant patients compression applied over a medicated bandage or dressing is appropriate. Once the ulcer has healed, maintenance of compression reduces the risk of recurrence.

Venous insufficiency

Chronic venous insufficiency in the limbs may result from thrombophlebitis causing oedema and dilated superficial veins. Stasis pigmentation, stasis dermatitis and stasis ulceration may follow as may the development of varicose veins. Post-thrombotic venous insufficiency may be reduced or prevented by means of suitable elastic support of the limb.

METHODS OF APPLYING COMPRESSION THERAPY

Bandaging

Adhesive or non-adhesive support and compression bandages, described in the previous chapter (see Ch. 33), may be used to apply differing degrees of compression to the limbs. Application of the appropriate compression requires nursing skill and is unlikely to be achieved by the patient at home.

Too tight a bandage will cause pain and possible damage to underlying tissues. Too loose a bandage is ineffective and may slip down the limb.

Compression hosiery

Elastic or compression hosiery has a number of advantages over limb bandaging:

1. Different degrees of compression can be applied by design and construction of different garments. This degree of compression will remain relatively constant during the life of the garment.

2. The compression can be graduated along the leg to produce maximum compression where required at the ankle with compression gradually reducing towards the thigh.

3. The patient is less dependent on skilled nursing time.

4. The garments can be designed to resemble conventional hosiery and thus improve patient compliance, particularly for long-term wear.

Types of hosiery available

The garments prescribed to apply therapeutic compression are below-knee stockings for lower limb disorders, and thigh stockings for more complete limb support (Fig. 34.1).

Graduated compression hosiery is classified by the degree of support provided. The mean compression applied to an average ankle is defined together with the change in compression along the leg (Table 34.1).

For support of soft-tissue sprains and strains, anklets and knee caps are available in Class 2 and Class 3 fabrics. The garments that may be prescribed on NHS forms are described in the Drug Tariff and are available for both male and female patients. Suspenders may be supplied with thigh-length garments prescribed for men and suspender belts are also available.

Other garments available for purchase but not allowed on NHS prescription include support tights and waist-length stockings for women and support socks for men. These garments may provide relief from leg discomfort but do not provide the precise therapeutic compression required for diagnosed pathological conditions.

THE ROLE OF THE PHARMACIST

The pharmacist may offer a complete service in measuring, fitting and supplying compression hosiery. The

Table 34.1 Classification of graduated compression hosiery

Class 1: Mild support or light compression	Indicated for prophylaxis during pregnancy and for the treatment of early varices Mean ankle compression 14–17 mmHg
Class 2: Moderate support or medium compression	Indicated for varices of medium severity and varicosis during pregnancy; for ulcer treatment and prevention of recurrence and mild oedema Mean ankle compression 18–24 mmHg
Class 3: Strong support and compression	Indicated for gross varices and gross oedema: for post-thrombotic venous insufficiency; for ulcer treatment and the prevention of recurrence Mean ankle compression 25–35 mmHg

(Drug Tariff 1988 and BS 6612:1985)

garment manufacturers usually provide size charts for standard product ranges. The measurements required for stockings include foot length, the circumference of the slimmest part of the ankle, the widest part of the calf and around the thigh for thigh-length garments. Measurements are best made as early in the day as possible when postural oedema is minimal and with the patient seated. For non-standard sizes a made-to-measure facility is available. Whenever possible the fitting of the garment should be demonstrated in the pharmacy. The technique of fitting elastic hosiery differs from that for conventional hose and defective patient

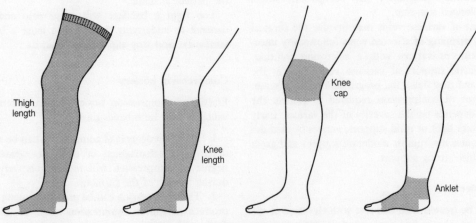

Fig. 34.1 Types of support stocking

technique may limit the benefit of the therapy and the life of the garments. Manufacturers may offer hosiery fitting training for pharmacists and assistants.

Garments prescribed on NHS prescription must conform to Drug Tariff specification and the prescriber must include on the prescription the quantity of garments (single or pair), the article required including accessories such as suspenders and the compression (Class 1, 2 or 3). A prescription charge is payable for each garment (ie. two charges for a pair of stockings) unless the patient is exempted from payment (see Appendix 2). Patients will generally require two pairs of stockings in use to allow for wearing, washing and drying. With careful handling and laundering compression hosiery should retain its elasticity for several months.

Since therapy with compression hosiery is usually maintained for long periods the pharmacist may find the keeping of patient records advantageous. An occasional check to ensure that the patient's measurements have not changed will be required. The patient can be reminded to renew the hosiery at suitable intervals and stock control is facilitated. In addition, patient compliance is improved and any problems experienced by the patient with the hosiery may be discussed on a regular basis.

BIBLIOGRAPHY

Drug Tariff current edition HMSO, London (updated monthly)
McCreedy C 1988 Elastic hosiery on the NHS. Pharmaceutical Journal 240: 412–413

NPA Guide to the Drug Tariff 1987/88 National Pharmaceutical Association, St Albans
Scurr J 1988 Why use elastic hosiery? Pharmaceutical Journal 240: 410–411

35. Stoma care and incontinence appliances

D. M. Collett

Introduction

A stoma is an opening in the abdominal wall created surgically in order to allow the outflow of intestinal contents or urine. The patient rarely has complete voluntary control over the outflow. This is usually collected into an ostomy appliance for disposal at regular intervals.

Urinary incontinence is the involuntary loss of urine via the urethra both day and night and may be a symptom of a variety of underlying conditions. A wide range of products and appliances are available to allow the patient to cope with the problem of incontinence.

The pharmacist can make a valuable contribution to the overall care of the ostomy patient and incontinence sufferer in supplying appliances, associated products and medicines, and in providing sympathetic and informed advice.

This chapter provides a brief description of the different types of ostomy, the main classes of appliance and some of the associated products. The major types of incontinence aids and appliances are also described in this chapter. It should be remembered that only those appliances listed in the Drug Tariff may be prescribed on NHS prescription

STOMA CARE

There are three main types of stoma: ileostomy, colostomy and urostomy. The outflow from the three types differs and therefore the appliances worn and the associated problems experienced by the patient vary.

Main types of ostomy

Ileostomy (Fig. 35.1)

The reason. An ileostomy is usually created in patients with an inflammatory disease of the large bowel (such as ulcerative colitis or Crohn's disease) or in patients with colonic or rectal cancer. The terminal ileum is separated from the colon and brought through

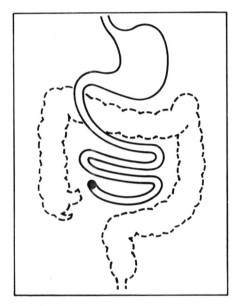

Fig. 35.1 Ileostomy. (Reproduced with permission from the author and the *Pharmaceutical Journal* (Watkins 1987))

a small opening in the abdominal wall to form a short 'spout'. The large bowel may be removed or in some cases allowed to remain inactive in order to allow healing of the inflamed tissue with eventual surgical restoration of normal bowel function.

The patient (known as the ileostomist). The ileostomy patient is typically a young adult, physically and sexually active. The life-expectancy after surgery is good and they should be encouraged to lead full and active lives.

The appliance. The effluent from an ileostomy has a liquid consistency and is rich in digestive enzymes. The appliances are attached to the abdomen by means of a ring of adhesive which fits over the stoma 'spout' allowing the effluent to be collected in a drainable plastic bag. The lower end of the bag is closed by a clip which may

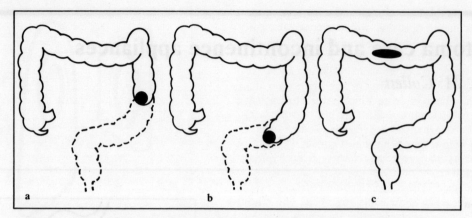

Fig. 35.2 Colostomies. **a**, Descending colostomy, **b**, Sigmoid colostomy, **c**, Temporary loop colostomy (Reproduced with permission from the author and the *Pharmaceutical Journal* (Watkins 1987))

be removed to allow the bag to be emptied when necessary. The appliance can be left in place on the abdomen for several days in order to minimize soreness of the skin caused by constant changing of adhesive bags.

Colostomy (Fig. 35.2)

The reason. Colostomies may be created for patients with spinal injuries or acute bowel obstruction but are most frequently created for patients suffering from cancer of the colon, rectum or anus. The diseased portion of the large bowel is removed and an opening created through the abdominal wall for exteriorization of the ending of the remaining bowel. The amount of bowel removed depends on the extent of the disease. A descending colostomy is formed from the decending colon and a sigmoid colostomy from the sigmoid colon. Sometimes a 'temporary' colostomy may be created in the transverse colon. In this case the opening is 'double barrelled' since both cut ends of the colon are brought to the surface. The lower bowel is allowed to rest and normal function may be restored eventually. More rarely, a temporary opening may be created in the ascending colon.

The patient (the colostomist). The colostomy patient is typically an elderly adult (over 60 years) and the life-expectancy may be reduced by recurrence of the disease.

The appliance. The effluent from a colostomy will depend on the amount of remaining bowel and varies from semi-liquid from ascending and transverse colostomies to soft semi-solid from a descending colostomy and firm from a sigmoid colostomy. Most colostomists use a closed pouch which fits around the stoma and is attached to the abdominal skin by means of an adhesive ring. The pouch is removed and replaced when full.

Patients with temporary transverse or ascending stomata may use drainable pouches.

Urostomy (Fig. 35.3)

The reason. A urostomy is created in order to divert the flow of urine from the kidneys away from the urinary bladder. This procedure most commonly follows removal of the urinary bladder in the surgical treatment

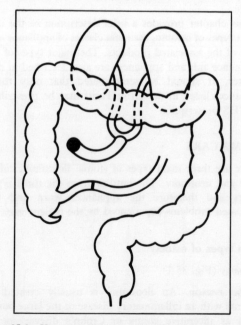

Fig. 35.3 Urostomy (ileal conduit). (Reproduced with permission from the author and the *Pharmaceutical Journal* (Watkins 1987))

of cancer of the bladder, urethra and sometimes of the cervix and uterus. Patients with unmanageable incontinence due to anatomical or neurological deficiencies may also require a urostomy. As an emergency procedure the ureters may be brought to the surface of the abdominal wall but more usually the ureters are implanted into a piece of ileum which is used to create a stoma in the abdominal wall. This ileal conduit acts merely as a drainage tube, the remaining ileum is reconnected and normal bowel function continues.

The patient (the urostomist). There is no 'typical' urostomy patient.

The appliance. The urine which flows from a urostomy is collected in a drainable bag. This, like other ostomy appliances, is fixed to the abdominal skin by means of an adhesive ring which surrounds the stoma. Urine collects in the bottom of the urostomy bag and should be prevented by means of a non-return device from irritating the stoma. The bag may be emptied when required by means of a drain tap which may also be connected via additional tubing to a larger receptacle for night-drainage purposes. The bag usually remains attached to the abdominal skin for several days before being replaced.

Types of stoma appliance

There are two major types of stoma appliance: one-piece and two-piece products.

One-piece stoma appliances (Fig. 35.4)

In this type of appliance the skin adhesive is an integral part of the appliance. The adhesive ring is protected by a removable cover which is peeled off prior to application. This has the advantage of simplicity and may be suitable for patients with limited manual dexterity. The main disadvantage is that the repeated removal of the

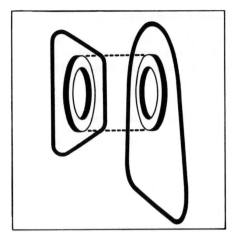

Fig. 35.5 Two-piece appliance. (Reproduced with permission from the author and the *Pharmaceutical Journal* (Watkins 1987))

adhesive from the skin may lead to soreness, skin breakdown and eventual reduction in the adhesiveness of the device.

Two-piece stoma appliances (Fig. 35.5)

The two components are:

A base plate or flange which adheres to the abdominal skin surrounding the stoma and may remain in position for several days. The flange provides a means of attachment for the pouches.

A pouch which fastens on to the flange. It can be changed as necessary without removing the flange. This type of appliance requires more manual dexterity than the one-piece type. However, providing that the material of the base plate is hypo-allergenic, irritation is minimal and damage to the surrounding skin is limited by the fact that only infrequent removal is required.

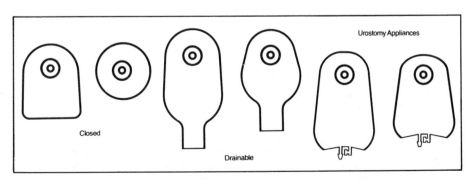

Fig. 35.4 One-piece appliances. (Reproduced with permission from the author and the *Pharmaceutical Journal* (Watkins 1987))

The range of stoma appliances

A glance at the relevant section (Part IXc) of the current Drug Tariff will indicate the large range of stoma appliances and accessories available. The main choices are listed below.

1. *Closed, drainable or with a drain tap*

Depends on the type of effluent — semi-solid, semi-liquid or urine.

2. *One-piece or two-piece*

Both one-piece and two-piece appliances are available as closed pouches (permanent colostomy), drainable pouches (ileostomy or temporary colostomy) and pouches with a drain tap (urostomy).

3. *Clear or opaque*

Clear pouches are preferred postoperatively, for patients with poor eye sight and where there is a need to be able to see the contents. Opaque pouches may be more acceptable to patients for routine use.

4. *Pouch size*

Drainable pouches (both ileostomy and urostomy) are available in large or small sizes to suit the lifestyle and stature of the patient. The smaller sizes may be more discrete for social use, especially with smaller patients. For colostomists with a predictable emptying pattern very small 'mini' pouches are available. These pouches have no actual capacity but cover and protect the stoma and may be used for several hours by patients with a continent stoma or for short-term activities such as sport.

5. *Stoma size*

The adhesive seal incorporated in the appliance (one-piece products) or in the flange (two-piece systems) should fit as closely round the stoma as possible to protect the surrounding skin against the effluent faeces or urine. However, it is essential that the stoma is not constricted in any way as this may result in necrosis of the tissue. The size of the orifice in the adhesive seal must therefore be chosen carefully to fit neatly but easily round the stoma. Most product ranges include appliances with pre-cut holes in a number of standard sizes and other appliances with 'starter holes' that can be enlarged and cut to shape for irregular stomata.

6. *Type of adhesive or backing*

Different products utilize different materials to provide an adhesive seal with the skin. One of the older materials is karaya gum. Newer products include compounds based on gelatin, pectin and carmellose sodium. Patients who react to one type of adhesive may benefit from transfer to a less allergenic product. In some cases the addition of an extra skin protective wafer may allow a potentially irritating appliance to be used.

Stoma care accessories

Belts

Some patients feel more confident if the appliance is held in place by a belt in addition to the adhesive seal. Belt loops are provided on a number of pouches and the corresponding belts may be prescribed on NHS prescription if listed in the Drug Tariff.

Pouch covers

Washable cotton covers are available for a number of appliances. These reduce the noise which plastic appliances may create and also add to the comfort and cosmetic appeal of the appliance.

Flatus filters

Flatus may be a problem, particularly for colostomists wearing closed appliances. Several manufacturers produce flatus filters which allow the escape of the flatus through activated charcoal to reduce odour. Alternatively the patient may be able to release the flatus from a two-piece system without changing the whole appliance.

Deodorants

A number of deodorant products are available for placing within the stoma appliance and include solutions, powders and gel formulations. Aerosol atmospheric deodorants may also be used when emptying the appliance.

Irrigation appliances

Some colostomists achieve continence by adopting a daily irrigation technique. Warm water instilled into the colon stimulates peristalsis and faecal evacuation. The necessary apparatus is listed in the Drug Tariff and is available on NHS prescription.

Adhesives and adhesive removers

Some patients may additionally secure their appliance with adhesive tape or may apply extra adhesive to the skin. Some adhesive products are applied by brush, others are formulated as pressurized spray applications. Removal of the adhesive often also requires a special solvent spray.

Skin protectives, fillers and cleansers

Patients are usually advised to cleanse the area around the stoma with warm water since detergent and disinfectant products may cause irritation. Dusting powder is useful to ensure that the area is completely dry before an attempt is made to attach the adhesive to the skin surface. A barrier cream is useful to protect sensitive or excoriated skin. Any creams used should be massaged into the skin and the area wiped dry before application of the adhesive. Powders, pastes and gels containing karaya and other adhesives are also available to aid adhesion and reduce leakage, particularly if the skin is uneven or creased.

Prescriptions for stoma appliances

After surgery to create the stoma, the patient should leave hospital with a 'take-home supply' and with written details of their equipment which will enable their general practitioner to write prescriptions for further supplies. The pharmacist obtains stoma-care products from general or specialist wholesalers or sometimes directly from the manufacturer. Maintenance of patient records will enable the pharmacy to maintain a stock of regularly prescribed items since it would be impracticable to carry the complete range of possible combinations of appliance. Continuity of supply is essential for the patient and the provision of a prompt and reliable service will be much appreciated.

Medicines for the ostomist

The ostomist may require medication to modify bowel function, either to control diarrhoea or to relieve constipation. This should usually be carried out under medical supervision, although the patient may learn to manage the medication to produce an effluent of appropriate consistency. Whenever possible, dietary modifications should precede drug therapy and the patient should be discouraged from the indiscriminate use of over-the-counter (OTC) medication.

Intestinal transit time will be markedly changed and drug absorption may be difficult to predict, particularly if part of the ileum has been removed.

Enteric-coated and sustained-release formulations are unsuitable for stoma patients, and other dosage forms such as gelatin capsules may be unsatisfactory. Oral methods of contraception may be unreliable. Side-effects of drugs such as diarrhoea or constipation (especially with opiate analgesics) may be exaggerated in the shortened bowel. The patient will be very aware of any changes in the colour or consistency of the effluent and should be warned if such changes are predicted. Electrolyte balance may be a problem, especially in ileostomists. Excessive dehydration should be avoided and the patient is particularly vulnerable to potassium depletion, especially if diuretic therapy is prescribed. Sustained-release potassium supplements cannot be used and liquid formulations are to be preferred.

Ostomy patients frequently experience problems with the skin surrounding the stoma because of faecal or urinary irritation, allergy to the adhesive or soreness because of frequent dressing changes. The pharmacist may offer short-term advice but referral to a stoma-care nurse for longer-term management is advisable.

Other problems

Leakage

This may occur if the patient has an inappropriate appliance, is not fitting the appliance correctly, is unable to achieve a good seal between the adhesive and the skin, or very occasionally because the device is faulty. The pharmacist is in a unique position to offer advice since the patient (or representative) is seen regularly when appliances are collected from the pharmacy.

Diet

Patients are usually encouraged to eat a varied diet which incorporates some but not too much fibre. Foods which are found by the individual to cause problems should be avoided. The addition of yoghurt or buttermilk to the diet may help to reduce faecal odour and excessive wind.

Disposal

The contents of used appliances should be emptied and the bag rinsed. After suitable wrapping the appliance can be placed with the domestic refuse. Recently a 'flushable' colostomy bag has been produced but it would be unwise to attempt to flush away conventional plastic bags. Alternative 'dirty dressings' or 'waste disposal' services may be provided in some local areas.

Psychological problems

The ostomy patient, especially in the early days, has a number of problems to face. A normal physiological function has been replaced by an 'abnormal' procedure which may be perceived as dirty, smelly and generally unclean. The patient may feel socially unacceptable and isolated from help and may try to cope alone with the various problems that occur.

The pharmacist can contribute significantly to the restoration of the ostomist's health and morale by providing simple advice, prompt supply of appliances and an empathic approach to the patient and his problems.

Additional sources of help

General practitioner:

— for access to support services
— for problems with drug therapy
— for prescribed products

Stoma-care nurse:

— for pre-operative advice
— for postoperative care
— for advice in the community on home use

The names of stoma-care nurses and their designated areas are listed by the Royal College of Nursing.

Self-help organizations for general advice and support. Each ostomy type has its own organization with publications, local meetings and visitors who can identify with the patient's problems.

Stoma appliance manufacturers. The appliance manufacturers produce both product-specific and general literature for health-care professionals and also advisory booklets for patients and can prove an invaluable source of information.

AIDS FOR URINARY INCONTINENCE

Incontinence in its various forms is a common problem. Because of the perceived social stigma many sufferers deny themselves access to treatment. The pharmacist may be able to identify possible sufferers and to provide confidential and discrete help.

Types of urinary incontinence

Overflow (or dribble) incontinence

In this condition the bladder leaks constantly as a result of an obstruction of the urethra or because of a neurological deficiency.

Stress incontinence

This is more common in females as a result of relaxation of the pelvic floor muscles due to childbirth or ageing. The result is a leakage of urine on exertion or straining, e.g. coughing, sneezing, laughing or hurrying.

Urge incontinence

Insufficient warning of an urgent need to void urine results in this type of incontinence. In the elderly or disabled, a reduction in mobility and manual dexterity compounds the problem.

Neurogenic bladder

Dysfunction of the bladder may result from abnormality, injury or disease of the brain, spinal cord or local nerve supply to the bladder. Patients affected include those with spina bifida, paraplegia and quadriplegia, multiple sclerosis and stroke.

Types of incontinence appliance

The type of appliance selected depends on the type of incontinence experienced, devices suitable for dribble incontinence would not cope with sudden voiding of large volumes. The sex of the patient is highly significant since most of the devices designed for use in the male are totally unsuitable for the female.

Drainable dribbling devices

These are suitable for men with very light overflow incontinence and consist of a small collecting bag held in place by leg straps and waist straps together with adhesive strips or tape.

Incontinence sheaths

These consist of a soft latex sleeve worn over the penis and held in place by adhesive. Urine, collected continuously, is channelled into a drainage bag to be emptied when necessary. The device may be left in place for 2 or 3 days although problems may arise because of allergy to the adhesive. The sheath is unsuitable for severely disturbed patients and users must have adequate eyesight and manual dexterity.

Urinal systems

These are complex body-worn systems which include a sheath retained in position by waist and groin straps. Specialist measuring and initial fitting is advisable.

Urethral catheters

These are tubes introduced into the bladder in order to withdraw urine and are of two types, indwelling and intermittent. The risk of urinary infection is increased by catheterization.

Indwelling catheters (Foley catheters) have a self-retaining balloon incorporated in the tip which is inflated after insertion into the bladder. Male and female versions are available and the outflow is collected in a drainage bag.

Intermittent catheterization may be used by patients to empty their own bladder several times daily and thus retain some 'control' over the process.

Suprapubic catheters

These are inserted into the bladder via the abdominal wall and are associated with less urinary infection than urethral catheters. Once the entry channel is established, the catheter can be changed by a nurse in the home. The outflow is collected in drainage bags.

Drainage bags

Leg bags. These are worn on the leg and may be attached at various positions and by various mechanisms to suit the patient. They are used to collect the urine from incontinence sheaths and from indwelling catheters in either sex.

Suspensory systems. These are drainage bags carried by a waist support which allows a greater weight to be accumulated before emptying than do the leg supports. They are also more discrete for female patients.

Night drainage bags. These provide a greater capacity for night-time collection of urine and may be connected via the usual daytime system or directly to the catheter or incontinence sheath.

Accessories

A number of accessory products are available for use with the appliances described above. These include tubing, connectors, incontinence belts and incontinence sheath adhesives and fixing strips. Pharmacists should check that all accessories are compatible, e.g. same tubing connection, and also, for NHS prescriptions, that the item is listed in the current Drug Tariff. Some of the products described under stoma care, adhesives, deodorants, etc. may also be of value to incontinence sufferers.

Absorption products

A wide range of absorption items are available for sale by the pharmacist but this type of product is not available on prescription. Items include pads with or without waterproof backing, and pants with pouches and with integral washable pads. Product literature can be obtained from the manufacturers and from organizations concerned with the welfare of the disabled.

The role of the pharmacist

Urinary incontinence is a symptom which may present in a variety of forms requiring different approaches to treatment. A discrete display of incontinence aids together with information leaflets and the offer of confidential advice may encourage patients to seek help from the pharmacist in the community. In some cases surgical correction of anatomical problems may be possible, e.g. an enlarged prostate gland. The treatment of chronic infection may help, as may re-training exercises for the bladder or pelvic floor exercises. Anticholinergic drugs may benefit some patients if the side-effects are tolerated. Sufferers should be advised to seek medical help and reassured that, should complete resolution of the problem not prove possible, a variety of aids are available to enable them to cope.

BIBLIOGRAPHY

British National Formulary 1988 16th edn. British Medical Association and Royal Pharmaceutical Society of Great Britain, London (updated twice yearly)
Brown D 1988 Incontinence aids: (1) prescription items. Pharmaceutical Journal 240: 247–249
Brown D 1988 Incontinence aids: (2) OTC items. Pharmaceutical Journal 240: 440–442

Drug Tariff current edition HMSO, London (updated monthly)
NPA Guide to the Drug Tariff 1987/88 National Pharmaceutical Association, St Albans
Norton C 1988 Catheters and aids for urinary incontinence. Pharmacy Update 4: 315–317
Watkins D K 1987 Ostomy care and the pharmacist. Pharmaceutical Journal 238: 68–71

36. Medical gases

D. M. Collett

A number of substances in the gaseous state are administered by inhalation to achieve therapeutic effects, i.e. anaesthesia, analgesia, stimulation and maintenance of respiration and oxygen therapy (Table 36.1).

Medical gases are usually packed in metal cylinders designed to withstand pressures significantly greater than the gases contained under pressure within. Cylinders should be stored, handled and used in accordance with a strict code of practice prepared by the British Standards Institution (BS 1319) in order to minimize any risks associated with their use.

Since the cylinders are similar in appearance each type of gas is given a colour coding (Table 36.2) for ready identification. The cylinders also bear the chemical symbol or name of the gas.

In hospitals, medical gases may be distributed by pipeline to wards and theatres from a central store. The pharmacist generally accepts responsibility together with other hospital personnel for the provision of medical

Table 36.1 Medical gases and their uses

Carbon dioxide (CO_2)	5–7% mixture in oxygen is used to induce or improve respiration
Cyclopropane (C_3H_6)	Potent gaseous anaesthetic
Helium (He)	More diffusible than air. 1 vol. He + 2 vol. air or 21 vol. O_2 + 79 vol. He is used to aid patients with respiratory difficulties
Nitrous oxide (N_2O)	Gaseous anaesthetic. 50% mixture with O_2 is used as obstetric analgesic
Oxygen (O_2)	Used to treat hypoxaemia of various causes At sea level maximum concentration is 60% in inspired air For chronic obstructive airways disease, maximum 24–28% advisable.

Table 36.2 Medical gases cylinder colour codes

Gas	Colour	State in cylinder
Carbon dioxide	Grey	Liquid
Cyclopropane	Orange	Liquid
Helium	Brown	Gas
Nitrous oxide	Blue	Liquid
Oxygen	Black body, white top	Gas
Oxygen/carbon dioxide	Black body, grey and white top*	Gas
Oxygen/helium	Black body, brown and white top*	Gas
Oxygen 50%/nitrous oxide 50%	Blue body, blue and white top*	Gas

* In four equal segments, two of each colour

gases within the hospital and will operate within strict local and national guidelines.

Domiciliary oxygen therapy may be prescribed for patients requiring intermittent or long-term oxygen therapy and an oxygen cylinder service is provided by pharmacists in the community.

OXYGEN THERAPY

Benefits and risks of oxygen therapy

The value of increasing the oxygen concentration in the inspired air of patients with obstructive lung disease is to reduce the effort of breathing necessary to achieve a given degree of oxygenation and to relieve respiratory distress. In the long term the survival time of patients with advanced bronchitis and emphysema may be increased by oxygen therapy.

However, a distinction must be made between patients suffering from hypoxia (lack of oxygen) and those suffering from hypoxia with hypercapnia (lack of oxygen with retention of carbon dioxide).

In the normal subject, respiration is stimulated by the accumulation of carbon dioxide (hypercapnia) but in patients with longstanding disease causing chronic hypercapnia, the respiratory centre may become insensitive to carbon dioxide accumulation. In such patients respiration is driven by hypoxia and the administration of high concentrations of oxygen will depress this hypoxic drive and may lead to respiratory failure.

The aim of therapy is therefore to administer sufficient oxygen to relieve respiratory distress without inducing respiratory failure. In order to minimize the risks of administering too high a concentration of oxygen in the home, domiciliary apparatus is designed to deliver a maximum concentration of 28% oxygen in inspired air, although for some patients a concentration above 24% may be excessive. Ideally the appropriate concentration should be determined in hospital where blood gas analysis is available before domiciliary treatment is initiated.

Patients and their relatives should be made aware of the fire risks resulting from oxygen therapy and should be discouraged from smoking for medical as well as safety reasons.

Domiciliary oxygen therapy

Some patients with acute or chronic respiratory diseases causing hypoxaemia may be given oxygen therapy at home.

Intermittent oxygen therapy

The requirement for oxygen may be intermittent, e.g. for asthmatic patients during an acute attack. Patients with advanced irreversible airways obstruction may benefit from administration prior to and after exercise to improve mobility and quality of life. Such patients are usually supplied with oxygen in cylinders.

Long-term oxygen therapy (LTOT)

Other patients with chronic severe obstructive airways disease may require almost continuous oxygen therapy (at least 15 hours per day) in order to prolong survival or to relieve distress in terminal lung disease. For these patients a *concentrator* (see later in this chapter) is the preferred source of oxygen.

THE ROLE OF THE PHARMACY OXYGEN CONTRACTOR

The supply of oxygen cylinders to NHS patients in the community is provided from pharmacies on the Family Practitioner Committee (FPC) list of approved contractors. The pharmacist receives remuneration to stock and supply on loan the appropriate equipment (cylinders, head sets, masks and cylinder stands). Only the equipment listed in the Drug Tariff (Part X) is available for supply to NHS patients at home and is prescribed by the patient's general practitioner on FP10 prescription forms (see Appendix 2). The patient's representative should be responsible for collection of replacement cylinders if possible, although the pharmacist would normally undertake the first supply in order to set up the equipment and to counsel the patient or the carer in the appropriate and safe use of the apparatus. In many cases the patient is unable to arrange for transport of cylinders and the pharmacist will continue to collect and deliver equipment for the appropriate remuneration. This contact with the patient allows the pharmacist the opportunity to ensure that the equipment continues to be used as prescribed and also to offer advice on other medication the patient may be taking.

When the patient's requirement for the oxygen therapy ceases either because of recovery or death the equipment should be returned to the pharmacy or collected by the pharmacist when notified.

Equipment supplied on loan from the pharmacy

Cylinders

Oxygen BP for domiciliary use is usually supplied in 1360 litre (48 ft^2) quantities, although smaller sizes of cylinder may be supplied if specifically prescribed. For some patients smaller 'portable' cylinders may be more appropriate but these must be prescribed by size, i.e. 170 litre (36 gal) and not by reference to 'portability'. The older heavy steel cylinders require the support of a cylinder stand which is also supplied by the pharmacist in the interests of safety unless an alternative form of securing the cylinder is available. The lighter cylinders do not normally required additional support.

Oxygen sets (headsets)

The headsets that may be supplied on NHS prescription are lightweight, single-unit sets. Two specifications are described in detail and illustrated in the Drug Tariff. Essentially, the control head comprises a valve which reduces the gas cylinder pressure, a contents (pressure) gauge, a flow rate selection device and an outlet carrying the male side of a bayonet connection. The head is fitted with a standard bull-nosed cylinder adaptor designed for finger tightening and incorporating a neoprene O-ring washer. Although spare washers are provided with the set it is recommended that these are replaced only by the pharmacist and that the patient is discouraged from attempting any modification to the apparatus. A key spanner to open the cylinder valve and tubing to connect the outlet to the mask are packaged with the headset.

Oxygen masks

Masks supplied for domiciliary oxygen therapy are of two types, constant performance and variable performance. One constant performance-type mask is supplied as part of each complete headset pack. Masks are considered to be disposable, i.e. returned masks are not re-issued to another patient, but the mask may be used by an individual patient for several months.

Constant-performance masks

Two constant-performance masks, the Ventimask Mk IV 28% and the Intersurgical 010 Mask 28%, are described and illustrated in the Drug Tariff. These are designed to deliver a concentration of oxygen in air of 28% over a wide range of settings and irrespective of variation in breathing patterns. For patients with chronic obstructive airways disease (described above) the 28% maximum concentration reduces the danger of removing the hypoxic drive and causing fatal carbon dioxide narcosis. Nevertheless, patients and their carers should be advised to seek medical help if unusual drowsiness or confusion occurs. The appropriate flow rate for this type of mask is 2 litres per minute (the medium setting on the control head).

Variable-performance masks

These are designed to allow the delivery of higher concentrations of oxygen to patients with acute conditions and a previously healthy respiratory system.

The medium head setting (2 litres per minute) provides 25–30% oxygen and the high setting (4 litres per minute) provides up to 40% oxygen. The actual concentration will vary with the patient's breathing pattern. It must be emphasized that such concentrations in a patient with chronic obstructive airways disease could be fatal. Two variable performance masks, the Intersurgical 005 Mask and the MC Mask, are described and illustrated in the Drug Tariff.

Oxygen concentrator therapy

An oxygen concentrator is a device which removes nitrogen and some other gases from atmospheric air and delivers oxygen-enriched gases to the user. A small electric compressor is used to draw air through a series of filters and then over zeolite molecular sieve beds to remove nitrogen. The separation of the gases depends on the differences in molecular diameter of oxygen and nitrogen and their relative speeds of passage through the sieve bed. Two columns of molecular sieves are included within each concentrator and the flow is constantly switched between the two so that one is operating while the other is being regenerated. The product of the concentrator is a mixture of 95% oxygen with 5% argon which has a similar molecular size and passes at the same rate as oxygen. The argon has not been shown to produce any adverse effects in patients using concentrator generated oxygen.

For patients requiring long-term oxygen therapy (LTOT), an oxygen concentrator may provide a cheaper and more convenient source of therapy than oxygen from cylinders.

Those patients for whom concentrator therapy is considered to be appropriate are those receiving oxygen for 15 hours a day over a long period or requiring the equivalent of 21 cylinders or more per month. In no circumstances should concentrators be considered for patients using oxygen for less that 8 hours per day. The use of oxygen for such long periods requires a considerable amount of commitment to compliance on the part of the patient and this should be assessed before the concentrator is prescribed.

Oxygen concentrators may be prescribed on NHS prescription forms and are distributed by selected local suppliers. They are not supplied through pharmacies. The patient is also supplied with either a nasal cannula or variable-performance face-mask and a humidifier if required. (Constant-performance face-masks are not designed to operate with concentrators.) Installation of a concentrator is carried out by an engineer provided by the supplier and an outflow is usually provided at two separate outlet points to provide a daytime and night-time supply.

The advantages of the concentrator for the patient include greater mobility around the home, the opportunity to eat and talk while therapy is delivered through a nasal cannula and freedom from anxiety about cylinder supplies. In some cases a back-up supply of oxygen cylinders is considered appropriate but this too is provided by the concentrator supplier and only exceptionally from a pharmacy.

BIBLIOGRAPHY

Axon S 1987 Providing an oxygen service. Pharmaceutical
Journal 239: 733–734
BOC Ltd 1981 Medical gases. Gases Division, BOC Ltd,
Guildford
BOC Ltd 1988 Guide to the safe use of medical gas
cylinders. Gases Division, BOC Ltd, Guildford
British National Formulary 1988 16th edn. British Medical
Association and Royal Pharmaceutical Society of Great
Britain, London (updated twice yearly)

British Pharmacopoeia 1988 HMSO, London
Drug Tariff current edition HMSO, London (updated
monthly)
NPA Guide to the Drug Tariff 1987/88 National
Pharmaceutical Association, St Albans
O'Sullivan J 1988 Oxygen concentrators. British Journal of
Pharmaceutical Practice 10: 395–400
Rose G 1987 Oxygen concentrators in the home.
Pharmaceutical Journal 239: 776–777

PART 6

Relating to the patient

37. Patient compliance and counselling

M. H. Jepson

Introduction

It will be apparent from other chapters of this book that the essential role of the practising pharmacist, especially in community and hospital pharmacy, includes far more than the accurate distribution of medicinal products correctly labelled. Appropriate advice and counselling by the pharmacist can encourage patient compliance through a better understanding by the patient of their medication, thereby improving therapeutic efficacy and the patient's well-being.

Patient compliance or adherence may be defined as the extent to which a patient takes or uses their medication, in accordance with the medical or health advice given. The person's behaviour, and acceptance of associated dietary or lifestyle factors may often be involved. However, the definition is intended to be neutral in not implying fault where there is non-compliance.

Non-compliance from the doctor's point of view may extend to the failure to keep an appointment and non-participation in a screening programme which may relate back to a patient's behaviour and acceptance of health-care advice.

Patient compliance from the pharmacist's point of view is largely dependent upon the communication of information necessary for the correct use of medication in association with supportive advice or counselling.

Communication may be defined as the means by which information is passed from a sender to a receiver. It is important to ensure that the information received (and understood) is the same as that sent.

Counselling often involves the giving of advice and making certain that the advice is understood after listening sympathetically to the patient's doubts, problems or viewpoint. A suitable environment is very important for effective counselling.

PATIENT COMPLIANCE

Compliance and the extent of non-compliance

An examination of compliance rates derived from a number of studies (Sackett and Snow 1979), summarized in Table 37.1, shows great variation from which it must be inferred that it is most unwise to generalize about the reasons for non-compliance.

The wide range of compliance rate for a particular situation may be partly explained. Although the compliance in keeping appointments for disease screening initiated by health professionals is often below 50%, it rises markedly where children are involved. Where the appointment is initiated by the patient for treatment, compliance again rises.

Patients on short-term medication tend to show greater compliance than those on long-term therapy, as might be expected. In a study of over 2300 men in Sweden (Hedstrand and Aberg 1976) surveyed for hypertension, the rate of compliance, i.e. remaining in

Table 37.1 Patient compliance rates

Compliance in	Compliance rate
Keeping appointments for disease screening	10–65% (8 studies)
Keeping appointments for treatment	55–84% (7 studies)
Short-term medication for illness prevention (immunization)	60–64% (2 studies)
Short-term medication for treatment or cure	77–78% (2 studies)
Long-term medication for illness prevention	33–94% (15 studies)
Long-term medication for treatment or cure	41–69% (8 studies)

(Source: Sackett and Snow 1979)

care and on therapy, after a 3-year period fell from 94% at the end of the first year to 34% at the end of the third year. The rates of compliance with different long-term medication for different illnesses in different situations seems to approximate to 50%.

However, average rates of compliance can also be very misleading and Gordis et al (1969) has shown that children on long-term oral penicillin prophylactic treatment for rheumatic fever can be subdivided into three groups; one-third take almost all the medication, one-third of the patients take almost no medication and the remaining third are scattered in between. This is not a normal distribution and although other studies have reported similar results it remains to be seen whether or not this distribution can be claimed to represent a general pattern for medication compliance.

Compliance and patient perceptions

As indicated in the previous section, compliance is subject to great variation as well as to many variables. Research has not identified one general specific cause for non-compliance, nor does it seem possible to identify a special type of patient who lacks compliance (Stimson 1974). Importantly, the active participation of the patient in his own treatment can be influenced by factors which either inhibit and limit or enhance and promote compliance.

Among *inhibiting factors* are: (a) personal characteristics, such as overdependency or despair, and (b) social and cultural factors, such as illness as an excuse, or fatalism.

Limiting factors overlap with inhibiting factors, and include: length of illness; social isolation; poverty; lack of appliances; anxiety and wrong information.

The key factor to promoting the patient's participation in his/her own treatment is *motivation*. As is to be expected most of the *promoting factors* are the opposite to those with inhibit or limit. The way in which the patient perceives the meaning and purpose of life and his/her resulting lifestyle are most important influences. The acceptance of being ill or handicapped or disabled, former experience of illness, and attitude are characteristics which encourage the patient to take part actively in his/her own treatment.

In practical terms, the pharmacist may find that non-compliance is directly related to or affected by one or more of the following:

1. Difficulty in keeping to dosage regimen because of lifestyle. For example, liquid medicines may not be as easily taken in some work situations as a tablet. Many patients find it easier to remember to take medicines at mealtimes than say an hour beforehand. If remembered later, the patient may be inhibited from taking that particular dose at all.

2. The drug regimen is too complex and not properly understood. A classic example is illustrated below:

PREDNISOLONE REDUCING DOSAGE SCHEDULE.
GEORGINA ALLEN
On days 1 to 5, take TWO tablets from bottle A morning and night, then from days 6 to 10, take TWO tablets in the morning and ONE at night from bottle A, then from days 11 to 15, take TWO in the morning from bottle A. Do not take any tablets from bottle B on days 1 to 5, then on day 6 take FOUR at night with tablet from bottle A, then on day 7 take THREE at night from bottle B, TWO at night on day 8 from bottle B, ONE at night on day 9, and no tablets from bottle B on day 10. On day 11 start again with FOUR tablets from bottle B, THREE tablets from bottle B on day 12, TWO tablets from bottle B on day 13, ONE tablet from bottle B on day 14 and no tablet from bottle B on day 15.

Bottle A contains prednisolone 5 mg tablets and bottle B contains prednisolone 1 mg tablets. Thus on days 1–5, a total of 20 mg prednisolone is to be taken, 19 mg total on day 6, 18 mg total on day 7, 17 mg on day 8, 16 mg on day 9, 15 mg on day 10, 14 mg on day 11, 13 mg on day 12, 12 mg on day 13, 11 mg on day 14 and 10 mg on day 15.

The patient, aged 79, has haemolytic anaemia induced by methyldopa, and this is the reason for this treatment. She also has Parkinsonian tremor, and hypertension and mild congestive failure for which she is taking six other drugs. It is hardly surprising if there is a compliance problem. A steroid-reducing dosage schedule like this, intended to allow the adrenal cortex to normalize, is enough to daunt the most alert and intelligent.

This example also illustrates another common contributor to non-compliance, namely that of multi-drug therapy. It has been frequently shown that patients taking three or more drugs concurrently, tend to have compliance problems.

What action might the pharmacist take in a situation such as that above? He/she may be able to design a chart to help the patient who is required to take up to 17 tablets a day. If the patient is not living alone, it may be possible to recruit a member of the family to help with the medication schedule. Different types of container for different tablets or capsules may be helpful too.

However, in this particular case it would be sensible to refer to the prescriber and discuss just how critical the reducing dose steps are likely to be. Many clinicians for example, consider it satisfactory to reduce the dose of prednisolone by 5 mg every 5–7 days down to 5 mg daily, which should then be reduced slowly and which will result in a much simpler reducing dosage schedule. The importance of active communication between pharmacist and prescriber, pharmacist and patient should be obvious.

3. A lack of confidence in either prescriber or medication.

4. The influence of incorrect and conflicting information or ideas supplied by the patient's family, relatives and friends about either the medication or condition being treated, or both.

Child-resistant containers

Child-resistant containers seem to have contributed often unnecessarily to non-compliance. During the decade in which child-resistant closures and containers (see Ch. 8) have been available, patients, especially among the elderly, have had problems in opening containers fitted with child-resistant closures. Disappointingly, many more people have experienced difficulty than need have done. Some studies have shown that even among the elderly, including those with mild or moderate arthritis, providing the patient is properly shown by demonstration followed by the pharmacist's supervision, the vast majority of patients and customers can open and effectively reclose the three common types of child-resistant containers currently available. It has to be admitted that further counselling may be necessary in order to persuade some patients that such containers are desirable and have contributed significantly to the improvement in child mortality figures due to accidental poisoning.

Compliance and the pharmacists' contribution

Dame Cecily Saunders, Founder of the Hospice Movement, on the subject of pain relief said: 'It is the intelligence with which you give it — not the drug that counts — it equals compassionate competence.'

As the involvement of the pharmacist in the primary health care team is increasingly recognized, the importance of communication with the patient cannot be over-emphasized. The right information at the right level is the most important constructive influence on compliance which the pharmacist can make. Information which should be considered as important by the pharmacist to convey to the patient includes:

a. The pharmaceutical form of the medicine and its identity.
b. The intended use and expected action.
c. The method of use.
d. The dosage or amount to be used.
e. The frequency and correct time(s) of administration or use (administrative schedule).
f. The maximum dose in 24 hours.
g. The duration of treatment.
h. Side-effects to be minimized by the patient.
i. Side-effects to be referred to the doctor.
j. Medicines, food or activities the patient has to avoid during treatment.
k. Action to be taken in the event of a missed dose.
l. The storage of medication.
m. The discarding of unused medicine beyond a specified 'expiry' date.
n. The arrangement for further supplies and, where the pharmacist is counter-prescribing or responding to symptoms described by a patient.
o. The aim of the treatment.

This last point should be considered with caution in regard to prescribed medication as it is then primarily a professional matter between prescriber and patient. Patient confidentiality, as well as the patient's confidence in the prescriber, must be respected and not impaired. The pharmacist must be selective both with the extent of the information conveyed, the order and the method used as will be made more apparent later in this chapter.

It would thus be usually inappropriate to counsel or advise a patient on all the headings listed which can cover information at least as diverse as that in a product data sheet. The attention, understanding and memory of most patients would soon be overstretched, unfounded anxieties might be aroused and the time required be considerable and impractical.

What is essential, is for the pharmacist to ensure that the patient knows and understands sufficient for the effective and safe use of the medicine supplied. The pharmacist who is able to develop a rapport with customers and patients who regularly come to the pharmacy, who can establish in the minds of customers and patients, professional confidence in a stable and familiar and unthreatening environment, has the opportunity to contribute increasingly to the user's confidence in the medication supplied.

COMMUNICATION

Fletcher (1973) has identified the following characteristics of successful communication:

1. The purpose of communication is not just to deliver a message but to effect a change in the recipient, in respect of his knowledge his attitude and eventually his behaviour.

2. The value of communication is to be judged not on its purpose or content, but on its effect on the recipient.

3. Good communication is difficult.

4. Communication must be matched to the knowledge, social background, interest, purposes and needs of the recipient.

5. Communication is effected not only by words, which must have the same meaning for giver and receiver, but also by attitudes, expressions and gestures.

6. If communication is to change behaviour, the required change in the recipient must be seen by him to have more advantages than drawbacks.

7. To make sure that communication has succeeded, information about its effect ('feedback'), both immediate and subsequent, is needed.

8. Communication demands effort, thought, time and often money.

If these characteristics of successful communication are achieved, the extent of non-compliance can be influenced and reduced.

Much work has been done and ingenuity used to support verbal communication and medicine labels. One manufacturer (Warner-Lambert) has made generally available braille labels for blind patients reproducing simple directions like 'one to be taken three times a day' on semi-rigid plastic strips approximately 107 mm × 29 mm. The braille markings are superimposed over large print lettering which may be sufficiently clear for partially sighted patients. Leaflets, both product specific and to help patients to know how to use particular forms of medication presentation, e.g. eye ointments or nasal drops, have been devised. The design of special treatment packs, calendar packs and medication dose compartment aids, suitably labelled, have all been aimed at stimulating patient motivation to try to improve compliance through a better understanding by the patient of their own treatment.

Additional information on leaflets

Why leaflets? Leaflets have a place in the communication of information to patients which is too detailed to include on the medicine label, whether dispensed or sold.

Many leaflets include illustrations which may be especially helpful and easier to comprehend by the poorly sighted and those with a literacy or language difficulty. The physical dimensions of many containers are insufficient to allow such information as is necessary to be affixed to the surface in a size which is easily read. The leaflet should not be seen as an alternative to either a label or to oral advice but rather as complementary and at best a very useful supplement to these essential and main means of communication. The advantages of leaflets are mainly to do with the less restrictive space limits than those of a label and associated ease of readability and illustration potential. They are also more permanent than the spoken word and can referred to later by the patient or product user. Their main disadvantages are obvious, a leaflet can become detached from the product to which it applies and unlike verbal advice it is not interactive, or in computer jargon 'user-friendly'.

A wide variety of leaflets have been produced mainly by manufacturers of proprietary products principally as package inserts for the information of users. In packages of prescription medicines these were often written for the prescriber or pharmacist and included data sheet style information but including some information relevant to patient use. For bulk dispensing packs some manufacturers have produced pads of leaflets written specifically for patient guidance and information. Unfortunately there is no co-ordination between manufacturers of similar products in the design and continuing availability of useful information leaflets of this type.

The most satisfactory of the leaflets of the patient package insert (PPI) type are supplied with unit pack items, such as pressurized inhalers. They are usually very well produced, often with some colour printing and frequently include step-by-step graphic illustrations to aid comprehension. It is nevertheless very important for the pharmacist to have studied such leaflets prior to giving medicines out to patients and for him/her to be in a position to go through the salient points of the leaflets with surety and to ensure that the patient understands their medication, especially when supplied for the first time. It has been found in some cases that this type of leaflet is far too detailed to be meaningful to some patients, especially the elderly, without careful detailing by the pharmacist. Either the patient has forgotten what was written at the start of the leaflet by the time the end of the leaflet has been reached, or the patient 'switches off' before reaching the end. In practice, it has been found that a limit of five or six main points summarized on a leaflet achieves the maximum effect. The example shown in Figure 37.1 has been found to be useful for pressure-pack inhalers and often complements the manufacturer's leaflet. The single illustration on the

NOTES FOR THE PATIENT

HOW TO USE THE INHALER:

To get the maximum benefit from your inhaler, make sure that you follow these simple instructions:-

(1)   Always shake the inhaler before use.

(2)   Breathe out as fully as you can just before placing the mouthpiece in position.

(3)   Tilt your head back slightly so that the medication ends up in your lungs, *NOT* your mouth.

(4)   Now suck in air (if your inhaler is the pressurized type, you should spray it *at the same time*), and continue to inhale so that the medication is taken deep into your lungs.

(5)   Hold your breath for as long as possible then breathe out slowly.

It may help to first go through this procedure, without activating the inhaler, until you feel confident about it.

Always make sure that the inhaler is thoroughly dry before and dried after use. The mouthpiece may be detached and washed after use but *DRY THOROUGHLY*

KEEP ALL MEDICINES OUT OF THE REACH
OF CHILDREN

Pharmacy Practice Group
University of Aston in Birmingham ©8098

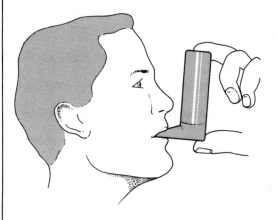

Fig. 37.1   Example of a simple leaflet intended to aid patient counselling. It is not intended as an alternative to a manufacturer's more detailed product-specific leaflet

back of the leaflet emphasizes the advantageous slight tilt back of the head and the 'upright' position of the pressure pack.

Leaflets intended to inform the patient or purchaser are mainly of two types:

1. Those which identify possible side-effects, foods or other medication which is contraindicated, dosage advice, warning about misuse, risks, storage, etc.

2. Those which attempt to ensure the proper and effective administration of a particular form of drug presentation, e.g. suppositories or eye ointment.

A number of investigations have studied the need for, and the format, wording and range of such leaflets, in an attempt to effect some degree of standardization and even rationalization of patient advise leaflets. Too many variations or a different pad of leaflets for each dispensary medicine would create problems. The Royal Pharmaceutical Society's treatment card, produced

jointly with the British Medical Association for patients on monoamine oxidase inhibitor (MAOI) drugs, and the Society's treatment card for patients on oral anticoagulant therapy have each fulfilled an important need. Mr Roland Moyle (1977), then the Minister of Health, said

The Medicines Commission has stressed the importance of written information to patients to supplement oral advice from the doctor and pharmacist and to remind the patient on how to take the medicine and on actions to avoid. Warning cards and leaflets issued by pharmacists when appropriate are an important means of communication and will continue to be so even when unitpack dispensing becomes the rule rather than the exception.

In the UK, 'actions to avoid' have been mainly accommodated by the development of a range of 29 'Cautionary and Advisory Labels for Dispensed medicines'. These are included in the British National Formulary and are described in Chapter 10 of this book.

Leaflet design and wording

Attention must be given when designing a leaflet to ensure that sentences are short and that technical 'jargon' is avoided. Phrases like 'one drop to be instilled into the conjunctival sac' are better replaced by 'put one drop in each eye'. The philosophy of the Plain English Campaign is relevant to more than just income tax and other official forms! Some words and phrases are more easily substituted than others. 'Thinly' may be considered to be more widely understood than 'sparingly' where the latter word is generally used in relation to the application of topical steroid creams and ointments. It is not, however, easy to find an entirely satisfactory word for 'discard' when giving advice about the disposal of an expired medicinal product. 'Do not use after . . .' is negative and does not discourage keeping the medicine while 'Throw away . . .' may be seen as an unfortunate choice of words.

Other design factors which should be considered are page and type size, line spacing, margins, contrast and colour, illustrations or graphics as well as, inevitably, cost. Type size variation and contrast can aid readability.

A current fallacy seems to exist that typewritten and machine-produced labels, as now required on all dis-

pensed medicines, have eliminated unreadable directions on labels. On the contrary there are too many labels produced with typeface lettering which is too small and/or too faint and is unnecessarily difficult to read or even actually unreadable by many elderly patients. Leaflets can be designed to avoid many of these problems.

Figure 37.2 illustrates the information which can be condensed onto a leaflet 105 mm × 150 mm (i.e. A6) with the text on the front and a simple illustration on the back. Other examples include the Royal Pharmaceutical Society's monoamine oxidase inhibitor (MAOI) card (Fig. 37.3) and their more elaborate anticoagulant treatment card (Fig. 37.4).

For those who may not speak, write or read English there are obvious additional difficulties. In many cases, patients with this disadvantage are accompanied to their doctor's surgery and later to the pharmacy by a family member who does understand English. Sometimes, however, it is a very young member of the family who has to act as interpreter and the quality of translation due to a child's inexperience may be less than satisfactory. Unfortunately some studies have shown that many elderly immigrants unable to speak any English are frequently also illiterate in their own language. In such

---

NOTES FOR THE PATIENT

HOW TO USE YOUR EYE OINTMENT

(1)   First wash hands and then gently clean the eyelids.

(2)   Next, gently pull the lower lid downwards, and direct your gaze upwards.

(3)   *Carefully* place a thin line of ointment along the inside of the lower eyelid. Avoid touching the eyelid with the tube nozzle if possible.

ILLUSTRATION OVERLEAF

(4)   Next close your eye, and move the eyeball from side to side. *Gentle* massage will also help to spread the ointment.

Initially your vision may be blurred, but will soon be cleared by blinking. *DO NOT RUB THE EYE AT THIS STAGE*

Be sure to complete the course of the treatment as directed.

Do not share the eye ointment with anyone else.

Store in a cool dark place

KEEP ALL MEDICINES OUT OF THE REACH OF CHILDREN

Pharmacy Practice Group
University of Aston in Birmingham © 8093

How to use your Eye Ointment

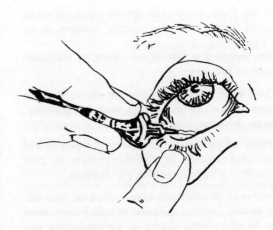

Fig. 37.2   Patient information leaflet

TREATMENT CARD

Carry this card with you at all times. Show it to any doctor who may treat you other than the doctor who prescribed this medicine, and to your dentist if you require dental treatment.

INSTRUCTIONS TO PATIENTS
Please read carefully
While taking this medicine and for 14 days after your treatment finishes you must observe the following simple instructions:-

1 Do not eat CHEESE, PICKLED HERRING OR BROAD BEAN PODS.

2 Do not eat or drink BOVRIL, OXO, MARMITE or ANY SIMILAR MEAT OR YEAST EXTRACT.

3 Do not take any other MEDICINES (including tablets, capsules, nose drops, inhalations or suppositories) whethar purchased by you or previously prescribed by your doctor, without first consulting your doctor or your pharmacist.

  NB *Treatment for coughs and colds, pain relievers, tonics and laxatives are medicines.*

4 Drink ALCOHOL only in moderation and avoid CHIANTI WINE completely.

  Keep a careful note of any food or drink that disagrees with you, avoid it and tell your doctor.

Report any unusual or severe symptoms to your doctor and follow any other advice given by him.

| M.A.O.I. | Prepared by The Pharmaceutical Society and the British Medical |

Association on behalf of the Health Departments of the United Kingdom.

Fig. 37.3 MAOI Treatment Card

cases the otherwise excellent multilanguage leaflets produced by some pharmaceutical companies (Fig. 37.5) and by some health authorities may be of little value and the pharmacist must be alert to ensure that some alternate means is used to ensure that the patient is not left in ignorance about his or her medicine and its regimen.

It must however be re-emphasized that only if the content of a leaflet or warning card is drawn to the attention of the patient by the pharmacist, is the information likely to be of most effect.

Mechanical compliance aids

For difficult cases of non-compliance often aggravated by forgetfulness, especially in the elderly, the community or hospital pharmacist may find it helpful to introduce the patient to one of the special medicine packaging devices now available. These compliance aids vary considerably in the sophistication of their design and cost.

A simple plastics extrusion with four compartments in line, labelled for example: 'morning', 'noon', 'evening' and 'night' with a transparent sliding lid top with space for the pharmacist to insert the patient's individual label is available (Beehive Industries, Watford).

Other aids which have been the subject in some cases of published research assessment include:

1. The 'Dosett' dispensing device (Astra Pharmaceuticals) consists of four compartments per day, with 7 days' capacity on the one tray. Braille markings to help blind patients are included.

2. The 'Medidos' device (Age Concern, England) consists of a separate tray, with adjustable divisions, for each day. The daily trays fit into a plastic wallet designed to take either a week's supply or enough for a weekend. The latter is particularly useful for mental hospital patients who are able to go home at weekends.

3. The 'Ezydose' devise (Pharmaceutical Packaging) consists of a compact seven-sided, seven-compartment 'pill minder', with just one compartment per day.

A number of other devices available are generally more applicable where an elderly infirm patient is visited regularly by a community nurse who can prepare the patient's medication on a labelled tray which may include liquid medicines already measured out in dispensing cups. Such cups, complete with lids, are available in different colours and capacities from several sources.

Warning

Pharmacists should exercise professional judgement when supplying mechanical compliance aids or counselling patients in their use. Although the devices may be of considerable benefit, a number of problems may arise. The device may not provide adequate protection from the environment or from access by children. Medicines may not legally be dispensed into daily dose reminders unless the labelling regulations can be fulfilled (see Ch. 10). Whoever is responsible for transferring medicines from the dispensed container into the compliance aid should be reliable and competent.

Family support

Where it is possible to involve, the support of other members of a patient's family who can give encouragement, improve understanding and, if necessary, supervise the taking or using of medication, compliance will invariably improve, at least in the short term. Such involvement is most helpful and virtually essential where compliance aids such as those described above require regular refilling.

Communication — summary

To use a medicine effectively and safely the patient needs certain basic information:

a. How and when to take/use the medicine.
b. How much to take/use.

ADVICE FOR PATIENTS ON ANTICOAGULANT TREATMENT

Always carry this card with you and show it to your doctor or dentist when obtaining treatment. Show it to your pharmacist when you are having a prescription dispensed and when purchasing medicines. As the pharmacist can advise you, it is in your own interest that you purchase all medicines from a pharmacy. Also show it to anyone giving treatment which may result in bleeding.

NAME OF YOUR ANTICOAGULANT

adjusts your anticoagulant dose. Aspirin may be an ingredient of other medicines, so when purchasing medicines always tell the pharmacist that you are taking an anticoagulant. Some other medicines may also interfere with the action of your anticoagulant so when you see the doctor who adjusts your anticoagulant dose always tell him about any new treatments or medicines and mention any changes, even a change of dose. If you have any doubts about your medicines ask the pharmacist or doctor.

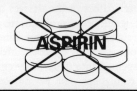

TREATMENT

The success of your treatment depends on your taking the correct dose of anticoagulant, which varies from person to person. The dose is decided by the clinic doctor after testing your blood.

TAKING YOUR TABLETS

Remember the name and strength of the anticoagulant you are taking and always take the correct dose. Take your tablet(s) at the same time(s) each day. If necessary, use a calendar and mark off each dose by a line through the date. In this way you will be unlikely to miss a dose.

Sun Mon Tue Wed Thu Fri Sat
1 2 3 4 5 6 7
8 9 10 11 12 13
15 16 17
22

Always make sure that you have at least a week's supply of tablets in hand so that you will not run short.

NEVER miss a dose; if you do, don't take a double dose to make up for it, but tell the clinic

BLOOD

Blood does not usually clot (coagulate) within the blood vessels. When this happens (and it may do so following illness or operation), anticoagulants are used to treat or prevent the condition by reducing the clotting power of the blood to safe levels.

FOOD AND ALCOHOL

Keep to your normal diet and do not make big changes. You may drink moderate amounts of alcohol; do not make big changes in your food and alcohol consumption.

PREGNANCY

Oral anticoagulants taken in the early weeks of pregnancy carry a small but proven risk of damaging the unborn child. If you are a woman of childbearing years receiving oral anticoagulants, you should not embark upon a pregnancy without consulting your doctor who will be able to decide whether or not you should discontinue the anticoagulant treatment. If you find that your period is two weeks overdue and you consider that you may

doctor when you next go for a blood test. If more than one dose is missed, contact your general practitioner as soon as you can for advice.

ILLNESS OR BLEEDING

In the event of illness, bleeding or apparent severe bruising, consult your general practioner immediately. If you consult another doctor who might not know that you are having anticoagulant treatment, you must tell him, especially if an operation is necessary. Always tell your dentist.

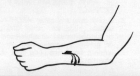

OTHER MEDICINES

Aspirin and some other pain relieving medicines affect the clotting power of blood. You should not take them unless they have been prescribed for you by the doctor who

be pregnant while taking anticoagulants, you should make an early appointment to see your doctor.

Published by the Pharmaceutical Society of Great Britain, 1 Lambeth High Street, London SE1 7JN. Printed July 1983.

The Society acknowledges the co-operation and sponsorship of Duncan Flockhart & Co. Ltd., Geigy Pharmaceuticals and WB Pharmaceuticals Ltd.

KEEP YOUR TABLETS IN A SAFE PLACE WELL OUT OF THE REACH OF CHILDREN

Fig. 37.4 Anticoagulant treatment card folds to 100 mm × 70 mm

c. How long to continue.

d. What to do if he/she forgets to take/use the medicine.

e. What to do if something goes wrong.

f. Is it safe to drive?

g. Is it safe to take alcoholic drink?

Additional information to that on the label conveyed orally by the pharmacist, supplemented by auxiliary labels and leaflets also explained by the pharmacist, will improve the patient's knowledge.

Information (patient education) and the patient's motivation will generally result in improved compliance.

COUNSELLING

This term has been used increasingly to describe the sympathetic interaction between pharmacist and patient, or customer, which may go beyond the conveying of straightforward information about the medication and how and when to use it.

Much greater attention is being paid to counselling and training for counselling, especially by the health-care professions. This is especially so since there has been a greater awareness of and attention given to holistic health, concerned as it is with the integrated health and well-being of the person as a whole. While there are

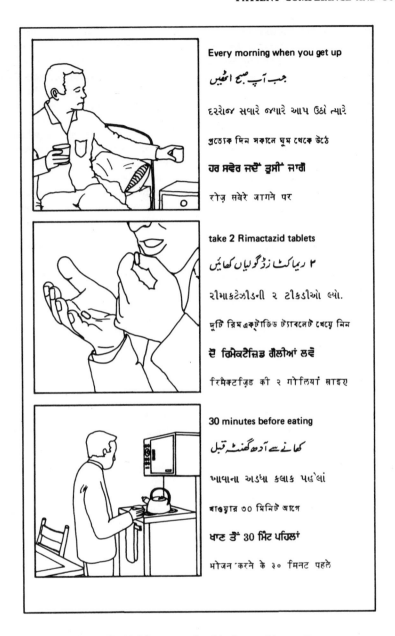

Fig. 37.5 Multilanguage visual leaflet to aid compliance

many forms of counselling it is generally a way of relating to a person in need of guidance, using understanding, sympathy and sincerity. Most counsellors are eclectic, drawing from different types of counselling such as 'behavioural' (which is concerned with modifying behaviours from the unacceptable to the acceptable) and 'humanistic' (which is more concerned with personal growth and human potential) (Murgatroyd 1983).

Although the pharmacist is often conscious how time-consuming successful counselling can be, even to establish an initial pharmacist–patient relationship, he/she must place sufficient emphasis upon watching and listening patiently to the patient.

Counselling may be described succinctly as helping people to help themselves. The importance of listening to and understanding the patient cannot be over-emphasized. Simple facts clearly expressed are fundamental to successful counselling.

'If pharmacists in community practice do not spend more time educating patients on the medication they are taking, they run a serious risk of becoming redundant in ten years time' (Clayton 1983). This may be something of an overstatement but with the advent of unit pack dispensing, the pharmacist has the opportunity to devote more time to communication and counselling which he should recognize as a professional priority.

It is generally accepted that pharmacists should not only advise both doctors and patients about prescribed medicines but monitor adverse drug reactions, consult with doctors about prescribing and dispensing procedures, advise members of the public about 'over-the-counter' (OTC) medicines and expand the primary health care role of giving advice to patients in response to the description of symptoms. Pharmacists may also contribute to health education, take part in diagnostic screening procedures and provide domiciliary pharmaceutical services. Counselling is the cornerstone of all these facets of the pharmacist's role when relating to the individual patient or customer.

At the present time, patient medication records (see Ch. 38) are not usually accessible to the community pharmacist in the UK and it has yet to become commonplace to build up patient prescription records either on file cards such as those available from the National Pharmaceutical Association (NPA) or on pharmacy labelling microcomputers. The pharmacist in this situation must be particularly cautious when giving advice. How much information a pharmacist should give to a patient requires particular tact when the pharmacist is confronted with the common prescription enquiry 'What is the medicine for?'. Not only has the pharmacist no access to the patient's medical notes but he does not know how much the patient has been told by his/her doctor. Confidence in the doctor must be preserved and it is usually wise to counter the question by a question such as 'what did your doctor say it was for?' or 'What did you go to the doctor for?'. From the answer it is often possible to reassure the patient and the opportunity is provided for the pharmacist to disseminate to the patient, receptive to receive, further advice on how and when to take or use their medication.

It must be emphasized again that usually for counselling to be most effective a rapport between pharmacist and patient needs to have had time to develop.

Patient education

It is generally considered that patient education is the most important variable affecting compliance. Information provided to the patient concerning medication must be understood. Faulty comprehension has been reported to contribute to some two-thirds of compliance problems (Ellis 1979). Where the medication has been prescribed, information provided by the pharmacist must reinforce and complement the prescriber's directions. According to Peterson (1981) most patients are only able to recall about a third of what has been told to them and it is recommended that when counselling the more important points should be given initially and finally as recall of interviewing items has been shown to be erratic (Warden-Flood 1984). Among factors which has been found to decrease effective interaction between patient and doctor and thus equally handicap counselling by a pharmacist are:

1. The patient is too fearful or nervous to ask questions.
2. The patient is unwilling to ask questions for fear of appearing ignorant.
3. The patient is confused by a spate of medical terminology or jargon.
4. The patient does not appreciate the importance of the information conveyed.
5. The doctor or pharmacist lacks the time or devotes insufficient time to explain instructions adequately to the patient.
6. The consultation is awkwardly terminated, for example by the prescriber writing a prescription or the pharmacist placing the medication in a bag and handing it to the patient.

The pharmacist has the opportunity and responsibility, where such deficiencies exist in the patient–doctor relationship, to ensure that the patient understands all immediately relevant information relating to the prescribed medication regimen. The pharmacist should use, as appropriate, suitable verbal, written or audiovisual communication techniques (as described previously) in order to inform, educate or reinforce the knowledge of the patient about his/her medication.

The effectiveness of patient counselling depends on many variables detailed below.

Environment

Space, furnishing, privacy and noise can be significant influences. Few community pharmacists in the UK presently, have a separate counselling room or booth. Many however do have a quiet end of a medicine counter or prescription reception point. Even a reduction in lighting at one end can convey an impression of greater privacy. The counter itself can be a serious barrier and inhibit the patient from being communicative or being receptive to information. It is often important to go round the end of the counter to talk privately. Alternatively, the dispensary may be more suitable for counselling discretely on such matters as the use of pessaries or suppositories.

Pharmacies which have established counselling facilities engender and experience a heightened awareness by the public of the pharmacist's professional contribution to primary health care.

Personal

To most people, a clean white lab. coat or uniform or smart business-like dress gives a professional image which helps to put the patient at ease and conveys confidence. It is important that the pharmacist can be distinguished from dispensing technicians and assistants. Name badges which include the word pharmacist and the official green cross symbol for pharmacy can be most helpful.

The pharmacist's behaviour will also subconsciously as well as consciously contribute to the ease and effectiveness of communication and counselling. An awareness of the non-verbal aspects of communication is very important to the work of the pharmacist as far as both perceiving signals from the patient and conveying appropriate signals back to the patient.

What are these non-verbal forms of communication? They include such factors as body contact, proximity, relative positioning, gestures, facial expressions, eye movement, posture, head movement and, as referred to above, appearance. Physical positioning is important, the pharmacist should be a comfortable distance from the patient, not too close so as to threaten him and not too far away to make a quiet conversation ineffective. The pharmacist's voice level should be kept low and personal. Avoid speaking down to the patient while at the same time trying to speak in a manner, and using a vocabulary, which will be understood. Eye contact is also important but should not be too excessive such that the patient feels both stared at and uncomfortable. Both verbal tics, for example, repeatedly saying 'you know' or 'OK' and physical tics, such as repeatedly scratching the nose or ear, should be avoided as they are irritating and distract the concentration of the patient.

The pharmacist should aim to be friendly (a smile helps), sincere and sympathetic. At least appear to have time and, most important of all, be willing to listen (Howells 1984). The major self-limiting factor determining whether and indeed how much patient counselling actually happens in practice in community pharmacy is time. With increasing emphasis on the counselling role, restructuring of the work load will be necessary to free the pharmacist for this important activity.

Counselling — summary

The pharmacist involved in counselling patients must both watch and listen carefully, paying attention to non-verbal aspects such as facial expression, posture and body movements. Any irrational fears about a treatment must be considered and preferably discussed before factual information is conveyed.

Counselling which is likely to influence compliance is generally helped by the continuity and quality of the patient–pharmacist relationship. It is often not realized that a quality relationship can be built up in a short time if sympathetic face-to-face contact occurs and an interest in and empathy for the patient exists.

BIBLIOGRAPHY

Bazire S 1984 An assessment of the 'Dosett' compliance aid in psychiatric patients. British Journal of Pharmaceutical Practice 6: 316–20

Clayton B 1983 Counsel or become redundant. Australian Journal of Pharmacy 64: 894

Ellis B 1979 Patient counselling by pharmacists. Proceedings of General Hospital Pharmacy 5: 1–42

European Public Health Committee Final Report 1980 The patient as an active participant in his own treatment. Council of Europe, Strasbourg

Evison R, Veitch G B A 1985 Towards effective communication. Pharmaceutical Journal 234: 833–836

Feetham C L, Kelly D 1982 An assessment of a new compliance aid: the 'Medidos'. British Journal of Pharmaceutical Practice 4: 5–12

Fletcher C M 1973 Communication in medicine. Nuffield Provincial Hospitals Trust, London

Gordis L, Markowitz M, Likenfeld A M 1969 Why patients don't follow medical advice: a study of children on long term antistreptococcal prophylaxis. Journal of Pediatrics 75: 957–968

Haynes R B, Taylor D W, Sackett D L (eds) 1979 Compliance in health care. John Hopkins University Press, Baltimore

Hedstrand H, Aberg H 1976 Treatment of hypertension in middle-aged men. Acta Medica Scandinavica 199: 281–288

Howells K 1984 Non-verbal communication — an introduction. Pharmaceutical Journal 233: 647–648

Jones I F 1985 Medicines for the elderly: dispensing and compliance. Pharmaceutical Journal 235: 516–518

Morrow N C, Hargie O D W 1985 Interpersonal communication. (1) Introduction. (2) Nonverbal & explaining skills. (3) Questioning skills. Pharmaceutical Update 1: 161–165, 206–210, 255–257

Murgatroyd S 1983 Counselling and the doctor. Journal of the Royal College of General Practitioners 33: 323–325

Peterson G M 1981 The pharmacist's role in patient counselling. Australian Journal of Pharmacy 62: 749–750

Porter A M 1969 Drug defaulting in a general practice. British Medical Journal 1: 218–222

Report 1984 Guide to cautionary and advisory labels for dispensed medicines. Pharmaceutical Journal 232: 321–326

Report 1984 Working party on pharmaceutical education and training. Pharmaceutical Journal 232: 495–508

Sackett D L, Snow J C 1979 In: Haynes R B, Taylor B W, Sackett D L (eds) The magnitude of compliance and non-compliance in health care. John Hopkins University Press, Baltimore pp 14–18

Stimson G V 1974 Obeying doctor's orders — a view from the other side. Social Science and Medicine 8: 97–104

Walker R, Wright S E, Aitchison L 1985 Saccharin — a urinary tracer to monitor patient compliance. Pharmaceutical Journal 235: 592

Warden-Flood J 1984 Handbook for Patient Medication Counselling. Australian Pharmaceutical Society, Canberra, Australia

Anon 1981 What should we tell patients about their medicines? Drug and Therapeutics Bulletin 19: (19) 73–74

Anon 1985 What can we expect the label to tell the patient? Drug and Therapeutics Bulletin 23: (22) 87–88

38. Patient medication records

J. A. Rees

In recent years, there has been a trend towards community pharmacists maintaining patient medication records (PMRs). This trend has been encouraged by the Royal Pharmaceutical Society who have recommended the use of PMRs in both the Interim report of the working party on general practice pharmacy and the Guide to self-assessment of professional practice.

PMRs have been developed to assist the pharmacist in detecting and preventing drug-related problems. The background to the development of PMR is as follows: There is an increasing number of NHS prescriptions dispensed per year with a concomittant increase in the number of prescriptions per head of pupulation. This increase is the result of an ever-increasing pressure being put on doctors from people seeking or demanding medication. The nation's expectation of health, including relief from pain and disease is increasing. Under this sort of pressure, it is highly likely that doctors will make mistakes from time to time, more due to the speed at which they work than from lack of professional knowledge or care. Also, the drugs being prescribed are powerful substances which may interact with other drugs or other substances, such as food, to cause adverse drug reactions. These reactions may be of minor importance or they may be quite serious perhaps causing iatrogenic disease in the patient. Certainly 3–5% of hospital admissions are claimed to be due directly or indirectly to an adverse drug reaction. Whilst, in hospital 10–25% of patients experience some sort of drug reaction, which may prolong their stay.

Besides doctor-prescribed medication, patients may also take dentist-prescribed medication which may interact with each other and with over-the-counter (OTC) medicines.

Also of importance is the usage by the public of OTC medicines. This usage is considerable and it is claimed that 60% of dose units are OTC medicines. Thus, the likelihood of OTC medicines interacting or interfering with any prescribed medicine being taken by the patient concurrently should not be overlooked.

In order that the pharmacist does not dispense a possible drug interaction, it is essential that the pharmacist knows what other medications either prescribed or self-administered are being taken by the patient, as well as other relevant information about the patient, such as drug sensitivities. PMRs have been set up by pharmacists to enable them to monitor patient medication and hopefully to detect and prevent drug-related problems. Some pharmacists have claimed that it is only at a pharmacy that a totally comprehensive medication profile could be set up.

The PMR would normally include all the drug treatment being taken by the patient including OTC medicines bought at the pharmacy or elsewhere. Other information recorded, if known, would include the patient's name, address, date of birth, telephone numbers, GP, drug history, any reported hypersensitivities and current medical problems including chronic illness.

The value to the patient of PMRs is that at the time of dispensing the pharmacist is able to review the current drug treatment along with other important information, such as age, medical condition and hypersensitivities, so as to be able to detect possible drug interactions, contraindicated treatment and undue frequency or inconsistency of prescribing. Also, when medicines are counter-prescribed or sold over the counter for patients, PMRs will help the pharmacist to offer more appropriate advice. It has been suggested that PMRs promote patient compliance and health education.

Two-card system

The first British study on PMRs described a system which necessitated the utilization of two cards: a so-called 'Personal Medicine Record' used and retained by the patient and a second card which was filed in the pharmacy (Shulman et al 1981). Both cards are essentially the same, giving the name and address of the patient, names of drugs, dosage, quantity and date of dispensing.

In addition, the patient's card includes written advice so that the patient shows it: to his GP or on admission to hospital; to his dentist if treatment or an anaesthetic is needed; or to the pharmacist when presenting each prescription and before purchasing home remedies.

Information for completing entries on the card is obtained by interviewing the patient and recording data from the prescriptions. However, it must be pointed out that this means of elucidating a patient's medical history and drug sensitivities is by no means 100% accurate, since the patient is often unaware of all the details of their own past medical history and medication.

'Special cautions', for example, diabetes, penicillin allergy, monoamine oxidase inhibitor therapy should also be recorded on the front of the patient card and at the top of the pharmacy card. Changes in drug dosage or strength should be recorded only after the patient had been consulted to check that the change was intentional.

Shulman et al (1981) studied the feasibility of a PMR system. Over a 3-year period PMRs were maintained for selected patients on long-term multiple-drug therapy and all patients on long-term medication, such as psychoactive drugs, steroids, antihypertensives or cardiovascular drugs. The study detected potential adverse drug reactions and mistakes on prescriptions and highlighted cases where advice was given to the patient by the pharmacist to reduce the likelihood of an adverse drug reaction. Also, the study recorded several cases where an OTC sale was refused because of possible adverse drug reactions with prescribed medicine.

The success of a two-card system depends on patient acceptance of the card and on he/she presenting it on each occasion to doctors, dentists and pharmacists. If the card is not presented when a prescription is dispensed, the information on the card cannot be updated. Various reasons were given by patients for not presenting the card with the prescription. However, it is disturbing to note that nearly 50% of patients who did not present their cards with the prescriptions were apathetic. The efficiency of the system lies ultimately with the patient.

If PMRs are not to become obsolete, it is important that the pharmacist convinces the patient that compliance with the drug regimen is essential. In order to do this, the pharmacist must be prepared to give the patient the necessary information about the drug treatment and explain why the medication should be taken as prescribed.

One-card system

At the request of the Royal Pharmaceutical Society, who are aware that some pharmacists were maintaining individual PMR systems, the NPA have made available a standard system of cards. This is a one-card system. The card being kept at the pharmacy for use by the pharmacist when dispensing, counter prescribing or selling OTC medicines. These cards, one of which is shown in Figure 38.1, are designed to fit into a standard filing box.

Both the Royal Pharmaceutical Society and the National Pharmaceutical Association (NPA) suggest that

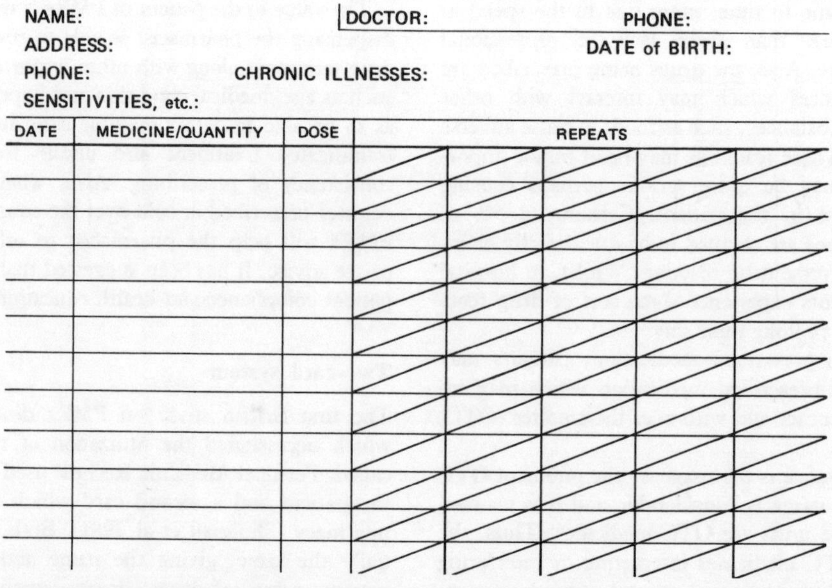

NAME:		DOCTOR:		PHONE:		
ADDRESS:				DATE of BIRTH:		
PHONE:		CHRONIC ILLNESSES:				
SENSITIVITIES, etc.:						

DATE	MEDICINE/QUANTITY	DOSE	REPEATS			

Fig. 38.1 NPA Patient Medication Record Card. (Reproduced with permission from the National Pharmaceutical Association)

pharmacists should normally inform the patient that records are being kept and that the pharmacist should take adequate precautions to ensure the confidentiality of the PMRs.

The one-card system is obviously cheaper and quicker than the two-card system but it only works properly if the patient returns to the same pharmacy; 80% of people regularly return to the same pharmacy for their dispensed medicines.

Advantages of card-based PMRs

Poston & Shulman (1985) have surveyed the use of PMRs in the UK and found that their use helped to correct errors, particularly omissions and to provide a base for giving patient advice. However, of much greater importance was the contribution of the record system to the detection of errors that would otherwise have been overlooked. In many cases these errors might have led to problems for the patients concerned. The problems detected in this study by the use of PMRs, over a 4-week period are shown in Table 38.1.

Other studies in which pharmacists have maintained PMRs has shown their usefulness in studying drug

Table 38.1 Problems detected by use of patient medical records

Problem	No.	%
Error in dose	24*	29
Error in drug	18	22
Error in strength	9	11
Error in form	6	7
Error in quantity	5	6
Error in appliance	3	4
Repeat prescription, too soon	3	4
Others (frequency less than 2)	15	18
Total	83	101†

* 12 from one pharmacy.
†Error from rounding.
(Reproduced from Poston and Shulman (1985) with permission from the *Pharmaceutical Journal*)

usage and costs within various age/sex groups of a community as well as the differences in prescribing costs between doctors within a group practice (Rees & Baumgard´ 1983, Baumgard et al 1984). An additional advantage to pharmacists is that knowing the pattern of drug usage in a community pharmacy could lead to better and more rational stock control.

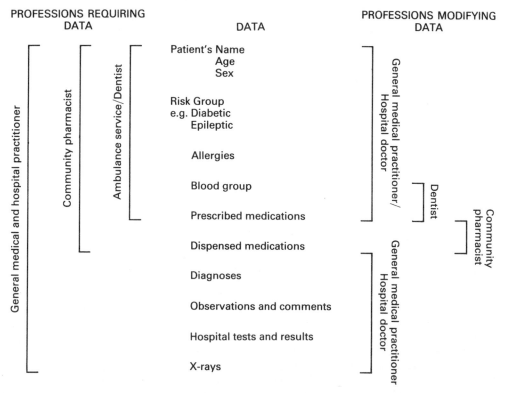

Fig. 38.2 Potential patient data utilized by health-care professionals. (Reproduced from Stevens (1984) with permission from the *Pharmaceutical Journal*)

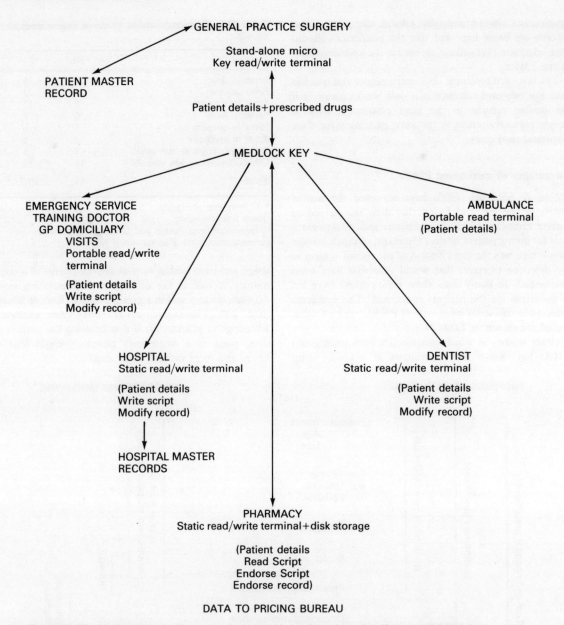

Fig. 38.3 The Medlock system. (Reproduced with permission from the author (Stevens 1984) and the *Pharmaceutical Journal*)

Computerized PMR systems

Manual systems of record keeping are labour intensive, time consuming and require storage space. Patient medication records kept on a computer system significantly reduce the time required by manual systems and provide all the previously stated benefits and more. On a computer system it is possible to have automatic drug interaction warnings.

Computerized patient medication records are developing along two main approaches. Both approaches involve the introduction of patient-retained medication records and close links between the doctors' surgeries and pharmacies (King 1982, Stevens 1984).

One of these approaches involves pharmacy-held records in combination with patient-held record cards. The new patient card is in the initial stages of development and uses a plastic wallet in to which a duplicate label of the dispensed medicine is stuck. The labels will be cancelled to show they are duplicates. The second stage is a fully computerized record system which will include details of current and past medication, drug interactions and hopefully any details of OTC medicine purchased. Ideally in this system there would be computer links between the doctor's surgery and the pharmacy with the object of creating detailed and rapidly accessible records — as well as making prescription information available to the pharmacy.

The ultimate objective would be a patient flow pattern as follows:

1. Patient checks in at surgery reception.

2. Receptionist keys in patient's name and address and consulting doctor.

3. Patient records appear on doctor's VDU.

4. Doctor has options to add to or amend records.

5. Doctor has option to prescribe, to authorize repeats and to record special 'notes' for the pharmacy (for example, 'Patient does not know he has cancer').

6. Prescription file and special notes file transferred to pharmacy.

7. Prescription prints out at pharmacy.

8. Patient collects medicine and receives medication record.

9. Patient collects authorized repeats direct from pharmacy at required intervals.

10. On collection of last repeat, either (a) the patient is advised to make a surgery appointment at least 1 week before medicine runs out or (b) the surgery is notified and an appointment card is sent to the patient by post.

The other approach to computerized PMR involves a patient-retained medication record which was based on a British prototype medical record system, Medlock. This patient-retained PMR contains only selected information, which can be dumped from a master patient record held at the doctor's surgery. The patient record system remains under the control of the GP and data held on the patient-retained medication records may only be accessed with the active consent of the patient. The computer system of medical records at the doctor's surgery remains secure and the ethical and technical difficulties of sharing patient data between other people besides the doctor and patient is overcome. Various aspects of the system are illustrated in Figures 38.2, 38.3 and 38.4.

The present Medlock system includes the use of a smart card token, as opposed to the original key-shaped token. The smart card contains a full page of information about the patient which is of use to the various

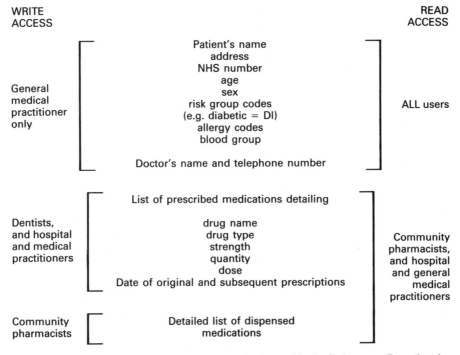

Fig. 38.4 The projected structure of the patient-retained record in the final system. (Reproduced from Stevens (1984) with permission from the *Pharmaceutical Journal*)

potential users. In addition to the personal details, full information on some 400 individual drug prescription items or purchases can be stored on each card. On presentation by the patient, the card is inserted into a read/write device connected to a suitable host computer.

The national acceptance of a patient card record would permit the maximum utilization of essential patient information by all the professions charged with health care. The equipment required by Medlock individual users would be cheaper than any alternative

method of providing a national record system. The provision of card readers at the surgery or pharmacy would permit the patient to check that all details of the record were correct, a facility that would be hard to provide in any other data-processing system.

In conclusion, in the space of just a few years PMRs have developed from manual card systems to sophisticated computerized systems. The pace of development has been rapid and the results exciting. What is now required is patient, doctor and pharmacist acceptance of them.

BIBLIOGRAPHY

Baumgard L, Frank P, Rees J A, Shearer K 1984
Comparison of prescription costs within a group practice.
British Medical Journal 289: 1196–1197
Chemist and Druggist (1984) 107.
King R 1982 Computers in pharmacy. Pharmaceutical
Journal 228: 4
Poston J W, Shulman S 1985 Patient medication records in
community pharmacy. Pharmaceutical Journal
234: 442–443
Rees J A, Baumgard L 1983 British Journal of
Pharmaceutical Practice 5: 6–13

Rees J A, Baumgard L 1984 J. Soc. Admin. Pharm.
2: 29–33
Shulman J I, Shulman S 1979 Operating a two-card
medication record system. Pharmaceutical Journal
222: 554–556
Shulman J I, Shulman S, Haines A P 1981 Journal
of the Royal College of General Practitioners
31: 429–434
Stevens R G 1984 Patient-related medical records.
Pharmaceutical Journal 232: 570–573

39. Responding to symptoms

C. Edwards

Introduction

The general public has self-medicated for longer than doctors have existed. Today, the public are better informed about health and disease and, as a result of powerful advertising, are persuaded to buy a great variety of remedies to relieve the symptoms of self-limiting illness. Nevertheless, there is still a need for professional advice and guidance in treating those maladies which seem too trivial to consult the doctor about. This is a role which the pharmacist has adopted over many years and indeed is an activity which is as old as the profession itself. A working party of the Royal Pharmaceutical Society published a report in 1981 on the 'response to symptoms in general practice pharmacy' which provided guidelines on the kinds of symptoms which required medical referral. By introducing a limited prescribing list of drugs in 1985, the government of the day has encouraged the public to purchase medicines to treat trivial disorders rather than obtain them on prescription. Thus the pharmacist is expected to respond to requests from the general public regarding the evaluation of symptoms and their treatment. This activity is *counter-prescribing*.

The objectives of this chapter are:

1. To provide some knowledge base of symptoms and their causes.
2. To differentiate where possible, potentially serious disorders requiring medical attention from more trivial illnesses which may be treated with over-the-counter (OTC) medicines.
3. To rationalize where appropriate the choice of OTC medicines.

Should pharmacists diagnose?

It may be argued that pharmacists who attempt to diagnose illnesses are exceeding their competence and treading on territory which traditionally belongs to the doctor. Furthermore, pharmacists do not have the facilities, equipment or expertise for physical examination of the patient. However, at the level at which the pharmacist is responding to symptoms, i.e. as a first-line adviser as to whether a sign or symptom presented to him represents a self-limiting trivial illness or a possibly more serious one, he is merely acting as an informed, intelligent professional who is unlikely to produce worse results than a patient who self-diagnoses and self-medicates. The pharmacist is acting as a screen, sieving out those patients who should perhaps seek medical advice. Obviously, at this level there will be overlap with the patients who visit their general medical practitioner with trivial symptoms. Sophisticated equipment, knowledge and physical examination are not necessary at this level of the diagnostic process. So pharmacists, in evaluating symptoms, are merely making an informed judgement on their severity and are excluding potentially serious pathology, before providing appropriate advice or symptomatic relief with OTC medicines. Cases which present any possibility of major problems requiring either medical appraisal or more potent medicines are referred to the doctor. In this process, therefore, pharmacists are collaborating with doctors rather than usurping part of their role and indeed should be reducing the workload of the doctor, allowing him more time to devote to patients who require his medical expertise.

Responding to the patient

Some useful general principles for consideration when responding to the patient are given below.

Reassurance

It should be remembered that patients frequently require only reassurance about their symptoms. A sympathetic ear, a little time and a kind word may do more good than any medicine that is recommended. The placebo effect should not be underestimated. It is a powerful tool which can be genuinely used toward the good of the patient.

Taking a history

Whilst it is important to listen to information volunteered by the patient, it is also necessary to ask the right questions which will allow differentiation of the likely causes of the patient's problem. The major part of this chapter aims to assist in asking the right questions.

Observation of any physical abnormalities

Unless it is entirely inappropriate, following or alongside the history, any lesion which is apparent visually should be observed, e.g. any tenderness or pain assessed by both touch and by the appearance and demeanour of the patient, etc. Nothing should be taken for granted.

Exclusion of any necessity for medical referral before recommending any treatment

A patient's condition can change, often rapidly and sometimes for the worse. It is good practice therefore to ask the patient to return for reassessment or to see a doctor if his symptoms change or worsen. This is particularly true for young children.

Explanation to the patient

Where possible, the cause of the symptoms should be explained to the patient and how the treatment will work. If the specific underlying cause is not clear, but there is no need for medical referral, at least the patient can be reassured that the illness will probably resolve itself and that symptoms can be relieved.

Advice to the patient to see the doctor if the condition does not improve

Although the time-scale depends on the particular condition being assessed, pharmacists should remember that they can only alleviate symptoms and the patient will return to good health, with or without his help if the illness is 'trivial', within a few days. Should this not occur, then the initial assessment may have been wrong or the patient's illness may have developed further revealing signs and symptoms which were not apparent at the initial interview.

Elements of diagnosis

The decision to refer a patient or not rests, in part, on pure commonsense. One important question to ask oneself is 'Does the patient look ill?'. If a patient has a hangover headache and gastrointestinal upset from a generous amount of food and drink the night before, he will look and feel quite dreadful. However, because his symptoms can be easily related to the likely cause and we know that they will resolve spontaneously there is no cause for concern. On the other hand, someone with the same presentation of symptoms with no obvious cause will be classed as ill and should be referred. An easy rule of thumb is to say 'If I was this patient, would I, with my knowledge, go to the doctor?'.

An important question to ask the patient when assessing the seriousness of an illness is 'How long have you had the symptoms?'. Someone with minor abdominal discomfort or pain continuing for several weeks, which has not become worse, is unlikely to suffer if the pharmacist decides to counter-prescribe symptomatic treatment for a few days, to try out a simple remedy. However, someone who presents with a problem which is only of several minutes' or a few hours' duration places the pharmacist in some difficulty because with only such a short history to assess, he cannot always easily judge whether the patient is going to become better or worse over the next few hours. In such a case, he must base his decision of whether to refer or not on the answers to questions posed to attempt to differentiate the cause or likely pathology.

Following the above line of questioning the pharmacist should ask whether the patient has already self-medicated and whether any relief was obtained. This may help in deciding whether any further OTC medication is going to help or whether more potent remedies and medical follow-up are required.

In view of the increasing incidence of iatrogenic disease, the patient should always be asked if he is taking any medicines which may have caused the symptoms. This is particularly appropriate with gastrointestinal symptoms and headaches.

The next line of questioning should be designed specifically to exclude serious pathology before instigating OTC treatment. The pharmacist should have a checklist of possible diagnoses in his mind for the symptoms presented and, by a series of pertinent questions, should be able to exclude any major disease states.

RESPIRATORY TRACT DISORDERS

Coughs, colds and sore throats are common symptoms which in the vast majority of cases are accompaniments of self-limiting trivial illness, usually a bacterial or viral infection, which will run their own course with no serious consequences.

Cough

In the case of cough, the following warning signs will usually require medical referral:

— Wheezing (as occurs in asthma).
— Shortness of breath (as may occur in asthma, bronchitis and congestive heart failure for example).
— Pain: on coughing or on breathing.
— Diabetic patients with severe symptoms (these patients are more susceptible to infections, pneumonia, etc. and require special care).
— Elderly patients.
— Children under 9 months, especially if irritable and not feeding.
— Symptoms persisting longer than 10 days, and not getting better.
— Patients with a history of chronic bronchitis, if symptoms seem severe.
— Cigarette smokers, if they have had frequent coughing on previous occasions (may indicate a chronic bronchitis or emphysema).
— Patients with a raised temperature who feel ill.
— Patients with green/brown sputum during the day (signifies infection; discolored sputum in the morning only signifies concentrated nasal secretions or non-infected bronchial tube secretions).

Sore throat

Sore throats may be due to a streptococcal or viral infection. Streptococcal throats usually present themselves with fever, exudate visible on the back of the throat, and enlarged and tender cervical lymph nodes.

Sore throats superseded by rhinorrhoea and nasal congestion indicate infection by the common cold virus. Sore throats with no associated symptoms of the common cold may be due to other viruses such as herpes which produces mouth ulcers and cold sores. Viral sore throats produce inflamed cervical lymph nodes.

Sore throats of longer than 4 days' duration should be referred, since antibiotic therapy may need to be started (streptococci can rarely cause rheumatic fever and kidney infections).

Any difficulty in swallowing, persistent hoarseness, or noisy breathing requires medical referral.

Rhinorrhoea and nasal congestion

The main symptoms of the common cold are rhinorrhoea (excessive nasal secretions) and nasal congestion, often accompanied transiently by a sore throat early on and sometimes followed by a cough. The latter two symptoms may be caused by postnasal drip, when excessive secretions in the nose pass down into the oropharynx and irritate the throat and upper trachea.

Other symptoms accompanying respiratory tract infections

Sinus pain

Sinusitis is an infection of the sinuses which are extensions of the nasal airways and which are lined with a similar mucous membrane to the nasal mucosa. The sinuses are vestigial air spaces, which in our ancestors and predecessors in the evolutionary tree, were probably associated with a well-developed olfactory function. When the mucosa of the sinuses is infected and inflamed it can cause severe pain and sometimes dizziness. Sinusitis can be confirmed by palpation of the skin above the frontal and maxillary sinuses (over the eyebrows and below the cheek bone), when pain or tenderness will be elicited.

Earache

Earache may complicate a sore throat. Infection in the pharynx will easily spread up the eustachian tube to the middle ear, causing otitis media, a very painful condition and particularly distressing in young children. Although the cause may be viral, medical referral is required to allow antibiotics to be considered for a possible bacterial cause.

Myalgia

Generalized muscle aching or pain is often an accompanying feature of viral or bacterial infection. However, specific joint pain is not indicative of respiratory tract infection.

Rash

In children particularly, symptoms of a cold accompanied by a rash may indicate one of the childhood infectious diseases such as measles, German measles or perhaps chickenpox. It should be remembered, however, that antibiotics prescribed for infections may sometimes cause a skin rash.

Treatment

Cough

Having confirmed that a patient requires only symptomatic relief for a cough, the pharmacist has two types of treatment at his disposal.

Expectorants (see Table 39.1). Expectorant drugs act by stimulating secretion from the mucus-secreting glands in the lungs. Excessive secretion means that copious amounts of fluid mucus can be coughed up and thus this will act as a vehicle to remove any irritant or infected material in the sputum. Thick, tenacious mucus is liable not only to become infected but to cause obstruction in the bronchioles. Thus the production of a watery mucus by stimulating the mucous glands allows removal of the causative agents of a cough as well as facilitating easier breathing. Most of the expectorant agents are thought to act on the lungs indirectly by primarily stimulating the glands in the gastric mucosa and this initiates a reflex whereby the glands in the respiratory tract are stimulated.

This efficacy of expectorants is a controversial issue, especially since few clinical studies are documented. Nevertheless, a patient with a cough expects something and the placebo effect of a cough remedy is substantial. Perhaps one of the best expectorants is water. When taken orally it will hydrate the tissues of the body, including the lungs and thus facilitate secretion of thin mucus. When inhaled as steam, it provides local hydration of the upper airways and gives a soothing relief of symptoms.

Cough suppressants (see Table 39.1). Cough suppressants are effective agents. They act centrally by depressing the cough centre in the medulla. Antihistamine drugs are effective cough suppressants. Most antihistamines do however have intrinsic anticholinergic activity which tends to dry up secretions and although this is a useful property when drying up nasal secretions it can sometimes be a disadvantage when lung secretions are reduced (see 'Expectorants' above).

Polypharmacy. There are many proprietary cough products which contain several drugs (see Table 39.1). These should be evaluated carefully by pharmacists. For example, a mixture of an expectorant agent with an antihistamine drug or cough suppressant or perhaps even a mixture of all three should be viewed suspiciously because of the pharmacological and physiological antagonism which is likely to exist.

Sore throat

Sucking a lozenge can soothe a sore throat. The mechanism of action however, probably lies in the secretion of saliva which coats a raw, inflamed mucosa and offers symptomatic relief. The efficacy of the numerous antibacterial agents often formulated into sore throat products in the clinical situation is difficult to assess in view of the fast self-resolving nature of most sore throats and the fact that many, if not most, are caused by viruses.

Common cold products

The common cold remedy is a multi-million pound market and this emphasizes the public's desire for symptomatic relief, particularly of rhinorrhoea and nasal congestion. There are many efficacious products available. They contain one or more of the following:

Decongestants. These are mainly sympathomimetic agents such as phenylephrine, ephedrine and phenylpropanolamine. They may be formulated for oral use or for local use as nasal sprays and drops. Sympathomimetic agents may aggravate or predispose to hypertension and should not be used by hypertensive patients in the oral form. Local use is safer since vasoconstriction at the site of application reduces the effect on the systemic circulation. Nasal drops and sprays should not be used for periods longer than 1 or 2 weeks because they may cause a rebound congestion (rhinitis medicamentosa).

Antihistamines. Most antihistamine drugs have anticholinergic activity and will dry up the excessive nasal secretions associated with the common cold. Care must

Table 39.1 Drugs used in cough medicines

Drug	Effect
Codeine Dextromethorphan Morphine Noscapine Pholcodine	Centrally acting cough suppressants
Brompheniramine Chlorpheniramine Diphenhydramine Promethazine Triprolidine	Antihistamines (cough suppressants; anti-secretory)
Ephedrine Pseudoephedrine Theophylline	Bronchodilators
Acetic acid Ammonium salts Guaiphenesin Ipecacuanha Liquorice Sodium citrate Squill Terpin hydrate	Expectorants

be taken with their use because of sedative effects experienced with many.

Analgesics and antipyretics. Aspirin and paracetamol are effective for the relief of headache, myalgia and fever which may accompany the common cold.

Vitamin C. Ascorbic acid is reputed to relieve the severity and shorten the duration of the common cold. However, a daily dosage of several grams is required and this is not found in the combination products available.

GASTROINTESTINAL SYMPTOMS

Indigestion

Indigestion may present as heartburn. This is a symptom characterized by a sensation of burning or pain in the chest and acid-brash in the mouth, particularly after meals. It is often related to position — being worse on lying down flat or bending over. It is due to reflux or acid from the stomach into the oesophagus. Alternatively indigestion may present with abdominal symptoms. Typically there will be a feeling of fullness in the abdomen, tenderness or pain. The symptoms will be related to food — either made worse or sometimes relieved by it. This characterizes a gastrointestinal complaint. Symptoms not related to food will usually be found to originate from sources outside the gastrointestinal tract. Indigestion may be transient and self-resolving but it may be an early symptom of more progressive illness such as peptic ulceration. Transient indigestion is usually caused by some insult to the stomach such as overindulgence with food or drink (especially alcoholic) or spicy foods. It is exacerbated by cigarette smoking. The pharmacist should remember that many drugs can cause digestive upset and these should be enquired for. Persistence of symptoms for more than a few days may indicate that the patient is developing a peptic ulcer — either gastric or duodenal — and he should be referred.

Abdominal pain

Pain may be due to ingestion of some irritant but it may also indicate an infection of the stomach (gastritis) or the intestine (enteritis) or both (gastroenteritis). This will often be associated with vomiting and diarrhoea. The syndrome is of colicky pain in the midline of the abdomen with vomiting or diarrhoea. When properly treated, the condition is short-lived.

Warning signs

Any symptoms of troublesome indigestion or abdominal pain in a person aged over 40 years who has had no previous history of a gastrointestinal complaint may in a few cases indicate a serious problem, e.g. gastric carcinoma.

Any patient who has lost weight rapidly over the past few weeks (without dieting) should be referred because of the possibility of gastric carcinoma.

Persistent vomiting or diarrhoea require a medical opinion. Blood in the vomitus or the stool requires that the patient should be referred.

Treatment of indigestion

The basic first-line approach to indigestion is to give antacids. In the correct dosage they are effective, although this may mean that large doses are required. However, generally speaking antacids are not absorbed and hence no toxic effects are evident even with high doses, provided that the period of usage is short. One exception to this is sodium bicarbonate which is absorbed and although harmless in normal dosage, might cause an alkalosis in large, prolonged doses and should also be avoided by patients on salt-restricted diets for whom additional sodium ions would be inappropriate.

Most proprietary antacids contain magnesium or aluminium compounds or a mixture of both. They are effective and safe. Magnesium may cause diarrhoea and aluminium, constipation. Calcium compounds such as calcium carbonate are present in some antacid mixtures. Calcium can caused a rebound effect and instead of neutralizing any excess acid, it may actually stimulate gastric acid secretion. It is thought to do this by stimulating gastrin, a local hormone which acts on the acid-secreting cells in the gastric mucosa.

Several studies have attempted to compare the efficacy of antacids in vitro by examining their acid-neutralizing properties (see Fordtran et al 1973, Jones et al 1977, Barry & Ford 1978, Duffy et al 1982, Woolfson et al 1985). Although useful, care must be taken when extrapolating the results of these tests to the in vivo clinical situation. For instance the, in vitro test should be designed so that acid is pumped continuously into the reaction to reproduce the effects in vivo. Also, although it is natural to assume that antacids relieve the symptoms of indigestion and peptic ulceration by neutralizing excess acid and increasing the gastric pH, this may not be the whole story, since many patients with gastric ulcers for instance, do not secrete excess acid. Finally in vitro tests do not take account of the presence of food in the stomach. If antacids are taken on an empty stomach, gastric emptying is rapid and the majority will be discharged within 30 minutes. However, if antacids are taken an hour after meals the presence of food delays the emptying of the gastric contents, allowing more time for antacid to react. If taken with meals, more antacid is required because food will stimulate acid secretion. Thus antacids are best given 1 hour after meals for optimal efficacy.

Constipation

Some people become obsessed with the normalization of their bowel movements and it is commonly believed by the lay public that bowels must be opened once a day without fail. This is of course not the case and people's habits vary considerably. Thus anyone complaining of constipation should be questioned as to how the bowel habit has changed and whether there has really been an abnormally long time since the last movement.

Warning signs

Pain, especially persistent, may need medical investigation. Blood observed in the faeces (if passed) or around the anus may be harmless due to tearing of the mucosa but if persistent or excessive may indicate haemorrhoids or damage higher in the bowel.

Treatment

The cause of constipation, if discovered, can be removed and no treatment will be necessary. Enquiry about drugs being taken, diet, reduced fluid intake and exercise may suggest possible triggers. In pregnancy, high levels of progesterone in the body will result in relaxation of smooth muscle including that of the bowel and constipation is commonly seen. It may also be caused by iron, changes in diet, lack of exercise or the enlarged uterus causing compression of the large bowel. It is necessary to relieve it since otherwise haemorrhoids may develop.

The gentlest laxatives are the bulk-forming agents such as ispaghula husk and sterculia.

Increased fibre in the diet and an increased fluid intake will be useful advice to the patient. For rapid evacuation, magnesium sulphate is useful. Stimulant laxatives such as senna may also be recommended.

Liquid paraffin and products containing it have fallen out of favour because it tends to leak from the anus and also from the oesophagus into the trachea and lungs.

Diarrhoea

Diarrhoea may be a concomitant symptom of an abdominal disorder but generally speaking uncomplicated diarrhoea is transient and self-limiting. It should be remembered that, like other abdominal illnesses, it is often caused by insults to the digestive system such as

food, drink or medication and certainly, in the latter case, removal of the cause may be necessary.

Adults

Provided that the warning signs below are heeded and that a sensible time duration is decided upon by the pharmacist, after which he will make a medical referral, symptomatic treatment will suffice.

Warning signs requiring medical referral

1. Recent overseas travel to countries where dysentery, cholera, etc. may be endemic requires medical intervention.
2. Blood or mucus in the stool.
3. Longstanding or recurrent episodes.
4.. Weight loss — either short term or long term may reflect carcinomas or malabsorption syndromes such as coeliac disease.
5. Dehydration, particularly if vomiting is present.
6. Severe vomiting accompanying diarrhoea may represent a serious underlying disorder.

Treatment. There are numerous over-the-counter remedies for diarrhoea ranging from generic mixtures such as Kaolin and Morphine Mixture BP to ethical tablet formulations. Medicines containing codeine or morphine are well-known bowel sedatives and can be recommended. Drugs such as loperamide will also relieve acute diarrhoea. Another approach is to use bulking agents such as ispaghula husk which will often absorb excess water in the colon and help form a semi-solid stool. The use of absorbents such as kaolin may allow stools to be formed by absorbing water but their efficacy is not proven. Above all, patients should be reminded to drink copious fluids to counteract that lost. If diarrhoea does not improve within 48 hours a medical opinion should be sought.

Diarrhoea in children

As with all disorders, diarrhoea causes particular concern when it occurs in children, especially babies and toddlers. It can manifest as either acute or chronic diarrhoea. Acute diarrhoea is often caused by infection and may be associated with fever and vomiting. The problems which ensue are a result of dehydration and electrolyte loss. Chronic diarrhoea may point to malabsorption (e.g. coeliac disease, cow's milk protein intolerance) or simply toddler's diarrhoea which is benign and self-limiting.

Treatment. Chronic diarrhoea requires a medical opinion to establish the cause. Acute diarrhoea can be treated symptomatically, provided that the child is reasonably well and active. A child who looks and behaves 'sick' should be referred.

Babies should be given no milk for 24 hours. They should receive either a homemade solution of glucose in water (one level 5 ml spoonful in 100 ml water to be sipped slowly for every watery stool that has been passed) or a readymade proprietary glucose-electrolyte mixture. Glucose acts as a carrier for electrolyte absorption in the gut and thus facilitates sodium absorption which allows water to be absorbed too. After 24 hours, quarter- or half-strength feeds may be reintroduced, doubling up in a further 24 hours until normal feeding is resumed. It should be remembered that when the bowel is inflamed, enzyme secretion from the mucosa will be impaired and hence lactose will not be split into its component monosaccharides and absorbed. It will thus remain in the bowel and act as an osmotic purgative and hence aggravate the situation. Older children may be symptomatically treated with adsorbents such as kaolin mixture.

Vomiting

Vomiting is usually short-lasting, benign and needs no treatment, except for rehydration and rest. Frequent vomiting lasting more than 24 hours and which is not improving requires a medical opinion. Otherwise resting the stomach (by fasting) for a day or so should allow it to rid itself of the causative toxin and promote healing. Vomiting with diarrhoea is often caused by viral infections which are common in the spring and autumn.

Warning signs requiring referral

— Blood in the vomitus.
— Projectile vomiting (e.g. vomiting forcefully as if under pressure, particularly important in babies).

SKIN DISORDERS

Acne

Acne vulgaris is a common skin complaint which flourishes in adolescence. It causes great cosmetic concern to young patients and consequently the number of acne products on the market are legion. An understanding of the pathology assists in rationalizing treatment as well as educating the patient.

The sebaceous glands (Fig. 39.1) become overactive secreting excessive amounts of sebum. An attractive theory is that this is due to changing testosterone metabolism in both males and females. Triglycerides in the sebum are split by bacteria to form irritant fatty acids. Sebum escapes from the glands to the surface of the skin up the shaft of a hair follicle. The shaft of a hair follicle, being a continuation of the outermost layer of the skin, is lined with cells of the stratum corneum which are keratinized. The fatty acids irritate these cells, causing an inflammatory reaction and the lumen of the hair shaft becomes narrowed. A similar inflammation occurs on the surface of the skin around the hair follicle. Sebum cannot escape and a white plug — a whitehead — is seen on the skin. Eventually this becomes blackened (probably by oxidation) to form a comedone or blackhead — giving the typical presentation of acne. If the hair shaft ruptures beneath the surface, then the inflam-

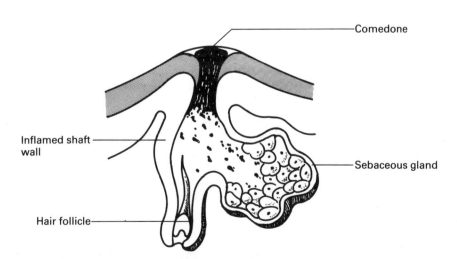

Fig. 39.1 The pilo-sebaceous unit in acne vulgaris

matory process spreads under the skin and then infection may become a complication, resulting in red, raised papules and pustules. Acne lesions occur on the face, and upper chest and back.

Treatment

Although accepted as a fact of life by some, the lesions can be unsightly and some sympathetic explanation of the disorder is called for. Healing is a slow process and will occur naturally. Medication is hardly curative but will help prevent scarring and stop lesions developing. Frequent washing with soap and water will remove keratin and sebum from the skin surface. Sunlight is usually helpful but diet plays a dubious role. Picking the lesions may cause scarring and squeezing erythematous lesions too enthusiastically, especially if there is no head (as in a pustule), will merely cause subsurface damage and spread the lesions into deeper skin layers.

Time-honoured preparations containing sulphur, resorcinol and salicylic acid exist. Some products contain benzoyl peroxide, which is both an antibacterial agent and a peeling agent. It acts as a keratolytic, stripping the outer layers of the skin and hence removing the comedones. Because it is initially irritant, especially on the face, it is wise to start with a concentration of 5% applied once daily, gradually increasing to twice daily and if tolerable then moving onto a 10% preparation. There are numerous washes, spirits and abrasives available designed to strip the keratin and to dry excess sebum. All have their place and individual patients should be treated according to the severity of the lesions, their skin sensitivity and tolerance. It should always be remembered, as with any skin complaints, that sometimes sensitivity may develop to the medication, making the condition appear worse.

Eczema

Eczema is an inflammatory disorder of the skin involving the epidermis in particular. It is virtually synonymous with dermatitis. Eczema is a group of several diseases which result in redness of the skin (erythema). Swelling with vesicle formation, and scaling and cracking may also occur. This causes severe itching and scratching, producing thickening of the skin (lichenification) and sometimes infection.

Atopic eczema

Atopy is an inherited predisposition to develop asthma, hay fever and eczema. Atopic eczema usually begins in infancy between 2 and 6 months of age but it may appear later in life. There is usually a family history of atopy. Classically it affects the face initially and then spreads to the flexures of the wrists, knees and arms. It is a dry, irritating rash.

Seborrhoeic eczema

There are two types of seborrhoeic eczema — an infantile and an adult form. Infantile seborrhoeic eczema usually presents as a red rash with intense scaling on the scalp (cradlecap) at about 2 months of age. It may spread to the face, particularly the eyebrows, and behind the ears, and then to the axillae, the napkin area and trunk. Infection may occur in intertrigenous areas.

The adult form of the disorder principally affects the face, presenting as a red, scaly rash.

Primary contact eczema

Primary contact eczema is caused by irritation of the skin by such insults as detergents, mineral oils, chemicals, acids and alkalis. It is an occupational hazard and is easily recognizable in some circumstances by its sudden appearance in association with use of the offending irritant and the pattern produced (corresponding to the skin exposed to the irritant).

Allergic contact eczema

Some chemicals are skin allergens and will sensitize susceptible individuals who, on future contact, will have an allergic reaction manifested as eczema, either at the location of the previous sensitization or spread elsewhere on the body. Common skin allergens include nickel in jewellery, chromate in cement, dyes, chemicals in rubber, cosmetics and some plants such as the primula. Often the site of the rash and a brief history regarding usage of potential allergens will elucidate the diagnosis.

Discoid (nummular) eczema

Discoid eczema presents usually initially in adults as coin- or disc-shaped lesions, a few centimetres in diameter, on the extensor surface of the limbs, e.g. the forearm. It can be distinguished from tinea corporis, because in the case of eczema the erythema is consistent throughout the lesion, whereas with tinea, central clearing is seen with marked red margins.

Treatment

Eczema can be a stubborn condition, liable to relapse, but symptomatic treatment is available. If the lesion is dry, then bland hydrating emollients such as emulsifying ointment, aqueous cream and various proprietary products will do no harm and often much good. Pruritus can be alleviated by oral antihistamines which are particularly useful in allergic contact eczema.

Obviously protection of the skin from any irritants is essential and may involve wearing gloves or other protective clothing or even changing occupations. Infants may be sensitized to the lanolin in wool and if affected will benefit from cotton clothing.

The skin of eczema patients is very sensitive and they should be advised to avoid or minimize the use of perfumed soaps, bubble baths and detergents. Dermatologists often prescribe the use of emulsifying ointment in the bath to prevent the skin from dying out. Proprietary oil-based products for use in the bath are available. Topical medication may cause of exacerbate a sensitive skin and pharmacists should enquire from manufacturers whether products contain sensitizers such as lanolin or preservatives such as parabens.

In several countries, topical hydrocortisone is available. This is an efficacious treatment for mild dermatitis and there are few reported adverse effects. In the UK, proprietary brands of hydrocortisone cream and ointment (maximum concentration 1%) may be sold for the treatment of allergic contact dermatitis and irritant dermatitis. The products should be applied sparingly, avoiding the eyes and face, anogenital region and broken or inflamed skin.

Napkin dermatitis

Napkin rash is a common affliction in babies. It is diagnosed by the mother and the pharmacist rarely has the opportunity to see the lesions. Napkin rash may be caused in one of two ways. First, poorly rinsed napkins after washing may cause irritant sensitizing chemicals or detergents to be retained, which on contact with the skin cause an eczematous reaction. Secondly, urea in the urine may be broken down by urease present in bacteria in the stool. Thus unchanged napkins will harbour faecal bacteria. The urea degrades to form ammonia, which is a very irritant chemical. The net result is an erythematous rash where the napkin or the urine is in contact with the skin. This means that the inside of skin folds in the groin are spared and this serves to differentiate napkin dermatitis from seborrhoeic eczema where all the napkin area, including skin folds, are involved. Since the affected area is usually covered by a napkin and then contained in plastic pants, there exists a warm moist environment ideal for colonization of bacteria and fungi. Secondary infection should therefore be borne in mind, particularly

from candida and bacteria. Infected lesions may weep, will contain pustules and scaling may be present.

Treatment of napkin rash

Prophylaxis. General measures of hygiene obviously will go some way towards preventing napkin rash. For example, regular napkin changes, minimizing the contact time between skin, urine and faeces are advisable. Should soiling of the skin occur, the mother should be advised to scrupulously clean away all traces of urine and faecal matter, especially in the skin folds. If this is not done then a vicious cycle of irritation will develop and the rash will be extremely difficult to clear. Air should be allowed to circulate around the napkin area by removing the napkin and leaving the baby to lie or sleep with no occlusion over the sensitive areas. Rinsing the napkins in a final solution of an antiseptic solution, such as 1% cetrimide, may reduce bacterial action and reduce the consequences on the skin. However, if the rash is thought to be caused by detergents, special care in rinsing napkins after washing should be stressed to the mother.

Barrier creams containing dimethicone are effective in protecting the skin from irritants and are therefore good prophylactic agents for napkin dermatitis.

Management of the rash. When a rash is present, the skin will be sore and sensitive. Careful hygiene as described under prophylaxis is therefore important again in this situation. However, barrier creams should not be used to treat napkin rash. A water-miscible cream rather than an ointment base is best, because it can be rubbed into the skin and will allow access of air to the skin and drainage of water from the skin, thus drying the lesion and reducing the risk of infection. There are many products on the market containing antibacterial agents and these are to be recommended in a suitable base. If infection is suspected, as in a worsening rash, the presence of weeping lesions or pustules and crusting, then a short course of treatment with an antifungal/antibacterial agent is best such as topical clotrimazole or miconazole.

Fungal infections

Candidiasis

Candidiasis is caused by a yeast-like organism, *Candida albicans*, which may infect the mouth, alimentary canal, vagina or the skin. It is a commensal organism which under certain circumstances overgrows and causes symptoms. It is common in intertrigenous areas (where skin folds overlap, creating a warm moist environment) such as the axillae, the genitalia, submammary areas and finger and toe clefts. Candida often infects eczemas and particularly napkin dermatitis. It presents as a red rash which itches and may become scaly and blistered.

Treatment. There are several OTC antifungal creams which are effective in candidiasis, such as clotrimazole and miconazole. Treatment should be continued for at least a week after symptoms clear.

Ringworm (tinea)

The ringworm or tinea infections which will present to the pharmacy will be caused mainly by various species of *Trichophyton*, a fungus.

Tinea pedis. Better known as 'athlete's foot', this form of tinea invades the moist warm environment of the foot, particularly between and underneath the toes. It causes itching and may be seen as an erythematous rash but may become white and macerated, particularly if sweating is a problem. It is transmissible by contact with changing room floors which may be contaminated by a sufferer walking barefoot.

Resistant cases may become secondarily infected with candida or even bacteria.

Treatment of simple cases is with any of the proprietary topical products containing such antifungal agents as tolnaftate, undecylenic acid, the undecanoates and chlorphenesin. However, clotrimazole and the imidazole antifungal agents such as miconazole and econazole are effective against trichophyton, candida and some Gram-positive bacteria, and therefore give a broader spectrum of cover.

Patients should be told to apply an antifungal cream twice daily and to continue for at least 1 week after lesions disappear, to avoid recurrence. Footwear should be liberally dusted with antifungal talc to prevent re-infection and to dry up perspiration. Regular washing and attentive drying of the feet is essential, especially to prevent relapses.

Tinea corporis. Body ringworm (tinea corporis) presents typically intially as a single round lesion. It may be seen on the trunk or the limbs. The lesion is red, itching and on careful examination the margin is seen to be well defined, sometimes raised and redder than the central portion of the lesion. The lesion spreads outwards, and red margin advancing and leaving a healing centre behind. This distinguishes it from a discoid eczema, where the lesions are consistently red throughout with no angry margin. The lesion will usually self-resolve but the use of an antifungal cream may be useful if the lesion spreads.

Tinea cruris. Tinea cruris is a ringworm infection of the groin, more commonly seen in males than females. It is also known as 'Dhobie itch' and presents as a well-defined erythema with intense pruritus. Treatment is with antifungal agents as described under 'Tinea pedis'.

Scabies

Scabies is an infestation of the skin by a mite, *Sarcoptes scabei*. The female mite burrows into the skin to lay eggs. These burrows are grey in colour and can be seen on the skin by the experienced or alert eye, but often a magnifying glass is needed (since they are only a few millimetres long) and sometimes they are difficult to see. They appear initially on the hands — particularly between the fingers and thumb and finger, on the wrists, and also on the feet. An itchy rash develops and the lesions spread up the limbs to the rest of the body, particularly affecting the genitalia, female breasts and the buttocks. The face is not affected in adults although it may be involved in infants.

The offending mite can survive for at least a few hours outside the body but it is generally said that transmission only occurs on close personal contact, especially with bedmates. Infection from clothes, bedlinen and lavatory seats is generally believed to be unlikely but is theoretically possible. The eggs hatch and grow over 3 weeks, males and females mate and the females burrow again to restart the cycle.

Scabies should be considered in any patient who presents with an itchy rash especially if other members of the household are affected or the patient gives a history of working closely with known sufferers.

Treatment

The most commonly used ascaricide is benzyl benzoate application but proprietary lotions of gamma benzene hexachloride are equally effective and often less irritant. The treatment should be applied to the whole body from the neck downwards, after a hot bath. It should be left on for 24 hours. After a bath the whole procedure is repeated. Other close contacts of the patient should be treated because even if they are asymptomatic they may be incubating eggs in their skins.

The itchy rash is caused by an allergic reaction to the mite. Thus, although the treatment will kill the mite, symptoms may still persist for a week or two. These should be alleviated by oral antihistamines and/or the use of calamine lotion or topical hydrocortisone or similar mild steroids. The patient should be told this, otherwise he may attempt to repeat the treatment which in excess will itself cause irritation of the skin and a vicious cycle may develop.

Care should be taken that persistent scratching does not cause infection of the skin. If this is the case, topical steroids alone are contraindicated and an antibiotic cream is required.

Lice

Head lice

Head lice are common in children and spread easily in the school community. Head lice bite the scalp and cause an irritant reaction. The female louse lays eggs close to the scalp on hair shafts. The egg capsules or nits eventually become visible as the hair grows. The lice are believed to be spread by direct contact. There is a controversy over whether they can be spread by contact with hair brushes, since the brushing of hair will usually damage the nit or louse and hence brushes (and combs) will only bear non-viable remnants of the creatures.

Treatment. Fine tooth combs alone are ineffective in eradicating infestation since the eggs are laid close to the scalp and are inaccessible. However, lotions containing gamma benzene hexachloride, malathion or carbaryl are effective if left on the scalp for 2 hours. This long contact time is more effective than the shorter time which a shampoo is allowed to stay in contact with the scalp during normal washing routine.

Pubic lice

Pubic lice cause itching in the genital areas and can be treated similarly to head lice.

Body lice

Body lice are seen in unkempt individuals with poor standards of hygiene. The lice reside in clothes and bed-linen and bite the skin causing a red, irritating rash. Creams or lotions containing malathion or gamma benzene hexachloride are effective and infested clothing and linen should be washed.

Warts

Warts are benign tumours of the epidermis caused by a virus infection. The virus penetrates the skin in susceptible individuals and the epidermal cells thicken and multiply to form the characteristic outgrowth. A wart on the sole or heel of the foot is called a verruca. The latter is painful because of the pressure exerted on it so that the wart is forced inwards into the skin. Warts can be transmitted by contact but only individuals with an inborn susceptibility will incubate the virus.

Treatment

Warts will resolve spontaneously if left alone as the body forms antibodies to the virus. However, this can take from 6 months to 2 years. Sufferers like to treat themselves, usually for cosmetic reasons. Keratolyic solutions or paints are useful, such as salicylic acid in concentrations up to 50%. Podophyllin is also present in some proprietary products. These solutions are caustic to normal skin and hence care should be taken in their use. They act by stripping the keratin layers of the skin and should be applied for 24 hours and then the wart pared with a pumice stone or file. Although such treatment will not remove the wart, it does enhance the appearance of the lesion.

Counselling is important — patients should be told that it will take a long time to remove the wart. There is controversy over the spread of verrucae in swimming pools. Some authorities say that the virus will survive in a moist warm floor and will be picked up and will grow on a person susceptible to warts. However, many dermatologists claim that the virus is so deep-seated in the skin when there is visible skin thickening, that it does not make contact with the surface on which the foot treads. Indeed, it is more likely that the virus is spread in this way only from infected feet incubating the virus which are at an asymptomatic stage.

Haemorrhoids and genital itching

Any suspicion of haemorrhoids must be referred for medical investigation. Similarly, any perivulval or perianal skin irritation should be followed up by the patient's doctor. Blood in the stool can be caused by disorders other than haemorrhoids and, similarly, pruritus around the anus could be due to other causes such as threadworm and bowel disease. Perivulval irritation may be due to a bacterial or fungal skin infection or if there is a discharge from the vagina, there may be vaginal infection, and this needs to be investigated.

Treatment

If a patient can assure you that they are suffering from symptoms of previously diagnosed haemorrhoids then the best treatment is anal hygiene. After defaecation the perianal area should be cleaned and washed with water and soft tissues. Otherwise small amounts of faecal matter will irritate the sensitive lesions further. Various OTC products are available but hygiene and regular bathing are the cardinal treatments. If particularly itchy, topical mild steroids would be prescribed by the doctor in many cases for short periods.

Women present with perivulval itching quite commonly in pharmacies. Although topical local anaesthetics are available and will alleviate symptoms, they will not remove the cause and an antifungal product will probably be better, although medical examination is desirable, especially if the problem is recurrent.

It should be remembered that local anaesthetics, such as lignocaine and its analogues are skin sensitizers and care should be taken to ensure that no more harm is caused to a sensitive skin area of this type when recommending treatment.

HEADACHE

Headache is a common complaint. Patients in pharmacies do not often ask for advice since many analgesic products are widely advertised household names. However, headache can be a symptom of serious pathology as well as a minor illness. In most cases the causation of a headache will not be ascertained, but when asked for advice the pharmacist may wish to approach the problem by considering the types and causes of headaches some of which are listed in Table 39.1.

The relationships between symptoms (site, intensity, description, duration, onset and other factors) and possible types of headache are given in Table 39.3.

To elicit the severity of the cause of a headache, the patient should present his symptoms in his own words and the pharmacist should assess whether the patient appears ill from general observation.

Questions should then elicit other signs and symptoms.

Table 39.2 Types and causes of headaches — italics indicate referral necessary

1. Tension	e.g. Muscular, stress and 'psychogenic' headaches
2. Vascular	Migraine, cluster headaches, *hypertension, temporal arteritis*, influenza/fever
3. Cerebral haemorrhage	*Intracerebral, subdural* and *subarachnoid haemorrhage, aneurysms*
4. Space-occupying lesions (SOL)	*Tumours* and *abscesses*
5. Infections	*Meningitis* and *encephalitis*
6. Miscellaneous	*Trauma*, sinusitis, hangover, *dental pain, trigeminal neuralgia, eye strain, shingles, glaucoma* and *cervical arthritis*, iatrogenic, hormonal (females)

Treatment

Having eliminated any potentially serious pathology, the cause of headache should be identified where appropriate. For example, many drugs may produce

Table 39.3 Relationship between symptoms and possible type of headache

Symptom	Possible type
Site	
Frontal, occipital, 'like a tight band round the head', neck muscles	Tension
Hemicranial	Migraine, shingles
Face	Sinusitis, cluster, trigeminal neuralgia
Eye	Vascular, glaucoma
Temples	Temporal arteritis
Intensity	
The intensity of the pain serves as a general guide to determine when mild OTC analgesics will be effective and, in conjunction with duration, whether referral is necessary. A headache which is getting worse after treatment with OTC analgesics for 1 week should be referred to the doctor	
Description	
Throbbing, pounding	Vascular
Duration	
A headache lasting more than 7 days, if the patient has pain at the time of presentation, should be referred.	
Onset	
Was onset:	
Post-injury?	Trauma
Related to drug therapy?	Adverse effect of drugs (ask i.e. oral contraceptives, if appropriate)
Accompanying symptoms	
Concomitant factors, e.g.:	
Drowsiness	Space-occupying lesion (SOL) or head injury
Disorientation	SOL or head injury
Slurred or otherwise impaired speech	Head injury
Unsteady gait	SOL or head injury
Numbness or weakness	SOL or head injury
Vomiting	SOL or head injury
Fainting	Possible systemic causes
Symptoms of a head cold	Sinusitis, viral infection
Pyrexia	Viral infection
Toothache	Dental origins
Assymetry of pupils	Head injury

Table 39.3   Relationship between symptoms and possible type of headache (*cont'd*)

Symptom	Possible type
Enquire regarding:	
Vision — blurred	Migraine, glaucoma, eye injury
Stiff neck	Meningeal infection
(Ask patient to put his chin on his chest. If this causes pain, as does turning the head from side to side, referral is necessary)	
Aggravating factors	
Painful to the touch	Shingles, trigeminal neuralgia
Related to posture	Hypertension, SOL, sinusitis
Foods, e.g. chocolate, coffee	Migraine
Hunger, exercise	Migraine
Radiation	
Spreading to neck	Muscle spasm, meningitis
Spreading to other muscles in body	Viral infection
Incidence/frequency	
A pattern of occurrence in females during the menstrual cycle	Hormonal cause, induced by oral contraceptive
Previous episodes, unresponsive to OTCs	Refer
Relieving factors:	
Analgesics	Possibly trivial if not recurrent
Lying down	Tension, hypertension
Dark	Migraine

headache as an adverse effect. Hormonal imbalance in a woman due to either endogenous hormones or oral contraceptives may cause headache and in patients with migraine, trigger factors such as stress, exercise, some foods or alcohol may cause an attack.

If the causative factors cannot be found or removed, recourse to the simple OTC analgesic remedies can be made. The simple over-the-counter analgesics are aspirin, paracetamol, codeine and combinations thereof. Ibuprofen, which like aspirin is anti-inflammatory, is very effective too especially in toothache, menstrual pain and where there is an inflamed component. Usually combination products are considered to be more potently analgesic than single drugs but basically the response is good with any of these drugs, provided that the dose is adequate.

Aspirin and the non-steroidal anti-inflammatory drugs (NSAIDs) are contraindicated in patients known to have peptic ulcers and are best avoided in any patient with 'gastric' symptoms. Clearly, any history of sensitization to aspirin means that other NSAIDs are contraindicated too.

SYMPTOMS IN THE EYE

Treatment of eye disorders by pharmacists is perhaps one of the more controversial areas of counter-prescribing, because sight is such a treasured sense and any lapse in responsibility might have dire consequences, at worst blindness.

The facts are, as with any other condition elsewhere in the body, certain conditions of the eye need urgent medical attention, otherwise the consequences may be serious. Caution is therefore commendable but should not serve to exclude the treatment of trivial symptoms which do not represent any major pathology.

In order to appreciate the significance of signs and symptoms in the eye, a brief consideration of the basic anatomy and physiology of the pertinent components is necessary. Consider Figure 39.2.

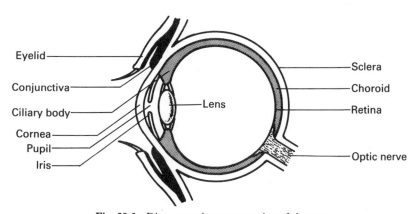

Fig. 39.2   Diagrammatic representation of the eye

Light enters the eye through the pupil, which is that part of the lens which is not covered by the iris. The shape of the lens can be altered by the ciliary body which will contract and relax and allow focussing of the incoming light rays onto the retina. The cornea is a transparent 'window' in front of the lens and iris. The conjunctiva is a thin membrane which covers the white of the eye but does not overlie the cornea and also folds around to line the inner surface of the eyelids.

Inspection of the normal eye

Visual inspection of the healthy eye reveals:

1. Clear, bright, round pupils, equal in size and shape in both eyes.
2. By shining a pen torch, the ciliary reflex causes the pupils to contract. Pupil size should decrease equally in both eyes and the shape remain round.
3. The conjunctiva covering the inside of the eyelid should be pink and that covering the white of the eye should not be injected, i.e. no, or few, blood vessels showing.

EYE DISORDERS

Red eye

There are four main causes of red eye of which the pharmacist should be aware:

1. Conjunctivitis.
2. Iritis.
3. Glaucoma.
4. Subconjunctival haemorrhage.

Of these, conjunctivitis is the most common and can be treated by the pharmacist. Subconjunctival haemorrhage is less common but normally requires no specific treatment. The other two disorders require medical attention.

1. Conjunctivitis

Inflammation of the conjunctiva manifests itself as red conjunctiva lining the eyelids and over the white of the eye. This will usually be obvious to the observer by the pink-red appearance of the normally white sclera. On everting the lower eyelid the conjunctiva will be seen to be redder than normal. Both eyes are commonly affected. The patient will complain of itching, grittiness, prickling, soreness on the surface of the eye, but not of real pain. Real pain, e.g. throbbing, knife-like, sharp pain felt within the eye, is indicative of serious pathology and will not be due to conjunctivitis. The conjunctiva is a covering membrane and if inflamed will manifest only as a superficial uncomfortable feeling which causes the patient to rub the eye. Thus, on questioning, the pharmacist must discern between this type of irritation and a more fundamental pain.

On inspection the pupils should appear normal (round and of equal size in both eyes). They should be bright and if a light is shone into the eye the ciliary reflex should be normal.

Finally because the conjunctiva is not located within the normal light pathways, vision will not be affected.

Causes

Conjunctivitis may be caused by allergy or infection. The symptoms of both types are generally the same.

Allergy. By taking a history, the possibility of an allergic factor or a contact irritation may be elicited. Allergies, such as hay-fever, often manifest themselves as conjunctivitis and if the patient suffers from seasonal rhinitis or asthma then he/she may be predisposed to allergy. Obviously seasonal environmental factors such as pollen can be identified as a likely cause in the summer months, but may be less likely at other times of the year. Eye cosmetics may be a cause. Also exposure to other irritants which may cause either a true allergic reaction in the conjunctiva or a simple physical irritation should be enquired for, such as chlorine in swimming pools (common cause in children) and dust or chemicals in the atmosphere.

Infection. Infection of the conjunctiva may be caused by Gram-positive organisms such as staphylococci, streptococci, Gram-negative bacteria such as *Haemophilus influenzae* and more rarely, pseudomonas, *Escherichia coli*, or viruses. Infection may be discerned by the discharge of pus which collects in the corner of the eye and which causes the eyelids to stick together, particularly on awakening. This is the only sign by which the pharmacist can positively identify infectious conjunctivitis.

Treatment

Allergic conjunctivitis. The causative factor (if known) and the patient should be separated. Symptomatic treatment using eye drops containing antihistamine and/or sympathomimetic (vasoconstrictor) drugs is effective, giving prompt relief in most cases.

Relief is best maintained by the instillation of eye drops on an hourly basis.

Oral antihistamine drugs will be more suitable only if symptoms of allergy occur elsewhere, such as in the nose.

Infective conjunctivitis. Antibacterial eye drops or ointments are required to be instilled hourly for optimal effects. Although clinical evidence is lacking, the in vitro spectrum of some of the antibacterial agents available in OTC eye products such as dibromopropamidine, propamidine, gramicidin and aminacrine would indicate that they should be effective in most cases of infected conjunctivitis.

Sympathomimetic agents will also give symptomatic relief as in allergic conjunctivitis. Obviously viral infections will not be influenced by antibacterial agents.

Eye ointments are useful for night-time application.

If the type of the conjunctivitis cannot be determined, then treatment of both types, with both drops and ointments, is both wise and safe.

If the patient suffers from photophobia, sunglasses will reduce glare. Eye patches, besides being cosmetically less acceptable, are not advisable because secretions and pus will not be allowed to drain away and infection will flourish.

Prognosis

Conjunctivitis is usually a self-limiting condition and will normally completely resolve without treatment in less than 7 days if caused by infections or within 1 or 2 days if allergic.

Symptoms which are not beginning to improve within 3 or 4 days may require a medical opinion.

2. Iritis

Iritis (uveitis) is an inflammation of the iris. One eye only may be affected. There is some redness but it differs from conjunctivitis in that it is painful. Because the iris is inflamed, vision may be worsened. On inspection, the iris and pupil may appear hazy. This is due to inflammatory exudate in the anterior chamber causing the humour to be unclear.

The iris may adhere to the lens so that the pupil does not appear round, but has an irregular shape. Iritis should be regarded as a medical emergency and, if suspected, urgent referral made.

3. Glaucoma

Glaucoma is caused by a reduction in the normal drainage of the aqueous humour from the eye, resulting in raised intraocular pressure. This may cause pain, especially in so-called acute or narrow angle glaucoma where the onset is sudden and severe. In chronic or open angle glaucoma the onset is insidious and pain not always appreciated.

There may be some redness of the eye and one or both eyes may be affected. On inspection the pupil and iris will become hazy because of corneal oedema caused by increased pressure forcing fluid into the cornea so that it changes from a transparent window to a blurred one. This also causes vision to be blurred or affected in some other way; in chronic glaucoma, tunnel vision may occur. Patients may see coloured lights or halos around lights at night. The pupils may appear normal in shape but may sometimes be semi-dilated and fixed, i.e. showing no response to light. Pupils may even be oval in shape. Glaucoma is a serious condition and any suspicion of it requires early medical referral.

4. Subconjunctival haemorrhage

A subconjunctival haemorrhage commonly appears as a red spot in the sclera, caused by a burst blood vessel. It occurs more frequently in older patients than in the young, but is generally painless, harmless and of no consequence. It resolves itself like a bruise anywhere else in the body over 1 or 2 weeks. No treatment is necessary, but reassurance about no underlying causes should be given. If, however, the patient has suffered a blow to the head or other symptoms which might be related to possible trauma, then medical referral is advisable.

The eyelids

Sty

A sty is an infection (often staphylococcal) of a hair follicle at the base of an eyelash on the eyelid margin. It is painful for 1 or 2 days causing inflammation of the affected area of the eyelid and then points through, or near to, the base of the lash, bursts and exudes pus.

Treatment is by a hot compress to enhance pointing of the sty. No other treatment is usually necessary, since the condition will resolve itself spontaneously.

Chalazion (internal sty)

This is an inflammation of the meibomian glands on the underside of the eyelid — frequently the upper one. It is due to infection and presents as an irritation, and when the eyelid is everted, an 'angry' locus of inflammation can be seen. This may eventually form a hard, red lump, palpable when running the finger over the eyelid. Normally chalazia subside and require no treatment, except reassurance. They may flare up from time to time and sometimes require surgical removal.

Blepharitis

Blepharitis is a chronic inflammation of the glands at the eyelid margin, around the eyelash roots. It may be allergic in origin and spread to cause conjunctivitis, but often, only the lid is inflamed. Squamous blepharitis is a form of seborrhoeic dermatitis usually associated with seborrhoea (greasiness) on the face and scalp, commonly accompanying dandruff. It may become infected. Often crusty scales form on the lid margin.

Treatment. If not severe, bathing any scales off with a diluted neutral pH shampoo such as a baby shampoo will be useful. This may be followed by the use of antibacterial and/or antihistamine eyedrops (see 'Conjunctivitis' earlier in this chapter).

Final comment

Inflammation of the skin around the eyes may give rise to symptoms in the eye. The pharmacist should always be on guard against such secondary involvement, where treatment of the primary disorder is paramount. Examples of such instances are cellutitis of the face and shingles, the latter affecting the face and scalp and tracking along the optic nerve to involve the eye. Both of these conditions require medical referral.

BIBLIOGRAPHY

Anon 1981 Response to symptoms in general practicé pharmacy. Pharmaceutical Journal 226: 14–18
Balon A D J 1985 Response to symptoms. Pharmaceutical Journal 234: 532–536
Barry R E, Ford J 1978 Sodium content and neutralising capacity of some commonly used antacids. British Medical Journal 1: 413
Duffy T D, Fawzi S Z, Ireland D S, Rubinstein M H 1982 A comparative evaluation of liquid antacids commercially available in the United Kingdom. Journal of Clinical and Hospital Pharmacy 7: 53–58
Edwards C 1986 Pharmacist's Therapeutic Reference. Medical News Group, Tower House, Southampton Street, London
Edwards C, Stillman P 1982 Minor illness or major disease. Pharmaceutical Press, London
Fordtran J S, Morawski S G, Richardson C T 1973 In vivo and in vitro evaluation of liquid antacids. New England Journal of Medicine 288: 923–928

Godding E W 1976 Constipation and allied disorders. Pharmaceutical Press, London
Handbook of Non-prescription Drugs 1986 8th edn. American Pharmaceutical Association, Washington DC, USA
Jones B, Rhodes M, Rhodes J 1977 Which antacid? An assessment of liquid antacids. Practitioner 219: 559–562
Li Wan Po A 1982 Non-prescription drugs. Blackwell, Oxford
Morley A, Blenkinsopp J, Nicholls J R, Nicholls J L 1985 Choosing an antacid. Pharmaceutical Journal 235: 156–157
Royal Phamaceutical Society of Great Britain 1985 Council statement on responding to symptoms. Pharmaceutical Journal 235: 242–246
Woolfson A D, McCafferty D F, Scott M G, Weir A 1985 Comparison of liquid antacids available on the NHS. Pharmaceutical Journal 235: 108–109

40. Diagnostic tests

D. M. Collett

The pharmacist, particularly in the community, may be involved with the provision of a diagnostic testing service and with the sale or supply of various diagnostic test kits. A wide range of diagnostic tests may be purchased for use by non-trained individuals in the home. The pharmacist acting as a supplier of such testing devices has a responsibility to counsel the purchasers on the conduct of the test and the interpretation of the result obtained. A number of diagnostics are supplied to patients on prescription and, as with other medicinal products, the pharmacist should provide appropriate advice when dispensing these preparations. Pharmacists in the community may offer diagnostic testing as a professional service which may be linked to the provision of advice on health care. Some of the tests that are sold, supplied or provided by the pharmacist are outlined in this chapter.

MEASUREMENT OF BODY TEMPERATURE

Most community pharmacies sell clinical thermometers for the measurement of body temperature in the home. Temperature-sensitive strips for application to the body surface may be safer and more convenient for use in children.

Fertility or ovulation thermometers with an accuracy of 0.1°C are used to measure basal body temperature in the female. The regular recording of basal body temperature (measured on waking but before any kind of activity) may be used to detect the occurrence of ovulation. A small decrease in temperature usually occurs on the day of ovulation. On the following day a rise of up to 1°C occurs and this higher temperature persists until the onset of menstruation. This information may be used to establish the fertile phase of the menstrual cycle in an attempt to achieve conception or alternatively as a contraceptive method. Fertility thermometers may be supplied on an NHS prescription. Special charts for recording the basal body temperature are usually supplied by the prescribing doctor although

the pharmacist may be asked for further advice. Medicines containing certain drugs, e.g. antipyretic, antibiotic or hypnotic drugs, may mask physiological changes in body temperature and patients taking such drugs require counselling.

MEASUREMENT OF BLOOD PRESSURE

The community pharmacist may become involved in the measurement of arterial blood pressure by providing a professional blood pressure measuring service, by siting an automatic apparatus for the unassisted use by patients in the pharmacy, or by selling equipment for patients to use in their own home.

Arterial blood pressure is usually measured indirectly. Arterial occlusion is produced by an inflatable cuff placed around the upper arm and connected to a pressure-measuring device. The cuff is inflated to a pressure above the expected systolic blood pressure and the pressure gradually released. Blood flow sounds are detected by means of a stethoscope or microphone placed over the brachial artery. The first appearance of an intermittent sound (tapping) corresponds with the systolic blood pressure and the disappearance of the intermittent sound indicates the diastolic pressure.

Types of equipment

Mercury sphygmomanometer

The pressure in the inflatable cuff is measured by means of a mercury manometer and the blood flow sounds are detected aurally by means of a stethoscope placed over the brachial artery. This is generally accepted to be the most accurate method with trained personnel.

Aneroid sphygmomanometer

The pressure is measured by an aneroid manometer instead of the mercury column. Regular recalibration is necessary to maintain accuracy over a period of use.

Electronic sphygmomanometer

An aneroid manometer is also used but pressure readings may be converted to a digital display. Blood flow sounds are detected electronically by means of a microphone placed over the brachial artery. This type of equipment may be sold for use by a patient self-monitoring blood pressure in the home.

Automatic sphygmomanometer

Coin-in-the-slot machines have been developed whereby the patient places the arm into a fixed cuff. The machine sequence is initiated by the coin, the cuff is inflated, the blood flow sounds are recorded electronically and the readings may be displayed or printed out for the patient to retain.

Any equipment that is used or recommended for use by a pharmacist should be accurate and reliable under the conditions of use. Detailed guidelines have been prepared by the Royal Pharmaceutical Society for pharmacists in the UK who provide a blood pressure measurement service in the pharmacy. The pharmacist making the measurement should be competent in the use of the apparatus and the unsupervised use by patients of automatic sphygmomanometers should be discouraged. Measurements should preferably be made in a room where confidentiality can be maintained and where the environment minimizes the stress on the patient.

Interpretation of the readings

Hypertension, i.e. a raised arterial blood pressure, reduces life expectancy although the patient may remain free of symptoms for many years. The condition is often detected as a result of a routine check and results in the physician prescribing antihypertensive therapy. The pharmacist who provides a primary screen must decide which patients should be referred for medical investigation and which can be declared to be 'normotensive'. Arterial blood pressure increases with age and therefore each age group has a 'normal range' for blood pressure. The Royal Pharmaceutical Society's guidelines include a list of readings of diastolic blood pressure above which medical reference is advised. These guideliness would usually apply to measurement used as a screen for the detection of hypertension and would not necessarily be relevent to a patient already being treated with antihypertensive therapy.

Pharmacists should consult with local doctors in drawing up a list of readings considered to be the upper limits of 'normal'. It is generally agreed that a single high reading is of little significance because of the many factors that can influence the blood pressure. The measurement should be repeated at least twice before the patient is referred to the doctor. Care should be taken at all times to avoid alarming the patient or damaging the relationship between the patient and the doctor.

PREGNANCY TESTING

Most pregnancy tests depend on the detection of human chorionic gonadotrophin (HCG) in the blood or urine. HCG is secreted soon after implantation of the fertilized ovum and can be detected in blood and urine within a week of ovulation. This substance is not detectable in the urine of healthy non-pregnant females and may be considered to be a specific test for pregnancy in the early months of gestation. Early detection depends on highly selective immunochemical tests based on the production of monoclonal antibodies specific for HCG. The reaction between HCG in the urine and the monoclonal antibodies may be visualized in a number of ways, e.g. by agglutination of coated latex particles or gold sol particles to produce a detectable physical or colour change.

Although tests for HCG are regarded as specific for pregnancy in healthy females, certain tumours are associated with high levels of HCG secretion in the nonpregnant state. Conversely, pregnancies in which the embryo becomes embedded outside the uterus (ectopic pregnancy) are often associated with low levels of HCG secretion.

Sale of pregnancy testing kits

Pharmacists in the community may sell pregnancy test kits for use by women in the home. Pharmacists should have an understanding of the products sold in the pharmacy in order to offer advice to purchasers if requested. The purchaser should be treated with confidentiality and advised to seek medical advice whatever the result of the test.

Provision of a pregnancy testing service

The Council of the Royal Pharmaceutical Society has issued guidance to pharmacists offering a pregnancy testing service in the UK. The pharmacist is advised to obtain a signed and dated confirmation of the request for testing, to retain a record of the test and the result for at least 1 year and to provide a written confirmation of the result to the patient. In communicating the result the patient should be advised that a test for urinary gonadotrophin has been found to be positive or negative and the patient further advised to seek medical advice.

Facilities for carrying out the test

Any tests involving handling of body fluids should be carried out in an area totally separate from that used for dispensing and high standards of hygiene maintained. The materials used should be of reliable quality and stored and handled as recommended by the manufacturer. Specimens collected should be carefully labelled to avoid possible confusion.

Possible interference with the test

Early morning samples of urine should be collected into clean containers. Detergent or disinfectant present in the collection vessel may interfere with the test. The presence in the sample of drugs excreted into the urine may also produce false results and should be considered when the sample is accepted for testing.

OVULATION TESTING KITS

Conception is most likely to occur if intercourse takes place near to the time of ovulation. Various methods have been used to predict or detect ovulation, the use of the basal body temperature method is described above. A surge of luteinizing hormone (LH) from the anterior pituitary gland precedes ovulation by approximately 36 hours. Like human chorionic gonadotrophin (HCG), LH is secreted into the blood and urine and may be detected in the urine by means of a specific monoclonal antibody test.

Various test kits for LH are available for sale from pharmacies for use by women to detect the pre-ovulatory LH surge and hence to predict the time of ovulation approximately 24 hours later. A series of tests are carried out on early morning urine samples for 6 or 7 days in the middle of the cycle. The days chosen vary according to the normal cycle length and are explained in the literature supplied with the test. Detection of ovulation does not guarantee that conception will occur and the pharmacist should be able to provide further advice and explanation if required.

DIABETIC TESTING

Diabetes mellitus is a disease characterized by hyperglycaemia and glycosuria. Traditional tests for the adequacy of control of hyperglycaemia have involved the measurement of the glucose that appears in the urine. While testing of urine is relatively convenient, the information gained is limited and is a poor reflection of the blood glucose concentration at the time of the urine test. Tests designed to measure the glucose concentration directly from a drop of capillary blood are considered by most clinicians to offer better diabetic control.

For patients with Type 1 diabetes mellitus who are at risk from ketoacidosis, tests for detecting ketones in urine are also available.

Most diabetic patients take responsibility for monitoring of their own glucose levels and the consequent adjustment of their therapy. The test kits are prescribed or recommended by the physician and are usually supplied from the pharmacy. Newly diagnosed diabetics are likely to be under hospital care but the community pharmacist is involved in the long-term care of diabetic patients in the community.

Most tests for glucose in body fluids involve the generation of a colour which is compared against a standard colour chart and a qualitative or quantitative inference made. The accuracy of the test depends on the competence of the patient to perform the test in accordance with the manufacturer's instructions and the ability of the patient to read and interpret the result. The pharmacist is in a unique position to advise diabetic patients in the correct use and interpretation of the test. It should be noted that tests produced by different manufacturers require different techniques and produce different end points. Elderly diabetics especially those with impaired vision and patients with defective colour vision may experience particular problems. Several manufacturers have produced 'glucose meters' which read the results of a particular test but are not interchangeable with tests of a different manufacturer. These meters are available for purchase by diabetic patients and may also be provided on loan from some hospitals or through charitable organizations.

OTHER SCREENING TESTS

With the increasing availability of relatively simple test kits for a number of constituents of body fluids pharmacists may consider providing a multicomponent testing service. Members of the public are increasingly aware of the existence of substances such as cholesterol and triglycerides and wish to be reassured that their levels are 'normal'. Such testing is of little value without appropriate clinical support and pharmacists would be well advised to liaise closely with community physicians before undertaking the provision of a general screening service. In particular, the local concensus of the 'normal' range of test results should be determined since this may vary from area to area.

Concluding comment

The pharmacist has an important role in the sale, supply and provision of diagnostic tests and in so doing may make a valuable contribution to primary health care in the community in liaison with other members of the health-care team.

BIBLIOGRAPHY

Drug Tariff 1988 HMSO London (updated monthy)
Edwards C, Stillman P 1980 Blood pressure measurement. Pharmaceutical Journal 224: 246–248
McCreedy C 1987 Blood pressure measurement in the Pharmaceutical Journal 239: 468–470, 481
Pharmaceutical Society 1979 Guidelines on blood pressure measurement in the pharmacy (Council Statement). Pharmaceutical Journal 222: 179
Pharmaceutical Society 1987 Pregnancy testing in pharmacies (Council Statement). Pharmaceutical Journal 238: 345
Royal Pharmaceutical Society of Great Britain 1988 Medicines and ethics — a guide for pharmacies, No. 1, RPSC, London (updated twice yearly)

Relating to the prescriber

41. Therapeutics in practice

S. A. Hudson   R. W. Walker

Therapeutics has evolved from a practised art into a scientific discipline based on the understanding and the measurement of drug effects in clinical practice. The more knowledge that exists about a drug and how it acts, the greater the attention that must be given to ensure that it is prescribed and administered for optimum effect. To achieve this optimum effect in an individual patient, a number of decisions must be made.

The need for drug treatment must first be established, thereafter the appropriate drug, dose, route, form, frequency and duration of treatment must be determined. The drug must be administered appropriately and its beneficial effects and adverse effects monitored. A vast amount of pharmacological, pharmaceutical, therapeutic and toxicological information is available on individual drugs which may be relevant to these decisions. The pharmacist must be able to evaluate and assess the relative importance of this information in order to advise the physician appropriately. Pharmacists may also be involved in pharmacokinetic and adverse reaction monitoring, thereby adding to the clinical observations made by the prescriber. The response of the pharmacy profession to these new challenges has become identified with term *clinical pharmacy*; an approach to the practice of pharmacy which steers the attention of the pharmacist to the patient as much as to the properties of the chosen pharmaceutical product.

Limitations on pharmacological knowledge

All newly developed medicines must secure a *product licence* from the Committee on Safety of Medicines (CSM) before they can be marketed in the UK. The CSM requires evidence of safety, quality and efficacy before a product license can be granted. However, all medicines existing at that time received a product licence of right when the 1968 Medicines Act was implemented. The Committee on Review of Medicines (CRM) was established in 1974 to scrutinize the quality, efficacy and safety of all products that had been granted a license of right. Under an EEC Directive this review should be completed by 1990, thereby offering some guarantee of reliability for all medicines on the UK market.

Pharmacological knowledge on a drug accumulates initially during the various phases of clinical trial research involved in the development of a new drug (Table 41.1). Premarketing trials in patients may demonstrate adequate effectiveness of a new drug in a particular condition, but clinical trials comparing the new drug with other forms of drug treatment are necessary to establish its relative merits and disadvantages. However, comparative trials with a similar drug are often not conducted until the drug has been in widespread use.

At the time a drug is granted a product licence, it may have been studied in a few hundred or a few thousand patients (Phase 3 trials). However, it is not until the drug becomes widely used in patients of various ages and clinical condition that uncommon adverse effects become apparent.

There is therefore a degree of uncertainty about the initial information on a drug that is available to the prescriber. A further limitation on the application of pharmacological knowledge to the care of patients is the uncertainty, even with established drugs, that is associated with predicting the response to treatment in individuals suffering from widely different disease states which vary in nature and extent. Therapeutics is about managing this uncertainty by the adoption of a rational approach to drug treatment.

Table 41.1 Stages in the study and development of a drug

Phase 1 Studies in human volunteers
Phase 2 Studies in small groups of highly selected patients
Phase 3 Premarketing clinical trials
Phase 4 Postmarketing trials and surveillance during general use

Sources of individual variation in response to drugs

Variation in the nature and degree of the therapeutic and toxic responses to drugs between patients is a reflection of human diversity. Genetic, environmental and pathological factors play an important part in determining the way an individual responds to a drug. Few of these factors are understood. Even fewer factors can be identified or measured in a way which provides a practical means of predicting how suitable a drug might be for an individual patient or predicting the dosage regimen that is most appropriate.

Emphasis is often placed on the disposition of a drug in the body as a source of human variability in response to treatment. These pharmacokinetic factors involved in interpatient variability deserve to be studied and defined since they can be determined in a patient through the measurement of plasma drug concentration. The application of these principles of clinical pharmacokinetics to pharmacy practice will be considered in Chapters 42 and 43.

The most important sources of pharmacological variation undoubtedly lie in genetic differences at a biochemical level or at the drug receptor and in the conditioning imposed on pharmacological responsiveness by concurrent disease. These pharmacodynamic sources of variability determine the degree of therapeutic effect and determine the likelihood of unwanted drug effects oc-

curring during treatment. The occurrence and nature of adverse drug reactions are discussed in Chapter 44. It is inevitable that the pharmacodynamic determinants of drug action are much more difficult to measure than those due to pharmacokinetic variability. In Tables 41.2 and 41.3 respectively, examples are used to illustrate some pharmacokinetic and pharmacodynamic sources of variation in drug response.

Table 41.3   Examples of factors that may effect the pharmacodynamic response to a drug

Factor	Examples
Ageing	Increased responsiveness to warfarin; increased sensitivity to drug-induced sedation/confusion and seizures; increased risk of certain adverse drug reactions, e.g. postural hypotension, parkinsonism and dyskinesias, glucose intolerance
Immaturity	In babies: poor development of beta-adrenoceptors in the lungs and reduced responsiveness to sympathomimetic bronchodilators; increased sensitivity of CNS effects of drugs (e.g. sedation, seizures); susceptibility to dose-related shock caused by chloramphenicol
Gender	Drug-induced lupus erythematosus and dyskinesias are more likely in women; men gain more benefit from the antithrombotic action of aspirin
Disease process	In chest disease: increased risk of respiratory depression from CNS drugs; reduced penetration of drugs administered by inhalation In liver disease: increased sensitivity to CNS drugs; increased sensitivity to anticoagulation In heart disease: increased sensitivity to drugs affecting cardiac rhythm or contractility; increased sensitivity to fluid retention due to drugs
Tolerance	Chronic treatment with some drugs may selectively diminish response; e.g. opioids, some hypnotics and anxiolytics, sympathomimetic agents and some vasodilators. Acquired resistance of tumour or micro-organism to chemotherapy
Drug interaction	One drug may interfere with the activity of another either directly (agonist/antagonist) or indirectly (the effect of one drug mitigating or augmenting the therapeutic or toxic effect of another)

Table 41.2   Pharmacokinetic sources of variation in clinical response to a drug

Absorption	Variations in environment at site of absorption (e.g. digestive process and gastrointestinal motility, tissue pH and blood flow to site of i.m. injection). Biopharmaceutical differences between drug products
Distribution	Variations in protein and tissue binding, body composition, drug concentrations in body fluids and at receptor sites
Renal excretion	Variations in glomerular filtration, tubular reabsorption and secretion
Hepatobiliary elimination	Variations in biliary excretion and gastrointestinal deconjugation or degradation
Hepatic metabolism	Variations in microsomal enzyme activity, hepatic conjugation mechanisms and liver blood flow

Note: pharmacokinetic variations may represent a function of natural human diversity, they may be imposed by concurrent disease states or may arise from drug interactions

Drug manufacturers attempt to take into account the unpredictability of an individual patient's response to a drug by advising a dosage range based on clinical experience at the time the drug is licensed and these recommendations are updated periodically. This experience is embodied in the data sheet of the drug protect. The data sheet dosage guidelines are accompanied by a specification of disease categories and risk factors (contraindications and precautions) known to have a bearing on the response to the drug. In practice information from the drug's data sheet should be considered carefully in conjunction with information from other sources of literature available to the prescriber and the pharmacist. First-line sources of prescribing information may help in the selection of a starting dose and dose regimen which may then need to be re-evaluated periodically as the patient is re-assessed. The use of important sources of drug information is considered in Chapter 45.

Decisions in drug therapy

In prescribing a drug for a patient, a doctor strives to obtain the optimum therapeutic benefit to the patient at minimum risk of unwanted effects. A wide choice of medicines is available to the prescriber and for each agent a large, expanding volume of information exists. The selection of the most appropriate therapeutic agent and dosage regimen for a particular patient requires a rational approach and the application of the basic principles of therapeutics summarized below:

1. Clinical assessment of the impact of illness on the patient.

2. Arrival at an accurate diagnosis.

3. Identification of disease process or symptoms which realistically are amenable to drug treatment.

4. Contemporary appreciation of available effective pharmacological options.

5. Assessment of the patient as an individual in terms of the presence of factors likely to influence drug action (age, body, weight, disease processes).

6. Evaluation of the benefits and risks associated with the drug treatment options.

7. Definition of short- and long-term goals of treatment and end-points for the monitoring of efficacy and toxicity. Wherever possible end-points which are relevant to the clinical expression of disease activity should be sought.

8. Consideration of the implications of the required speed of onset of action, the importance of precise control of dosage and patient compliance on the route of administration.

9. Selection of agent of choice, dosage regimen and route of administration.

10. Monitoring of outcome in terms of defined therapeutic end-points and possible unwanted effects of predefined stages after the start of drug treatment. Periodically review the relationship between the benefits achieved and the cost of drug therapy in terms of undesirable effects, inconvenience and expense.

This process frequently requires access to detailed information on clinical efficacy, precautions and contraindications, dosage, adverse effects and pharmacokinetics (Fig. 41.1).

In practice, information from the medical and scientific literature is often useful in guiding the choice of therapeutic agent and its dosage. However, since patients may show great individuality in the way they respond to a particular drug, careful evaluation of response to a prescribed therapy and periodical re-evaluation of its effectiveness are important. Therapeutic response may be judged in terms of subjective end-points such as relief of symptoms, or objectively by monitoring clinical measurements resulting directly from the disease process such as X-ray findings, joint movements, psychiatric rating scales. Laboratory markers, for example haematological measurements, microbiological analysis, serological tests or plasma enzymes, are also useful end-points but may be inferior to clinical measures if they are not clearly related to disease activity. In some cases, for instance in the prevention of seizures using anticonvulsants, clinical or biochemical end-points of the effectiveness are sparse or absent and an intermediate end-point (such as plasma drug concentration) has to be used.

The physician's diagnosis and clinical assessment from observation, examination and obtaining a history is essential to the process of deciding optimum drug treatment. One of the earliest examples of the use of a potent pharmaceutical preparation serves to illustrate the factors involved in prescribing decisions. The use of digoxin to treat atrial fibrillation and left ventricular failure relies on subjective assessment of the patient's symptoms. The pulse rate, blood pressure, reduced evidence of oedema especially on examination of the chest, relief from breathlessness and tolerance to exercise are major indicators of benefit from the drug. However, subjective physical assessment of patients is only a limited guide to digoxin therapy since the detection of its cardiotoxicity is unreliable. Excessive doses of digoxin are mainly recognized by gastrointestinal, psychiatric or visual side-effects. Objective evidence from an electrocardiogram or plasma drug measurement

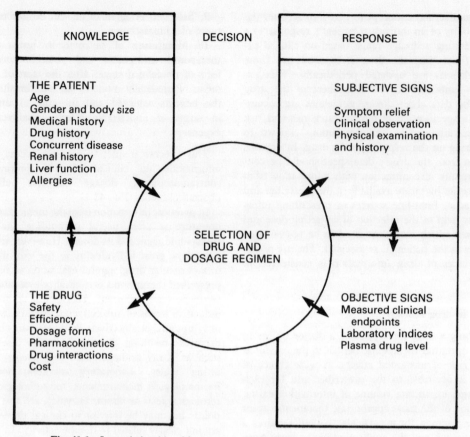

Fig. 41.1 Interrelationship of factors contributing to the selection of drug therapy

is often necessary to provide confirmation of digoxin toxicity.

The large amount of pharmacological research of digoxin over many years has not altered the fact that therapeutic decisions about the use of the drug still rely largely on subjective physical assessment of the patient. The main contribution of pharmacological studies has been the recognition of objective measures which contribute to the cardiotoxicity of digoxin, such as the plasma drug concentration and a low plasma potassium concentration. This knowledge has provided the basis for reducing the risk of toxicity by adjustment of the dose of digoxin in accordance with renal function, by monitoring the drug concentration in plasma and by the use of potassium supplements.

In spite of all of these pharmacological considerations, the major source of variation in drug response stems from the uncertainty of whether or not the patient is taking the drug as advised. This question of patient compliance is discussed fully in Chapter 37. Consideration of the behaviour of the patient and his or her

attitude to the prescribed medication must not be allowed to escape the attention of the prescriber or the pharmacist whenever an explanation is sought for a patient failing to respond to treatment.

Responsibility and behaviour in prescribing and dispensing

In practice when prescribing a drug for a patient, doctors must rely not only on their own knowledge and experience but also on that of others. This combination of knowledge and experience of a particular drug gives the prescriber confidence in the medication and guides decision making. The conservatism inherent in the therapeutic practice of many doctors is worthy of encouragement since it often forms the basis of good prescribing practice. The careful prescriber favours the use of tried and trusted medication over the latest novel compound of which there is high expectation but an inadequate 'track record' as regards clinical superiority in terms of effectiveness or safety over established treatments.

The contribution of the pharmacist to drug therapy

The pharmacist not only prepares and supplies medicines but also provides doctors, patients and other health-care staff with information and advice. He is obliged under common law and in line with professional conduct to satisfy himself that the medication as prescribed does not present undue hazard to the patient. To carry out this obligation the pharmacist must concern himself with dosage, dosage form, precautions and contraindications. The pharmacist also has a professional and indeed a moral obligation to satisfy himself that as far as possible the patient receives drug treatment that is prescribed in a way likely to prove effective. The pharmacist cannot therefore escape from being drawn into the consequences of the doctor's action.

Close professional contact between doctors and pharmacists usually leads to a climate of mutual respect and understanding. Under these circumstances the pharmacist is able to satisfy his legal, professional and moral obligations by making contributions to the process of decision making that are described by Figure 41.1 and listed on p. 381. These contributions may include drug knowledge, some interpretation of the signs of response and the monitoring of compliance. The pharmacist relies on a constructive interaction with the prescriber in order to discharge his legal and professional responsibilities thoroughly. Most doctors and pharmacists experience an unwritten code of behaviour which tends to ensure that the interests of each are respected. Should, on occasion, this code of behaviour break down, clearly the patient's well-being will be placed at risk.

The tradition of pharmacy practice is one of a complex professional relationship between pharmacist and physician, involving the exchange of advice and information on the technicalities of drug therapy and the individual needs of patients. For such a relationship between two independent professionals to succeed, there must be mutual recognition of skills, duties and responsibilities in order to achieve co-operation in the interests of the patient.

The tradition of independence is more marked in community practice than in the institutionalized setting of hospital practice. This independence of the community pharmacist inevitably imposes the problem of remoteness on the doctor–pharmacist relationship, whilst at the same time, the location of the pharmacy in the community ensures that pharmacy services are readily accessible to the patient. The result is a pharmacist–patient relationship which is unique in its assets and its

complications. Although the contributions to drug therapy made by the community pharmacist and the hospital pharmacist differ in their emphasis, they are similar in their intention.

The services of the pharmacist may have a decisive or a modifying influence on the patient's drug therapy in a variety of ways. Working in either a community or hospital setting, the pharmacist is involved at several important stages of drug therapy. Although the hospital pharmacist is in a better position to collaborate directly with the prescriber and other members of the health-care team, the community pharmacist may also be able

Table 41.4 Pharmaceutical contributions to drug therapy

Stage of drug therapy	Collaborative contribution	Independent contribution
1. Presenting complaint	Drug history from patient interview	Assessment of symptoms in community practice Medical referral where appropriate
2. Management strategy	Advice on treatment options, clinical and pharmaceutical factors influencing response	Provision of drug information. The monitoring of contraindications, drug interactions and allergies
	Assistance in defining benefits and risks of treatment options. Advice on specific end-points of efficacy and toxicity such as plasma drug concentration	Consideration of OTC treatment options in response to symptoms in community practice
3. Prescription	Advice on dose, dose form, route, formulation and cost. Advice on prescribing policies	Confirmation that dosage and dose form are appropriate
		Patient education and instruction on their medication
		Correction of ambiguities and illegalities
		Recommendation of OTC medication in response to symptoms
4. Assessment of response	Interpretation of symptoms in terms of effectiveness and possible toxicity of drug treatment	Counselling of patient to identify poor compliance and signs of unwanted effects of drug therapy
	Documentation of adverse drug reactions	

to develop services in co-operation with local prescribers. The use of pharmacy-based patient medication records provides the community pharmacist with a facility for identifying medication problems such as poor compliance, contraindications, adverse reactions and interactions. These developments in pharmacy services both require and create close working relations with prescribers. Regardless of whether practice is based in the community or in the hospital, pharmacy may make contributions to decisions affecting drug therapy which are dependent or independent of the prescriber. Table 41.4 summarizes some of the points at which these professional contributions are made.

The modern practice of pharmacy must place a priority on identifying and meeting the therapeutic needs of the patient. Clinical pharmacy can be seen simply as a redefinition of the traditional role of both community and hospital pharmacists towards patient care in line with the increasing complexity of modern drug treatment.

FURTHER READING

Goodman Gilman A, Goodman L S, Rall T W, Murad F 1985 The pharmacological basis of therapeutics, 7th edn. Macmillan, London

Barrett C W, Vere D W 1979 The interface between pharmacy and medicine. Journal of Clinical and Hospital Pharmacy 4: 159–165

Katcher B S, Young L Y, Koda-Kimble 1983 Applied therapeutics. The clinical use of drugs, 3rd edn. Applied Therapeutics, Spokane

Rogers H J, Spector R G, Trounce J R 1985 A textbook of clinical pharmacology. Hodder and Stoughton, London

42. Practical pharmacokinetics

S. A. Hudson   R. W. Walker

The principles of pharmacokinetics are important to the practice of therapeutics since they can be used to help explain the time-course of drug action. For many drugs it is possible to establish a relationship between the plasma concentration and the time of onset and duration of pharmacological response. Under these circumstances, an understanding of the pharmacology and toxicity of a drug is incomplete without a knowledge of its pharmacokinetic characteristics. Members of the same pharmacological drug group can display different pharmacokinetic properties which may confer therapeutic advantage or disadvantage. A sound knowledge of pharmacokinetic principles is therefore essential in the promotion of rational drug therapy.

A descriptive appreciation of pharmacokinetics is helpful in the interpretation of the clinical response to a drug. Similarly, a level of mathematical appreciation is necessary if pharmacokinetic data are to be used to assist dosage selection. When therapeutic drug monitoring is practised, drug concentration data from an individual patient are manipulated in order to optimize dosage.

The rationale for therapeutic drug monitoring is discussed in more detail in Chapter 43. The reader is referred to Part 2 of the companion volume (Aulton 1988) for an introduction to bioavailability and further details of drug absorption and elimination.

BASIC CONCEPTS AND FIRST PRINCIPLES

Drug distribution

Plasma concentration data can be described most simply in pharmacokinetic terms after administration of a drug by rapid direct intravenous injection. The human body is chemically and physically complex. Consequently, the distribution of a drug throughout its fluids and tissues occurs in a complex and selective fashion and is a dynamic process which continues through to an apparent equilibrium. After equilibrium, the drug concentration most relevant to the pharmacological effect is the concentration at the site of action. However, this site is not usually amenable to direct sampling. Fortunately, once drug distribution has reached equilibrium, changes in concentration at the site of action are generally reflected by changes in blood concentration. Since blood is convenient to sample, pharmacokinetic studies are often based on the examination of changes in drug concentrations in whole blood, plasma or serum.

The various rates at which a drug may partition from the blood into other body fluids and tissues can be explained mathematically by imagining that the drug acts as if it were being distributed into only a small number (often less than three) of different theoretical spaces or *compartments*. This mathematical device is drawn up merely to permit the most simple equation necessary to be used to describe the movement of drug into and away from the blood. This device may be understood by considering each theoretical compartment as a group of tissues which are similarly perfused by blood and which are penetrated by the drug to the same extent. Each compartment occupies a theoretical volume in which the drug 'appears' to be distributed. This volume does not necessarily correspond to any actual body space and so usually has no physiological meaning (see below). Two commonly used compartment models in pharmacokinetics are the *one-compartment* and the *two-compartment* open models illustrated in Figures 42.1 and 42.2.

A simple one-compartment model can be applied to many drugs and used in practice to derive pharmacokinetic information useful in dosage adjustment techniques. However, the drug distribution characteristics which are described by the two-compartment model are also important because they carry practical implications, particularly after the rapid intravenous administration of some drugs.

Apparent volume of distribution

The volume of distribution is a mathematical proportionality constant which serves to relate the amount of

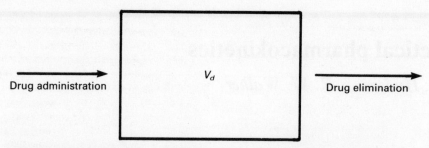

Fig. 42.1 One-compartment open model. Drug is assumed to be rapidly distributed throughout the body (apparent volume of distribution = V_d) and elimination occurs from the same pool of drug

drug in a body compartment to its concentration in that compartment. The body compartment therefore appears to occupy a calculated volume. This volume may approximate to some defined physiological space but more often does not. For example, the apparent volume of distribution of a large polar molecule which is not extensively bound to plasma proteins, such as the aminoglycoside antibiotic gentamicin, has a mean apparent volume of distribution of approximately 16 litres in a 70 kg adult. This volume is similar to that of extracellular fluid (interstitial fluid + intravascular volume) and reflects the predominant extracellular location of this drug in the body. On the other hand, the volume of distribution for warfarin is around 6 litres in

a 70 kg adult. Warfarin is extensively (99%) bound to plasma albumin and the volume of distribution reflects the location of albumin within the intravascular space (around 5 litres/70 kg). Therefore the concentration of warfarin in plasma is relatively high. In contrast, digoxin has an apparent volume of distribution of over 600 litres, is poorly bound to plasma proteins and highly bound to skeletal muscle. Over 99% of digoxin is located outside the vascular space and, consequently, the concentration in plasma is relatively low. Mean values for volumes of distribution of drugs are usually derived from studies of adults of normal build and expressed in the literature in terms of body weight as litres/kg. Standardization of volumes of distribution in terms of body weight may be useful to aid the adjustment of estimates for small deviations in the body size of normal adults. However, large inaccuracies may result if these standardized values are applied indiscriminately to subjects of abnormally small or large body size (such as children and obese individuals). Some apparent volumes of distribution (V_d) are given in Table 42.1.

Fig. 42.2 Two-compartment open model. Drug is administered to and eliminated from the 'central' compartment (V_1) and is partitioned with a second 'peripheral' compartment (V_2). There is significant time for equilibration to occur as the drug is distributed between V_1 into V_2. During this time partitioning of drug between tissue compartments occurs and drug is eliminated from V_1. Partitioning of drug between V_1 and V_2 results from the differences in drug penetration of the tissues due to the drug's solubility characteristics and because of variations in perfusion of tissues by blood. At equilibrium, a steady-state apparent volume of distribution (V_{ss}) represents the sum of V_1 and V_2

Table 42.1 Volume of distribution (V_d) and plasma protein binding of some drugs

Drug	V_d l/70 kg	% protein bound
Amitriptyline	60	97
Atenolol	50	<5
Carbenoxolone	7	99
Chloroquine	>10 000	55
Diazepam	120	95
Digoxin	>600	25
Gentamicin	16	25
Lignocaine	65	90
Nortriptyline	2000	95
Paracetamol	60	25
Phenobarbitone	35	50
Propranolol	180	90
Salicylate	12	80
Theophylline	35	60
Warfarin	6	99

Knowledge of a drug's apparent volume of distribution is sometimes useful in calculating loading doses and in predicting the plasma concentration after a single dose as the following examples (Examples 42.1, 42.2) illustrate.

Example 42.1

What peak plasma concentration might be obtained after administering a single dose of 120 mg gentamicin intravenously to a 70 kg man?
From the literature, gentamicin V_d = 0.25 l/kg
$\qquad$ = 17.5 l/70 kg
Gentamicin pharmacokinetics may be simplified to a one-compartment model.

Plasma concentration after 120 mg i.v. =	C_p	= Dose/V_d
		= 120/17.5
Peak plasma concentration		= 6.8 mg/l

Example 42.2

What dose of aminophylline should be given to achieve a plasma theophylline concentration of 15 mg/l in a 60 kg woman?
Aminophylline is approximately 85% theophylline
From the literature, theophylline V_d = 0.45 l/kg
$\qquad$ = 27 l for a 60 kg woman

Plasma concentration	C_p	= Dose/V_d
Dose theophylline		= $C_p \times V_d$
		= 405 mg
Dose aminophylline		= 405/0.85
		= 476 mg

A dose of 475 mg is required

Changes in plasma drug concentration

When plasma is sampled after a rapid direct intravenous injection of a drug and the drug concentrations plotted against time, a curve is usually obtained which can be rendered rectilinear by transformation of the concentrations to a logarithmic axis. This linear transformation is obtained by plotting log concentration against time or, more conveniently, by using semi-logarithmic graph paper. The semi-logarithmic plot of the concentration data may reveal one, two or more distinct linear phases and each phase requires an exponential function to describe mathematically the decline in plasma drug concentration. Each linear phase also corresponds to the movement of drug between theoretical body compartments.

For practical purposes the decline in plasma concentration for most drugs can be described adequately by up to three exponential functions. The majority of drugs appear to follow a monophasic (one-compartment model) or biphasic (two-compartment model) decline from plasma. In situations where one phase of a biphasic curve is small by comparison to the other phase, it may be possible to simplify a two-compartment model into a one-compartment model for practical convenience without loss of clinical significance.

Log-linear decline in plasma concentrations is a reflection of the drug movement away from plasma according to the laws of a first-order rate process (see companion volume, Aulton 1988, Ch. 7). In a first-order process, the amount of drug to undergo reaction per unit time is higher at higher drug concentrations. At high drug concentrations more drug will be absorbed, distributed, metabolized or excreted from that compartment in a time interval than at lower concentrations. The concentration of drug being distributed or eliminated from the body is constantly changing (decaying) and, according to the laws of a first-order process, at any point in time a fixed fraction of that concentration will be processed.

The behaviour of most drugs conforms to the principles of a first-order process at doses used in clinical practice. These drugs are said to display linear pharmacokinetic characteristics. For a minority of drugs, the processes of distribution and/or elimination of a drug do not consistently conform to this type of behaviour within the dose range encountered in practice. These drugs are said to display dose-dependent or non-linear pharmacokinetics. This form of pharmacokinetic behaviour is usually the result of an aspect of drug distribution or elimination being subject to the laws of a zero-order rate process. The phenomenon may occur after overdosage of a drug whose means of elimination becomes saturated at high doses (e.g. salicylate intoxication). It may occur in the normal therapeutic dose range of a drug and so be important in the routine clinical use of a drug (e.g. the metabolism of phenytoin). Non-linear pharmacokinetics and zero-order rate processes are discussed separately later in this chapter.

Drug elimination

As a consequence of plasma concentrations generally conforming to a first-order rate process, the fixed fraction of drug leaving the plasma at any point in time is known as the rate constant and is measured as a fraction of drug per unit time (often per hour). After rapid direct intravenous injection, a monophasic decline in plasma concentrations indicates that distribution of a drug is occurring at a rate so rapid as to be undetectable from the plasma concentration data. The single rate constant that describes the plasma concentration–time curve repre-

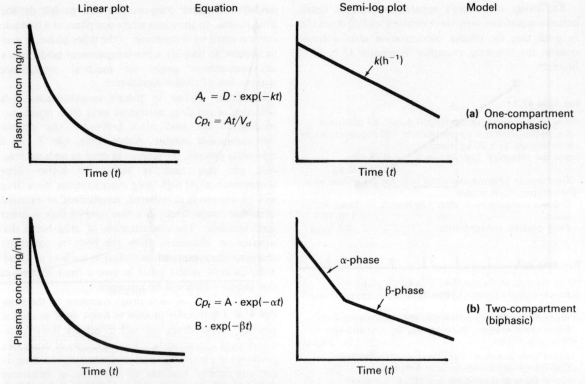

Fig. 42.3 Comparison of one- and two-compartment models. Rapid direct intravenous administration of (a) a drug conforming to a one-compartment model, and (b) a drug-conforming to a two-compartment model.

A_t = amount of drug in the body at t hours after injection (mg).
Cp_t = plasma concentration at time t.
D = dose administered (mg).
k = elimination rate constant (h^{-1}).
V_d = apparent volume of distribution of a single compartment (litres).
$\exp$ = base of natural logarithms = 2.72.

sents elimination of the drug from the body (by biotransformation or excretion) and is known as the elimination rate constant 'k'. The equation which describes the change in plasma concentration or amount of the drug in the body with time is indicated in Figure 42.3. A consequence of monophasic log-linear decay of the drug from plasma is that the amount or concentration of drug in plasma will halve over the course of a fixed time interval leading to the concept of half-life '$t_{\frac{1}{2}}$' of a drug. The relationship between elimination rate constant and half-life is shown in Figure 42.4 and illustrated by Example 42.3.

The term e^{-kt} represents the fraction of a drug amount or concentration that remains after a period of decay of 't' hours. This fraction is sometimes referred to as the 'fraction remaining' term and is often found in pharmacokinetic expressions. It can be calculated readily if k and t are known (Example 42.4).

Example 42.3

The half-life of a drug is the time taken for the amount of drug present in the body to be halved.

Therefore after one half-life ($t_{\frac{1}{2}}$) following intravenous administration of D mg

$$
\begin{aligned}
\text{Amount in body at time } t, A_t &= D \cdot \exp(-kt_{\frac{1}{2}}) \\
\text{But } A_t &= 0.5\,D \\
\text{Therefore } \exp(-k \cdot t_{\frac{1}{2}}) &= 0.5 \\
-k \cdot t &= \ln 0.5 \\
&= -0.693 \\
k &= 0.693/t_{\frac{1}{2}}
\end{aligned}
$$

Example 42.4

How much of a 10 mg intravenous dose of atenolol will remain in the body 5 hours after administration in a patient with normal renal function?

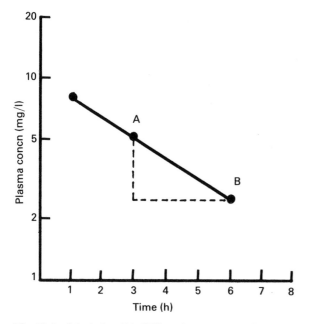

Fig. 42.4 Calculation of half-life and rate constant from semi-log plot. Plasma concentrations after i.v. injection of gentamicin 120 mg.

Method 1: by inspection. Take two concentration points on the graph (A and B) which differ by a factor of 2. The interval between them is the half-life, $t_{\frac{1}{2}} = 3$ hours.

Method 2: by calculation of slope.

Slope $= -k/2.303$

Take any two points on the line (e.g. A and B)

Slope $= (\log A - \log B)/3$

Converting to natural logs ($\times 2.303$):

$k = (\ln A - \ln B)/3$
 $= (1.6 - 0.9)/3$
 $= \mathbf{0.23\ h^{-1}}$

$t = 0.7/k$
 $= 0.7/0.23$
 $= \mathbf{3\ h}$

From the literature, $t_{\frac{1}{2}} = 6$ h, $V_d = 50$ l for a 70 kg patient
$k = 0.693/t_{\frac{1}{2}} = 0.115\ h^{-1}$

$\exp(-kt)$	$= \exp(-0.115 \times 5)$	
	$= 0.56$	
Fraction remaining	$= 0.56$	
Amount remaining	$= 5.6$ mg	
Plasma conc. at 5 hr	$= 56/50$	
	$= \mathbf{0.11\ mg/l}$	

Since e^{-kt} represents the fraction of drug remaining after a period of decline from plasma, it follows that the fraction lost during this period can be expressed by the term $1 - e^{-kt}$ as indicated in Figure 42.5.

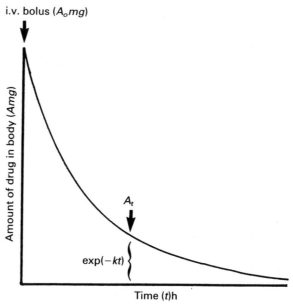

Fig 42.5 Fraction of drug remaining after direct i.v. injection. Estimation of amount of drug in the body (or plasma concentration) at any time after drug administration can be made by using the 'fraction remaining' term $\exp(-kt)$.

$$At = A_o \cdot \exp(-kt)$$

It follows that the fraction of drug eliminated in this time period is $1 - \exp(-kt)$.

It is clear that 90–95% of a drug will be eliminated after 3–4 half-lives (see Table 42.2). This rule of thumb is often useful in practice, for instance when considering how long it will take for a drug to be removed from the body (e.g. when discontinuing one drug and starting the administration of another which may interact).

Table 42.2 Change in fraction of drug remaining in the body with time

Time elapsed (half-lives)	% Drug in body	% Drug removed
0	100	10
1	50	50
2	25	75
3	12	88
4	6	94
5	3	97
7	1	99

It is useful to remember that 90–95% of a drug is removed after about 3–4 half-lives

3.3	10	90
4.4	5	95

Clearance

The body can be thought capable of removing a drug completely from the plasma at a rate which can be expressed as a fixed volume of plasma cleared of blood per unit time. The more efficiently the drug is removed from the body the greater the elimination rate constant, the smaller the half-life and the larger the volume of plasma that can be cleared of drug per unit of time. Excluding the effects of disease, drug interaction and environmental factors, drug clearance from plasma tends to be constant for a given drug in any one patient. The size of the clearance value for a drug is a useful pharmacokinetic parameter but does not define the fraction of administered dose that will be removed from the body over a particular time period.

Consider two drugs such as the beta-adrenoceptor antagonist atenolol and the aminoglycoside gentamicin. Both drugs rely almost entirely on glomerular filtration by the kidney for their removal from the body. Only a small fraction of the dose is reabsorbed or secreted by the renal tubule so that in both cases the healthy kidney is capable of clearing all drug from the plasma filtrate. The clearance of both drugs therefore approximates to a glomerular filtration rate which is about 6–8 litres per hour for a healthy adult. However, atenolol differs from gentamicin in being about three times less concentrated in the plasma (V_d atenolol = 0.75 l/kg: V_d gentamicin = 0.25 l/kg). The rate of elimination of atenolol is approximately three times smaller than that of gentamicin and the half-life about three times longer (atenolol k = 0.12 h^{-1}, $t_{\frac{1}{2}}$ = 6 h; gentamicin k = 0.36 h^{-1}, $t_{\frac{1}{2}}$ = 2 h). The clearance of a drug (Cl) can be thought of as a volume (litres), which represents the fraction of the drug's volume of distribution that is cleared per hour. Hence $Cl = k \cdot V_d$. Drugs with a high clearance may be eliminated slowly if their volume of distribution is large.

Clearance is important because it is less misleading than k or $t_{\frac{1}{2}}$ as a measure of ability to eliminate a drug. For instance, two patients may be equally efficient at clearing their plasma of drug but may be of different body size and have different volumes of distribution. Clearance of drug will be similar in both patients but the elimination rate will be smaller in the larger patient due to less of the drug being present in the plasma. Similarly the larger patient will show a longer half-life of the drug.

In practice this phenomenon is a possible source of variation in the half-life of the drug between patients. For example, obese patients have a higher distribution volume than the non-obese, particularly for lipophilic drugs such as the benzodiazepines. The clearance of diazepam is similar in normal and obese individuals but the volume of distribution may be over twice as large in the obese. The result may be more than a doubling of diazepam plasma half-life in obese patients.

The relationship between clearance, elimination rate constant and volume of distribution is explored in more detail under 'Dosage regimens' below (p 391).

Since most drugs depend both on metabolism and on renal excretion for their removal from the body, drug elimination can often be resolved into a non-renal (or metabolic, k_m) and a renal (k_r) component. Each component will have its own rate constant and clearance (Cl_m and Cl_r) which are additive, so the $k = k_m + k_r$ and $Cl = Cl_m + Cl_r$. The relationships k_m/k and k_r/k (or Cl_m/Cl and Cl_r/Cl) quantify the fraction of drug metabolized and the fraction renally excreted unchanged respectively (Example 42.5).

Example 42.5

After intravenous administration the anti-arrhythmic drug quinidine has an apparent volume of distribution of 35 l/70 kg, a metabolic clearance of 4.2 l/h and a renal clearance of 1.1 l/h. What are the drug's metabolic (k_m), renal (k_r) and total (k) elimination rate constants? How much of the drug is excreted unchanged in the urine?

$$Cl = Cl_m + Cl_r$$
$$Cl = 4.2 + 1.1$$
$$= 5.3 \text{ l/h}$$
$$k = Cl/V_d$$
$$= 5.3/35 = 0.15 \text{ h}^{-1}$$
$$k_m = 4.2/35 = 0.12 \text{ h}^{-1}$$
$$k_r = Cl - Cl_m = 0.03 \text{ h}^{-1}$$

Cl_r/Cl and k_r/k both represent the fraction excreted unchanged in the urine:

$$= 1.1/5.3 = 0.21$$
$$= 21\%$$

Two-compartment pharmacokinetic characteristics

The biphasic decay of plasma concentrations exhibited by some drugs (as shown in Fig. 42.3) is of particular relevance to the intravenous route of administration. Even when the duration of the early distribution (α) phase is small compared with the terminal (β) phase, the biphasic decay may lead to transiently high plasma concentrations after rapid direct intravenous injection. With some drugs (e.g. aminophylline and lignocaine) possible toxic effects such as seizures and cardiac arrhythmias may be produced. For example, immediately after intravenous injection of lignocaine the apparent volume of the central compartment (V_1) is about 30 l, and over about

30–40 minutes the drug distributes into a final V_d of about 90 litres. This rapid three-fold dilution of the drug during distribution renders its half-life of pharmacological action after direct intravenous injection short, requiring a repeated dose within 20 minutes. Emergency bolus doses of the drug need to be relatively small but repeated frequently, based on calculations involving the smaller distribution volume, whereas maintenance doses of the drug, which are administered by continuous infusion, are relatively large and are based on the larger (equilibrated) distribution volume. This pharmacokinetic phenomenon often explains recommendations for some intravenous drugs with a narrow therapeutic index to be administered over a minimum time period (perhaps 15–60 minutes) or in a minimum volume of carrier solution (perhaps 50–250 ml). The latter can be readily achieved by dilution of a drug in an appropriate small volume infusion solution if compatibility allows.

A second consequence of two-compartment model characteristics is the demand it may place on plasma sampling in therapeutic drug monitoring. For example, digoxin pharmacokinetics require a two-compartment model to describe the decline of plasma concentrations after oral or intravenous administration. The distribution half-life of digoxin is approximately 1 hour and the terminal half-life is about 40 hours. The pharmacological and toxic effects of digoxin are related only to the plasma concentration during the terminal phase. Plasma must therefore be sampled after equilibration (after about 6 distribution half-lives, beyond 6 hours after oral or intravenous administration of the drug). Failure to adhere to this sampling procedure will invalidate any attempt to interpret the digoxin concentration in the blood sample. Other examples of the importance of sampling time in therapeutic drug monitoring are considered in more detail in Chapter 43.

DOSAGE REGIMENS

Drugs tend to be prescribed in dosage regimens (i.e. the rate of drug administration in terms of dose quantity and dose interval) that are chosen from what is conventionally accepted and not always from what appears rational in pharmacokinetic terms. The dosage regimen of an established drug product arises from a combination of manufacturer's recommendation (based on the product licence application) and prescribing custom and practice from years of clinical usage. For some drugs a relationship between the plasma drug concentration and pharmacological response has not been clearly demonstrated and knowledge about the mode of action and fate in the body is incomplete. There is an inevitable reliance on customary prescribing practice and observed clinical response takes precedence over pharmacokinetic theory in the selection of dosage regimens. Drugs with pharmacological actions which do not correlate with their plasma drug concentration include those with irreversible (non-competitive) actions and those with active metabolites.

Dosage regimes are discussed further in Chapter 11 of the companion volume (Aulton 1988).

Drug accumulation

When plasma concentrations are known to correlate with the response to a drug, a pharmacokinetic approach to dosage regimen design may be useful when treating individual patients.

Continuous infusion and the chronic administration of a drug by multiple dosing are ways of achieving a sustained therapeutic effect which usually involves some degree of drug accumulation. Drug accumulation ceases during the regular administration of a drug once a 'steady state' has eventually been achieved. Modification of the dosing schedule of a multiple dose regimen (the rate of drug administration in terms of dose quantity and dose interval) determines the degree of drug accumulation, the intensity of drug effect and any fluctuation in response during the time interval of each administered dose.

Continuous drug infusion

Drug accumulation is readily illustrated during continuous intravenous infusion. A constant infusion delivers drug to the body in a fixed quantity per unit of time. Assuming distribution occurs rapidly, the body responds to the drug it receives by eliminating a fixed fraction of the amount of drug in the body at any time. With time the amount of drug in the body rises, the rate at which the drug is metabolized or excreted also increases until drug is eliminated at the same rate at which it is being administered. At this point of equilibrium a 'steady state' has been reached and the amount of drug in the body, and consequently the plasma drug concentration, remain constant (see Figure 42.6(a)).

At steady state the amount of drug cleared from the body, which is determined by the product of the steady-state plasma concentration and the clearance, $Cp_{ss} \times Cl$, equals the infusion rate. If the clearance of a drug is known then the Cp_{ss} can be calculated from infusion rate/Cl.

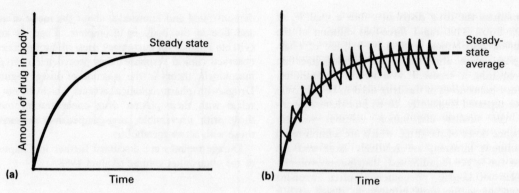

Fig. 42.6 Comparison of the changes in amount of drug in the body during continuous infusion (a) and multiple intermittent intravenous injection (b) showing the accumulation of drug towards a steady state

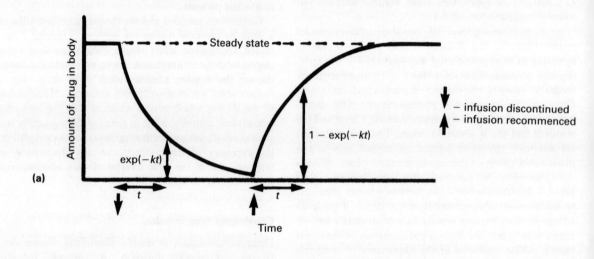

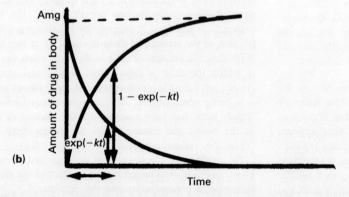

Fig. 42.7 (a) Infusion discontinued and recommended; In maintaining a constant amount of drug (*Amg*) in the body (steady state) the processes of drug removal and accumulation act simultaneously and so must be equal and opposite. Note that the shape of the downward 'decay' curve complements the shape of the upward 'accumulation' curve. (b) i.v. loading dose sustained by a continuous infusion.

When the infusion is stopped the amount of drug in the body decays according to the usual pattern of first-order elimination. It can be seen from Figure 42.7(**a**) that, at steady state, the tendency for a drug to accumulate and for it to decay can be imagined to be occurring simultaneously and therefore, mathematically, these two processes are complementary. From Figure 42.7(**a**), at time 't' hours after discontinuing an infusion the fraction of the previously constant steady-state amount of drug in the body is $\exp(-kt)$; whilst the fraction of steady state achieved at any time 't' during accumulation is $1 - \exp(-kt)(1 - e^{-kt})$.

Suppose the plasma concentration at time 't' hours after commencing a constant rate infusion is found to be 9 mg/l and the value of $1 - \exp(-kt)$ is calculated to be 0.75. It follows that the steady-state plasma concentration that will be achieved can be calculated to be $9 \times 1/0.75 = 12$ mg/l. The factor $1/(1 - \exp(-kt))$ extrapolates any plasma concentration on the accumulation curve to its steady-state value.

The relationship between drug decay and accumulation is further illustrated in Figure 42.7(**b**) by imagining an intravenous loading dose and a constant infusion of drug commenced simultaneously at a rate designed to sustain a constant amount of drug in the body A. At any time 't' thereafter, the amount of drug in the body which is due to the loading dose will be $A \times \exp(-kt)$, and therefore the amount due to the infusion will be $A \times (1 - \exp(-kt))$.

After a continuous infusion has been allowed to run for 3.3 half-lives, $\exp(-kt)$ equals 0.1 and so $1 - \exp(-kt)$ equals 0.9 indicating that 90% of steady state has been reached. Similarly 95% of steady state is reached after 4.4 half-lives. Steady-state is more or less achieved after about 4–5 half-lives regardless of how frequently or in what does the drug is administered. This practical rule reflects the complementary relationship between the rates of decay and accumulation of a drug. Doubling the dose or infusion rate simply doubles the amount of drug which accumulates in the body, without affecting the time at which steady state is achieved.

Intermittent regular administration

A situation analogous to constant infusion occurs with the administration of regular multiple intermittent doses of a drug (Figure 42.6(**b**)). In this case, although fluctuations of the amount of drug in the body occurs due to drug elimination between doses, the average amount of drug in the body between doses is constant at steady state (Figure 42.6(**b**), 42.8). After regular drug administration in Figure 42.8 it can be seen that the degree of accumulation expressed as a factor of the dose ad-

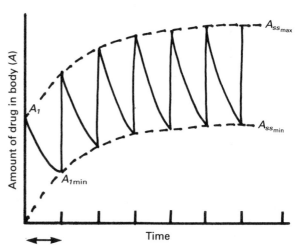

Fig. 42.8 Drug accumulation during multiple i.v. doses. A drug is administered intravenously as D(mg) every T(h). On multiple dosing a pattern of peak and trough variation in amount of drug in the body is achieved. After every dose each successive trough amount of drug in the body is the same fraction $(\exp(-kT))$ of each preceding peak amount. Immediately after the first dose, the amount of drug in the body (A_1) equals the dose (Dmg). The degree of accumulation of the steady-state peak $(A_{ss_{max}}:D)$ equals that for the trough $(A_{ss_{max}}:A_{lmin})$. A_{lmin} occurs at T hours after the first dose and represents a fraction $(1-\exp(-kT))$ of the steady-state trough. The value of $A_{ss_{min}}$ will therefore be $A_{lmin} \times 1/(1-\exp(-kT))$. It follows that $A_{ss_{max}}$ will equal $D \times 1/1-\exp(-kT))$.

The factor $1/(1-\exp(-kT))$ is known as the accumulation factor of a drug regimen.

Amounts of drug in the body:

Steady-state maximum $A_{ss_{max}} = D \times$ accumulation factor

Steady-state minimum $A_{ss_{min}} = D \times$ accumulation factor $\times \exp(-kT)$

ministered is dependent on the rate of drug elimination and the dose interval.

When a drug is required to be absorbed after administration, incomplete or slow absorption from an oral, parenteral or rectal dose form can greatly modify the size and time of attainment of peak plasma concentrations (Figure 42.9). Under these circumstances, analogy with intermittent intravenous injection to estimate plasma concentration fluctuations during the dose interval is likely to be inaccurate, particularly when absorption is slow or incomplete. Plasma concentration predictions may still be inaccurate even when bioavailability is complete, but the error will tend to be small when a drug's rate of absorption greatly exceeds its rate of elimination (see '1. Drug absorption' under 'Pharmacokinetic influences on dosage regimen design' p 396).

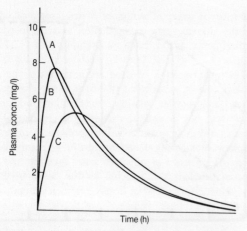

Fig. 42.9 Influence of rate of oral absorption on peak plasma concentrations of a short half-life drug. 100 mg of drug X ($t_\frac{1}{2}$ = 3 h): A, Direct i.v. administration; B, oral administration, absorption is complete and occurs in about 1 hour (k_a = 2.4 h^{-1}); C, oral administration, absorption is complete and occurs in about 4 hours (k_a = 0.6 h^{-1})

Notwithstanding these limitations, two methods for estimating the accumulation factor are described.

Method 1

The accumulation factor for a dose regimen can be calculated from $1/(1 - e^{-kt})$ as shown in Figure 42.8 (where k is the elimination rate constant and T is the dose interval). This factor is useful in practice for predicting steady-state peak and trough plasma concentrations of different dose regimens. In Table 42.3 accumulation factors have been calculated for different values of dose interval and elimination rate (expressed as half-life).

Method 2

For some practical pharmacokinetic considerations a simple estimate of the accumulation factor of a dose regimen may be helpful in considering different drug regimen options (combinations of dose and dose interval). This second method of estimating the accumulation factor applies the clearance concept.

At steady state the rate of drug administration expressed as dose (D) per number of hours dosage interval (T) (D/T) equals the rate of drug elimination. The rate at which drug is eliminated is obtained from the product of the mean steady-state plasma concentration ($Cp_{ss_{av}}$) and the clearance (Cl), $Cp_{ss_{av}} \times Cl$. If the clearance of a drug is known, the $Cp_{ss_{av}}$ of a dose regimen can therefore be estimated by calculating $D/(Cl \times T)$.

An alternative way of expressing this relationship is in terms of drug half-life. If $Cp_{ss_{av}} = D/(Cl \times T)$, then, since $Cl = k \times V_d$, the mean amount of drug in the body at steady state ($A_{ss_{av}}$) is equal to $D/(k \times T)$. Since $k = 0.693/t_\frac{1}{2} = 1/1.44 t_\frac{1}{2}$, $A_{ss_{av}}$ can be expressed as $1.44 \times D \times t_\frac{1}{2}/T$.

Once $A_{ss_{av}}$ or $Cp_{ss_{av}}$ is known it is possible to estimate the size of peak and trough. If half-life is at least as large as the dose interval, the accumulation factor is at least 2 (see Table 42.3). When the accumulation factor exceeds 2, $Cp_{ss_{av}}$ approximates to the plasma concentration at the midpoint of the dose interval. At steady state, by definition, the quantity of drug eliminated from the body during a dose interval equals the dose administered. It follows that approximately half the dose will be eliminated before the midpoint of the dose interval and half afterwards. $Cp_{ss_{max}}$ is thus approximately $Cp_{ss_{av}} + (0.5D/V_d)$ and $Cp_{ss_{min}}$ approximates to $Cp_{ss_{av}} - (0.5D/V_d)$. Similarly, $A_{ss_{max}}$ can be estimated from $A_{ss_{av}} + 0.5D$ and $A_{ss_{min}}$ from $A_{ss_{av}} - 0.5D$, remembering that, as described above, $Cp_{ss_{av}} = D/(Cl \times T)$ and $A_{ss_{av}} = 1.44 \times t_\frac{1}{2}/T$. As long as the half-life of the drug is at least as large as the dose interval, the error in estimating peak and trough concentrations during regular multiple intravenous doses is no more than 10% with this method.

Table 42.3 Accumulation factors. The half-life of the drug and the size of the dosing interval determine the degree of accumulation during regular administration

| Dosing interval T(h) | Half-life $t_\frac{1}{2}$ (h) | | | | | | | | | | | |
	2	4	6	8	10	12	16	20	24	36	48	72
4	1.2	2.0	2.7	3.4	4.1	4.8	6.3	7.8	9.2	13.5	18	26
6	1.1	1.5	2.0	2.5	2.9	3.4	4.8	5.4	6.3	9.2	12	18
8	1.0	1.3	1.7	2.0	2.4	2.7	3.4	4.3	4.8	7.0	9.2	13.5
12	1.0	1.1	1.3	1.6	1.7	2.0	2.5	3.0	3.4	4.8	6.3	9.2
24	1.0	1.0	1.1	1.1	1.2	1.3	1.5	1.8	2.0	2.7	3.4	4.8

Accumulation factor = $1/(1 - \exp(-kT)) \simeq (1.44 \times t_\frac{1}{2}/T) + 0.5$.

Dosage regimen design

Drugs which accumulate appreciably during the administration of dosage regimens used in clinical practice include those drugs with a half-life which is long in relation to the dose interval. In the same way that it will take 4–5 half-lives to reach steady state on any dose regimen, it will also take this length of time before the body is exposed to maximum amounts of the drug. For many drugs this time period coincides with the attainment of therapeutic or perhaps toxic effects.

A carefully estimated loading dose is the most appropriate way of removing the time lag and achieving a rapid therapeutic response. The loading dose may be given (acutely) as a single large dose. In theory the loading dose should be equivalent to the steady-state maximum amount of drug in the body after multiple dosing. For example, digoxin usually has a half-life of around 40 hours and is given in a maintenance dose of around 0.25 mg daily. The accumulation factor under these circumstances is around 3 and this helps explain the recommended acute loading dose being at least 0.75 mg for rapid digitalization. For some drugs where large single doses produce adverse effects or where a degree of tolerance to the drug needs to be allowed to develop, pharmacokinetic theory does not match usual practice (see Example 42.8 below).

Loading doses of drugs may be administered as a series of augmented maintenance doses for the first few dosing intervals. With digoxin, digitalization can be achieved by administering 0.5 mg for 2–3 days before reverting to a lower maintenance dose.

For drugs with a narrow therapeutic margin the fluctuations of drug concentrations in the body during a dose interval may be critical to the therapeutic and toxic response to the drug. Drugs in this category include most anticonvulsants and some chemotherapeutic agents, theophyllines, antibiotics and anti-arrhythmic agents. For such drugs estimation of the peak and trough plasma concentration fluctuation may be required. Assuming a drug shows linear pharmacokinetics, a reduction or increase in the dose will alter proportionately the peak and the trough plasma concentrations although the ratio of peak:trough will remain constant. On the other hand, changing the dose interval inversely affects the mean steady-state plasma concentration but alters the ratio of peak:trough. Therefore, when adjustment of a dosage regimen involving a change in the dose interval is required, pharmacokinetic calculations may be particularly helpful.

The degree of drug accumulation may help to explain the time of onset of action of a drug regimen, drug toxicity due to tissue accumulation and the need for loading doses, as illustrated by Examples 42.6, 42.7 and 42.8.

The quantification of drug accumulation is of particular practical value when variations in the elimination rate of a drug affect plasma concentration fluctuations in a way that is clinically significant, predictable or measurable. A frequent practical application of the use of pharmacokinetic calculations in dosage manipulation is in the presence of impaired renal function and this type of problem is considered further below in 'Pharmacokinetic influences an dosage regimen design'.

Example 42.6

What loading dose and infusion rate should be used to administer aminophylline to a 60 kg woman? (The target plasma concentration (C_p), is 15 mg/l theophylline. Assume $V_d = 0.45$ l/kg and half-life is 8 hours. Aminophylline is approximately 85% theophylline)

$$
\begin{aligned}
Cl &= k \cdot V_d \\
&= 0.7 V_d/t \\
&= 2.4 \text{ l/h} \\
Cp_{ss} &= \text{infusion rate}/Cl \\
&= 15 \times 2.4 \\
&= 36 \text{ mg/h theophylline} \\
&= \textbf{42 mg/h aminophylline}
\end{aligned}
$$

The loading dose can be calculated most easily from the volume of distribution (27 litres).

$$
\begin{aligned}
\text{Loading dose} &= C_p \times V_d \\
&= 15 \times 27 \text{ mg theophylline} \\
&= \textbf{475 mg aminophylline}
\end{aligned}
$$

Example 42.7

Spironolactone is a potassium-sparing diuretic with an action mediated mainly through its active metabolite, canrenone, which has a half-life of around 20 hours ($k = 0.035$ h^{-1}). What oral loading dose is appropriate for a dosage regimen of spironolactone of 25 mg q.d.s.?

$$
\begin{aligned}
\text{Accumulation factor} &= 1/(1 - \exp(-kT)) \text{ or } (1.44 \times 20/6) + 0.5 \\
&= 1/(1-\exp(-0.035 \times 6)) \\
&= 5.3
\end{aligned}
$$

Amount of drug in body at steady state
$$
\begin{aligned}
&= 5.3 \times 25 \\
&= 133 \text{ mg}
\end{aligned}
$$

Loading dose $= \textbf{125 mg}$

A delay of 2–3 days in the onset of maximum diuresis from spironolactone has been observed and may, in large part, be shortened by the use of a loading dose.

Example 42.8

What degree of fluctuation in the amount of phenobarbitone in the body during a dose interval would be expected from a dose regimen of 30 mg t.d.s.? (Phenobarbitone half-life is approximately 100 hours, $k = 0.007$ h^{-1})

Accumulation factor $= 1/(1-\exp(-kT)$ or $(1.44 \times t_{\frac{1}{2}}/T) + 0.5$
$= 1/(1-\exp(0.007 \times 8)$ or $(1.44 \times 100/8) + 0.5$
$= 18.4$

Maximum amount of drug in body at steady state $= \mathbf{552\ mg}$

Minimum amount of drug in body at steady state $= 555 \times \exp(-kT)$ or $552 -$ Dose
$= \mathbf{552\ mg}$

Assuming bioavailability (% absorbed orally) is constant at all doses, the theoretical loading dose is about 500 mg phenobarbitone. In practice, 500 mg as a single prophylactic dose would be considered hazardous, although the drug may be administered in a dose of up to 600 mg in 24 hours for the acute management of epileptic seizures.

Drug accumulation on a three times daily regimen exposes the patient to a gradually increasing amount of drug in the body over the 3 weeks required to establish steady state. During this period some tolerance to the sedative effects of the drug is acquired.

PHARMACOKINETIC INFLUENCES ON DOSAGE REGIMEN DESIGN

The therapeutic effectiveness of any drug treatment depends not only on the appropriateness of the drug selected but also on how it is prescribed in terms of dose, dose frequency and route of administration. A knowledge of the pharmacokinetic characteristics of a drug can act as a guide to the choice of the most rational dose regimen and the route of drug administration. For drugs with a narrow therapeutic index, a specific knowledge of the pharmacokinetics of a drug in a patient, derived from plasma drug concentration determinations, may enable a more precise dosage regimen to be designed for that individual (see Ch. 43).

Route of administration

1. Drug absorption

Drug absorption after oral, sublingual, rectal, topical and intramuscular administration is an important source of pharmacokinetic variation between patients and may influence the time of onset, intensity and duration of action of a drug. The process of absorption can contribute significantly to the inaccuracy of pharmaco-kinetic predictions because it is difficult to quantify from routine plasma concentration data.

There are three major components to the process of drug absorption; the delay in the start of absorption (lag time), the rate and the extent of absorption (bioavailability). After oral administration, the lag time is influenced by both the dissolution rate of solid oral dose forms and the gastric emptying rate. Both parameters may be greatly influenced by the presence of food. See also Part 2 of the companion volume (Aulton 1988) for more information on drug absorption.

The *extent of absorption* of a drug (F) is of practical importance when formulation differences between commercial preparations contribute to variable oral absorption or because variations in physiological factors alter drug absorption. Such factors include blood flow to the gut, the effects of food, drugs or changes in the gastrointestinal environment. For most drugs variations in formulation are much less important than physiological factors in influencing the extent of absorption. However, for a few drugs the extent of absorption is low (50–75% or less), e.g. thyroxine, erythromycin stearate, benzylpenicillin, metformin, frusemide, captopril, levodopa, iron, propantheline and emepronium. In these cases oral absorption may be sensitive to formulation changes such that bioavailability between brands may vary sufficiently to be of clinical significance. The systemic availability of a drug is also determined by the extent of metabolism during 'first pass' through the liver or during contact with the gut wall (see below).

The rate of oral absorption can vary greatly even in the same patient, depending on such variables as posture, time of day and presence of food. Drug absorption is often a first-order process and can be characterized by an absorption rate constant (k_{abs}) and a half-life ($t_{\frac{1}{2}abs}$). For example, a drug with a k_{abs} of 0.02 min^{-1} (1.2 h^{-1}) has a $t_{\frac{1}{2}abs}$ of 35 minutes. The absorption process for this drug is 90% complete after 3.3 absorption half-lives, that is after about 2 hours. In practice, the variability of $t_{\frac{1}{2}abs}$ is large even in the same patient. The absorption

Table 42.4 The effects of reduction in absorption rate on the peak plasma drug concentration

Fraction of normal absorption rate	Elimination half-life (h)				
	1	2	4	8	24
Half	20%	15%	10%	7%	3%
Quarter	40%	30%	25%	17%	10%
Eighth	60%	50%	40%	30%	17%

For drugs with different elimination half-lives, the table shows the percentage reduction in peak plasma concentration that would result from reducing the rate of oral absorption to one-half, one-quarter or one-eighth.

rate may influence the intensity of action of a short half-life drug (<8 hours) as indicated in Table 42.4. The effect of a reduction in drug absorption rates on the peak plasma drug concentration achieved is shown for drugs with different half-lives. The peak plasma concentration of very short half-life drugs (<2 hours) may be reduced by more than 25–50% if the rate of absorption is reduced by more than 50%. The drug illustrated in Figure 42.9 has a half-life of 3 hours. The peak plasma concentration obtained after administration on the slowly absorbed oral formulation is almost half that seen after rapid direct intravenous administration. The areas under each plasma concentration curve are comparable, indicating a similar biovailability in each case.

It is common for a drug which has a short distribution phase to give rise to transiently high plasma concentrations after intravenous administration (see two-compartment model, Fig. 42.2) but not after oral or intramuscular administration. The apparent absence of this phase after oral or intramuscular administration is due to distribution occurring simultaneously with the absorption process. This phenomenon is an explanation of why acute reactions to some drugs are more common after intravenous than after oral or intramuscular administration.

Controlled drug dissolution to produce slow absorption of a drug can be achieved by various oral and intramuscular formulation designs which enable larger than usual doses of drug to be administered with a sustained and prolonged therapeutic action. The ideal slow-release product should make drug available for absorption at a constant rate. In practice this objective is difficult to achieve and most oral sustained-release tablets or capsules only approach this ideal. Drugs with half-lives longer than 12 hours are unlikely to benefit from formulation into oral sustained-release dosage forms.

2. First-pass metabolism

Biotransformation of some drugs occurs extensively before they enter the main 'systemic' circulation because of metabolism during transfer through the gut wall (e.g. methyldopa, salbutamol) or during first passage through the liver (e.g. morphine, hydralazine, triazolam, hydralazine, chlormethiazole, organic nitrates and propranolol). Drugs highly 'extracted' by the liver during first pass have a low systemic bioavailability. Several drugs, including lignocaine, undergo extensive first-pass hepatic extraction such that the oral route is an ineffective means of administration. Any variation in the extent of first-pass extraction can provide an important source of differences in bioavailability. First-pass extraction tends to be affected by liver blood flow and is normally decreased by food (e.g. with propranolol and hydralazine). For some drugs first-pass metabolism is saturable and bioavailability is increased when a larger proportion of drug escapes extraction because of rapid absorption (e.g. aspirin and ethanol). For other drugs presystemic metabolism is reduced in the elderly or in liver disease such as hepatic cirrhosis (e.g. most opioids, triazolam, chlormethiazole). First-pass metabolism may result in different drug:metabolite ratios after oral compared with non-oral administration (e.g. propranolol). For drugs with active/toxic metabolites, the result may be variations in clinical effect according to the route of drug administration.

3. Other routes of administration

Drug absorption from the sublingual, rectal, topical or inhalation route may partially avoid presystemic metabolism and so may be an effective route of administration for drugs which undergo high hepatic extraction (e.g. nitrate anti-anginal agents, some opioids). Unintended systemic absorption after topical application or inhalation of some drugs may lead to unwanted effects from relatively small doses of drug (e.g. absorption from ·timolol eye drops or from nebulized salbutamol). The effectiveness of absorption by the rectal route is affected by the local retention of the dosage form.

Intramuscular administration is a practical means of administering a drug in patients unable to take medication orally because of disturbance of structure or function of the gastrointestinal tract or due to illness or loss of consciousness. It may be an unpredictable route of administration if blood supply to the site of injection is compromised (e.g. in shock) or in obese patients. Some drugs tend to be precipitated at the injection site because of the buffering effect of tissue fluid (e.g. digoxin, phenytoin, diazepam) which consequently reduces their effectiveness by this route.

The parenteral route may also be of value to sustain the action of a drug by the use of depot intramuscular injections or continuous intravenous or subcutaneous infusions. Short half-life drugs are particularly suitable for continuous infusion (e.g. heparin, insulin, dopamine, nitroprusside), since the infusion rate can then often be accurately titrated to therapeutic response. A similar result can be achieved by the topical administration of drugs that are effectively absorbed through the skin. Drugs such as glyceryl trinitrate have a half-life of a few minutes but a sustained therapeutic effect can be achieved by application to a prescribed area of skin which permits continuous administration at constant rate. This 'rate controlled' administration of a drug produces a more or less constant amount of drug in the body at any time and is analogous to continuous infusion. The 'infusion' rate of a drug absorbed topically is governed by the surface area of the skin to which drug is applied.

Dose regimen design in renal failure

Reduction in a patient's glomerular filtration rate (GFR) may be temporary (acute) or permanent (chronic). Mild to moderate renal failure is not uncommon in the elderly in particular and the effects of age alone mean that GFR is usually reduced by one-third by the age of 70 and one-half by the age of 80 years. Renal failure may affect the pharmacokinetics of drugs in different ways through associated metabolic disturbances. Most importantly, the loss of renal function drastically impairs the clearance of drugs that are substantially excreted unchanged in the urine. The result is an increase in accumulation of the drug in the body and an increased risk of toxicity unless the dosage is adjusted to compensate for loss of kidney function.

The degree of impairment of renal function (uraemia) is assessed in terms of GFR or creatinine clearance (normally 90–125 ml/min in an adult). Measurement of the clearance of several exogenously administered marker substances which rely exclusively on renal filtration can be used to estimate GFR. However, simpler endogenous markers such as plasma urea and creatinine are more convenient for routine use. Plasma urea is a readily available screening test for impaired renal function. The increase in plasma urea (reference range 2.5–5 mmol/l) is inversely related to GFR, but is unreliable and inaccurate due to tubular reabsorption of urea and the interference of factors such as liver function, diet, changes in extracellular fluid volume and gastrointestinal bleeding.

The most useful endogenous marker of GFR is creatinine, a product of muscle metabolism which is produced at a constant rate and eliminated almost wholly by filtration through the kidney. Creatinine clearance (Cl_{cr}) can be determined from plasma creatinine and urinary creatinine excretion which normally necessitates reliable 24-hour urine collection. The latter requirement is a serious practical disadvantage and source of error.

Alternatively, Cl_{cr} can be estimated from the plasma creatinine concentration if the patient's muscle mass, which varies according to age, gender and weight, is taken into account. In a young adult the normal plasma creatinine is 60–90 μmol/l for women and 80–110 μmol/l for men. The plasma creatinine is inversely proportional to changes in GFR. However, plasma creatinine may be deceptively low in elderly, frail or muscle-wasted individuals. For example, a plasma creatinine of 110 μmol/l in a 80-year-old 55 kg woman may represent an actual Cl_{cr} of 30 ml/min.

If plasma creatinine is constant (that is, renal function is stable) it may be used to estimate Cl_{cr} using either a nomogram (Siersbaek-Nielsen 1971) or an equation derived empirically (Cockroft & Gault 1976). The following equation of Cockroft and Gault is convenient and reliable when compared to other methods of interpreting plasma creatinine in adults:

In women,

$$Clcr \ (ml/min) = \frac{(140 - age) \times bodyweight \ (kg)}{plasma \ creatinine \ (\mu mol/l)} \quad (42.1)$$

For men, multiply right hand side by 1.23.

An alternative formula incorporating height must be used in children (aged 2–16 years), for example

$$\frac{Cl_{cr} \ (ml/min)}{1.73 \ m^2)} = \frac{40 \times height \ (cm)}{plasma \ creatinine \ (\mu mol/l)} \quad (42.2)$$

The estimate of creatinine clearance in this equation does not hold for children under 2 years and is expressed in terms of adult body surface area (BSA). To calculate actual Cl_{cr} the value for Cl_{cr} must be adjusted downwards according to the child's BSA.

The relationships between creatinine clearance and plasma creatinine in these equations do not hold if renal function (and plasma creatinine) is changing. For example, if there were a sudden drop of GFR to 20% of its normal value (to 25 ml/min) an increase in half-life of creatinine would be expected, from the normal 5 hours to around 25 hours. As with a drug there would be a period of equilibration of creatinine lasting 3–4 half-lives, in this case about 3–4 days, before the plasma concentration rose to properly reflect the reduced renal function.

Reductions in Cl_{cr} have particular implications for the renal component of a drug's clearance. The fraction that renal clearance represents of a drug's total body clearance is indicated by the proportion of a dose normally eliminated unchanged in the urine. For any drug, knowledge of the fraction of the systemically available dose that is excreted in the urine in unchanged form (F_e) can often be obtained from standard texts (e.g. Goodman and Gilman 1985).

The patient's Cl_{cr} can be expressed as a fraction of normal Cl_{cr} (R_f). Normal Cl_{cr} for a 70 kg adult (1.73 m² BSA) is usually taken to be 100–120 ml/min. For patients markedly smaller or larger than 70 kg, Cl_{cr} can be adjusted in proportion to BSA from a nomogram or equation using height and weight (The Extra Pharmacopoeia 1982). Since, in general, BSA varies according to body weight$^{0.7}$, the factor (body

Table 42.5 Degree of accumulation due to renal failure

Fraction excreted unchanged in the urine (F_e)	Fraction of normal renal function (R_f)				
	0.05	0.1	0.25	0.5	0.75
0.05	1.1	1.1	1.1	1.1	1.0
0.1	1.3	1.3	1.2	1.1	1.1
0.25	1.9	1.8	1.6	1.3	1.1
0.5	3.5	3.1	2.3	1.6	1.2
0.75	5.2	4.3	2.8	1.7	1.3
1.0	20	10	4.0	2.0	1.3

Dosage adjustment as fraction = 1/degree of accumulation in renal failure

Fractional dosage adjustment $= (1 - F_e) + F_e \cdot R_f$

$weight/70)^{0.7}$ may be a simpler method of adjusting the Cl_{cr} to take into account body size.

The degree of drug accumulation that is attributable to the change in renal function can be calculated, as indicated in Table 42.5, from a knowledge of F_e. Assuming no change in volume of distribution as renal function declines, the degree of accumulation is also the factor by which half-life is increased and clearance is decreased in renal failure. The reciprocal of the degree of accumulation represents the fraction of the usual dose of the drug which is required to compensate for the loss of GFR, as follows;

Dosage adjustment factors $= (1 - F_e) + (F_e \times R_f)$

It can be seen from Table 42.5 that drug accumulation due to loss of renal function leads, theoretically, to no more than a two-fold increase in the amount of drug in the body as long as F_e is <50% and Cl_{cr} is >50% of normal. Therefore, in general, one would anticipate that dosages should require reduction below 50% of those used in the presence of normal renal function if the drug in question is more than 50% excreted unchanged in the urine and renal function is reduced to less than 50% of normal.

From Table 42.5 it can also be seen that relatively small changes in the absolute value of GFR in severe renal failure cause dramatic increases in the accumulation of drugs highly dependent on the kidney for elimination.

The fractional dosage adjustment allows the rate of drug administration to be reduced by adjustment of the dose and/or the dose interval. The decision whether to change dose, dose interval or both is dependent on the relative practical importance of the steady-state peak, trough or average plasma concentration of a drug with respect to its therapeutic or toxic effects. Dosage regimen adjustment in renal failure is illustrated by Example 42.9.

Example 42.9

Disopyramide is an anti-arrhythmic agent normally administered in an oral dose of 100 mg four times daily. What dose regimen should be prescribed to a 60-year-old patient, weighing 73 kg with a plasma creatinine of 120 μmol/l?

(F_e for disopyramide is 60%, $t_{\frac{1}{2}} = 8$ h, $k = 0.09$ h^{-1})

Estimation of Cl_{cr} (Cockroft and Gault) $= 60$ ml/min

$R_f = 60/120 = 0.5$

Fractional dose adjustment necessary $= (1 - F_e) + R_f F_e$ $= 0.7$

Usual daily dose of 400 mg disopyramide needs to be reduced to $400 \times 0.7 = 280$ mg. Should this dose be prescribed as 100 mg t.d.s. or 150 mg b.d.?

Estimation of usual peak and trough fluctuations of drug in the body in absence of renal failure on 100 mg q.d.s.

Accumulation factor $= 1/(1 - \exp(-kT))$
$= 2.4$

$A_{ss_{max}} = 2.4 \times 100$
$= \textbf{240 mg}$

$A_{ss_{min}} = 240 \times \exp(-kT)$ or 240 − Dose
$= \textbf{140 mg}$

The effect of renal failure in this patient is to reduce k by 0.7 and so $k = 0.06$ h^{-1}.

Accumulation factor $= 1/(1 - \exp(-kT))$
$= 3.3$

$A_{ss_{max}} = 3.3 \times 100$
$= \textbf{330 mg}$

$A_{ss_{min}} = 330 \times \exp(-kT)$ or 330 − Dose
$= \textbf{230 mg}$

Now compare the effects of 100 mg t.d.s. with 150 mg b.d. in the patient in renal failure: 100 mg t.d.s.

Accumulation factor $= 2.6$
$A_{ss_{max}} = \textbf{260 mg}$
$A_{ss_{min}} = \textbf{160 mg}$

150 mg b.d.

Accumulation factor $= 2.0$
$A_{ss_{max}} = \textbf{300 mg}$
$A_{ss_{min}} = \textbf{150 mg}$

Since 100 mg t.d.s. in renal failure is the regimen most closely matching the effects of 100 mg q.d.s. with normal renal function, 100 mg t.d.s. is recommended.

Oral bioavailability is assumed to remain constant throughout. Although these calculations help to justify the selection of a dose regimen, pharmacological complications are added by the presence of the N-desalkyl metabolite of disopyramide which accounts for 20% of the dose, exerts anticholinergic effects and is renally excreted. The possible accumulation of this metabolite in renal failure and its potential to displace parent drug from plasma protein binding sites add uncertainty to the dose regimen and are additional reasons for closely monitoring the effects of the drug in this patient.

Table 42.6 Some drugs largely dependent on the kidneys for excretion

Acyclovir	Gold
Amiloride	Lithium
Aminoglycosides	Metformin
Atenolol	Methotrexate
Baclofen	Nadolol
Captopril	Nalidixic acid
Carbenoxolone	Primidone
Cephalosporins	Nitrofurantoin
Chlorpropamide	Nomifensine
Cimetidine	Penicillamine
Digoxin	Penicillins
Disopyramide	Phenazopyridine
Enalapril	Ranitidine
Ethambutol	Tetracycline
Flecainide	Thiazide diuretics
Flucytosine	Triamterene
Frusemide	Trimethoprim

In practice, this kind of dosage adjustment calculation can only provide an estimate of the dose required since it takes no account of active or toxic metabolites, no account of any change in drug absorption, volume of distribution, protein binding, biliary excretion or drug metabolism that may occur in renal failure, and no account of any changes in tissue responsiveness to a drug that may result from uraemia. Patients in severe renal failure (Cl_{cr} <10 ml/min) may require peritoneal dialysis or haemodialysis, procedures which will each have their own influences on the clearances of different drugs.

With these limitations in mind it is evident that, in many circumstances, pharmacokinetic calculations can only provide guidance on dosage adjustment in renal failure. Pharmacokinetic calculations are most helpful in guiding dosage adjustment in mild/moderate renal failure (Cl_{cr} 15–75 ml/min) which is an inevitable consequence of the ageing process and which may accompany a range of different disease states. Actual dosage recommendations for a particular drug need also to take into account studies of clinical response to the drug in patients with renal failure.

Table 42.6 lists some drugs which are largely dependent on the kidneys for excretion.

Protein binding

The extent to which drugs are bound to plasma proteins varies and pharmacological effects that are related to drug concentration in plasma are usually associated with the unbound fraction. When the degree of protein binding is high (>80%), minor changes in the fraction bound (due to the effects of disease, age or other drugs) may produce relatively large changes in the proportion of unbound drug.

In therapeutic drug monitoring it is the total concentration of drug in plasma that is most readily measured. Knowledge of the extent of protein binding of a drug in an individual patient is not usually available. The practical consequences of protein binding are still largely unknown for many drugs. Acidic drugs (such as warfarin, phenytoin, valproate, sulphonylureas, phenylbutazone) tend to be bound to sites on plasma albumin. Some basic and neutral drugs (notably propranolol, lignocaine, quinidine, some tricyclic antidepressants and chlorpromazine) are bound to alpha-1 acid glycoprotein (AAG). Some drugs are bound both to albumin and to AAG (e.g. disopyramide). Basic drugs may, to a lesser extent, also be bound to plasma lipoproteins and globulins. The fraction of bound drug varies with the concentration of these proteins in plasma and changes in other plasma constituents which may displace the drug (e.g. metabolic acids and fatty acids which may accumulate during fasting and may accompany diseases such as renal failure and diabetes). Plasma albumin is decreased if dietary asborption is decreased (malnutrition, some gut diseases), if albumin synthesis is impaired (liver disease), or if albumin is lost in the urine (some renal diseases affecting the glomerulus). Plasma albumin is often reduced in the elderly.

Plasma AAG is increased by some enzyme inducers, by traumatic conditions (including major surgery) and various acute and chronic disease processes (such as myocardial infarction, renal transplant, inflammatory bowel disease and malignancy). Reduction in AAG are associated with pregnancy and the use of oral contraceptives. An exaggerated pharmacological response may arise from a reduction in the binding of some highly bound drugs (warfarin, phenytoin, valproate) due to changes in plasma albumin or because of displacement by other drugs or endogenous compounds such as bilirubin. The clinical consequences of alterations in the fraction of drug bound to AAG are not well established for many drugs.

Non-linear pharmacokinetics

If the dose of a drug is increased, the pathways of elimination from the body may become overwhelmed. This saturation phenomenon is particularly true for drugs which undergo enzymic biotransformation. For most drugs saturation of elimination occurs only after very large doses and is not encountered within dose ranges used in clinical practice. For a few drugs, saturation of metabolic pathways occurs with therapeutic doses and consequently the rate of drug elimination from the body no longer represents a fixed fraction but a fixed amount of drug per unit time. Drug elimination therefore reverts from a first-order to a zero-order rate process. Common examples of drugs undergoing this process of saturation include ethanol and phenytoin. The practical implication is that with high doses the plasma drug concentration may continue to rise without reaching a steady state. Even at doses of these drugs which permit a steady state to be established, the plasma drug concentration may increase disproportionately to the dose. For instance in the case of phenytoin, a 33% increase in daily dose, from 300 mg to 400 mg, may produce as much as a 100% increase in plasma concentration.

The saturation of elimination mechanisms cannot be described by the first-order concepts of half-life, clearance and elimination rate constant. Characterization of a zero-order rate process depends on the determi-

nation of V_{max} (the maximum rate of elimination of the drug) and K_m (Michaelis–Menton constant). These variables represent the maximum amount of drug that may be removed from the body per unit time (V_{max}) and the plasma concentration (K_m) at which drug elimination proceeds at half the maximum rate. In practice these two pharmacokinetic parameters can be estimated in a patient if two steady-state plasma drug concentrations are measured on two different dosage regimens.

For some drugs (e.g. sodium valproate, disopyramide) the fraction bound to plasma protein may vary with concentration and these drugs appear to show non-linear pharmacokinetic behaviour if total drug concentration is interpreted without respect to the degree of protein binding.

BIBLIOGRAPHY

Aulton M E (ed) 1988 Pharmaceutics: the science of dosage form design. Churchill Livingstone, Edinburgh
Cockroft D W, Gault M H 1976 Prediction of creatinine clearance from serum creatinine. Nephron 16: 31–41
Evans W E, Jusko W J, Schentag J J 1986 Applied pharmacokinetics, 2nd edn. Applied Therapeutics, Spokane
Goodman Gilman A, Goodman L S, Rall T W, Murad F 1985 The pharmacological basis of therapeutics, 7th edn. Macmillan, London
Greenblatt D J, Shader R I 1985 Pharmacokinetics in clinical practice. WB Saunders, London
Kampmann J, Siersbaek-Nielsen K, Kristensen M et al 1974 Rapid evaluation of creatinine clearance. Acta

Medica Scandinavica 196: 517–520
Levy R H, Bauer L A 1986 Basic pharmacokinetics. Therapeutic Drug Monitoring 8: 47–58
Martindale, see Reynolds J E F
Morris M C Allanby C W, Toseland P et al 1982 Evaluation of a height/plasma creatinine formula in the measurement of glomerular filtration rate. Archives of Diseases of Childhood 57: 611–615
Reynolds J E F (ed) 1989 Martindale, The Extra Pharmacopoeia 1989 29th edn. Pharmaceutical Press, London
Winter M E 1987 Basic clinical pharmacokinetics, 2nd edn. Applied Therapeutics, Spokane

43. Therapeutic drug monitoring

S. A. Hudson   R. W. Walker

Drug assay technology is now sufficiently advanced for it to be possible to measure the plasma concentration of the majority of drugs used in clinical practice. However, the routine monitoring of plasma drug concentrations (*therapeutic drug monitoring*) is of proven clinical value for only a few drugs. This chapter will identify when it is appropriate to utilize therapeutic drug monitoring and to indicate limitations in the interpretation of the drug levels obtained.

It is generally only of value to monitor the plasma level of a drug when there is a direct correlation with its pharmacological or toxic effect. However, even if this relationship exists, it may still be unnecessary to carry out therapeutic drug monitoring if observation or measurement of the pharmacological effect of the drug is a convenient, obvious and direct way to monitor the outcome of treatment, e.g. with diuretics, anticoagulants and hypnotics.

The following guidelines indicate that therapeutic drug monitoring is appropriate if a drug displays:

1. A narrow therapeutic index.
2. Non-linear pharmacokinetics.
3. Large inter-individual pharmacokinetic variability.
4. Major side-effects related to the plasma concentration of the drug, together with a poorly defined clinical onset and end-point.
5. A steep dose–response relationship.

It may also be useful to measure the plasma concentration of a drug:

1. To confirm adequate dosage.
2. To identify non-compliance.
3. If the patient exhibits signs of possible drug toxicity.
4. When a patient responds poorly to therapy.
5. If a patient has a disorder that may alter drug disposition.
6. When a possible drug interaction is suspected.

Sample collection

Careful attention to the timing and practicalities associated with blood sample collection are required in order to facilitate correct interpretation of the results of therapeutic drug monitoring. The pharmacist is infrequently in a position to collect the blood sample, but may often be asked to provide advice to medical staff on the time a sample should be drawn.

The blood sample collection time is determined by the formulation of the drug, the route of administration, the dosage regimen and the clinical question to be answered. Moreover, interpretation of the results and therapeutic guidance can only be offered if the time of drug administration and its relationship to the collection of the plasma sample is known. The measured plasma drug level is useless and misleading if the timing of sample collection is not precisely known relative to the dosage schedule.

If a drug has only recently been introduced into a patient's treatment regimen or the dosage has been changed, the average steady-state plasma concentration corresponding to the dosage schedule employed may not have been reached. This early sampling of plasma may therefore produce misleading plasma drug concentrations. The time necessary to achieve steady-state plasma levels depends on the drug's elimination half-life. Once treatment has been continued for four to five times the elimination half-life of the drug the average-steady state plasma concentration will be more than 90% attained. Ideally, it is at this time that the plasma drug concentration should be measured (Fig. 43.1).

Unless a drug is administered by continuous intravenous infusion, a single steady-state plasma concentration will not be achieved. In practice the plasma concentration will rise and fall over a given dose interval. In particular, fluctuations of the plasma concentration between doses of drugs with a short half-life or over the course of a long dose interval may be con-

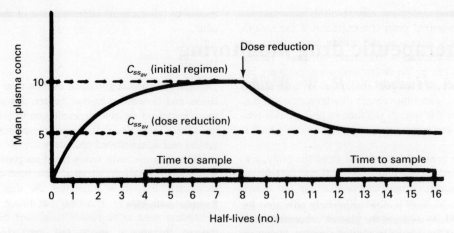

Fig. 43.1 Average plasma concentrations achieved during multiple dose therapy with a hypothetical drug administered at intervals equivalent to its half-life. Average steady-state levels ($C_{ss_{av}}$) are more than 90% achieved after 4 half-lives. When the dose is reduced by 50%, 4 half-lives are again required before the new $C_{ss_{av}}$ is achieved. Blood samples for therapeutic drug monitoring should ideally be drawn at steady state

siderable. The plasma concentration that is measured will be dependent on the time the sample is drawn relative to the last dose. In general, plasma concentrations are most useful and reliable when they are determined in the elimination phase (Fig. 43.2) immediately prior to the next dose (trough level). If the sample is drawn during the absorption phase or before distribution is complete a misleading low or high plasma concentration may be obtained. However, with drugs such as theophylline, a knowledge of the peak plasma concentration may be required, usually because it is directly related to the efficacy and toxicity of the drug. In these situations factors such as slow or delayed absorption can significantly delay the time to peak concentration. The

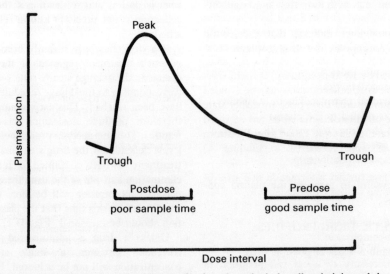

Fig. 43.2 Plasma concentration–time profile for a hypothetical orally. administered drug at steady state. Samples drawn in the latter part of the elimination phase (predose) are usually the most useful, consistent and reliable. Samples drawn to monitor the peak plasma concentration (postdose) are susceptible to variability in the rate of drug absorption and to the greater rate of change in plasma concentration that occurs during the elimination of high plasma concentrations

variation in drug absorption may result in important errors in the measured peak concentration if the sample is inadvertently drawn at the wrong time. After intravenous administration the time to peak plasma concentration can be predicted with some accuracy because the risk of variable absorption is eliminated. Unfortunately, with other routes of administration, e.g. oral, intramuscular, rectal, the time to peak plasma concentration is often subject to marked variation and is unreliable.

If the drug is rapidly eliminated from the body, e.g. gentamicin, both trough and peak levels may be relevant to dosage regimen design. In this example the trough level should be drawn immediately before the administration of the next dose. Because of gentamicin's initial short phase of distribution a sample drawn 30 minutes after the end of a 30-minute intravenous infusion or 15 minutes after a 60-minute infusion, will represent an equilibrated peak plasma concentration.

The peak plasma concentration of most drugs administered by mouth is often achieved within 1–2 hours post-administration when absorption and distribution are complete. However, for drugs with a long distribution phase a blood sample drawn before equilibration is complete will produce a misleadingly high concentration. For example, in the case of digoxin it is not possible to interpret the level of the drug from a sample drawn less than 6 hours after oral or intravenous administration, i.e. before distribution is complete.

Up to this point we have assumed that blood samples are drawn at steady state. In practice it may be useful to draw a sample after the first dose of the drug in order to predict the eventual steady-state drug concentration. If the predicted steady-state concentration is high, side-effects related to the drug concentration may be avoided by reducing the administered dose prior to steady state being reached. The pharmacokinetic equations required to predict steady state levels from blood samples drawn after the first dose were presented in Chapter 42 (Fig. 42.8).

The reader will find further information in Part 2 of the companion volume (Aulton 1988).

PHARMACOKINETIC DRUG PROFILES

A full appreciation of the pharmacokinetics of an individual drug is necessary to allow interpretation of plasma drug concentration data. In this section, a summary of important pharmacokinetic parameters will be presented for a selection of drugs routinely monitored in practice. The data relates, unless stated otherwise, to the oral (digoxin, phenytoin and theophylline) or in-

travenous (gentamicin) administration of the drug to an adult.

Digoxin

Digoxin is a cardiac glycoside used to treat atrial fibrillation and congestive cardiac failure. Its absorption is incomplete and variable depending on the choice of formulation (Table 43.1). It is generally prescribed as oral tablets and administered once daily.

Numerous methods, many based on predictions from a patient's creatinine clearance, have been developed to assist the clinician in estimating the digoxin requirements of each patient. It is clear that dosage adjustments of digoxin need to be closely monitored because of its narrow therapeutic index and marked interpatient variability. However, these factors, together with conflicting data on the effect of various disease states, contribute to the overall poor predictability of the

Table 43.1 Digoxin pharmacokinetic profile ·

Clinical use	Atrial fibrillation Congestive cardiac failure	
Absorption	60–70% (tablets) 70–80% (elixir)	
Volume of distribution	500–600 l/70 kg normal renal function 250–350 l/70 kg impaired renal function	
Elimination	75–80% renal excretion of unchanged drug 25–20% hepatic metabolism (increased in renal impairment)	
Half-life	Adults 40 h normal renal function >120 h impaired renal function	
Time to steady state	5–7 days of chronic administration (normal renal function) Longer in impaired renal function	
Usual sampling time	6 h after oral administration	
Plasma concentrations	0.9–2 µg/l therapeutic range >2 µg/l potentially toxic concentrations	
Factors affecting plasma concentrations		
Disease	Malabsorption syndromes	↓ absorption
	Renal impairment	↓ clearance
	Congestive cardiac failure	↓ clearance
	Hypothyroidism	↓ clearance
Drugs	Antacids	↓ absorption
	Verapamil	↓ clearance
	Amiodarone	↓ clearance
	Spironolactone	↓ clearance
	Quinidine	↓ clearance

methods available. To evaluate adjustments in the daily maintenance dose of digoxin, plasma levels should be determined at steady-state conditions. Moreover, because of digoxin's long half-life of distribution, samples should not be drawn until at least 6 hours after administration, at which time the plasma concentration reflects the maximum cardiac response.

Digoxin does not provide a good example of a drug suited to predictive pharmacokinetic modelling. Several studies have, however, demonstrated that the judicious use of therapeutic drug monitoring can significantly

Table 43.2 Gentamicin pharmacokinetic profile

Clinical use	Antibiotic
Absorption	Poor oral bioavailability Intravenous administration: complete absorption
Volume of distribution	10–20 l
Elimination	85–95% renal excretion of unchanged drug
Half-life	1.5–4 h normal renal function
Time to steady state	7.5–20 h normal renal function
Usual sampling time	
Peak	30 min after 30 min infusion 15 min after 60 min infusion
Trough	Immediately before next dose
Plasma concentrations	
Peak	5–12 mg/l
Trough	<2 mg/l Sustained concentrations above the recommended peak and trough levels are associated with nephrotoxicity and ototoxicity

Factors affecting plasma concentrations		
Disease	Dehydration	↓ Volume of distribution
	Obesity	↑ Volume of distribution
	Burn patients (acute)	↓ Volume of distribution
	Renal impairment	↓ Clearance
	Congestive cardiac failure	↓ Clearance
	Fever	↑ Clearance
Drugs	Carbenicillin	Inactivation in vitro and in vivo
	Ticarcillin	Inactivation in vitro and in vivo

reduce the incidence of adverse effects and provide valuable information to the overall clinical assessment and treatment of a patient.

Gentamicin

Gentamicin (and other aminoglycosides) is a bactericidal antibiotic which is valuable in the treatment of serious and often life-threatening Gram-negative infections. It is poorly absorbed from the gastrointestinal tract and is, therefore, usually administered parenterally by intermittent intravenous infusion. The selection of the dose and dosage regimen depends upon the causative infection, the renal function, concurrent disease state and weight of the patient.

Serious ototoxicity and nephrotoxicity have been frequently reported in patients receiving gentamicin. These adverse effects have been shown to correlate with such factors as age, renal function, cumulative dose, the duration of treatment and sustained elevations in peak and trough plasma gentamicin concentrations. Gentamicin is thus a good candidate for therapeutic drug monitoring.

Peak and trough gentamicin concentrations are frequently used to monitor and adjust a patient's dosage regimen (Table 43.2). However, dosage predictions are reliable only if the plasma samples are drawn under controlled conditions at a known time, if the dosage regimen received by the patient is accurately known and if the patient's renal function and the drug's volume of distribution do not change during therapy. Unfortunately, the volume of distribution of gentamicin often changes during therapy, making it difficult to accurately predict required dosage adjustments.

Overall, therapeutic drug monitoring of gentamicin and other aminoglycoside antibiotics is helpful in identifying the need for changes in the dosage regimen to optimize the therapeutic effect and to minimize the incidence of side-effects.

Phenytoin

Phenytoin is primarily used in clinical practice as an anticonvulsant agent. The activity of the drug increases as the plasma concentration rises. At a plasma phenytoin concentration of 15 mg/l the frequency of seizures is reduced in 85% of patients. Unlike most other drugs the dosage adjustment of phenytoin to achieve a target steady-state plasma concentration cannot be calculated by simple proportion. The hepatic metabolism of phenytoin is readily saturated so that a small adjustment to the maintenance dose can result in a disproportionately large change in steady-state plasma concentrations.

Table 43.3 Phenytoin pharmacokinetic profile

Clinical use	Epilepsy
Absorption	85–95% oral administration (variable depending on dosage form and manufacturer)
Volume of distribution	50 l/70 kg
Elimination	>95% hepatic metabolism <5% renal excretion of unchanged drug
Half-life (apparent)	30–100 h Half-life is not a useful parameter for drugs with dose-dependent pharmacokinetics. More useful terms are:- V_{max} 100–1000 mg/day K_m 1–12 mg/l
Time to steady state	8–30 days of chronic dosing
Usual sampling time	Immediately before next oral dose (trough)
Plasma concentrations	10–20 mg/l therapeutic range >20 mg/l potentially toxic concentrations

Factors affecting plasma concentrations		
Disease	Acute hepatitis	↑ clearance
	Chronic liver disease	↓ clearance
Drugs	Barbiturates (low concentration)	↑ clearance
	Carbamazepine	↑ clearance
	Alcohol	↑ clearance
	Barbiturates (high concentration)	↓ clearance
	Isoniazid	↓ clearance
	Cimetidine	↓ clearance

Phenytoin, therefore, exhibits non-linear pharmacokinetics (see Ch. 42).

Once treatment has been started with phenytoin, plasma steady-state concentrations may be seen in an adult after about 10 days (Table 43.3). However, because the rate of metabolism and apparent half-life of phenytoin vary at different plasma concentrations, in some patients it may take up to 4 weeks to achieve steady-state levels following a change in dosage. It should be clear, therefore, that it is inappropriate to state a value for the half-life of phenytoin. The availability of therapeutic drug monitoring has improved the use of phenytoin in the treatment of the epileptic patient. Plasma level monitoring has made it possible to obtain the maximum clinical effect, encourage the rational use of a single agent in the treatment of epilepsy, avoid dose-related

side-effects and assess compliance in patients receiving the drug. The majority of assay methods available monitor total plasma levels of phenytoin. It has been advocated that the free plasma concentration (8–10%), the true index of pharmacological activity, should be determined routinely since measurement of total plasma concentrations can only give an approximation of the 'free' fraction. However, regardless of the entity monitored, the plasma concentration must always be interpreted in the light of an assessment of the patient's clinical state.

Theophylline

Theophylline is a bronchodilator and respiratory stimulant used in the treatment of acute and chronic asthma. It is a drug with a narrow therapeutic index (Table 43.4) for which the benefits and risks associated

Table 43.4 Theophylline pharmacokinetic profile

Clinical use	Bronchodilator Prophylaxis in chronic asthma
Absorption	100% oral administration 90% rectal solutions Erratic: rectal suppositories
Volume of distribution	20–50 l/70 kg
Elimination	>90% hepatic metabolism <10% renal excretion of unchanged drug
Half-life	6–12 h
Time to steady state	1.5–2.5 days of chronic dosing
Usual sampling time	
Peak	4–7 h after oral sustained-release preparation (dependent upon product formulation)
Trough	Immediately before next dose
Plasma concentrations	8–20 mg/l therapeutic range >20 mg/l potentially toxic concentrations

Factors affecting plasma concentrations		
Disease	Cor pulmonale	↓ clearance
	Cardiac decompensation	↓ clearance
	Hepatic dysfunction	↓ clearance
	Acute pulmonary oedema	↓ clearance
	Sustained fever	↓ clearance
Drugs	Cimetidine	↓ clearance
	Allopurinol	↓ clearance
	Propranolol	↓ clearance
	Cigarette smoking	↑ clearance

with treatment correlate with the theophylline plasma concentration.

The absorption of theophylline is complete from the majority of formulations on the market. It is a drug with a short half-life (8 hours) which must maintain plasma levels within a well-defined therapeutic range to be effective. Fluctuations in plasma concentrations between doses of oral non-sustained-release dosage forms are likely to be excessive in most patients. The availability of oral sustained-release formulations has reduced the fluctuation in plasma concentrations and allowed longer dosing intervals.

Theophylline undergoes extensive hepatic metabolism to relatively inactive metabolites. It is therefore susceptible to disease and drugs which interfere with the activity of the liver. The potential wide variability in hepatic metabolism which exists between patients means that the use of fixed dosage regimens can result in potentially dangerous or ineffective plasma theophylline concentrations and should be discouraged. Theophylline dosage regimens should be individualized on the basis of plasma concentration monitoring.

Variable pharmacokinetics

In the practical application of pharmacokinetics there may be a need to base dosage predictions on average values for clearance, volume of distribution and half-life obtained from studies of particular patient populations. Knowledge of the normal distribution associated with such average values is required to appreciate the magnitude of variation in the patient population and thus the possible error that may be involved when data is used in an individual patient. It is also necessary to be aware of the many factors that may contribute to unexpected plasma drug concentrations being obtained and factors which alter the response to a specific drug concentration. Several factors relating to the four drugs discussed in the previous sections have already been identified.

A possible source of error in the interpretation of drug concentrations may be related to the decision to sample either plasma or serum. Undoubtedly the decision will rest with the laboratory responsible for the assay. However, most drugs appear to undergo minimal binding to the protein that forms the blood clot and results using plasma or serum are usually similar.

Plasma is obtained by centrifuging blood that has had coagulation prevented by the addition of agents such as heparin, EDTA, citrate or fluoride. The choice of the anticoagulant may affect the results of the assay. For example, fluoride inhibits serum cholinesterase which may cause in vitro degradation of acetylsalicylic acid; also

heparin is usually in the form of lithium heparin which may interfere with plasma lithium determination. In addition to the choice of anticoagulant, the selection of the blood collection tube may be important. Plastic blood collection tubes and stoppers can release plasticizers. These plasticizers have been shown to reduce the binding of some basic drugs to alpha-1-acid glycoprotein and result in apparently low total plasma levels of the drug due to the displacement of drug molecules which may then be taken up into red blood cells. Interactions between drugs may occur during storage and result in an apparent low drug plasma concentration on assay, e.g. carbenicillin interacts with gentamicin and results in a misleadingly low concentration of the aminoglycoside.

Factors inherent in the patient which may influence the pharmacokinetics of a drug include age, genetic predisposition, gender, body size and even posture. These factors may occur in combination with underlying disease states such as renal or hepatic disorders, altered metabolic status, gastrointestinal disease, or altered protein binding. In striving to identify patient-related problems, the possible influence of external factors should not be overlooked. These factors include cigarette smoking, diet and alcohol intake, variations in the physicochemical properties of the drug and its formulations, and the effect of concurrent drug administration (see Ch. 44).

Age

The influence of age is one of the principal factors which may contribute to interpatient variability in drug plasma levels and the response obtained to a given dosage regimen.

In the newborn infant there are many factors which will influence the pharmacokinetic profile of a drug, including the relatively high total body water, the low body fat content, immature renal and hepatic function, altered protein binding, and alterations in gastric acidity and motility. The neonate, however, cannot be considered to be in a subpopulation within which there are the usual interpatient variations in pharmacokinetic parameters. The first few months of life, especially for a premature infant, represent such marked physiological changes that the required dose relative to body weight for some drugs, e.g. gentamicin, may be 50% higher at 2 weeks of age than at 1 week of age. Therefore, before contemplating any pharmacokinetic intervention in the neonate, the investigator must be aware of the unique potential for variability which can arise.

As the child matures the problem of predicting the pharmacokinetic response to a drug is still not one of simply assessing the appropriate state of development in a linear progression to adult status. For some drugs the activity of certain metabolic pathways, such as conjugation and oxidation in children, may actually exceed adult values and necessitate the administration of higher doses, on a mg/kg basis, than those administered to adults. An example of this phenomenon is observed with theophylline, where the mean half-life of the drug in a child (4 hours) is less than half that seen in the adult (9 hours). In this case the adult half-life is often not achieved until adolescence. Dosage adjustments according to plasma concentration determination are required to compensate for this variable metabolic activity.

In the elderly patient there is an overall reduction in lean body mass and an increase in body fat. Cardiac output, organ and tissue blood flow, the concentration of plasma albumin, renal function and the activity of some drug-metabolizing enzyme systems all decline. It is not surprising, therefore, that age-related changes in the pharmacokinetic profile of some drugs have been reported. Moreover, it is difficult to predict the magnitude of change because of the continuous process of physiological change and the marked variation between biological and chronological age. Correction factors that are recommended for use in the elderly patient can only give an indication of the average dose required in this group of patients.

Genetic factors

Genetic factors probably contribute to the major inherent variability in human response to a given drug. Several of the genetic factors that have been identified are listed in Table 43.5.

Perhaps the best studied genetic factor is that associated with acetylator status. It is recognized that more than 90% of Canadian Eskimos and Japanese, 40% of Caucasians and 10% of Egyptians are fast acetylators, the remainder of these groups being slow acetylators. Acetylator status is particularly important in determining the response to drugs such as hydralazine, phenelzine, procainamide, dapsone, isoniazid, sulphasalazine and some sulphonamides.

With hydralazine, both bioavailability and the occurrence of side-effects are related to the degree of first-pass N-acetylation. On multiple dosing, fast acetylators demonstrate a bioavailability of 7% compared to a value of 40% in slow acetylators. Consequently, slow acetylators need to receive the drug in a smaller dose once daily, whilst fast acetylators require more frequent administration with a larger daily dose. Slow acetylators are also at greater risk from a hydralazine-induced systemic lupus erythematosus-like syndrome. The syndrome usually occurs in the slow

Table 43.5 Examples of known genetic traits which can alter the metabolism or action of a drug

	Condition	Drug(s) involved
Pharmacogenetic determinant of metabolism	Cholinesterase deficiency	Suxamethonium
	Lesch–Nyhan syndrome	Allopurinol; azathioprine; 6-mercaptopurine
	Hepatic N-acetyltransferase deficiency	Hydralazine; sulphadimidine; phenelzine
	Acatalasia	Hydrogen peroxide
	Methaemoglobin reductase deficiency	Sulphonamides
	Hydroxylase deficiency (specific deficiency for each drug)	Phenytoin Warfarin Debrisoquine
Pharmacogenetic determinant of drug action	Glucose-6-phosphate dehydrogenase deficiency	Nitrofurantoin; probenecid; quinine; sulphacetamide; sulphanilamide; vitamin K
	Unstable haemoglobins	Nitrofurantoin; probenecid; quinine; sulphacetamide; sulphanilamide; vitamin K
	Resistance to anticoagulants	Warfarin
	Malignant hyperpyrexia	Halothane; suxamethonium; nitrous oxide
	Glaucoma	Glucocorticoids
	Porphyria	Barbiturates; griseofulvin; oral contraceptives; sulphonamides; chlordiazepoxide; tolbutamide; methyldopa

acetylator after at least 6 months of treatment. Ideally the acetylator phenotype for each patient should be identified before receiving treatment. This can be determined readily by measuring the proportion of acetylated metabolite in plasma or urine after an oral dose of sulphadimidine (10 mg/kg) as the test substance.

Genetic factors are also known to be involved with various other abnormal drug responses including:

increased sensitivity to suxamethonium, barbiturate-induced porphyria, resistance to warfarin, nitrofurantoin-induced haemolysis, malignant hyperthermia associated with anaesthetic agents and steroid-induced glaucoma. These and other abnormal responses to drugs (see Ch. 44) contribute towards a better appreciation of the factors involved in variable drug response.

Gender

Gender may significantly influence the pharmacological response and pharmacokinetic profile of several drugs. The relative proportions of muscular and adipose tissue in men and women may be sufficient to alter the distribution and clearance of a drug from the body. When one superimposes surges of FSH, oestradiol and progesterone, as seen during various phases of the menstrual cycle, a further additional source of pharmacokinetic variation is added. Differences due to gender have been reported for several drugs including salicylates, hypoglycaemic agents, imipramine, diazepam, phenothiazines, and general and local anaesthetics. Pharmacokinetic studies need to recognize this potential source of variation and include groups matched for sex as well as age, together with information on the use of oral contraceptives or the stage of the menstrual cycle.

Posture

Several physiological functions are altered during bed rest when compared to the upright position. The rate of gastric emptying is reduced, particularly when a person is lying on their left side. However, the haemodynamic changes are perhaps the best studied. Cardiac output and liver and renal flow all increase during bed rest, whilst plasma volume and extracellular fluid volume decrease. Consequently, there is a trend for the plasma levels of drugs which undergo renal elimination to be lowest during the night. This effect is attributed to the increased renal blood flow which occurs during bed rest, although the influence of posture-induced changes in urine pH or urine flow cannot be discounted. Notable examples where decreased plasma levels have been observed during bed rest include amoxycillin, streptomycin, tetracycline, doxycycline, sulphamethizole and benzylpenicillin.

Hepatic blood flow is similarly related to changes in posture. Therefore, it would be expected that some hepatically metabolized drugs might also demonstrate diminished plasma levels during bed rest. However, although this effect has been demonstrated experimentally, few studies have been carried out to support this theory.

Social drugs

The concurrent intake of medication with social drugs such as alcohol, tea, coffee or cigarette smoking is often overlooked as a source of pharmacokinetic variability.

The chronic intake of alcohol induces hepatic drug metabolism. In contrast, the acute administration of alcohol has been shown to reduce the clearance of drugs such as diazepam, paracetamol and tolbutamide. The deep sedation observed following concurrent intake of diazepam and the acute administration of alcohol is partly the result of diminished clearance of the benzodiazepine.

Beverages such as tea and coffee are, by virtue of their caffeine content, potentially capable of influencing the pharmacokinetics of some drugs. The intake of coffee or caffeine has been shown to increase the bioavailability of paracetamol, dihydroergotamine, ergotamine and nitrofurantoin. However, it has not been possible to confirm the results of several studies on this subject, a factor which reflects the doubtful influence of beverage intake as a source of pharmacokinetic variability.

Tobacco smoke is known to contain more than 3000 chemicals, very few of which have been investigated for their effects on the body. The polycyclic hydrocarbons in cigarette smoke are known to be potent inducers of hepatic drug metabolism and have been reported to increase the elimination of several drugs, including diazepam, warfarin, theophylline, propranolol and pentazocine. These observations may be clinically significant since the increased elimination contributes to the apparent resistance of the heavy smoker to the effects of a given dose of a drug. The example with theophylline is perhaps the best documented, where the smoker may require an increase in dose to maintain therapeutic plasma levels.

Diet

Variation in the human diet presents a multitude of factors including nature of preparation, chemical composition, volume, time of consumption, etc., all of which can influence the pharmacokinetic profile of a drug.

The absorption of most drugs occurs from the proximal small intestine. Thus, any change in the stomach emptying rate is likely to affect the rate of drug absorption. In general, food reduces and large volumes of fluid accelerate the rate of stomach emptying. A prolonged residence in the stomach may increase the bioavailability of drugs that are absorbed over a small length of the intestinal tract, but may also be responsible for the increased degradation of acid-labile drugs such as some penicillins. Food-induced increase in intestinal motility may enhance contact between the drug and the intestinal epithelium and improve absorption or it may reduce absorption by speeding transit of the drug past the absorption site. In addition to these physiological factors food can also stimulate gastrointestinal tract secretions of digestive enzymes, acid and bile which in turn may influence the dissolution and absorption of a drug.

Components of the diet may interact directly with the absorption of a drug. The chelation of tetracyclines by calcium ions in dairy produce provides the basis for one of the best documented interactions. However, the reduced absorption of tetracycline is not solely due to the formation of insoluble chelates. The limited dissolution of tetracyclines at a food-induced gastric pH of 5–6, compared to dissolution at pH 1–3, also contributes to reduced drug absorption and emphasizes the potential complex nature of food–drug interactions.

High protein meals have been shown to significantly increase plasma concentrations of several drugs subject to extensive first-pass metabolism. The increased bioavailability of high extraction drugs such as propranolol and metoprolol has been attributed to food-stimulated elevation of hepatic blood flow, permitting the drug to pass rapidly through the liver and avoid hepatic removal. Several studies have, however, concluded that whilst food intake may enhance hepatic blood flow the postulated mechanism probably only makes a small contribution to the observed increase in bioavailability.

Many food–drug interactions have been reported to alter drug absorption (Table 43.6) but probably only a few of these are of clinical significance (Table 43.7). In

Table 43.6 Examples of oral drug administration where systemic absorption is delayed, reduced or increased by concurrent food intake

Delayed	Reduced	Increased
Amoxycillin	Amoxycillin	Canrenone
Aspirin	Ampicillin	Carbamazepine
Cefaclor	Aspirin	Chlorothiazide
Cephalexin	Atenolol	Diazepam
Cephradine	Benzylpenicillin	Griseofulvin
Cimetidine	Captopril	Hydralazine
Diclofenac	Cephalexin	Hydrochlorothiazide
Digoxin	Erythromycin stearate	Labetalol
Metronidazole	Hydrochlorthiazide	Lithium carbonate
Paracetamol	Isoniazid	Mebendazole
Quinidine	Ketoconazole	Metoprolol
Sulphanilamide	Penicillamine	Nitrofurantoin
Sulphafurazole	Phenoxymethylpenicillin	Phenytoin
Theophylline	Rifampicin	Propranolol
Valproic acid	Tetracycline	

Table 43.7 Examples of clinically relevant food–drug interactions

Drug	Bioavailability
Atenolol	↓ 20%
Captopril	↓ 42%
Isoniazid	↓ 50%
Ketoconazole	↓ 40%
Rifampicin	↓ 23%

general, interactions are dependent upon drug formulation characteristics, relative time of food and drug intake and the type of food ingested. Food–drug interactions are probably negligible if the drug is administered more than 2 hours before or after food ingestion.

A high ratio of protein to carbohydrate intake in volunteers on a fixed calorific diet has been demonstrated to increase the metabolism of theophylline, whilst a high ratio of carbohydrate to protein reduced metabolism. The ingestion of charcoal-cooked beef has been shown to enhance the metabolism of theophylline. This was attributed to the formation on the meat of polycyclic hydrocarbons which could stimulate hepatic cytochrome P-450 activity following ingestion. Similarly, the indole content of brussel sprouts and cabbage has been shown to be responsible for increasing the metabolism of theophylline.

Overall, the capricious nature of food–drug interactions often makes it difficult in practice to predict the extent of their contribution to observed pharmacokinetic variability.

The influence of fluid volume on oral drug absorption is more predictable than the effect of food. The ingestion of a large volume of fluid distends the stomach and stimulates gastric emptying. The administration of a drug with 200 ml water promotes the emptying of the drug from the stomach into the upper small intestine, faster than that observed following the ingestion of a small (< 25 ml) volume of fluid. Administration with 200 ml water, in general, improves dissolution characteristics, minimizes acid degradation of susceptible drugs and results in a more reproducible absorption profile.

Disease states

The response of an individual to a drug is the culmination of a series of interactions between the drug and various cells, tissues and organs of the body. It is inevitable, therefore, that if the ability to absorb, distribute, metabolize, or eliminate a drug is compromised by a disease state, there will be a marked change in the pharmacokinetic profile and subsequent response to a drug. Several disease states which can modify the pharmacokinetic profiles of digoxin, gentamicin, phenytoin and theophylline (Tables 43.1–43.4) have already been identified. The major identifiable disorders of organ function, which have a pronounced effect upon the pharmacokinetic profile of a drug, are those associated with renal and liver disease.

Renal disease

In normal renal function the fraction of drug or active metabolite that undergoes renal elimination is different for each drug, but it generally remains constant for the individual drug. Many drugs or their metabolites are extensively excreted by the kidney and their elimination rate reduced and half-life increased when renal function is impaired. The reduction in renal function may be directly related to pathological damage to the kidney or secondary to poor renal blood flow, e.g. following congestive cardiac failure or shock.

The degree of renal impairment can be determined by monitoring changes in endogenous creatinine clearance which correlate well with the glomerular filtration rate. As creatinine clearance declines, so usually does the renal clearance of a drug or its metabolites. Creatinine clearance determined from a 24-hour urinary excretion of creatinine, or more usually a clearance value estimated from a plasma creatinine determination, can be used to predict the dosage adjustment required (see Ch. 42).

In practice, it is oversimplistic to assume that the only effect of renal disease is to reduce the renal clearance of a drug. The absorption of some drugs may be reduced either by the elevated gastric pH, or by the nausea, vomiting, diarrhoea and oedema of the gastrointestinal tract which frequently accompany renal disease. Protein binding in renal disease, particularly of acidic drugs, may be reduced not only because of hypoalbuminaemia but also due to displacement by endogenous substances which accumulate in the plasma. This situation may lead to the volume of distribution of several drugs being increased in renal failure, e.g. clofibrate, frusemide, naproxen and phenytoin. In contrast, the displacement of digoxin from binding sites may reduce the apparent volume of distribution of the drug in renal failure.

Several studies have also shown that in the patient with renal disease the elimination of even some highly metabolized drugs may be increased e.g. phenytoin, or decreased, e.g. clonidine, propranolol and isoniazid.

Liver disease

Liver disease is not a single disorder which can readily be quantified. It usually encompasses a number of structural and functional conditions which range from reduced blood flow to the organ to cellular inflammation and necrosis.

The clearances of many drugs, but not all, that are metabolized by the liver are reduced in liver disease. An example of this complex situation is illustrated with the benzodiazepines. This group of drugs is very lipid soluble, highly bound to plasma protein and is metabolized before elimination. The clearances of diazepam and chlordiazepoxide are reduced in acute and chronic liver disease, whilst the clearance of lorazepam and oxazepam remain unchanged. Diazepam and chlordiazepoxide initially undergo oxidation before conjugation and renal elimination. In contrast, lorazepam and oxazepam directly undergo conjugation, a pathway which appears resistant to the effects of liver disease.

In liver disease, particularly cirrhosis, the ability to synthesize albumin is impaired. The low plasma albumin levels may change the volume of distribution, rate of metabolism and renal elimination of a drug. The volume of distribution of many drugs increases in patients with cirrhosis as observed with ampicillin, diazepam and propranolol. This increase in the volume of distribution cannot always be accounted for by reduced plasma protein binding. A change in the composition of the body such as the accumulation of ascitic fluid may also be responsible.

The disease state and its severity can have a pronounced effect upon the pharmacokinetic profile of a drug. There are inherent problems in predicting the influence of a specific disorder on the disposition of a drug, not least because the effects of disease states are difficult to quantify and rarely present in isolation. Patients frequently suffer from a wide array of clinical disorders which can contribute to a complex picture of observed pharmacokinetic variability.

FURTHER READING

Aulton M E (ed) 1988 Pharmaceutics: the science of dosage form design. Churchill Livinstone, Edinburgh

Evans W E, Jusko W J, Schentag J J 1986 Applied pharmacokinetics, 2nd edn. Applied Therapeutics, Spokane

Goodman Gilman A, Goodman L S, Rall T W, Murad F 1985 The pharmacological basis of therapeutics, 7th edn. Macmillan, London

Knoben J E, Anderson P O 1983 Handbook of clinical drug data, 5th edn. Drug Intelligence Publications, Illinois

44. Adverse drug reactions

S. A. Hudson   R. W. Walker

Throughout history there have been many reports of adverse reactions to drugs. Today's physician can prescribe from a wide selection of potent medicines which will provide effective treatment for the majority, but will predispose a few to serious unwanted and possibly harmful events. Such events are termed *adverse drug reactions* (ADRs) and are broadly defined by the the World Health Organization as 'any response to a drug which is noxious, unintended and, which occurs at doses used in man for prophylaxis, diagnosis or therapy'.

Interest in the monitoring of adverse reactions to drugs has, over the years, only made significant progress after a drug-related catastrophe has been identified. In the UK, the first committee of investigation into an ADR was probably that established in 1877 to investigate reports of cardiac arrest following the use of chloroform as an anaesthetic. In 1922, a similar formal enquiry was established to investigate the incidence of jaundice in patients treated for syphilis with salvarsan, an organic arsenical. This haphazard approach to the identification and documentation of adverse reactions was highlighted by the recognition of an association between congenital limb deformities (phocomelia) and thalidomide in the early 1960s. Thalidomide had, until then, been prescribed freely in the UK as a hypnotic. Its subsequent association with phocomelia when used during pregnancy was recognized by physicians world wide. The ensuing public outcry highlighted the inadequacies of existing drug legislation. It became clear that animal studies could fail to predict the toxicity of a drug. Moreover, human clinical trials could not detect adverse effects that occurred in less than 1% of those who received the medicine, simply because the trials probably only involved hundreds, as opposed to thousands of patients. In addition, the trials would have excluded certain categories of patients such as pregnant women, the elderly or the very young, i.e. individuals who may be most susceptible to a particular adverse reaction.

Regulatory authorities

In the UK The Committee on Safety of Drugs, the Dunlop Committee, was formed in 1963. The Committee operated under a voluntary agreement with the Association of the British Pharmaceutical Industry and the Proprietary Association of Great Britain. Both organizations agreed not to market a drug or subject it to clinical trial before receiving the approval of the Committee. The Committee on Safety of Drugs had no legal powers.

In 1971 The Committee on Safety of Drugs was disbanded and the Committee on Safety of Medicines (CSM) was founded in response to the Medicines Act of 1968. The Act introduced new regulations on the control of medicines, and in the CSM was vested statutory authority to advise health ministers on the licensing of drugs. The role of the CSM is to assess available data on new drugs before clinical trials and marketing are underway. Clinical trials can be carried out only when the manufacturer has obtained a clinical trial certificate for the drug from the licensing authority. The ministers responsible for issuing the certificate seek the advice of the CSM before reaching a decision. Similarly, the licensing authority will seek advice from the CSM before the medicine can subsequently be promoted, sold or supplied. It should be remembered that the CSM does not consider the comparative efficacy of a product, although it does assess efficacy in relation to safety.

Monitoring systems

The occurrence of ADRs is monitored by a system of centralized data collection. Prescribers are asked to report ADRs to the CSM by completing a standard report form ('Yellow Card'). Copies of these forms are bound into the current BNF and postage is paid by the CSM. Although the reports must be signed by a doctor, pharmacists may be involved in completing the report forms. In some other countries pharmacists may report directly and in both Canada and the USA patients themselves may report reactions. The 'yellow card' system is effective in detecting both common and rare adverse reactions and it operates from the first day a new drug is marketed. Reports relating to products introduced during the preceding 2–3 years, or occasionally even longer, are actively encouraged. Such products are marked with the symbol ▼ in the various prescribing guides (BNF, MIMS, Data Sheets). With older drugs all serious reactions should be reported even if these are well known. Unfortunately the system gives little indication of the incidence of an ADR because the number of patients exposed to the drug is unknown and not all adverse reactions are reported. Reports received are likely to be biased in favour of recognized and well-publicized ADRs.

Other monitoring schemes include postmarketing surveillance carried out by a DHSS-supported independent group and postmarketing surveillance carried out by the pharmaceutical industry.

With the increasing use of computer technology the potential exists for linking more directly prescribing data with medical data.

The role of the pharmacist in ADR monitoring

The appropriate therapeutic use of potent modern drugs involves the inevitable risk that some patients will develop an ADR. In addition to the consequent patient morbidity, the treatment of individuals suffering from ADRs costs the NHS tens of millions of pounds each year. Therefore, the effective involvement of a pharmacist in any ADR monitoring programme has the overall objective of minimizing patient morbidity and reducing NHS expenditure.

The involvement of community pharmacists in identifying ADR has been proposed by the Royal Pharmaceutical Society of Great Britain, but this has yet to be implemented.

Within the hospital sector medical staff are more likely to identify ADRs by virtue of their close patient contact. The pharmacist may identify potential ADRs

Table 44.1 Examples of drugs which could be used to alleviate the symptoms of an adverse drug reaction

Possible ADR	Prescribed therapy
Urticaria	Antihistamine
Dyspepsia	Antacid
Vomiting	Antiemetic
Fluid retention	Diuretic
Diarrhoea	Antidiarrhoeal agent
Constipation	Laxative

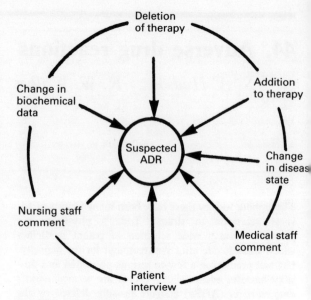

Fig. 44.1 Interrelationship of factors which may contribute to the identification of an adverse drug reaction

by noting changes in therapy including deletion of drugs which could be used to treat the symptoms of an adverse reaction (Table 44.1); noting changes in biochemical data; identifying changes in disease state; liaising with medical or nursing staff and responding to comments which may implicate an ADR; interviewing patients and discussing their therapy and associated problems (Fig. 44.1). It is the emphasis that the pharmacist places on drug therapy that is his greatest attribute in identifying an ADR. The pharmacist, by offering possible drug-related explanations for a patient's symptoms, may heighten the index of suspicion among medical and nursing staff that an ADR has occurred. The identification of adverse reactions is facilitated by understanding their aetiology and classification.

CLASSIFICATION OF ADVERSE DRUG REACTIONS

The common ADRs can readily be classified as being either Type A, which arise from the known pharmacological action of the drug, or Type B, which represent an abnormal or novel response to the drug (Table 44.2). Some adverse drug reactions (Type A or Type B) may be due to recognized genetic causes. However, regardless of the classification system used, its limitations can only be understood by appreciating that all adverse drug effects are the result of a complex interplay between the drug, the patient, the disease state and other known and unknown extrinsic factors (Tables 44.3, 44.4).

Table 44.2 Classification of adverse drug reactions

Type A	Type B
Quantitative variation in response to drug	Qualitative variation in response to drug
Dose related	Poor correlation with dose
Pharmacologically explicable	Inexplicable, often bizarre
Identifiable	Difficult to identify Mimic natural disease
Relatively common	Uncommon
Predictable	Unpredictable
Rarely fatal	Frequently serious

Type A reactions

Type A reactions are related to the known pharmacology of a drug and may be due to an excessive dose of the drug, an associated pharmacological effect or a pharmacological withdrawal effect.

Many ADRs are experienced by patients as a consequence of receiving an inappropriately high dose of a

Table 44.3 Factors which can influence the occurrence of adverse drug reactions

Drug	Physicochemical characteristics
	Pharmacokinetic profile
	Formulation, e.g. excipients
	Dose
	Route of administration
	Rate of administration
Patient	Age
	Sex
	Pregnancy
	Genetic factors
	Atopy
	State of nutrition
	Disease state
External factors	Concurrent drug therapy
	Alcohol intake
	Cigarette smoking
	Environmental pollutants
	Unknown (?) factors

drug. This problem of excessive dosage generally arises inadvertently, as a consequence of individual patient characteristics. The patient may in fact be receiving a standard dose, but the existence of renal or hepatic im-

Table 44.4 Examples of the association between various disease states, drug treatment and potential adverse drug reactions

Disease	Drug	Adverse effect
Cardiovascular disease		
Heart failure	β-blockers Tricyclic antidepressants	Aggravate heart failure
Hypertension	Carbenoxolone Oral contraceptives	Increase blood pressure
Gastrointestinal disease		
Peptic ulcer	Aspirin Corticosteroids Indomethacin	Increased risk of bleeding or perforation
Gastroenteritis	Oral contraceptives	Conception
Liver disease		
Prehepatic coma	Morphine Barbiturates	Encephalopathy
Hepatitis	Ergot drugs	Ergot poisoning
Renal failure	Aminoglycosides Digoxin Tetracyclines	Ototoxicity Digoxin toxicity Elevation of blood urea
Respiratory disease		
Asthma	β-blockers	Bronchospasm
Corpulmonale	Digoxin	Digoxin toxicity

pairment can reduce the clearance of the drug and result in excessively high plasma levels. The subsequent adverse effects observed are, therefore, an extension of the drugs own dose-related pharmacological or toxicological capabilities. Examples include the administration of digoxin, gentamicin or nalidixic acid to patients in renal failure, or the use of narcotic analgesics, phenytoin or ketoconazole in liver disease.

Particular caution is always required in the elderly and very young since they are liable to have reduced drug clearance when compared to the general adult population.

A change in drug formulation may result in an increase in the bioavailability of a drug and precipitate an ADR. This point has been well illustrated with the antiepileptic drug, phenytoin. When the excipient in phenytoin capsules was changed from calcium sulphate dihydrate to lactose, patients who received the 'new' formulation developed signs and symptoms of phenytoin toxicity consistent with the unexpectedly high plasma levels obtained. The incorporation of calcium sulphate dihydrate into the formulation was considered to have resulted in the formation of insoluble and unabsorbed phenytoin chelates, an effect not observed when lactose was used as the excipient (see also Ch. 19 in the companion volume Aulton 1988).

Problems associated with the use of phenytoin still arise in practice and further serve to illustrate the role of formulation and an inadvertent increase in drug dose as causative factors in ADRs. An epileptic patient may be stabilized on phenytoin capsules, which contain the active ingredient as phenytoin sodium. Should the patient be transferred to the same apparent dose as a suspension an increase in actual dose received will occur. The suspension is formulated with phenytoin and the capsule with phenytoin sodium, and 92 mg phenytoin is equivalent to 100 mg phenytoin sodium.

Few drugs have a single therapeutic effect on the body, the majority have several known pharmacological effects. Whilst a drug may be prescribed for a single pharmacological action, an associated pharmacological effect may precipitate an ADR. An oral antihistamine prescribed for pruritus may also cause the patient to experience its associated pharmacological actions of drowsiness and anticholinergic effects. Therefore, patients must be warned about the risk of driving or operating machinery and the increased depressant effect of alcohol. The anticholinergic effects such as dry mouth, blurred vision, gastrointestinal disturbance and urinary retention may also give the patient cause for concern. It is clear that even with antihistamines, many of which can be purchased by the public, a whole range of adverse reactions related to their additional pharmacological effects may be precipitated.

For several drugs, sudden withdrawal after prolonged use may contribute to a serious adverse reaction. Typical examples include clonidine, β-adrenoceptor blockers, benzodiazepines and glucocorticoids.

Clonidine, an antihypertensive agent, increases stores of neuronal catecholamines by inhibiting neurotransmitter release as a result of central stimulation of presynaptic α_2-adrenoceptors. The sudden removal of this inhibitory effect may release stored catecholamine, resulting in a pronounced sympathomimetic effect. This potential adverse effect can manifest itself even after the omission of a single dose. Consequently, the use of clonidine has declined, particularly where there may be any question of possible patient noncompliance.

A syndrome associated with the withdrawal of β-adrenoceptor blockers has also been described. Prolonged exposure to a β-adrenoceptor antagonist is thought to increase the number of postsynaptic β-adrenoceptors. Sudden withdrawal of the 'β-blocker', therefore, may result in a state of hypersensitivity to circulating endogenous catecholamines.

Perhaps one of the more established drug withdrawal syndromes relates to the supression of the hypothalamic-pituitory-adrenal (HPA) axis by the chronic administration of glucocorticoids. Suppression of the HPA has been reported following topical, inhaled, ophthalmic, rectal and systemic glucocorticoid therapy. Sudden withdrawal of the steroid may precipitate an acute adrenal crisis, resembling Addison's disease, in which the patient experiences weakness, malaise, despondency and hypotension. There is a need to gradually reduce the dose of the glucocorticoid over a prolonged period of time. The sudden withdrawal of glucocorticoids may also lead to reactivation of the underlying steroid responsive condition, e.g. chronic asthma.

A benzodiazepine withdrawal problem is now recognized. The existence of a benzodiazepine withdrawal effect is ironic considering these drugs were introduced to avoid the associated high risk of physical and psychological dependence seen with barbiturates. Benzodiazepine dependence tends to occur after treatment lasting several months or even years. When the drug is suddenly stopped a withdrawal reaction may occur. This reaction can involve a variety of non-specific symptoms including anxiety and dysphoria which may resemble the anxiety state for which the drug was prescribed. In order to avoid withdrawal symptoms, it is necessary to gradually reduce the dose of the benzodiazepine when a course of treatment has exceeded 3 months.

Type B reactions

The pattern of an allergic drug reaction is characterized by precipitation on re-exposure to even trace amounts of the drug. The allergic reaction is idiosyncratic in that it does not resemble the pharmacological action of the drug but has an immunological basis which may produce symptoms ranging from mild urticaria or pyrexia to serum sickness, blood dyscrasia or anaphylaxis which may be fatal.

Drugs such as protein or peptide hormones are macromolecules and are antigenic in their own right. Other drugs with a smaller molecular weight (less than 1000 Da) are not inherently antigenic, but may possibly be antigenic because of contamination with macromolecules which precipitate an allergic reaction. Alternatively, low molecular weight drugs or their metabolites can become antigenic by forming drug (hapten)–protein conjugates.

The severity of the allergic reaction is, in general, related to the route of administration. Anaphylactic reactions are more dramatic following parenteral than oral administration. However, the rapid and severe reaction which may rarely manifest itself following oral administration of penicillin preparations serves as a reminder of exceptions to the rule. It should be noted that patients known to be atopic, i.e. individuals with a history of immunological disorders such as eczema, hay fever and asthma, tend to be more susceptible to allergic drug reactions.

Allergic drug reactions can manifest themselves as any of a number of symptoms including, anaphylaxis, autoimmune reactions, Arthus-type and delayed-type hypersensitivity. The range of drugs involved in such reactions is diverse (Table 44.5).

The influence of genetic status on the pharmacokinetics of drugs has been discussed in Chapter 43, and the role of acetylator status in relation to the occurrence of a systemic lupus erythematosus-like syndrome to drugs such as isoniazid, hydralazine and sulphonamides reviewed. Genetic factors can also influence the risk of other adverse reactions. Pseudocholinesterase deficiency, glucose-6-phosphate dehydrogenase deficiency porphyria and glaucoma are notable examples.

One of the most common ADRs which occurs in the Western world and which is linked to a genetic factor is that associated with the metabolism of suxamethonium. Suxamethonium is a depolarizing neuromuscular blocking drug, with a duration of action of 3–5 minutes. Its action is rapidly terminated following hydrolysis by pseudocholinesterase enzymes found in the plasma and liver. Following reports of suxamethonium-induced apnoea in patients treated with the drug, a

Table 44.5 Examples of allergic drug reactions

Reaction	Drug
Anaphylaxis	Penicillins, demethylchlortetracycline, Vancomycin
Pyrexia	Penicillins, phenytoin
Haematological disorders	
Agranulocytosis	Sulphonamides, sulphonylureas, phenothiazines
Aplastic anaemia	Chloramphenicol
Haemolytic anaemia	Penicillins, cephalothin, sulphonamides, methyldopa
Hepatitis	Phenothiazines
Serum sickness	Penicillins, aspirin
Skin eruptions	
Urticaria	Aspirin, penicillins
Erythema multiforme	Sulphonamides, barbiturates, phenytoin
Photosensitivity	Sulphonamides, thiazides, phenothiazines, tetracyclines
Systemic lupus erythematosus-like syndrome	Hydralazine, isoniazid, phenytoin

plasma pseudocholinesterase polymorphism was identified. In fact, 1 in 3000 individuals have an atypical pseudocholinesterase which has a reduced ability to metabolize suxamethonium. The duration of action of suxamethonium may approach 3 hours in these susceptible individuals.

Glucose-6-phosphate dehydrogenase activity is required to stabilize red blood cells, particularly against the oxidative stress of drugs such as primaquine, sulphonamides, quinine and nitrofurantoin. There are more than 80 variants of glucose-6-phosphate dehydrogenase deficiency that are genetically influenced, they primarily affect males and render the individual vulnerable to drug-induced haemolysis. The enzyme deficiency is most common in those with either African or Mediterranean origins.

Other adverse effects which arise because of a genetic predisposition are indicated in Table 44.6. The majority of these adverse effects are uncommon in the UK.

Once a suspected adverse reaction has been identified a decision must be reached as to the degree of certainty to which the individual patient has suffered an ADR. In

Table 44.6 Examples of adverse drug reactions with a known genetic basis

Adverse effect	Gentically influenced variant	Drug
Systemic lupus erythematosus-like syndrome	Slow acetylation	Isoniazid, hydralazine, dapsone, sulphonamides, phenelzine
Prolonged muscle paralysis and apnoea	Pseudocholinesterase deficiency	Suxamethonium
Haemolytic anaemia	Glucose-6-phosphate dehydrogenase deficiency	Primaquine, sulphonamides, quinine, quinidine, nitrofurantoin
Malignant hyperthermia	Altered calcium regulation in voluntary muscle	Halothane, suxamethonium
Glaucoma	Trabecular meshwork outflow abnormality	Corticosteroid eye drops
Porphyria	Overproduction of δ-aminolevulinic acid synthetase	Barbiturate, dichloralphenazone, griseofulvin, sulphonylureas, chlordiazepoxide, phenytoin, oral contraceptives
Methaemoglobinaemia	Methaemoglobin reductase deficiency	Primaquine, chloroquine, dapsone

Table 44.7 Factors which classify the degree of certainty to which an adverse drug reaction may have occurred.

Factor	'Definitely'	'Probably'	'Possibly'
Onset related to time of administration	+	+	+
Follows a known response pattern	+	+	+
Recurs on rechallenge	+	−	−
Symptoms otherwise unexplained	+	+	−
Symptoms subside after discontinuation	+	+	+

many situations the adverse reaction cannot be distinguished in the clinic, in the laboratory or at post-mortem from an event which could have occurred spontaneously. Moreover, the problem of relating the adverse reaction to specific drug therapy may be compounded by the appearance of the reaction several years after treatment with a particular drug has been stopped (Table 44.7).

DRUG INTERACTIONS

The potential for drug–drug interactions to precipitate adverse effects is well documented and the majority should be recognized by the vigilant pharmacist. A drug–drug interaction may take the form of a pharmaceutical, pharmacodynamic or pharmacokinetic interaction which may either increase the toxicity or reduce the therapeutic efficacy of a drug. Drug–drug interactions are not classified as ADRs, although they do contribute to many, often avoidable, adverse drug effects.

Pharmaceutical interactions

Pharmaceutical interactions are related to the physicochemical properties of a drug and may involve a loss of potency, increase in toxicity or other adverse effect. Generally, these interactions arise outside the body and result in the inactivation of one drug. Examples include the inappropriate mixing of drugs in syringes, e.g. gentamicin and carbenicillin which inactivate one another, or the addition of an incompatible drug to an infusion fluid, e.g. an acid-labile penicillin to a low pH infusion solution such as dextrose.

Pharmacodynamic interactions

Pharmacodynamic interactions occur when two drugs act on the same pharmacological receptors, sites of action or physiological system to have similar or antagonistic pharmacological or toxic effects. Adverse pharmacodynamic interactions should easily be identified from a knowledge of the underlying pharmacological action of the drugs involved. Amongst the most serious adverse effects are drugs with a central nervous system depressant component. Examples include the concurrent administration of depressant drugs such as alcohol or antihistamines to patients receiving sedatives, hyponotics or anxiolytics.

Pharmacokinetic interactions

Pharmacokinetic interactions occur when one drug alters the absorption, distribution, metabolism or excretion of another. This may result in increased or reduced plasma levels with an associated enhanced or compromised pharmacological action. Pharmacokinetic interactions can be classified according to their site of interaction (Table 44.8).

Gastrointestinal absorption

Drug–drug interactions which affect absorption are a major problem with oral drug therapy. Drugs which alter gastrointestinal motility may affect their own absorption or that of another drug. Propantheline has an anticholinergic action and consequently reduces both intestinal motility and the rate of gastric emptying. This effect has been shown to result in reduced absorption rates for paracetamol, ethanol and hydrochlorthiazide. In contrast, metoclopramide accelerates the rate of gastric emptying and increases the absorption rates of paracetamol, ethanol and levodopa. Some drugs may themselves directly retard the absorption of other preparations. Antacids, in particular, have been shown to reduce the extent of absorption of several drugs including chlorpromazine, hyoscine, cimetidine, diflunisal, digoxin, indomethacin, levodopa, ranitidine and tetracyclines. Adsorbent agents such as kaolin-pectin, cholestyramine, cholestipol and activated charcoal have been shown to reduce oral drug availability.

Plasma protein displacement

Interactions which involve the displacement of a drug from protein binding sites have been shown to result in

Table 44.8 Classification of pharmacokinetic drug interactions according to their site of action

Site	Example of mechanism
Gastrointestinal tract	Absorption, adsorption
Plasma protein binding	Displacement
Tissue binding	Displacement
Hepatic metabolism	Induction, inhibition
Renal excretion	Competition for tubular secretion

a temporary elevation of free drug levels. The increased free drug levels have been considered to enhance the pharmacological effect of the drug or even precipitate a toxic adverse effect. Many drug displacement reactions have been described, particularly with the highly protein bound drugs phenytoin and warfarin. However, it is rare for such interactions to have clinical significance since compensation rapidly occurs with an increase in the clearance of the free drug, thus restoring the actual active plasma free drug concentration. Many reactions considered to be due to protein binding displacement and which have been shown to be clinically significant, have since been found to include an inhibitory metabolic component, e.g. phenylbutazone displaces racemic warfarin from albumin binding sites but also inhibits the biotransformation of its potent S isomer.

Far less information is available on tissue binding interactions. However, a two-fold increase in plasma concentrations of digoxin has been observed after administration of quinidine. The elevated plasma concentrations of digoxin have been attributed to non-cardiac tissue displacement of digoxin by quinidine.

Hepatic drug metabolism

The ability of some drugs to inhibit the hepatic metabolism of others has resulted in many serious adverse effects. Examples include haemorrhage due to the inhibition of the metabolism of warfarin by phenylbutazone or metronidazole; the reduced metabolic clearance and risk of bone marrow suppression with the cytotoxic drug azathioprine when administered concurrently with the xanthine-oxidase inhibitor, allopurinol; the inhibition of oxidative metabolism by the H-receptor antagonist, cimetidine, may lead to elevated plasma levels of many drugs including warfarin, theophylline, lignocaine, phenytoin, carbamazepine, and some benzodiazepines.

In contrast, some drugs can induce the metabolic clearance of others by enhancing hepatic microsomal enzyme hydroxylation. Barbiturates, phenytoin, carbamazepine, ethanol, rifampicin and griseofulvin are all potent inducers of hepatic P-450 microsomal enzymes. Several environmental pollutants, cigarette smoke and certain dietary components may also have this effect. The administration of a drug which induces microsomal enzyme activity is likely to gradually increase the clearance of other drugs metabolized by the P-450 enzymes over the course of 1–2 weeks. The overall effect will, therefore, probably be one of reduced efficacy, although if an active metabolite of the parent drug is responsible for the therapeutic effect, the inducer may augment rather than diminish the pharmacological action of the affected drug.

Renal excretion

Whilst the potential exists for one drug to affect the glomerular filtration, tubular reabsorption or active tubular secretion of another drug, clinically significant examples are rare.

Indomethacin administration can elevate lithium concentrations in plasma. This effect is thought to be modulated by inhibition of renal cyclo-oxygenase activity and a related reduction in glomerular filtration rate and creatinine clearance. Probenecid can inhibit the tubular secretion of sulphinpyrazone, indomethacin, penicillin and methotrexate. The combination of probenecid and penicillin may be used beneficially in practice to increase the half-life and effectiveness of penicillin. The secretion of digoxin by the distal nephron is reduced by spironolactone and results in a decreased renal clearance and elevated plasma digoxin concentrations.

A multitude of interactions are cited in the literature but many are unsubstantiated and likely to be irrelevant in clinical practice. Factors which diminish the clinical relevance of alleged drug interactions are listed as follows:

— Animal studies.
— Anecdotal reports.
— Single case reports.
— Unsubstantiated reports.
— Studies involving:
   Dosage regimens not used in practice.
   Infrequently prescribed drugs.
   Small number of subjects.
   No age control.
   No sex control.
   No control of additional drug intake.
   No control of social drug intake.

Interactions are likely to be important if they relate to drugs with a narrow therapeutic index such as digoxin, phenytoin, theophylline, warfarin, gentamicin and methotrexate. Wherever the control of a drug's dosage is critical, careful attention must be paid to the avoidance of drug interactions.

FURTHER READING

D'Arcy P, Griffin J 1987 Iatrogenic diseases, 2nd edn. Oxford University Press, Oxford
Davies D 1986 Adverse drug reactions, 2nd edn. Oxford University Press, Oxford
Goodman Gilman A, Goodman L S, Rall T W, Murad F 1985 The pharmacological basis of therapeutics, 7th edn. Macmillan, London
Inman W H W 1986 Monitoring for drug safety, 2nd edn. MTP Press, Lancaster
Stephens M D B 1985 The detection of new adverse drug reactions. Macmillan, London
Stockley I 1981 Drug interactions. Blackwell Scientific, Oxford
Veitch G B A, Talbot J 1985 The pharmacist and adverse drug reaction reporting. Pharmaceutical Journal 234: 107–109

45. Drug information and pharmaceutical advice

S. A. Hudson   R. W. Walker

The provision of information and advice to prescribers and patients is an important part of pharmacy practice. This professional service relies on a sound knowledge base coupled with interpersonal and problem-solving skills. These skills include the ability to clearly define a problem, to investigate information sources efficiently and to respond effectively with practical advice.

QUESTIONS AND PROBLEMS IN DRUG THERAPY

Once a decision has been taken by the doctor (to prescribe) and the patient (to co-operate), an experiment has been initiated. This experiment is a clinical trial of the drug involving one subject. The trial is carried out in the face of uncertainties about the drug's likely effects and its fate in the body together with doubts about the patient's physiological and psychological behaviour. Neither the prescriber nor the patient can be certain about the eventual clinical outcome.

The duration of the trial may be short term or long term depending on decisions made by the prescriber or the patient. Progress with the treatment on trial is monitored by the patient and guided by their subjective feelings, since the outcome cannot usually be measured objectively. Assessment must then rely on the patient reporting their symptoms. To add further complications, the experiment is often conducted without supervision, while the patient is at home, at work and at play.

The reliability of the trial requires pharmaceutical controls on the drug, the dose, the dosage form, and when and how it is administered. This concept of pharmaceutical control therefore extends beyond the idea of legal or economic regulation. It is concerned with the conduct of the experiment to ensure, in a scientific sense, that the known variables are taken into account and minimized wherever possible.

Either the pharmacist or the prescriber may decide to seek information from the other before carrying out

their role in the treatment process. Most people prefer to obtain advice from personal contact with those they regard as knowledgeable and helpful, rather than from print. The pharmacist must therefore be skilled at meeting requests for information or advice. The pharmacist's duty also involves responding in his own right to any indications of apparent or real medication problems that may affect the care of the patient. These problems may require investigation with the patient or the prescriber before the medication is dispensed. Questions or problems may also be raised as treatment continues. The pharmacist must therefore be accessible to be consulted and must also feel free to initiate any enquiries with the prescriber or the patient.

The hospital pharmacist

A variety of medication problems may be encountered by pharmacists in their role on the hospital ward. Several studies in the UK and USA have shown that problems of drug choice and dose selection are common, as are problems relating to drug administration, particularly when parenteral routes are involved. Questions relating to adverse drug reactions and drug interactions are also raised by medical and nursing staff on the ward. Examples of the types of medication problem encountered are:

1. Dose.
2. Dose regimen.
3. Drug administration (e.g. dilution of injections, alternative routes).
4. Drug choice (relative cost, efficacy and toxicity).
5. Unwanted effects.
6. Contraindications.
7. Drug interactions.
8. Special formulations (e.g. extemporaneously dispensed medicines, stability and storage).
9. New drugs.
10. Clinical trial evidence.

421

11. Cost.
12. Tablet/capsule identification.
13. Interactions with laboratory tests.

Participation in ward rounds or case discussions with medical staff can provide the pharmacist with background information about the patient's past and present condition, including clinical and laboratory investigations, and further management plans. In this situation the pharmacist can help identify or prevent drug-related problems and influence the prescribed drug regimen at the time decisions are taken. The recognition and investigation of medication problems requires knowledge of the drugs and the clinical condition involved. Additional information about drug treatment or the patient in question may be sought by a line of enquiry that is intended to identify, clarify and resolve any problems. The process of collecting data is helped by maintaining a patient record which includes relevant information from the patient interview (e.g. a drug history), discussion with medical or nursing staff and from clinical records. An example of a patient record card (medication profile card) is shown in Figure 45.1. Some important factors in identifying possible medication problems are:

1. Unusual doses.
2. Unusual indications.
3. Polypharmacy.
4. Extended treatment duration (e.g. antibiotics).
5. Missed doses.
6. Drugs which:
   a. Have low safety margin.
   b. Are monitored by clinical or laboratory measurements (e.g. plasma levels).
   c. Are newly marketed.
   d. Are under clinical trial.
   e. Could be treating adverse drug effects (e.g. change in bowel habit, allergies).
7. Patients who:
   a. Have disease that may affect drug handling.
   b. Are elderly or very young.
   c. Have physical abnormalities affecting drug handling (e.g. obesity, emaciation, surgery or marked disease of gastrointestinal tract).

The community pharmacist

Accessibility within the community allows the pharmacist to make an extensive and valuable contribution to health care. The problems encountered by the community pharmacist include not only those related to prescribed medicines but also those associated with the use of over-the-counter medicines and with general health education.

For geographical reasons the community pharmacist's relationship with the prescriber is often more remote than that of the hospital pharmacist. Since patients on chronic medication need not return to the same pharmacy, the opportunity for observing the outcome and following up any advice offered to the prescriber or the patient is limited. However, the maintenance of patient medication records for selected patients is a practical option in some pharmacies and provides a basis for monitoring drug therapy and identifying or preventing medication problems. These types of records are discussed in Chapter 38.

The emphasis of the community pharmacist's contribution to drug therapy is the relationship with the patient, since this is usually the main source of back-

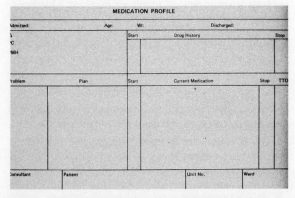

Fig. 45.1 Patient medication profile. The hospital pharmacist may need to maintain a brief record of the patient's clinical condition and drug therapy. This figure shows two sides of a standard 200 mm × 130 mm card format with relevant laboratory test results on the reverse. Abbreviations: △, diagnosis; PC, presenting complaint; PMH, past medical history; TTO, drugs 'to take out' at discharge

ground information to the prescription. A good patient interviewing technique is necessary to allow information about the patient's particular circumstances to be gathered in a brief conversation. At the same time the pharmacist must avoid being misled by the possibility that the patient's perception of their illness may be inaccurate and so may not be consistent with the doctor's record of their medical and drug history. Notwithstanding these limitations the community pharmacist must assemble a general impression of the clinical background to the patient's drug treatment. With this information professional judgement and discretion can be applied in deciding on the need for any further action, such as contact with the prescriber or the provision of advice to the patient.

Practical tips on the style of the patient interview are as follows:

1. The objective of the interview should be clear.
2. Suitable environment.
3. Patient should be put at ease.
4. Get quickly to the point. Efficient use of time without undue haste. Control direction by short questions:
   a. Open questions to gain insight into patient's feelings.
   b. Closed questions to obtain details.
5. Avoid making recommendations whilst gathering information.
6. Listen for facts. Avoid jumping to conclusions.
7. Avoid shifting from subject to subject.
8. Maintain objectivity.
9. Move from general to specific points.
10. Move from impersonal to personal questions.
11. Maintain eye contact. Avoid spending too much time on making notes.
12. Summarize to check facts.
13. Avoid ending abruptly. Convey reassurance and agree on any follow-up.

A plan of the patient interview to obtain drug history and clinical background can be summarized as follows:

1. Personal introduction.
2. State purpose of the interview.
3. Indicate time to be taken.
4. Allow patient to volunteer current problems.
5. Establish current medication list.
6. Establish current problem list.
7. Selective examination of each problem:
   a. Date of onset.
   b. Developments since onset.
   c. Precipitating or relieving factors.
   d. Present treatment (including OTC):
      i. Dosage changes.
      ii. Duration.
   e. Estimation of compliance
   f. Advice already received from the doctor or from others.
8. Impact of problem(s) on patient/family.
9. Other items of past medication.
10. Past untoward events associated with any medicine.
11. Identify serious misconceptions about drug therapy for clarification.
12. Identify particular needs of patient for further information or advice.
13. Nature and availability of support from relatives and friends.
14. Summarize and check major facts.
15. Provide any advice.
16. Thank you.

Several studies have indicated that patients are not well informed about the drugs they receive and generally want more information and advice. The types of drug information and advice for patients are discussed further under 'Communicating advice to patients' and this aspect of pharmacy practice is considered in more detail in Chapters 37 and 39.

The role of the community pharmacist in health education is increasing in importance and covers topics such as family planning, smoking and health, alcohol consumption, advice to travellers and nutrition. For these campaigns to be effective, community pharmacists must work closely with national campaign organizers, local general medical practitioners and other health-care workers. These health education campaigns have resulted in community pharmacies being recognized as information centres on matters of health education. To participate fully the pharmacist must be well informed, be capable of answering relevant questions and have the necessary literature at hand to support personal advice.

PROVIDING DRUG INFORMATION

The provision of drug information to prescribers and other health-care personnel requires skill in receiving and responding to enquiries made in person or over the telephone.

Handling enquiries

Whether an enquiry is received by telephone or in person the identity of the enquirer must first be established. The status of the enquirer gives some idea of their familiarity with pharmaceutical terminology and will govern the phrasing of the reply. The process of first receiving the enquiry is important. Is it a general question or does it relate to a specific patient? Any misunderstanding at this point can lead to unnecessary effort in researching a question which may not have properly addressed the real problem. Usually those seeking help do so after they have made an attempt to resolve the matter themselves. Drug enquiries therefore often represent questions that are somewhat removed from the problem that prompts them.

A common example of an enquiry is the question 'What are the side effects of . . . . .?', which may be an attempt to check whether a patient's symptoms are likely to be due to an adverse drug effect. In this case, rather than provide a list of drug effects of increasing obscurity, it is more appropriate to obtain a detailed description of the symptoms and identify all other drugs being taken, since any of these may also be candidates for investigation. Full appreciation of the problem allows the urgency of the enquiry to be assessed. The time available to provide an answer is likely to influence the extent of any search of the literature that may be necessary. An early grasp of the problem and its urgency allows the enquiry to be immediately referred to a specialist when appropriate. Where the enquiry relates to a particular patient background, clinical information must be obtained. Once the relevant question has been defined, it is necessary to identify what steps have already been taken by the enquirer to research the question. The level of detail needed in the answer should then be agreed, as well as when and how the response will be conveyed. Sometimes a written reply may be appropriate and if so, this should be established at the outset, since it will affect the time taken up with the enquiry.

These stages are summarized in Table 45.1.

Table 45.1 Handling drug information enquiries

The enquiry

Identify the:
  Name of enquirer
  Status of enquirer
  Question
  Underlying problem
  Relevant details (clinical background)
  Information sources already consulted
  Urgency
  Extent of detail required

The answer

Agree:
  The level of detail
  When it will be provided
  How it will be provided

Sources of drug information

Responding to an enquiry involves devising a strategy to search for information. All but the most straightforward problems require information from several sources, combined into a response that meets the individual need of the enquirer. The search strategy may include drug literature that is readily available on file or which is accessible via a database. Some problems are best dealt with through personal contact with information departments in the health service, the drug industry or professional organizations.

Literature sources can be grouped into three categories. General reference books (tertiary sources) are often on the front line, particularly in the dispensary. Journal review articles (secondary sources) can provide useful and often more detailed summaries of drug information; these are useful for keeping on file for ready access. Ultimately original articles such as clinical trials and case reports (primary sources) may need to be examined. A list of reference sources representing the minimum requirements for answering enquiries has been published by Drug Information Pharmacists in the UK (1984). This list is regularly updated and advice can be obtained from any of the drug information centres listed in the BNF. The continued development of computer-based information systems offers a solution to the problem of ready access to drug information in the dispensary.

Commonly used sources of drug information are summarized in Table 45.2.

The large number of journals in existence creates the need for abstracting and indexing systems to search the primary and secondary literature. Several abstracting services are available which provide a summary of the contents of a paper. They are partly an indexing system and partly a secondary literature source. These services include Pharmline, International Pharmaceutical Abstracts, Medline, Exerpta Medica and InPharma which are available in medical libraries, drug information centres and in some hospital pharmacies. Other methods of searching the literature involve using manual and on-line computerized subject indexing systems (e.g. Index Medicus, Medline); when the search is directed to a particular paper or a narrow field, an author index is useful (e.g. Index Medicus, Science Citation Index). A unique drug information system is provided by the Iowa Drug Information Service. This system comprises a database of complete copies of original published articles from approximately 150 journal titles on microfiche. With any database there is a time lag between the date an article is published and the time it appears in an index. The time lag for these different

Table 45.2   Commonly used sources of drug information

Primary literature	American Journal of Hospital Pharmacy★
	Annals of Internal Medicine★
	British Journal of Clinical Pharmacology
	British Medical Journal★
	Clinical Pharmacokinetics★
	Clinical Pharmacology and Therapeutics
	Clinical Pharmacy★
	Clinical Pharmacy and Therapeutics★
	Drug Intelligence and Clinical Pharmacy★
	European Journal of Clinical Pharmacology
	Journal of the American Medical Association★
	Journal of Pharmaceutical Sciences
	Journal of Pharmacy and Pharmacology
	Lancet★
	New England Journal of Medicine★
Secondary literature	Adverse Drug Reaction Bulletin
	British Journal of Hospital Medicine
	Drugs
	Drug and Therapeutics Bulletin
	InPharma
	Pharmaceutical Journal

★ These journals are also regular sources of secondary literature (review articles).

systems varies between 1 and 6 months. Each system has its own limitations and idiosyncracies based on the range of journals it chooses to cover and the indexing terminology (the thesaurus of drug and disease search terms) it adopts.

Limitations of the drug literature

Amongst the secondary literature sources summarizing the properties and merits of a drug is a wide variety of material produced by the pharmaceutical industry. While often providing useful factual information, such material may be wholly or partially promotional and requires critical examination. Similarly other secondary sources of information, such as independent review articles and leading articles (editorials), should be carefully scrutinized. Some are not as independent as they may at first seem, especially if there is commercial sponsorship. Even apparently unbiased reviews may contain inaccuracies or unsubstantiated opinions. A common problem with reviews occurs when one quotes another, without consulting the original data. In this way mis-conceptions and errors can be propagated in the literature.

There are estimated to be about 20 000 journals world-wide in the biomedical field. About 3500 of these are included in the Index Medicus indexing system. The mass of literature is huge and the number of journals is increasing. Research reports that show signs of incompetence or whose findings are trivial, although often rejected by the major journals, may eventually get published in a minor one. The size of the drug database therefore makes searching it increasingly cumbersome and its variable quality creates the need for careful evaluation.

The printed word conveys authority that may not always be deserved. Researchers may be inclined to underemphasize the uncertainties in their own methods and results. The enthusiasm to publish may lead authors to overvalue the importance of their work and the clinical impact of their findings. Since researchers and journals are more inclined to publish positive rather than negative findings, the literature as a whole may give an exaggerated impression of a drug's clinical effects. There is a lack of trials comparing different agents even though this type of trial is necessary to allow proper evaluation of new treatments. Manufacturers may be less enthusiastic to undertake a comparative trial, for fear that it may show negative findings or even provide evidence supporting a competitor. A trial against an inactive placebo is more attractive to commercial interests wishing to demonstrate the drug in a positive light.

When examining results from a literature search, citations from the major journals are first sought, since these journals usually seek criticism from an independent referee in judging material submitted for publication. However, even this procedure provides no guarantee of quality. Letters and some short communications are often published unrefereed.

Types of drug study

The purpose of publication is to allow experimental findings and interpretations about beneficial or detrimental effects of drugs to be examined. Conclusions can be drawn only from controlled studies. A controlled study is one which draws conclusions from observations about the effect of a drug by questioning whether the same effect is likely to occur without the drug. Case reports are anecdotal in that they describe findings in individual patients. They usually only serve to illustrate a supposed drug effect and are not, by themselves, conclusive nor do they allow generalizations to be made.

A series of cases presented as repeated examples of the same drug effect adds further weight to the idea that the drug is the cause. However, case reports only provide good evidence if their findings have been controlled in some way, for instance by showing that in each patient the observations can be related to the introduction and the discontinuation of the drug.

In a survey, although it may include a large number of subjects, the patients have usually been treated under normal practice circumstances, unrestricted by a formal protocol. Therefore the types of patients, when they were treated and the ways they were managed are largely unspecified and may vary widely. An uncontrolled trial is rather more rigorous in that it usually selects patients for inclusion and treats them according to a protocol drawn up in advance. However, it makes no reference to how the patients might have fared without the drug and so is unable to exclude interference from other factors. A prospective drug study is one which first identifies the subjects to be included, it prescribes a form of treatment and subsequently observes outcome by follow-up of the patient groups (cohorts). Control and treatment groups may be made up of different samples of patients studied concurrently. Where drug effects are known to be temporary and reversible (for instance, with analgesics), cross-over studies are often used. In a cross-over design the same sample of patients is assigned alternately to treatment and control groups, each patient acting as their own control.

A retrospective study gathers information after a period of drug treatment. A case-control study is a retrospective study frequently used in epidemiology. Subjects are identified who have already suffered a particular condition such as the symptoms of suspected drug toxicity. The proportion known to have taken the drug is then compared with that in another group of subjects free of the condition but who are otherwise similar (controls). The risk associated with taking the drug compared with not taking it (the relative risk) can then be calculated.

Evaluating clinical reports

Although small differences occur between different journals, papers publishing research findings generally conform to a traditional format as shown in Table 45.3.

A properly designed trial defines the types of patients making up the sample being studied. Randomly it assigns some to a control group and assesses subjects prospectively. Assessment is under 'double-blind' conditions whereby patients and investigators remain unaware of the results of the assignment. Measurements

Table 45.3 The format of a clinical/scientific paper

Title and authors	
Abstract	Summary of general method and findings but without method details or data. Reproduced on some databases (e.g. Medline). Keywords under which the article may be indexed (often chosen arbitrarily)
Introduction	Brief background to the problem, statement of the question addressed by the research. If the aim is vague at this stage it may later be reflected in a poor design
Subjects	Definition of the types of volunteers or patients and the method of assignment to experimental groups. Ethical considerations
Methods	Design, protocol, sample sizes, the treatment regimens, assessment/measurement (when, how and by whom?)
Results	Figures and tables. Statistical analysis
Discussion	Interpretation of findings in relation to original question. Reality of effect (statistical probability) considered separately from magnitude of effect. Comparison of findings with other reports. Theoretical considerations (confirmation of old ideas or presentation of new ideas). Appraisal of clinical/practical implications
References	

and observations are analysed by appropriate statistical methods. The results are interpreted into proven findings which form the basis of general conclusions about a drug.

The most common and important flaws in clinical reports involve the study design and incomplete descriptive details in the methodology. Surveys of published trials have shown that many are uncontrolled. In particular the description of the type of patients entered into a trial is often incomplete. Even in controlled trials, patients may be allocated to treatment in non-random fashion and it may be unclear whether patients and assessors were 'blind'.

Common statistical errors include the use of an inappropriate test of significance. Trials which report a 'negative' finding (the absence of a statistical difference between two treatments or between treated and control group) require particular attention since the study may have included too small a sample size to justify the conclusion.

Although surveys and case reports usually involve uncontrolled observations, they can provide useful information on the possible character of drug effects and the frequency of unwanted reactions. The reader will often need to judge the strength of an association between the findings described in the case report and drug administration, and should use the following criteria:

— Consistency.
— Timing.
— Dose gradient.
— Specificity.
— Mechanism.
— Analogy.
— Corroboration.
— Reproducibility.

Suspicions of an association may be heightened if the findings are consistent with a drug's known pharmacology and toxicology and if the timing of the observation closely follows starting and stopping the drug. Weight is added if a dose relationship (gradient effect) seems apparent or if the observation is a specific drug toxicity that rarely occurs as a separate pathological condition. The association is further strengthened if a mechanism can be proposed, if there are analogies with the established effects of other (perhaps related) drugs and if several authors have reported similar findings with the same drug (corroboration). Although often precluded by ethical considerations, if the phenomenon is reproducible on rechallenge with the drug a causal link becomes highly likely.

Although errors and omissions in clinical studies undermine confidence in the report, the author's conclusions may only need to be qualified rather than completely discounted. Published checklists are available and are useful aids when systematically evaluating clinical trial reports. It is also useful to follow criticisms of a paper which may occur in the correspondence columns of subsequent issues of the same journal.

Responding to enquiries

Having gathered and evaluated the drug information available on a subject a response to the enquiry is formulated. Where a specific clinical problem is involved, the information must be placed in context and the advice that is offered must take into account limitations imposed by the practical situation. If the reply is to be given orally, a series of written notes linking the relevant factual conclusions to the reference sources is useful. Brief notes help to organize thoughts, particularly when responding over the telephone. Methods of communicating information and of constructing a written report are considered later in this chapter.

Drug information centres

Drug information centres are based in the hospital service and have been established in the UK since 1970. There are now drug information centres in all major UK hospitals, usually attached to pharmacy departments. The drug information centres form a national network co-ordinated by 22 major units. This unique co-operative arrangement has allowed a national service to be developed which includes the provision of an abstracting scheme (Pharmline), new product evaluations, information bulletins and a national training scheme and procedure manual. Each major centre has developed specialist databases and local expertise in such areas as alternative medicine, drug use in nursing mothers, in pregnancy, renal disease and dentistry.

Drug information centres in the UK exist primarily to serve NHS personnel in hospitals and in the community. Unlike some centres in the USA they do not have the resources to provide a service to the general public. They are managed within the hospital pharmaceutical service and are staffed exclusively by pharmacists. The function of a drug information centre involves offering a query-answering service using an in-house system of tertiary and secondary literature and by access to an indexed primary literature database. A drug information service also involves publicizing news of recent developments, the training of pharmacists and the provision of drug information support to pharmacy services in hospital and the community. These functions require co-ordination with the pharmacy service and collaboration with local librarians, academics, clinicians and clinical pharmacologists.

Drug information centres are involved in general educational initiatives in drug usage. These areas of activity include the production of bulletins to doctors and pharmacists in hospitals and in the community. Drug information centres also act as central reference points for adverse drug reaction reporting and providing information for local drug formularies. Many of these activities involve the drug information pharmacist participating as a member of the local drug and therapeutics committee.

COMMUNICATING INFORMATION AND ADVICE

Communication skills are important in advising, reassuring and caring for patients. Good written and verbal communication between members of the health-care team determines the effectiveness of professional relationships and the co-ordination of activities. In pharmacy practice communication skills are important in responding to problems and enquiries and in persuading others to a point of view or a course of action. The pharmacist relies on effective communication to identify and help solve problems. Solving practical problems not only demands knowledge and judgement but also requires dealing with emotions and attitudes such as anxiety, embarassment, confidence, pride and feelings of status.

Successful communication requires conscious attention to accuracy and to being concise in an effort to explain or persuade. Communication skills can be acquired by experience or learnt by examining examples of failings and making a conscious effort to remedy them.

Failings in communication

Lack of success at trying to explain or persuade may become obvious during a conversation as we experience a feeling of being powerless to get our message across. At other times we are so involved in our efforts to make our point that we are blind to our failure. Successful communication relies on establishing and maintaining the receptiveness of those we are addressing. The detection, from signals fed back to us, of early signs of misunderstanding or loss of attention enables us to alter the delivery or content of the message accordingly.

Communication is improved by the development of rapport which is the emotional medium that encourages receptiveness and helps us to convey our ideas and feelings verbally. To establish rapport common ground may first need to be laid, for instance by engaging a common interest in solving a particular problem.

Errors of communication often involve loose or obscure terminology and the use of words that have several different meanings. Misunderstandings can arise from misjudgement of the emotional state of others and by misinterpretation of their intentions or motives. Simple misunderstandings and their consequences can grow when verbal messages are transmitted along a chain of individuals.

The time and place for the conversation must be appropriate if the pharmacist is to secure full attention. Apprehension about the topic of conversation may prompt avoidance or a change of the subject. People may behave on 'automatic pilot', particularly when busy, when they may be dismissive by unfairly prejudging a person or what they have to say. At such times for the sake of expediency we may place others into stereotypes or react to them on reflex without giving them a fair hearing. In conversation, by reacting before the other person has had time to finish we tend to hear only what we want to hear. Similar selfishness in conversation is displayed when, instead of properly listening to others, we switch the focus of the conversation onto ourselves and our own experiences.

If we let our emotions slip as we speak, attention will be diverted from the content of our message. Our emotions also tend to make us unreceptive to the feedback signals or lead us to misinterpret them. On the other hand, when we listen to someone who is in an emotional state, it is not helpful if we try to ignore their feelings or dismiss them with bland reassurances. It is important to try to stand back from the situation and avoid the emotional state being transferred from them to us, since this could result in a loss of control of the conversation.

The ideal message is:

— Relevant.
— Informative.
— Brief.
— Organized.
— Purposeful.
— Constructive.
— Justifiable.
— Valuable.

Effective communication relies on:

— Delivery.
— Reception of feedback.
— Listening.
— Enquiry.
— Anticipation.
— Tact.
— Assertiveness.
— Empathic responding.
— Responding to challenge.
— Patience and emotional objectivity.

Successful communication

Success in communicating requires attention to the content of the message and the manner in which it is delivered. Non-verbal projections of attitudes and feelings colour the message, strengthening or diluting its power. Elements of non-verbal communication include: eye contact; facial expression; tone of voice; personal manner; posture; proximity; and body gestures.

During the delivery, a good communicator will be sensitive to these non-verbal signs from his audience and seek indications of understanding and retention of interest. He will also concentrate on listening and will underline the non-verbal impression with consistent verbal responses (empathic responding). The composition and tactical delivery of the message is helped by anticipation of the likely response and any questions that may be raised. The aim is to avoid provoking an emotional response and losing control of the conversation. Maintaining an influence over the conversation involves conveying self-esteem and a sense of personal rights and values (assertiveness). We should be prepared to admit a lack of knowledge or understanding and to seek further explanation. Questions should be asked in a manner that shows intelligent curiosity rather than aggression. Questions should be met by rising to the challenge without feeling threatened.

Active listening

Pretending to listen, while continuing to think about other things, is a skilled habit. Taking the time and trouble to listen to others is essential to successful communication and requires active effort. Active listening involves the provision of verbal feedback. This demonstration of empathy helps someone deliver their message by showing attentiveness and understanding. Techniques of empathic responding include re-inforcing key statements by repetition. As we listen, we can test our grasp of someone's message by restructuring it, re-stating it, and making it available for correction. By empathic responding we should be able to show that we are listening and understanding without having to show agreement.

To summarize, active listening involves:

— Reinforcement.
— Reflection.
— Repetition.
— Restructuring.
— Questioning.
— Prompting.
— Linking.
— Probing.
— Pace and timing.
— Concern.

Empathic responses should be short and couched in non-emotive language so as to avoid diverting or interrupting the speaker. Although empathic responding is a way to demonstrate factual understanding, it also serves to generate trust by reflecting the other person's feelings.

Other responding techniques include trigger questions which prompt clarification or re-assertion to test a person's strength of feeling or confidence in a point of view. Empathic responding gives others a sense of whether their pace and timing are appropriate. It is also a way of showing concern in what they have to say and how they feel. For active listening to convey a sense of trust, it must encourage free expression of feelings by avoiding passing judgement. Any enthusiasm to dispense advice too early in a professional discussion should be tempered.

Assertiveness

Assertiveness is concerned with the giving and receiving of respect. It is a display of self-respect and personal rights, whilst acknowledging and not infringing the rights of others. Assertiveness is not aggression or arrogance since it does not seek to dominate and it recognizes the needs of others that may require compromises. Assertiveness accepts a compliment without embarrassment, whilst arrogance expects praise. Unlike passive behaviour, assertiveness does not fear the expression of feelings.

Assertive behaviour includes:

— Repetition.
— Seek restatement.
— Defer decision.
— Negotiation.
— Honest admission.
— Deflect criticism.
— Make enquiry.
— Disarm emotions.
— Seek a direct response.
— Short statements.

Assertiveness involves not being afraid to bring issues into the open. When under pressure, we should not be afraid to postpone decision making until we are ready. Fear of hurting feelings should not force us into agreeing with others. If we disagree with their suggestions, negotiating alternatives is a way of being assertive whilst still avoiding direct confrontation. We need not fear our critics but should feel free to accept criticism if we agree with it. We should reserve the right to examine criticism, or just acknowledge it without reaction, if we want to give it further consideration. Assertive attitudes can be developed by observing the following points:

1. Acknowledge criticism and praise but remain your own judge.
2. Do not feel you must justify your feelings.
3. Choose when to involve yourself with other people's problems.
4. Feel you can change your mind.
5. Accept that you can make mistakes.
6. Be prepared to admit lack of knowledge.
7. Feel able to express your feelings and beliefs without the consent of others.

8. Take responsibility for your own decisions.
9. Control how you spend your time.
10. Be guided by your own set of personal values.

Explaining and persuading

The product of effective professional communication is successful explanation or persuasion. For maximum impact the content of the message should be brief, relevant and should provide new information that is presented in an organized and constructive way. The message should have a purpose and should contain information that can be supported by evidence. The result will then be a contribution on which others place a value.

A good explanation will use terminology that is already acceptable to the audience or which has been clearly defined. Careful attention will be given to the information it contains. It will start simply, gradually introducing qualifying statements that show the bounds of knowledge of the subject. Theoretical arguments will be presented and facts identified. Examples and comparisons will be used to illustrate points and one concept will be linked to another. Major points will be emphasized throughout and summarized at the end.

Explaining involves:

1. Choice of vocabulary.
2. Accuracy of information content.
3. Simplicity. Gradual build up, define limits of knowledge.
4. Providing theoretical support.
5. Distinguishing fact from inference.
6. Examples as illustrations.
7. Comparisons as demonstrations.
8. Linking concepts.
9. Use of emphasis and repetition.
10. Summary.

The art of persuasion relies on combining skills of communication and explanation. Overcoming the natural reluctance of people to accept new ideas or to change their behaviour requires an approach that attracts trust and conveys credibility. Some techniques for successful persuasion are listed below:

1. Attention to personal manner and appearance.
2. Avoid an imposing or threatening attitude.
3. Reveal new information.
4. Provide interpretation and convey expertness.
5. Identify common ground first.
6. Start with less controversial points.
7. Avoid direct conflict, introduce new (related) ideas.
8. Acknowledge and respect opposing point of view.

9. Avoid casting blame/judging others.
10. Show patience and emotional detachment.
11. Do not be manipulated or diverted.
12. Be honest about your motives.
13. Explain carefully, without lecturing.
14. Show objectivity and an open mind.
15. Avoid relying on 'expert' opinion.
16. Avoid use of stereotypes.
17. Avoid exaggeration and use of extremes.
18. Recognize boredom, when to pause or lighten the atmosphere.
19. Recognize feelings. Don't rely on rational argument alone.
20. Settle by negotiation.

Report writing

Many of the principles of effective communication are relevant to the written as well as the spoken word. In providing professional information and advice a formal report may be required, particularly if a complex argument and supporting evidence are to be provided. In other circumstances a written response is preferred to ensure a legal or ethical position is presented as unambiguously as possible. The quality of presentation of a written report has a major impact on its ability to convince. A neat manuscript is unlikely to be an adequate cosmetic for a poorly researched answer; but a badly typed report certainly undermines confidence in an otherwise good piece of work.

The final report should be headed with a short relevant title, accompanied by a reference number to aid filing and retrieval. The text should be concisely written, adopting a simple clear style. Reference citations should include only those necessary to support the argument. Margins should be wide and paragraphs short. It is useful to compose a report in three sections.

The first section should be a brief introduction which may simply be a statement of the problem. Where appropriate the extent of the investigation may be summarized and any additional assistance from other sources may be acknowledged.

The body of the written report should include the findings with important statements clearly referenced, preferably by consecutive numbering. Particular care should be given to ensuring that factual information is accurate and statements are unambiguous. It is important not to make the report undigestible by overloading it with superfluous information.

The final section should briefly summarize and conclude by placing the findings in the context of the enquirer's underlying problem.

References should be in a uniform style (such as the widely used 'Vancouver' style, described in the British Medical Journal (International Committee of Medical Journal Editors 1982)), numbered and listed consecutively at the end of the report.

The enquirer should be encouraged to return any points that need further clarification or follow-up.

Communicating advice to patients

Drug information and pharmaceutical advice to doctors and other health-care workers must be soundly based on scientific knowledge and an understanding of clinical problems. Advice to patients on their medication must also be based on knowledge of the action of the drug. The information must be arranged in a priority order with emphasis on the most important aspects. The process of counselling patients therefore relies on the pharmacist having clear objectives in mind and a plan for presenting information to the patient. The types of information patients may require on their prescribed medicines are:

1. Indications.
2. Dose to be taken.
3. Frequency of dosing.
   Is timing crucial?
4. Administration in relation to food.
5. How to use special administration devices.
6. What to do if dose is missed.
7. Duration of therapy.
8. Side-effects
   a. How to recognize them.
   b. What to do about them.
9. How to recognize if the medicine is working.
10. Interference with alcohol, driving, hobbies.
11. Interference with oral contraception.
12. How to obtain more information.
13. What to do with tablets no longer required.

Some common faults encountered in advising patients are:

1. Making things too complex.
2. Using long words.
3. Providing too many facts.
4. Mixing fact and opinion.
5. Trying to be too brief or too simple.
6. Presenting information impersonally.
7. Speaking too quickly.

Patients often prefer personal advice rather than just written information. However, well-designed patient information leaflets are valuable as a guide and a supplement to the personal consultation. Patient counselling is discussed in detail in Chapter 37.

BIBLIOGRAPHY

Altman D G, Gore S M, Gardner M J, Pocock S J 1983 Statistical guidelines for contributors to medical journals. British Medical Journal 286: 1489–1493

Anon 1985 Reading between the lines of clinical trials. Drug and Therapeutics Bulletin 23: 1–8

Drug Information Pharmacists' Group 1987 Drug information procedure manual, Leeds

Drug Information Pharmacists' Group. Minimum recommended reference sources for answering enquiries. Pharmaceutical Journal 8: 721–722

Gardner M J 1986 Use of checklists in assessing the statistical content of medical studies. British Medical Journal 292: 810–812

Gore S M, Altman D G 1982 Statistics in practice. British Medical Association, London

Jones J K 1982 Criteria for assessing journal reports of suspected adverse drug reactions. Clinical Pharmacy 1: 554–555

Leach F 1986 A guide to evaluating drug advertisements. Pharmaceutical Journal 236: 172–173

McCabe J C, Richards R M E 1982 Drug information. In: Richards R M E, Lawson D H (eds) Clinical pharmacy and hospital drug management. Chapman & Hall, London, p 311

Pocock S J 1984 Clinical trials — a practical approach. Wiley, Chichester

Pocock S J 1985 Current issues in the design and interpretation of clinical trials. British Medical Journal 290: 39–42

Riegelman R K 1981 Studying a study and testing a test. Little, Brown and Co, Boston

Tindall W N, Beardsley R S, Curtiss F R 1984 Communication in pharmacy practice. Lea & Febiger, Philadelphia

Pharmaceutical Journal 8: 721–722

International Committee of Medical Journal Editors 1982 Uniform requirements for manuscripts submitted to biochemical journals. British Medical Journal 284: 1766–1770

Appendices

Appendix 1
Current UK pharmaceutical legislation

M. G. Aiken   A. L. G. Pugh

This appendix provides a brief but comprehensive summary of the major legislation affecting the sale and supply of medicinal products from a community pharmacy. It is not intended to replace other detailed sources of information on pharmaceutical legislation which are quoted in the reference list.

This summary aims to serve as:

— A clear introduction for the new student of pharmaceutical legislation.
— A basic guide for the student in the dispensing laboratory.
— An examination revision guide for pharmacy students.
— A revision summary for the pharmacist returning to community practice.

The reader is reminded that the law is constantly being changed and that frequently updated information sources such as those provided by the Royal Pharmaceutical Society should be consulted regularly.

The day-to-day professional work of a practising pharmacist involves many aspects of legislation. Medicines themselves are subject to the Medicines Act (1968) and the Misuse of Drugs Act (1971); the various National Health Service Acts cover aspects of pharmaceutical services, while the Health and Safety at Work etc. Act (1974) deals with a safe work environment for staff and patients or customers alike.

A brief outline of the relevant legislation is given in this Appendix. For further details the reader is referred to the specific Regulations or to Dale and Appelbe (1989), Pearce (1984) and to the Medicines, Ethics and Practice (Royal Pharmaceutical Society of Great Britain current edition).

The Law Department of the Royal Pharmaceutical Society may be consulted for up-to-date information and issues statements when appropriate on new and forthcoming legislation in the 'Pharmaceutical Journal'.

The sale and supply of medicinal products

This is governed by:

I. The Medicines Act, 1968 (and subsequent Regulations)

This defines General Sales List Medicines (GSL) and Prescription Only Medicines (POM). Medicines not defined as GSL or POM are classified as Pharmacy Medicines (P).

II. The Misuse of Drugs Act, 1971 (and Regulations, 1985)

Medicinal products that are liable to abuse are defined as Controlled Drugs (CD). The Act specifies Classes and penalties for offences while the Regulations classify Controlled Drugs into five Schedules.

THE MEDICINES ACT

Classes of medicines

General Sale List Medicines (GSL)

These are specified products that are considered safe enough to be sold without the supervision of a pharmacist.

Pharmacy Medicines (P)

These may be sold only from a registered pharmacy under the supervision of a pharmacist.

Prescription Only Medicines (POM)

These include:

1. Medicines containing one or more substances in the list (Schedule I, Part I to the Prescription Only Order). See below for exceptions.
2. Controlled Drugs. See below for exceptions.
3. Products in Part III, Schedule I to the Order.

4. Parenteral Products. Except insulin injections for human use.

Exceptions to 1 above. In some cases the classification of a medicine as POM or P depends on:

a. The quantity of the active drug in a dosage unit.

b. The concentration of the active drug in the medicine.

c. The quantity of the active drug in a recommended single dose.

d. The maximum quantity of active drug recommended to be taken in a period of 24 hours.

The terms *md* (maximum dose), *mdd* (maximum daily dose) and *ms* (maximum strength) are defined in the 'Medicines and ethics guide' (Royal Pharmaceutical Society of Great Britain 1988).

Exceptions to 2 above. Products containing no more than the specified strength of one only of six specified Controlled Drugs become Pharmacy Medicines. Details are provided in the 'Medicines and ethics guide' (Royal Pharmaceutical Society of Great Britain 1988).

THE SALE OR SUPPLY OF P AND GSL MEDICINES

Within the pharmacy there are few restrictions on the sale of GSL medicines. There are certain restrictions on the package sizes of some products, e.g. aloxipren, aspirin, paracetamol and salicylamide, which may be sold from non-pharmaceutical outlets.

Pharmacy medicines may only be supplied under the supervision of a pharmacist from a registered pharmacy.

The supply may be made at the request of the customer, at the recommendation of the pharmacist or in accordance with a prescription from a practitioner. There are no statutory requirements for prescriptions for P medicines although standard requirements for NHS prescriptions will apply.

THE SALE OR SUPPLY OF POM PRODUCTS

This is restricted to:

I. The supply to a patient in accordance with a prescription given by an appropriate practitioner (doctor, dentist, veterinary surgeon or veterinary practitioner).

POM prescription requirements

POM prescriptions must:

1. Be signed in ink by the issuing practitioner.
2. Be written in indelible ink (includes typing).

3. Indicate whether repeats are required.
4. Include the:
   a. Address of the issuing practitioner.
   b. Profession of the issuing practitioner.
   c. Name and address of patient (or owner of animal).
   d. Age of patient if under 12 years.
   e. Date of signing★ (valid for 6 months).

Private POM prescriptions must be retained for 2 years after dispensing unless repeatable (see below).

NHS prescriptions are sent for pricing (see Appendix 2).

Note that prescriptions for POMs that are also Controlled Drugs must fulfil the more stringent requirements of the Misuse of Drugs Act (MDA).

Repeatable prescriptions

NHS prescriptions may not be acted upon more than once. If indicated by the prescriber a private prescription for a POM may be dispensed on a specified number of occasions provided that the first supply is made within 6 months of the date of signing. If the number of repeats is unspecified the prescription may be dispensed only twice (i.e. one repeat) except for oral contraceptives which may be dispensed six times before the end of the period 6 months from the prescription date.

Records of POM prescriptions

A record must be kept for 2 years of all POM prescriptions unless:

1. Supplied on NHS prescription.
2. For oral contraceptives.
3. For Controlled Drugs (recorded elsewhere).

It is good practice to record the dispensing of all private prescriptions in a special register, giving each entry a reference number (see Ch. 9 and 10). The record should include:

1. Date of supply.
2. Name, quantity, form and strength of the POM.
3. Name, address and status of the prescriber.
4. Date on the prescription.
5. Name and address of patient (or owner of animal).

★ For NHS prescriptions the date may be the date of signing or the date before which the prescription may not be dispensed.

For second and subsequent supplies made on repeat prescriptions, a reference to the details recorded on the first supply is sufficient.

The prescription is retained for 2 years after the final repeat.

II. An Emergency Supply to a patient made at the request of a doctor

The pharmacist must be satisfied that:

1. The prescriber is genuine.
2. The reason for the request is valid.
3. A prescription will be provided within 72 hours.
4. The prescriber has indicated the directions.
5. The medicine is not in a disallowed category.

Records of Emergency Supplies made at the request of a doctor

In addition to the usual prescription records (see above), the pharmacist must record both the date on the prescription and the date on which it was received. This applies for both private and NHS prescriptions. The record must be retained for 2 years.

III. An Emergency Supply made at the request of a patient

This facility allows the pharmacist to supply up to 5 days' treatment (or smallest pack) in order to provide for a genuine emergency when a patient is unable to obtain a prescription immediately but has an urgent requirement for a POM regularly prescribed.

The pharmacist must be satisfied that:

1. There is an immediate need.
2. It is impracticable to get a prescription at once.
3. The medicine has been prescribed before.
4. The dosage is known.
5. The drug is not in a disallowed category, e.g. CD. (A special exemption is made for phenobarbitone and phenobarbitone sodium when used for the treatment of epilepsy).

The Royal Pharmaceutical Society gives the following guidance that the pharmacist should:

1. Consider the consequences of NOT supplying.
2. Identify the patient.
3. Identify and if possible contact the GP.
4. Check when the medicine was last prescribed.
5. Ask if the treatment has been discontinued.
6. Ask whether other medication is being taken. See BNF.

Note that:

1. Items last prescribed more than 6 months before the request would not be supplied except for the treatment of infrequently recurring illness.
2. Less than 5 days' supply may be made if sufficient.
3. The label must include the words 'Emergency Supply' in addition to the usual labelling for a dispensed medicine (see below and Ch. 10).

Records of Emergency Supplies made at the request of a patient

The record (to be retained for 2 years) must include:

1. Date of supply.
2. Name, quantity, form and strength of the POM.
3. Name and address of patient.
4. Nature of emergency.

It is also good practice to record the name and address of the GP.

IV. Sale to a practitioner (wholesale supply)

The pharmacist must be satisfied that the request is valid.

A record of the sale must be made unless a copy of the order or invoice relating to the sale is retained for 2 years or unless a separate record is made for the supply of a CD POM in the CD register.

The information which should be recorded includes:

1. The date of supply.
2. Name, quantity, form and strength of the POM.
3. Name, address, business or profession of the purchaser.
4. The purpose for which supplied.

V. Supply to other authorized persons

Persons subject to specific exemptions from the controls on sale or supply may also purchase those Prescription Only Medicines for which they are exempted. For details see the 'Medicines and ethics guide' (Royal Pharmaceutical Society of Great Britain 1988).

THE MISUSE OF DRUGS ACT

Categories of drugs

Schedule 1 (CD Lic)

Research purposes only. Possession and supply prohibited, e.g. cannabis, lysergide.

Schedule 2 (CD)

Fully controlled drugs, e.g. amphetamine, diamorphine, methadone. Must be kept in safe custody.

Schedule 3 (CD No Reg)

Less stringent control and no CD records necessary, e.g. pentazocine, phenobarbitone.

Schedule 4 (CD Benz)

Minimal control for benzodiazepine tranquillizers only, e.g. diazepam, lorazepam. POM regulations apply to sale or supply.

Schedule 5 (CD Inv)

Includes those preparations which because of their strength are exempt from all CD control except retention of invoices for 2 years. The preparations may be categorized as CD Inv POM, e.g. Chalk and Opium Mixture BPC 1973, or CD Inv P, e.g. Kaolin and Morphine Mixture BP, and the relevant POM or P regulations apply to sale or supply.

THE SALE OR SUPPLY OF SCHEDULE 2 AND SCHEDULE 3 CONTROLLED DRUGS

This is restricted to:

I. The supply to a patient in accordance with a prescription given by an appropriate practitioner

CD POM and CD No Reg POM prescription requirements

The prescription must be indelibly hand written, signed and dated by a valid prescriber and include:

1. Name and address of patient (or owner of animal).
2. Form of the medicine.
3. Strength of the preparation if appropriate.
4. Dose to be taken.
5. Total quantity to be supplied in words and figures.
6. The usual signature.

The prescription must also indicate:

1. The address of the prescriber which must be in the UK (all NHS prescribers are UK based).
2. For dental treatment only (if dental).
3. For animal treatment only (if vet).

Note that:

1. Requirements for POM prescriptions also apply.

2. Handwriting requirements may be waived for drug treatment centres.
3. Handwriting is not a requirement for prescriptions for phenobarbitone or phenobarbitone sodium.

Before dispensing the pharmacist must be satisfied:

1. That the prescriber is valid.
2. That the signature is genuine.
3. That the date is within 13 weeks.

The prescription must be dated at the time of dispensing and retained for 2 years. Repeats are not allowed.

Records of CD POM prescriptions

A special register of specified format is used for recording both the receipt and supply. A separate part of the register is used for each class of drug. The information which is recorded includes:

1. Receipt:
   a. Date received.
   b. Name and address of supplier.
   c. Amount received.
   d. Form in which received.
2. Supply:
   a. Date supplied.
   b. Name and address of recipient.
   c. Authority of recipient to possess.
   d. Amount supplied.
   e. Form in which supplied.

Entries should be made in chronological order on the day of the transaction. No alteration or cancellation is permitted, errors should be recorded as a marginal note and initialled. The register must be retained for 2 years after the last entry.

Note that no CD record is required for CD No Reg medicines but that POM regulations apply.

II. Sale to a practitioner of CD POM and CD No Reg POM

The pharmacist must be satisfied that the request is valid and that the purchaser is genuine.

A written requisition must be supplied and include:

1. The signature of the recipient.
2. The name, address, profession or occupation of the purchaser.
3. The total quantity of drug.
4. The purpose for which required.

A purchaser unable to collect the drug in person must

provide a messenger's authority to allow a third party to collect on his behalf.

All documents must be retained for 2 years and the transaction recorded in the CD register for CD POM.

III. Supply to other authorized persons

Certain authorized persons may also purchase specified CD POM or CD No Reg POM. For details see the 'Medicines and ethics guide' (Royal Pharmaceutical Society of Great Britain 1988).

LABELLING OF MEDICINES

All medicines must be labelled in accordance with the General Labelling Provisions (see the 'Medicines, Ethics and Practice (Royal Pharmaceutical Society of Great Britain 1988)).

All medicinal products for *retail* sale should carry a child warning label.

The labelling of dispensed medicines is discussed fully in Chapter 10 and includes items which are legally required and those which are included as good pharmaceutical practice. Minimum legal requirements are listed in the 'Medicines and ethics guide' (Royal Pharmaceutical Society of Great Britain 1988).

Labelling for sale

The Standard Labelling Particulars apply to medicines packaged for sale and include the following:

1. Name of product.
2. Pharmaceutical form.
3. The amounts of active and non-active ingredients or the source of an 'official' formula, e.g. BP (appropriate quantitative particulars).
4. Quantity in the container.
5. Directions for use. If not for sale directly to the public, i.e. if sold to a practitioner or as stock then 'to be used as directed by an appropriate practitioner' may be used.
6. Any special contraindications, precautions or warnings.
7. Storage requirements.
8. The expiry date.
9. The name and address of the supplier.
10. Product licence number PL. . . . .
11. Manufacturer's batch reference BN . . . .
12. Manufacturer's licence number ML. . . . . . or the name and address of the manufacturer.
13. Other particulars required by the product licence.

Special labelling requirements by legal class

GSL medicines

1. If containing aloxiprin, aspirin or paracetamol, with the warning label

> If symptoms persist consult your doctor

and the recommended dosage unless for external use.

2. These phrases must be enclosed in a ruled rectangle box
   a. If containing aloxiprin

> Contains an aspirin derivative

   b. If containing aspirin

> Contains aspirin

unless aspirin is included in the name of the product or the product is for external use.
   c. If containing paracetamol

> Contains paracetamol

unless paracetamol is included in the name of the product.
If more than one phrase applies they may be combined and surrounded by one rectangle.

3. If containing paracetamol

> Do not exceed the stated dose

placed near to the dosage directions.

P medicines

1. In a rectangle

> P

2. If containing aloxiprin, aspirin or paracetamol: as for 'GSL products' (see 2 above).
3. If exempt from POM control by reason of proportion or strength

> Do not exceed the stated dose

unless listed under 5 below.

4. If for the treatment of asthma or bronchospasm

> Warning. Asthmatics should consult their doctor before using this product

Does not apply to external products but does apply to nasal drops.

5. If containing any of a list of antihistaminics

> Warning. May cause drowsiness. If affected do not drive or operate machinery Avoid alcoholic drink

Does not apply to external products.

6. For external preparations that are liquids or gels

> For external use only

7. If containing hexachlorophane

> Not to be used for babies

POM sale labelling

1. In a rectangle

> POM

unless dispensed

2. Liquid and gel preparations for external use: as for 'P medicines' (see 6 above).

3. Products containing hexachlorophane: as for P medicines (see 7 above).

Labelling of ingredients for sale

The Standard Labelling Particulars apply with the exception of those which refer specifically to 'products', i.e.:

— Directions for use.

— Special precautions or warnings.
— Name and address of supplier.

Labelling of 'own-label' preparations

Medicines prepared in the pharmacy for retail sale must also be labelled with appropriate Standard Labelling Particulars and P label requirements. Since these products are not usually subject to a Product Licence those particulars which refer to such a licence are not applicable.

OTHER LEGISLATION

I. Poisons Act (and Rules)

This deals with the sale of non-medicinal poisons. These are substances which are included in either Part I or Part II of the Poisons List Order. There are 12 Schedules to the Rules: Schedule 1 is that covering the sale of certain poisons with respect to purchaser, storage and keeping of records.

Containers

These must be robust enough to eliminate the possibility of leakage in usual handling. Liquids, up to 1.14 litres, must be in ribbed containers.

Storage

Schedule 1 poisons must be kept in a safe place where no contamination of other goods or foods can occur.

Labelling

All poisons require: name, proportion of poison (if an ingredient), the word

> Poison

and the name and address of the seller.

For Schedule 1 poisons, the word must be in red or on a red background.

Alternative wordings are used for certain substances e.g.

> Caution. This substance is caustic.

on potassium and sodium hydroxide.

Sales of S1 poisons

These sales can only be made:

1. To a person known to the pharmacist to be a responsible person, when a signature in the Poisons Book is made.

2. If the proposed purchaser is not known to the pharmacist, then it is necessary to provide a Certificate for the purchase of a poison (Schedule 10), this is filled in by a householder, if this person is not known to the seller, then it is necessary to obtain an endorsement by the police officer in charge of a police station; again the Poisons Book is signed.

3. Users wanting poisons for trade, business or professional purposes may provide a signed order (to include name and address, business, etc., total quantity to be purchased and purpose for which the poison is required). An entry is made in the Poisons Book and the words 'signed order' entered in place of the signature.

Special restrictions are placed on certain poisons; e.g. strychnine, thallium salts and cyanides. See the 'Medicines, Ethics and Practice (Royal Pharmaceutical Society of Great Britain, current edition) (Pearce 1984).

II. Prescribed Dangerous Substances

These are subject to the Packaging and Labelling of Dangerous Substances Regulations. These bring together several EC Directives for a very wide range of potentially dangerous substances.

In general, the labelling (applicable to sales of such items from a pharmacy) requires:

1. Name of substance.
2. Name and address of manufacturer, or supplier.
3. Symbol(s) indicating the general risk(s) on an orange-yellow background.
4. Particular risks.
5. Safety precautions.

Substances included in the Poisons List, that are also 'prescribed dangerous substances', must be labelled according to these regulations and not to the Poisons Rules. Details are included in the 'Medicines and Poisons Guide' (Pearce 1984).

III. Spirits Regulations

The main application of the Spirits Regulations to pharmacy is in the sale of Mineralized Methylated Spirits and in the use of and supply of Industrial Methylated Spirits.

Mineralized Methylated Spirits (MMS)

MMS may be obtained without restriction from various types of supplier. Restrictions on sale in England are limited to a ban on sales during the hours between 10.00 p.m. on Saturday and 8.00 a.m. the following Monday. Additionally, in Scotland sales of MMS must be recorded in a special sales book and must not exceed 4 gallons (approx. 18 litres) unless sold by a wholesaler.

Industrial Methylated Spirits (IMS)

Application to receive supplies is made on Form Ex 225 (Customs and Excise) for use in pharmacy and a certificate of authority is issued.

The purchase of supplies is made with a written statement on headed notepaper, signed and dated and sent to the supplier. This covers one supply or a period of up to 12 months. Supplies of 20 litres or more must be obtained from a licensed or authorized methylator; less than 20 litres can be obtained from a pharmaceutical wholesaler.

Supplies can be used for:

1. Making articles in Appendix A of Customs and Excise Note 474.
2. Dispensing of IMS and articles made with IMS.
3. The making of other approved articles.
4. Sales to medical practitioners.

Dispensing. IMS and articles made with IMS may be supplied on a prescription signed by a medical practitioner which for the purposes of the Spirits Regulations includes a wide range of professions, i.e. doctors, dentists, nurses, chiropodists, veterinary surgeons, etc. No more than 3 litres may be supplied at any one time and a record should be made of private prescriptions. The label should include a

> Flammable

warning and

> For External Use Only

or

> Not To Be Taken

Sale. Sales of not more than 3 litres may be made to a practitioner on receipt of a written order.

Sales of up to 20 litres may be made to an authorized user on receipt of a signed written statement that he is authorized to receive. The statement will remain valid for 12 months. IMS must be labelled in accordance with the Classification, Packaging and Labelling of Dangerous Substances Regulations. In addition, the label should include

For External Use Only

or

Not To Be Taken

if for medical purposes.

The local Customs and Excise may require records to be kept.

IV. Health and Safety at Work, etc. Act (1974)

This replaces all other Acts relating to health and safety (e.g. Factories Act, Shops Act, etc.).

The intention is that all persons at places of work and members of the public visiting those places are covered with respect to health and safety. Health includes heating and lighting, washing facilities, first aid provision, while safety includes handrails on stairways, protective barriers around lift and hoist hatchways, protective clothing, instruction in safe handling of toxic materials and equipment, and fire drills.

Safety policies are set up, safety representatives appointed, and employers and employees both have responsibilities to each other to maintain and develop safe procedures. Inspection and enforcement are provided for by the Health and Safety Executive.

V. Consumer Protection Act 1987

Under this legislation the 'producer' of a product will be strictly liable for any injury caused by a defective product. In the case of the pharmacist this includes personal injury caused by the administration of a 'defective' medicine. Important implications of this legislation for the pharmacist include the need to retain complete records of the suppliers of all medicines and ingredients used in the manufacture of medicines, including batch identification, date of supply and date used. For further details the reader is referred to the Royal Pharmaceutical Society's Statement on 'Product liability and the pharmacist' (1988).

BIBLIOGRAPHY

British National Formulary 1988 16th edn. British Medical Association and Royal Pharmaceutical Society of Great Britain, London
Dale J R, Appelbe G E 1989 Pharmacy law and ethics, 4th edn. Pharmaceutical Press, London
Guide to the Controlled Drug Regulations 1988 Pharmaceutical Journal 240: 156–157
Own-label preparations and the law. 1987 Pharmaceutical Journal 239: 163–164

Pearce M E (ed) 1984 Medicines and poisons guide, 4th edn. Pharmaceutical Press, London (with cumulative amendments in the Pharmaceutical Journal)
Pharmaceutical Society 1988 Product liability and the pharmacist. Pharmaceutical Journal 240: 25
Royal Pharmaceutical Society of Great Britain 1988 Medicines, ethics and practice — a guide for pharmacists, No. 3. Royal Pharmaceutical Society of Great Britain, London (updated twice yearly) (use current edition)

Appendix 2
NHS dispensing

M. G. Aiken   A. L. G. Pugh

This appendix provides a brief guide to pharmaceutical services under the NHS and includes the types of prescription form, the necessary endorsements and the procedure for obtaining reimbursement from the Pricing Authority.

Pharmacists included on the Pharmaceutical List are contracted with the Family Practitioner Committee (FPC) to supply permitted drugs and appliances with reasonable promptness. The pharmacist must conform to a number of regulations with regard to the service provided. In turn the pharmacist receives payment for the supply of drugs, appliances, chemical reagents and for other aspects of the pharmaceutical service provided.

Details of current payments to Pharmacy Contractors are listed in the Drug Tariff.

Prescriptions

Payment will only be made in respect of prescriptions written on 'official' NHS forms. The official prescription forms currently in use are summarized in Tables A2.1–A2.5 and a facsimile of a standard FP10 form is shown in Figure A2.1.

As described in Chapter 9, the prescription form consists of three main sections; details of the medicinal

Table A2.1 NHS prescription forms issued in England and Wales (E + W)

Prescription code	Colour	Issued by	Purpose issued	Can it be dispensed in E + W?
FP10	White	GPs and dispensing doctors	Normal form	Yes
FP10(HP)	Peach	Doctor (clinic or hospital)	Outpatients	Yes
FP10(HP)ad	Red	Drug addiction clinic	For drug addicts	Yes
FP10MDA	Blue	GP	Installment dispensing for addicts only	Yes
FP10(D)	Green-blue	Dispensing doctor	For drug not in stock	Yes
FP10(S)	Buff	Medical officers and doctors in armed forces	For service personnel and dependants	Yes
FMED296	White	Army doctors	For army personnel	No
FP10DTS	White	Sampling officers of Drug Testing Scheme	Drug Testing Scheme	Yes
FP14	Yellow	Dentists	Normal dental form	Yes
FPBC10	Blue	Somerset Family Planning Depts	Contraceptives	Yes, return to Somerset AHA for payment. No Prescription Tax

Table A2.2 NHS prescription forms issued in Scotland (S)

Prescription code	Colour	Issued by	Purpose issued	Can it be dispensed in E + W?
GP10	White	GPs	Normal form	Yes
GP10A	White	GPs	Doctors stock order	No
GP10(S)	Buff	Medical officers and doctors in armed forces	For service personnel and dependants	Yes
GP10DTS	Pink	Sampling officers of Drug Testing Scheme	Drug Testing Scheme	No
GP14	Yellow	Dentists	Normal dental form	Yes
HBP	Blue	Hospital doctors	Outpatients	Yes
HBP(A)	Pink	Drug addiction clinics	For drug addicts	Yes

Table A2.3 NHS prescription forms issued in Northern Ireland (NI)

Prescription code	Colour	Issued by	Purpose issued	Can it be dispensed in E + W?
HS21	White	GPs	Normal form	Yes
HS47	Yellow	Dentists	Normal dental form	Yes
HS21MMS	White	Doctors with maternity services only	Maternity Medical Services	Yes

Table A2.4 NHS prescription forms issued in Isle of Man (IOM)

Prescription code	Colour	Issued by	Purpose issued	Can it be dispensed in E + W?
HS10	White	GPs	Normal form	Yes
HS10A	Pink	GPs	Form for patients exempt from prescription charges	Yes

Table A2.5 NHS prescription forms issued in Jersey (J) and Guernsey (G)

Prescription code	Colour	Issued by	Purpose issued	Can it be dispensed in E + W?
H9	White	Jersey	Normal form	No
(G) P S6	White	Guernsey	Normal form	No

product ordered, the patient identification and endorsement sections for the pharmacist.

The reverse of the form is composed of two main parts; important notes for patients and a declaration section for patients exempt from charges.

Prescription charges

Certain categories of patient are exempt from NHS prescription charges. These include children under 16 (under 19 if in full-time education), pregnant women

FRONT

BACK

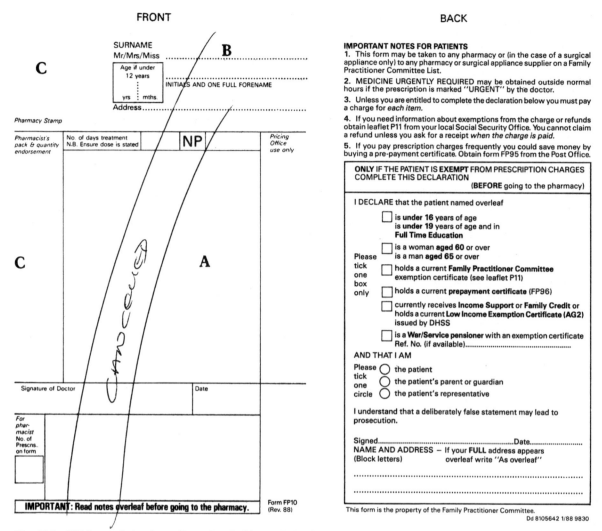

C

SURNAME
Mr/Mrs/Miss
B

Age if under
12 years
INITIALS AND ONE FULL FORENAME
yrs mths
Address

Pharmacy Stamp

Pharmacist's
pack & quantity
endorsement

No. of days treatment
N.B. Ensure dose is stated

NP

Pricing
Office
use only

C

A

Signature of Doctor   Date

For
phar-
macist
No. of
Prescns.
on form

IMPORTANT: Read notes overleaf before going to the pharmacy.

Form FP10
(Rev. 88)

IMPORTANT NOTES FOR PATIENTS
1. This form may be taken to any pharmacy or (in the case of a surgical appliance only) to any pharmacy or surgical appliance supplier on a Family Practitioner Committee List.
2. MEDICINE URGENTLY REQUIRED may be obtained outside normal hours if the prescription is marked "URGENT" by the doctor.
3. Unless you are entitled to complete the declaration below you must pay a charge for *each item*.
4. If you need information about exemptions from the charge or refunds obtain leaflet P11 from your local Social Security Office. You cannot claim a refund unless you ask for a receipt *when the charge is paid*.
5. If you pay prescription charges frequently you could save money by buying a pre-payment certificate. Obtain form FP95 from the Post Office.

ONLY IF THE PATIENT IS EXEMPT FROM PRESCRIPTION CHARGES COMPLETE THIS DECLARATION
(BEFORE going to the pharmacy)

I DECLARE that the patient named overleaf

☐ is **under 16** years of age
is **under 19** years of age and in **Full Time Education**

☐ is a woman **aged 60** or over
is a man **aged 65** or over

Please tick one box only

☐ holds a current **Family Practitioner Committee** exemption certificate (see leaflet P11)

☐ holds a current **prepayment certificate** (FP96)

☐ currently receives **Income Support** or **Family Credit** or holds a current **Low Income Exemption Certificate (AG2)** issued by DHSS

☐ is a **War/Service pensioner** with an exemption certificate Ref. No. (if available)

AND THAT I AM

Please tick one circle

○ the patient
○ the patient's parent or guardian
○ the patient's representative

I understand that a deliberately false statement may lead to prosecution.

Signed.....................................Date............
NAME AND ADDRESS – If your FULL address appears
(Block letters)   overleaf write "As overleaf"

....
....

This form is the property of the Family Practitioner Committee.
Dd 8105642 1/88 9830

Fig. A2.1   FP10 prescription form. (Reproduced with permission from the Family Practitioner Committee)

and mothers of babies under 12 months old, men over 65 and women over 60 years old. Patients with certain specified medical conditions, e.g. diabetes mellitus, are also exempted, as are persons holding DHSS certificates — mainly those on low incomes.

Prescription charges are payable by non-exempted patients and are collected by the pharmacist on behalf of the DHSS. A charge is made for each item prescribed including drugs, preparations, appliances, articles of elastic hosiery and oxygen equipment.

Details of relevant prescription charges are to be found in the current Drug Tariff and explained in the current NPA Guide to the Drug Tariff.

Prescription endorsement

Each prescription form is endorsed with the name and address of the pharmacy and date of dispensing (top left) and the number of prescriptions (items) on the form (bottom left) (Figure A2.1).

Details of the items supplied are entered in the left margin under 'pharmacists pack and quantity endorsement'. Details of required endorsements are given in the current Drug Tariff and explained in the current NPA Guide. It is sensible to endorse with as much information as possible since prescriptions not adequately endorsed will be returned from the Processing Division and payment delayed. It should be noted that if as few as 5% of submitted prescription forms are unendorsed, a complete month's forms may be returned. Examples of NHS endorsement requirements are shown in Table A2.6. For further details see the current Drug Tariff.

All prescriptions attract a professional fee per item dispensed. There are certain additional fees for which special endorsement is required (see Table A2.6).

Pack sizes and broken bulk

Pack size endorsement only applies to items listed as Drug Tariff Category C. If the pharmacist has little call for a product he will be paid for a small pack, but if demand is considerable his payment will be based on a pack size related to his overall demand. Where it is found that a smaller pack has been used and the demand for that medicine for the month (monitored by Processing Division) exceeds two-thirds of the larger pack size, a letter is sent to the pharmacist requesting that a larger pack be used in future. If this is ignored the pharmacist is eventually paid on the larger pack, if demand continues at a high level for that medicine.

If the quantity of a proprietary medicine ordered does not coincide with an original pack and the pharmacist, because of lack of demand, cannot readily dispose of the remainder, payment is made for the residue in the pack containing the quantity nearest to that ordered. The form must be endorsed 'claim broken bulk', 'residue claimed', or similar wording. The cost of the remainder is only paid if the claim is considered justified. If the same medicine is dispensed again within the next 3 months, the balance from the pack previously claimed for should be used up and further packs ordered and claimed for, if necessary. Records are kept by the Processing Division of 'broken bulk' claims and it is advisable for pharmacists to mark containers for which 'broken bulk' claims have been made with the date of claim.

Many proprietary medicines are now supplied as calendar packs (foil strips marked with days of the week). Pharmacists have the option of supplying these products:

Table A2.6 NHS prescription endorsement

Endorsement	Where used	Example
No endorsement	Category A and Category E drugs of Drug Tariff (1988) (A basic price is paid for Category A drugs by NHS; an extemporaneous fee is automatically paid PPA for Category E drugs)	Paracetamol Tablets BP, 500 mg (Category A) Potassium Citrate and Hyoscyamus Mixture BPC (Category E)
(In practice, many pharmacists still endorse Category E prescriptions, 'Extemporaneously prepared')		
Extemporaneously dispensed (Extemp. prep.)	Unit dose forms	Capsules Powders
This means prepared from suitable materials using skill/knowledge of pharmacist (fiat secundum artem)	Liquids	Special formula preparations, e.g. mixtures
	Liquids prepared by dilution	50% v/v Simple Linctus
	Ointments, creams, pastes	Dithranol Paste with 1% w/w hydrocortisone*
	Ointments, creams and pastes prepared by dilution with standard or proprietary ointments, creams or pastes	Diluted Betnovate ointment (ex pack size) 1/3*
No. or quantity dispensed	When prescribing is given by 'period of treatment', i.e. no. of days treatment ⑦	Terfenidine Tabs 60 mg, i.b.d., 1/12 (Endorse 56 Triludan, ex 60, or 56/60 Triludan)
Aseptically dispensed	Unit dose forms Non-unit dose forms	Some injections Some eye drops
Extemporaneous sterilization	Liquids, solids, semi-solids	Products requiring sterilization with a BP sterilization process, prior to issue
(For community pharmacies have adequate facilities for these processes)		

— either as exact amount ordered by doctor
— or to the closest number in complete strips

e.g. Tenormin 100 ordered.
　Pharmacist can supply:

either 100 tablets
or 7 × 14 tablets

　If unendorsed, the prescription will be priced on the basis of complete calendar strips supplied.

Out-of-pocket expenses

Occasionally, expenses (such as telephone, postage) are incurred in obtaining a medicine for an NHS prescription, and a claim can be made for these expenses, e.g. where specialized surgical appliances, which are not kept by local wholesalers, and which do not appear with a price in the Drug Tariff, have to be ordered direct from the manufacturer. Before making such a claim (and endorsing appropriately) the pharmacist should note:

　1. This does *not* apply to appliances and dressings with a price in the Drug Tariff, but does apply to oxygen and equipment (a special form is used for delivery of oxygen and equipment).
　2. The claim must be over a set minimum. The first part of any claim is not paid.
　3. The item must be specially obtained, not one that is frequently supplied by the pharmacist.
　4. Expenses cannot be claimed for visiting a patient's home to fit appliances, nor for telephone calls to doctors or dentists.

Bulk prescriptions

Certain items may be ordered in bulk for schools and institutions for 20 or more patients. Both the doctor and

Table A2.6　NHS prescription endorsement (Contd)

Endorsement	Where used	Example
Measured and fitted	Elastic hosiery, requiring measurement	Thigh stockings
	Trusses, requiring measurement	Spring truss
Pack size, broken bulk[†], out-of-pocket expenses[†] ([†]details in separate	Drug Tariff Category C products	Cimetidine tabs 200 mg, 120 (endorse Tagament 120/100) Hydroxycobalamine Injection BP, 10 (250 μg/ml) (endorse 2h × OP (5) Neocytamen)
Number of extra container supplied	If a liquid preparation has stability of less than 14 days, and more than 14 days supply is ordered	Merbentyl syrup 2.5 ml q.d.s. mitte 200 ml. (This involves mixing Merbentyl syrup (50%) with Syrup BP (50%))
	Claim in the example for TWO containers of 200 ml 50% Merbentyl Syrup	Diluted syrups usually only keep 14 days–20 days supply has been ordered Thus endorse — 2 × 200 ml supplied Extemp. prep. 200 ml Merbentyl Syrup (ex 500 ml) + Syrup BP 200 ml
CD or /CD/ (preferably in red)	Where the prescription is for a Controlled Drug	MST Continus Tablets, 10 mg Dexedrine Tablets
Time, and date of dispensing and if pharmacist is resident or non-resident at pharmacy	Prescriptions marked URGENT by prescriber or marked DISPENSED URGENTLY by pharmacist, and signed by the patient. They are dispensed at times when the pharmacy is not normally open, e.g. Bank holidays, or after 11 p.m.	Pharmacist is called out, often at request of prescriber, police, or hospital to dispense 'out of hours'. 'Urgent' fee is paid per form, not per item

(Where a pharmacy is opened at the request of the police to dispense an urgent prescription, and the patient does not turn up, urgent fees may still be claimed by submitting a written statement, verified by the police or hospital)

(*Note*: The materials used and the amounts should be endorsed on the form)

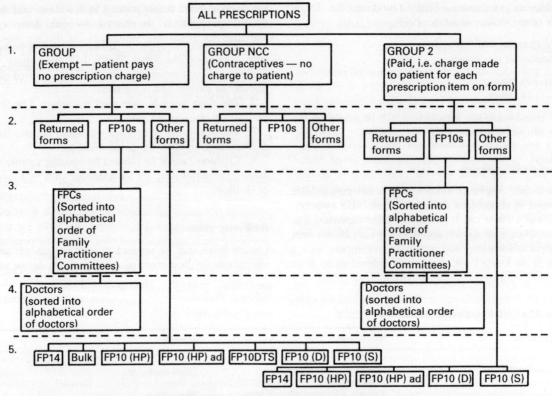

Fig. A2.2 Sorting of NHS prescriptions

the institution must be on the FPC list. The prescription is written on a standard FP10 form and states the name of the institution and number of patients in place of the patient's name. There is no prescription charge and payment will not be made if non-BNF medicines, Controlled Drugs, appliances or dressings are supplied. A container charge may be made. The prescription is endorsed 'bulk prescription' on the back of the form and sorted into Group 1 (Fig. A2.2).

Prescription sorting

After dispensing, stamping, dating and endorsement the prescriptions are filed, and at the end of each month sorted, packed and sent to the Processing Division as soon as possible. Packing must be done with care and a summary form of the number of prescriptions in each category (Form FP34(A)) is included. Details of the prescription sorting procedure are shown diagramatically in Figure A2.2.

Group NCC in Figure A2.2 contains FP10s for contraceptives only. Where an FP10 for a contraceptive also contains other items (e.g. paid items, Group 2) they are included in the other Groups as appropriate. If included

in Group 2, the contraceptive is counted as a 'no charge' item. Prescriptions for oxygen, hosiery, trusses and ostomy appliances are not sorted in a particular manner but are included with the appropriate Group. If the number of FP10s per doctor is 20 or less they may all be bundled together and put at the front of the FPC section.

Limitations for NHS prescribers

Appliances, dressings, etc.

The prescribing of the following items on NHS prescription is limited to those items listed in the current Drug Tariff: appliances, dressings, stoma appliances and accessories, urine drainage equipment, trusses, chemical and diagnostic reagents, oxygen therapy equipment.

Payment will not be made to the pharmacist for other items ordered and supplied.

Dental prescriptions (FP14)

Drugs that may be prescribed by dentists on NHS prescription are limited to those listed in the Dental

Practitioners Formulary (DPF) found in the Drug Tariff (Part XVII) and in the BNF

Schedule 3A (the 'Black List')

Drugs and other substances that may not be prescribed on NHS forms are listed in Part XVIIIA of the Drug Tariff. Drugs not allowed include some substances from the following groups: analgesics for mild to moderate pain, antacids, cough and cold remedies, laxatives, tonics and bitters, vitamins and benzodiazepine tranquillizers. Some products that are black listed under their proprietary name may be prescribed by generic name or by a British Approved Name. The proprietary product may then be supplied if this is the only preparation on the market or if the price does not exceed the tariff price. For guidance, disallowed products are marked NHS in the BNF.

Borderline substances

In certain conditions some foods and toiletries are considered to have the characteristics of drugs and may be prescribed on NHS prescription. The conditions and associated products so considered by the Advisory Committee for Borderline Substances (ACBS) are listed in Part XV of the Drug Tariff. The pharmacist will generally receive payment if these items are dispensed although the prescriber should endorse the form ACBS to avoid further investigation.

Facts and figures (from Pharmaceutical Services Negotiating Committee 1988)

Some 70% of the turnover of the average community pharmacist is derived from NHS dispensing. Over 350 million prescriptions are dispensed annually in England and Wales. The pharmacist charges the NHS for the cost of the medicine prescribed plus a fee for dispensing together with 5% of the drug cost (the on-cost)

Further information may be obtained from the Pharmaceutical Services Negotiating Committee, the National Pharmaceutical Association and the Prescription Pricing Authority.

REFERENCES

British National Formulary 1988 16th edn. British Medical Association and Royal Pharmaceutical Society of Great Britain, London (update twice yearly)
Drug Tariff current edition HMSO, London (updated monthly)

NPA Guide to the Drug Tariff 1987/88 National Pharmaceutical Association, St Albans
Pharmaceutical Services Negotiating Committee 1988 Pharmacy facts and figures, an essential guide to pharmacists' statistics. Pharmaceutical Services Negotiating Committee, Aylesbury

Appendix 3
Medical abbreviations

D. M. Collett

Introduction

In order to practice the clinical aspects of pharmacy the student must become familiar with the terminology of the physician. It is beyond the scope of this book to include definitions of medical terms, the reader is referred to one of the excellent medical dictionaries published. However, the following list of the more commonly used medical abbreviations is included as a guide to the physician's shorthand. It is not intended to be comprehensive and users should be aware of local variations in the use of terms and their abbreviations.

Some commonly used abbreviations for medical terms

Abbreviation	Term
Ab	abortion
Abd	abdomen
ADH	antidiuretic hormone
ADR	adverse drug reaction
A & E	accident and emergency
AFB	acid-fast bacillus
A/G	albumin/globulin ratio
Ag	antigen
ALL	acute lymphocytic leukaemia
AMI	acute myocardial infarction
AML	acute myelogenous leukaemia
A-R	apical-radial pulse
ASCVD	arteriosclerotic cardiovascular disease
AV	arteriovenous, atrioventricular
BaE	barium enema
BBB	bundle branch block, blood–brain barrier
BM	bowel movement
BMR	basal metabolic rate
BNO	bowels not open
BOR	bowels open regularly
BS	bowel sounds, breath sounds, blood sugar

Abbreviation	Term
BUN	blood urea nitrogen
Bx	biopsy
c̄	with
CA	cancer, carcinoma
CAPD	continuous ambulatory peritoneal dialysis
CAT	computer assisted tomogram
CC	chief complaint
CCF	congestive cardiac failure
CCU	coronary care unit
CHD	coronary heart disease
CHF	congestive heart failure
CNS	central nervous system
CO	cardiac output
C/O	complains of
COAD	chronic obstructive airway disease
COLD	chronic obstructive lung disease
COPD	chronic obstructive pulmonary disease
C & S	culture and sensitivity
CSF	cerebrospinal fluid
CSU	catheter specimen of urine
CVA	cerebrovascular accident
CVP	central venous pressure
Cx	cervical, cervix
CXR	chest X-ray
D	diagnosis
D & C	dilation and curettage
DD	differential diagnosis
DH	drug history
DM	diabetes mellitus
DNA	did not attend (outpatient)
DOA	dead on arrival
DOB	date of birth
DOE	dyspnoea on exertion
DTs	delirium tremens
DU	duodenal ulcer
D & V	diarrhoea and vomiting
DVT	deep vein thrombosis
ECG	electrocardiogram
ECT	electroconvulsive therapy

Abbreviation	Term	Abbreviation	Term
EEG	electroencephalogram	MI	mitral incompetence or insufficiency
EMS	early morning specimen	MI	myocardial infarction
ENT	ear, nose and throat	MIC	minimum inhibitory concentration
ESR	erythrocyte sedimentation rate	MS	mitral stenosis, multiple sclerosis
EUA	examination under anaesthetic	MSU	mid-stream urine specimen
FB	finger breadths, foreign body	N	normal
FBC	full blood count	NAD	nothing abnormal detected
FBS	fasting blood sugar	NBM	nil by mouth
FEV$_1$	forced expiratory volume in 1 second	NG	nasogastric
FFA	free fatty acids	NPN	non-protein nitrogen
FH	family history	NPO	nothing by mouth (non-peroral)
FROM	full range of movement	NS	nervous system
FUO	fever of unknown origin	NSR	normal sinus rhythm
FVC	forced vital capacity	N & V	nausea and vomiting
Fx	fracture	^{0}BS	absence of bowel sounds
GFR	glomerular filtration rate	o	absent
GI	gastrointestinal	O	oedema
GIT	gastrointestinal tract	O/A	on admission
GTT	glucose tolerance test	Obs-Gyn	obstetrics and gynaecology
GU	genitourinary	O/E	on examination
gyn	gynaecology	OOB	out of bed
Hb, Hgb	haemoglobin	OP	outpatient
Hct	haematocrit	OPD	outpatients department
HCVD	hypertensive cardiovascular disease	Para	number of pregnancies
H & P	history and physical	PBI	protein-bound iodine
HPI	history of present illness	PCV	packed cell volume
HTVD	hypertensive vascular disease	PDQ	at once
ICM	intracostal margin	PE	physical examination, pulmonary embolism
ICS	intercostal space		
ICU	intensive care unit	PERRLA	pupils equal, round, reactive to light and accommodation
ID	intradermal, initial dose		
Ig	immunoglobulin	PF(R)	peak flow (rate)
IHD .	ischaemic heart disease	PKU	phenylketonuria
IM	intramuscular	PM	post mortem
INR	International Normalized Ratio (prothrombin time)	PMH	past medical history
		PMT	premenstrual tension
IP	intraperitoneal, inpatient	PND	paroxysmal nocturnal dyspnoea
IPPB	intermittent positive pressure breathing	PO	oral (peroral)
IUD	intrauterine device	PR	rectal (per rectum)
IV	intravenous	Pt	patient
IVP	intravenous pyelogram	PT	prothrombin time
J	jaundice	PTA	prior to admission
JVP	jugular venous pulse	PUO	pyrexia of unknown origin
LA	local anaesthetic	PV	per vagina
LD	lethal dose	PVC	premature ventricular contraction
LE	lupus erythematosus	(R)	right
LVF	left ventricular failure	RA	right atrium, rheumatoid arthritis
LVH	left ventricular hypertrophy	RBC	red blood cells
MCH	mean corpuscular haemoglobin	RBS	random blood sugar
MCHC	mean corpuscular haemoglobin concentration	RCC	red cell count
		RF	rheumatoid factor
MCV	mean corpuscular volume	RHD	rheumatic heart disease

Abbreviation	Term
Rh	rhesus factor
ROS	review of symptoms
RS	respiratory system
s̄	without
S1	first heart sound
S2	second heart sound
SA	sino-atrial
SB	seen by, short of breath
SBE	shortage of breath on exertion
SBE	subacute bacterial endocarditis
SC	subcutaneous
SGOT	serum glutamic oxaloacetic transaminase
SGPT	serum glutamic pyruvic transaminase
SH	social history, serum hepatitis
SL	sublingual
SLE	systemic lupus erythematosus
SOA	swelling of ankles
SOB	shortness of breath
SOS	swelling of sacrum
STD	sexually transmitted disease
Sx	symptoms
T	temperature
T3	tri-odothyronine
T4	thyroxine

Abbreviation	Term
T & A	tonsillectomy and adenoidectomy
TB	tuberculosis
TBA	to be arranged or to be administered
TIA	transient ischaemic attack
TIBC	total iron binding capacity
TKVO	to keep vein open
TLC	total lung capacity
TPN	total parenteral nutrition
TPR	temperature, pulse, respiration
TTO	to take out (home)
Tx	treatment
UA	uric acid, urinalysis
UC	ulcerative colitis
U & E	urea and electrolytes
UTI	urinary tract infection
UR(T)I	upper respiratory (tract) infection
VD	venereal disease
VP	venous pressure
VS	vital signs
VT	ventricular tachycardia
WBC	white blood cell
WBS	whole body scan
WNL	within normal limits
WR	Wassermann reaction
XR	X-ray

BIBLIOGRAPHY

Harris J M 1983 Medical abbreviations. Brighton Polytechnic United Kingdom Clinical Pharmacy Association Brighton Polytechnic
Roper N 1987 Pocket medical dictionary, 15th edn.

Churchill Livingstone, Edinburgh
Steen E B 1984 Abbreviations used in medicine, 5th edn. Baillière Tindall, London

Appendix 4
Latin terms and abbreviations

D. M. Collett

Introduction

Prescriptions written in the UK should be written in English and the use of Latin is strongly discouraged. However, the use of some Latin terms persists and abbreviations are often used, especially to indicate the frequency of dosing.

The following lists include terms which may be encountered in current practice. For more comprehensive lists see previous editions of this book (Carter 1975) and the Pharmaceutical Handbook (Wade 1980).

Dosage forms

Latin name	Abbreviation	English name
Auristillae	aurist.	ear drops
Capsula	caps.	capsule
Cataplasma	cataplasm.	poultice
Collunarium	collun.	nosewash
Collutorium	collut.	mouthwash
Collyrium	collyr.	eye lotion
Cremor	crem.	cream
Guttae	gtt.	drops
Haustus	ht.	draught
Liquor	liq.	solution
Lotio	lot.	lotion
Mistura	mist.	mixture
Naristillae	narist.	nose drops
Nebula	neb.	spray solution
Oculentum	oculent.	eye ointment
Pasta	past.	paste
Pigmentum	pig.	paint
Pulvis	pulv.	powder
Pulvis conspersus	pulv. consp.	dusting powder
Trochiscus	troch.	lozenge
Unguentum	ung.	ointment
Vapor	vap.	inhalation
Vitrella	vitrell.	glass capsule (crushable)

Terms used in prescriptions

Latin	Abbreviation	English
ante cibum	a.c.	before food
ante meridiem	a.m.	before noon
ana	aa.	of each
ad	ad.	to
ad libitum	ad lib.	as much as desired
alternus	alt.	alternate
ante	ante	before
applicandus	applic.	to be applied
aqua	aq.	water
bis	b.	twice
bis die	b.d.	twice daily
bis in die	b.i.d.	twice daily
calidus	calid.	warm
cibus	cib.	food
compositus	co.	compound
concentratus	conc.	concentrated
cum	c.	with
dies	d.	a day
destillatus	dest.	distilled
dilutus	dil.	diluted
duplex	dup.	double
ex aqua	ex.aq.	in water
fiat	ft.	let it be made
fortis	fort.	strong
hora	h.	at the hour of
hora somni	h.s.	at bedtime
inter cibos	i.c.	between meals
inter	int.	between
mane	m.	in the morning
more dicto	m.d.	as directed
more dicto utendus	m.d.u.	to be used as directed
mitte	mitt.	send
nocte	n.	at night
nocte et mane	n.m.	night and morning
nocte maneque	n.p.	the proper name
nomen proprium	n.et m.	night and morning

455

Latin	Abbreviation	English
nocte	noct.	at night
omnibus alternis horis	o.alt.hor	every other hour
omni die	o.d.	every day
omni mane	o.m.	every morning
omni nocte	o.n.	every night
parti affectae	p.a.	to the affected part
parti affectae applicandus	part. affect.	to the affected part
partes aequales	p.aeq.	equal parts
post cibum	p.c.	after food
post meridiem	p.m.	afternoon
partes	pp.	parts
pro re nata	p.r.n.	when required
parti dolenti	part. dolent.	to the painful part
quater die	q.d.	four times daily
quater die sumendus	q.d.s.	to be taken four times daily
quater in die	q.i.d.	four times daily
quaque	qq.	every
quaque hora	qq.h.	every hour
quarta quaque hora	q.qq.h.	every fourth hour
	q.q.h.	every fourth hour

Latin	Abbreviation	English
quantum sufficiat	q.s.	sufficient
recipe	R	take
secundum artem	sec. art.	with pharmaceutical skill
semisse	ss.	half
si opus sit	s.o.s.	if necessary
signa	sig.	label
statim	stat.	immediately
sumendus	sum.	to be taken
ter	t.	thrice
ter de die	t.d.d.	three times daily
ter die sumendus	t.d.s.	to be taken three times daily
ter in die	t.i.d.	three times daily
tussis	tuss.	a cough
tussi urgente	tuss. urg.	when the cough troubles
ut antea	u.a.	as before
ut dictum	ut. dict.	as directed
ut directum	ut. direct.	as directed
utendus	utend.	to be used

Numerals

The *cardinals* in Table A4.1 refer to number and thus are translated, one, two, three, etc.

The *ordinals* refer to position and thus are translated first, second, third, etc.

The *adverbs* qualify verbs and thus are translated once, twice, three times, etc.

Table A4.1 Roman numerals: Roman symbol and corresponding Latin names for the cardinal and ordinal numbers and their adverbs.

Arabic number	Roman symbol	Cardinals	Ordinals	Adverbs
1	I	unus	primus, -a, -um	semel (once)
2	II	duo	secondus or alter	bis (twice)
3	III	tres, tria(n.)	tertius	ter (three times)
4	IV	quattuor	quartus	quater (four times)
5	V	quinque	quintus	quinquies
6	VI	sex	sextus	sexies
7	VII	septem	septimus	septies
8	VIII	octo	octavus	octies
9	IX	novem	nonus	novies
10	X	decem	decimus	decies
11	XI	undecim	undecimus	undecies
12	XII	duodecim	duodecimus	duodecies
14	XIV	quattuordecim	quartis decimus	quattuor-decies
15	XV	quindecim	quintus decimus	quindecies
20	XX	viginti	vicesimus	vicies
50	L	quinquaginta	quinquagesimus	quinquagies
100	C	centum	centesimus	centies

REFERENCES

Carter S 1975 Dispensing for pharmaceutical students 13th edn. Pitman Medical, London

Wade A 1980 Pharmaceutical Handbook 19th edn. Pharmaceutical Press, London

Appendix 5
Qualifications of practitioners

D. M. Collett

Introduction

The practising pharmacist receives prescriptions, requisitions and requests for the supply of medicines from a number of different types of medical practitioner. Before fulfilling such requests the pharmacist must be satisfied that the prescriber or purchaser is a genuine practitioner and legally entitled to prescribe or purchase the medicinal product requested. The restrictions on the sale and supply of medicinal products to various practitioners are summarized in Appendix 1. It is important to note that the definition of a 'practitioner' with respect to the Medicines Act (1968) differs from that of the Spirits Regulations (1983).

The various health-care professions maintain national registers of members qualified and entitled to practice and these are described briefly below.

A list of commonly encountered abbreviations for qualifications of practitioners follows. Note that the presence of 'qualifications' on a prescription or requisition does not give legal validity to the document unless the pharmacist is satisfied that the practitioner is duly registered and that the signature is genuine.

Chiropody

State registered chiropodists in the UK are qualified Members or Fellows of The Society of Chiropodists.

Dentistry

Dentists practising in the UK must be in the Dentist's Register maintained by the General Dental Council. Qualifications recognized for registration include Bachelor or Master of Dental Surgery and Licentiate in Dental Surgery.

Medicine

Doctors who practise as medical practitioners in the UK must be registered with the General Medical Council. Qualifications recognized for registration include: the degrees of Bachelor of Medicine and Bachelor of Surgery, Doctor of Medicine and Master of Surgery or Licentiate of the Royal College of Physicians of London and Member of the Royal College of Surgeons of England.

Nursing

The UK Central Council for Nursing maintains a professional register of various categories of enrolled or qualified general or specialist nurses.

Ophthalmics

Members or Fellows of the British College of Ophthalmic Opticians with a diploma in ophthalmic optics (optometrists) are registered by the General Optical Council.

Previous examining bodies were the British Optical Association and The Worshipful Company of Spectacle Makers.

Pharmacy

Pharmacists practising in the UK must be registered as Members or Fellows of the Royal Pharmaceutical Society of Great Britain. The degrees of Bachelor of Pharmacy or Bachelor of Science (Pharmacy) fulfil the academic qualifications necessary for preregistration training.

Veterinary medicine

Practising veterinary surgeons must be Members or Fellows of the Royal College of Veterinary Surgeons. A supplementary register of veterinary practitioners with no academic qualification but qualified to practice by experience was closed in 1966.

Abbreviations of commonly encountered qualifications

BCh	Bachelor of Surgery
BChir	Bachelor of Surgery
BChD	Bachelor of Dental Surgery
BDS	Bachelor of Dental Surgery
BM	Bachelor of Medicine
BPharm	Bachelor of Pharmacy
BS	Bachelor of Surgery
BSc(Pharm)	Bachelor of Science (Pharmacy)
ChB	Bachelor of Surgery
ChD	Doctor of Surgery
CM	Master in Surgery
ChM	Master in Surgery
DOpt	Diploma in Ophthalmic Optics
EN	Enrolled Nurse
EN(G)	Enrolled Nurse (General)
EN(M)	Enrolled Nurse (Mental)
EN(MH)	Enrolled Nurse (Mental Handicap)
FBCO	Fellow of the British College of Ophthalmic Opticians (Optometrists)
FBOA	Fellow of the British Optical Association
FChS	Fellow of the Society of Chiropodists
FRCP	Fellow of the Royal College of Physicians
FRCS	Fellow of the Royal College of Surgeons
FRCVS	Fellow of the Royal College of Veterinary Surgeons
FRPharmS (FPS)	Fellow of the Royal Pharmaceutical Society of Great Britain
FSMC	Fellow of the Worshipful Company of Spectacle Makers
LDS	Licentiate in Dental Surgery
LRCP	Licentiate of the Royal College of Physicians
LRCS	Licentiate of the Royal College of Surgeons
MB	Bachelor of Medicine
MBCO	Member of the British College of Ophthalmic Opticians (Optometrists)
MC	Master of Surgery
MCh	Master of Surgery
MChD	Master of Dental Surgery
MCPS	Member of the College of Physicians and Surgeons
MD	Doctor of Medicine
MDS	Master of Dental Surgery
MRCP	Member of the Royal College of Physicians
MRCS	Member of the Royal College of Surgeons
MRCVS	Member of the Royal College of Veterinary Surgeons
MRPharmS (MPS)	Member of the Royal Pharmaceutical Society of Great Britain
PhC	Pharmaceutical Chemist
RGN	Registered General Nurse
RM	Registered Midwife
RMN	Registered Mental Nurse
RNMH	Registered Nurse for the Mentally Handicapped
RSCN	Registered Sick Childrens Nurse
SCM	State Certified Midwife
SEN	State Enrolled Nurse
SRN	State Registered Nurse

BIBLIOGRAPHY

British Qualifications 1988 18th edn. Kogan Page, London
Roper N (ed) 1987 Pocket medical dictionary, 15th edn.
  Churchill Livingstone, Edinburgh

Appendix 6
The imperial system of weights and measures

D. M. Collett

The imperial system

The imperal system of weights and measures is no longer used in pharmacy and medicine in the UK but is still used for some trade and domestic purposes.

Measures of mass (weight)

Avoirdupois weights

1 pound (avoirdupois) (lb) is the imperial pound (as defined in the UK Weights and Measures Act, 1963). Other measures of mass are derived from the imperial standard pound:

— 1/16th part of imperial standard lb is 1 ounce (oz) (avoirdupois).
— 1/7000th part of imperial standard lb is 1 grain (gr).
— 437.5 grains = 1 ounce avoirdupois.

Apothecaries or troy weights

These are based on the grain (as defined above) and are as follows:

20	grains	form	1 scruple
60	grains	form	1 drachm
480	grains	form	1 apothecaries (or Troy) ounce
12 apothecaries (or troy) ounces	form		1 apothecaries (or Troy) pound

It should be noted that the grain is the same in both avoirdupois and apothecaries systems. Care should be taken to avoid confusing the avoirdupois ounce (conventionally designated ounce or oz) with the apothecaries ounce (oz troy).

Measures of mass and their symbols are summarized in Table A6.1.

Table A6.1 Measures of mass (weight)

Latin name	Symbol	English name	Equivalent (grains)
Granum	gr	grain	1
Scrupulus	Э	scruple	20
Drachma	ℨ	drachm	60
Uncia	oz	ounce (Avoirdupois)	437.5
Uncia	℥	ounce (Troy or Apothecaries)	480
Libra	lb	pound (Troy or Apothecaries)	5760
Libra	lb	pound (Avoirdupois)	7000

Measures of capacity (volume)

1 gallon (gal) is defined in the UK under the Units of Measurement Regulations 1976.

Other measures of capacity are derived from the gallon:

— 1/8th part of 1 gallon is 1 pint.
— 1/160th part of 1 gallon is 1 fluid ounce.
— 1/8th part of 1 fluid ounce is 1 fluid drachm.
— 1/60th part of 1 fluid drachm is 1 minim.

Measures of capacity and their symbols are summarized in Table A6.2.

Table A6.2 Measures of capacity (volume)

Latin name	Symbol	English name	Equivalent
Minimum	m	minim	
Gutta	gtt	drop	
Fluidrachma	ℨ	fl. drachm	60 minims
Fluiduncia	℥	fl. ounce	8 fl. drachms
Octarius	O	pint	20 fl. ounces
Congius	C	gallon	8 pints

Relation of weight to capacity (measured at a temperature of 62°F (16.7°C)

— 1 minim is the volume of 0.91146 grain of water.
— 1 fluid drachm is the volume of 54.688 grains of water.
— 1 fluid ounce is the volume of 437.5 grains of water or 1 ounce (avoirdupois).
— 109.71 (110) minims is the volume of 100 grains of water.

Metric equivalents of imperial quantities

In order to prepare imperial quantities of a preparation from a metric formula the following approximate equivalents may be used:

Required	Prepare
1 fluid ounce	30 ml
3 fluid ounces	100 ml
4 fluid ounces	120 ml
6 fluid ounces	200 ml
8 fluid ounces	240 ml
1 ounce (avoirdupois)	30 g
1 ounce (troy)	31 g

Preparation of percentage solutions

General formula for 1% weight in volume (w/v) solution:

Solid	1 oz (avoir)	4.375 grains	1 grain
Solvent to produce	100 fl. oz.	1 fl. oz.	110 minims

General formula for 1% volume in volume (v/v) solution:

Liquid	1 fl. oz	4.8 minims	1 minim
Solvent to produce	100 fl. oz	1 fl. oz	100 minims

Further types of calculation using the imperial system together with methods for converting from imperial to metric units may be found in Carter (1975).

REFERENCE

Carter S 1975 Dispensing for pharmaceutical students, 13th edn. Pitman Medical, London

Appendix 7
Homeopathic preparations

D. M. Collett

Homeopathy is a system of medicine that differs significantly from the orthodox medicine currently practised in the UK. This chapter outlines the types of preparation which may be prescribed by the homeopathic physician or recommended as 'counter-prescribed' homeopathic remedies.

In orthodox medicine, drugs are selected to reverse identified pathological changes or to produce effects that oppose unwanted symptoms. In homeopathy drugs are selected by observing their effects in healthy volunteers, a process known as 'proving'. Drugs producing a particular group of symptoms in the healthy 'provers' may then be used to treat a patient presenting with a similar group of symptoms. The word homeopathy (similar suffering) is descriptive of this underlying philosophy, 'let likes be cured by likes'.

In orthodox pharmacology the effects of a drug are generally related to the concentration of drug molecules at its site(s) of action. For most drugs, increasing the dose within a particular range increases both the therapeutically desirable effects and also the occurrence of unwanted adverse effects with ultimate toxicity.

In homeopathy the curative action of a drug is considered to be enhanced by dilution in a defined manner. Obviously any harmful effects are also decreased by dilution.

Homeopathic compounding

Solutions

Homeopathic medicines may be prepared from materials of vegetable, animal or mineral origin. The active principles are, when possible, dissolved in water, ethanol, or in a mixture of the two. For drugs of vegetable origin, the active ingredients may be extracted by pressing juicy plants, by maceration or by percolation of dry materials. The resulting solution containing the greatest concentration of the vegetable drug used in homeopathy is known as the 'mother tincture'. It is from this mother tincture

that liquid attenuations or dilutions are prepared. Mother tinctures of materials of animal origin such as snake venom and solutions of chemical materials may also be prepared.

Liquid attenuations (dilutions)

The mother tincture (symbol ϕ) is diluted with distilled water or ethanol in ten-fold or 100-fold stages to prepare what are described as 'potencies'. At each stage of the dilution process very vigorous mixing is applied, a procedure known as 'succussion'. This is believed to be an essential part of the process and is believed to involve some energy release or transfer. The series of decimal and centesimal potencies are described in Table A7.1.

Potencies on the centesimal scale are most common and 30c, 200c and 1000c (1M) are frequently used. From the homeopathic point of view the greater the

Table A7.1 Homeopathic dilutions or potencies

Decimal potencies	
First decimal potency (1x)	1 part of mother tincture with 9 parts diluent (1/10)
Second decimal potency (2x)	1 part of 1x with 9 parts of diluent (1/100)
Third decimal potency (3x)	1 part of 2x with 9 parts of diluent (1/1000)
Sixth decimal potency (6x)	1 part of 5x with 9 parts of diluent (1/1 000 000 ≡ 1M)
Centesimal potencies	
First centesimal potency (1c)	1 part of mother tincture with 99 parts of diluent (1/100)
Second centesimal potency (2c)	1 part of 1c with 99 parts of diluent (1/10 000)
Third centesimal potency (3c)	1 part of 2c with 99 parts of diluent (1/1 000 000 ≡ 1M)

461

degree of dilution the greater the potency of the resulting solution, although it is acknowledged that few if any molecules of the original substance may be present in these preparations.

Triturations

Since it is not possible to make a mother tincture of an insoluble substance an alternative method of 'potentization' is used. Triturations are prepared by grinding and mixing the insoluble drug (for at least an hour) with an inert powder, such as sugar of milk (lactose), in order to produce an intimate and uniform mixture. One part of the insoluble drug mixed with 99 parts of diluent produces a first centesimal (1c) potency in solid form. Further 100-fold dilutions to the third centesimal (3c) may be made. At this stage the insoluble drug is considered to be in a 'colloidal' state and capable of producing a stable homogeneous dispersion.

Liquid attenuations may then be prepared from the triturations by dissolving 1 gram of the 3c (equivalent to 6x) trituration in 10 ml of 95% ethanol to give a 7x product. Further liquid potencies are then prepared by serial dilution of this solution.

Homeopathic dosage forms

Solid dosage forms such as tablets, granules or powders are prepared from an inert substance such as sugar of milk (lactose) and then impregnated with a liquid tincture of prescribed potency so that they then take on its medicinal properties. These dosage forms are considered to be extremely delicate and should receive the minimum amount of handling.

Homeopathic prescriptions

Homeopathic preparations are described with the latin name of the drug. The pharmacist wishing to undertake dispensing of these preparations will therefore require access to a homeopathic pharmacopoeia or Materia Medica. Stocks of commonly used preparations may be purchased from specialist suppliers.

Abbreviations which are used on homeopathic prescriptions include those shown below:

φ or TM   for basic tinctures.
x or D or Dec.   for decimals (preceded by the number of the dilution).
c or cH   for centesimals (preceded by the number of the dilution). Because the potencies prepared on the centesimal scale are the most commonly prescribed, the letters 'c' or 'cH' are often omitted, thus Bryonia 3 is interpreted as the third centesimal potency of the substance Bryonia.
S.L. Saccharum Lactis   sugar of milk (lactose).

Homeopathic counter-prescribing

The system of homeopathic medicine is based on close observation of the patient's symptoms including behavioural patterns and physical type. The treatment offered is then specific to a group of symptoms in a particular patient rather than to a named disease or even to a general group of symptoms. Many patients find such homeopathic treatment beneficial and because of the low concentrations of drugs prescribed toxicity is rare. It is not likely however, that a self-selected purchase of a homeopathic product by a patient nor the recommendation of such a product by a non-initiated pharmacist would produce the benefit which might be derived from a full consultation with a homeopathic practitioner.

Pharmacists supplying homeopathic remedies should make the nature of the product clear to any potential purchaser and as with any sold or counter-prescribed orthodox medicine, advise the seeking of medical advice for persistent symptoms.

BIBLIOGRAPHY

Mitchell G R 1975 Homeopathy, the first authoritative study of its place in medicine today. W. H. Allen, London
The Pharmacist and Homeopathic Medicines 1981 The

British Homeopathic Association, London
Wade A 1980 Pharmaceutical handbook, 19th edn. Pharmaceutical Press, London

Appendix 8
Sources of information for compounding and dispensing

D. M. Collett

Competency in the use of information sources is an essential part of the practice of pharmacy. The following account summarizes the type of information to be found in the major pharmaceutical publications.

Students who are new to pharmacy are advised to become familiar with these different sources so that required information of various types can be readily retrieved.

Pharmacopoeias

These are officially published lists of drugs with directions for uses and standards of purity.

British Pharmacopoeia (BP)

The BP is published by HMSO Books (London) on the recommendation of the Medicines Commission pursuant to the Medicines Act, 1968. It is updated by addenda when necessary. This is primarily a book of standards of purity and strength for medical substances, products, dressings, etc., together with 'official' assays and tests. A formulary of dosage forms is included. Some 'official' preparations are defined in terms only of the principal ingredients while others have the full formula defined and in some cases the method of manufacture. Products suitable for extemporaneous dispensing are defined in terms of a full formula and often include the method of preparation. Information on storage, stability and labelling is also included.

There is also a British Pharmacopoeia (Veterinary).

British Pharmaceutical Codex (BPC) 1973

This provides a source of standards for some extemporaneous preparations not included in the BP and is now incorporated into the Pharmaceutical Codex.

Pharmaceutical Codex (PC) 1979

The PC is intended to be an encyclopaedia of drug information and includes entries on diseases and conditions, aspects of pharmaceutics, surgical dressings and veterinary information as well as the formulae for medicines.

European Pharmacopoeia (EP)

This is prepared under the auspices of the Council of Europe and was created to permit free circulation of drugs within the European Community. Its standards may take precedence over those of the BP. Edited monographs of the EP are reproduced in the current BP and certain official procedures, e.g. tests for pyrogens, are performed according to EP methods.

International pharmacopoeia

This is a publication of the World Health Organization providing recommended standards for international use.

United States Pharmacopeia (USP) and National Formulary (NF)

The official standard reference of the USA. There is a companion volume of dispensing information (USPDI).

Reference will be found in the Extra Pharmacopoeia (see below) to a number of other national pharmacopoeias.

Martindale: The Extra Pharmacopoeia

An authorative reference book on drugs and medicines in current use throughout the world. Martindale

463

provides detailed information on nomenclature, physical and pharmaceutical properties, adverse effects, actions and uses, etc. It is also available as an 'on-line' database and is accessible via the Prestel telephone system.

Pharmaceutical Handbook

This is a companion volume to the Extra Pharmacopoeia. It is described as a reference manual for practitioners and students of pharmacy and the allied professions.

The Handbook is a mine of useful information on such diverse subjects as 'The preparation and supply of medicines', 'Methods of sterilization', 'Bites and stings', 'Removal of stains', 'Computers and their applications' and 'Nomenclature of organic compounds'. The section containing miscellaneous data including catheter gauges, paper sizes, desirable body weights and calculation of body surface areas provides useful and readily accessible data relevant to pharmacy.

British National Formulary (BNF)

A joint publication of the British Medical Association and Royal Pharmaceutical Society of Great Britain (updated twice yearly).

The BNF is intended to be a pocket book for rapid reference and as such is an invaluable initial information source.

General guidance for prescribers is provided together with the special requirements of particular groups of patient, e.g. the very young, the elderly, pregnant women and patients with renal or hepatic failure.

The main text contains notes on drugs and preparations classified under the diseases and conditions that they are used to treat. Information on the indications, contraindications, cautions, side-effects and doses are given for each drug listed. An indication of the legal category and any restrictions on prescribing of particular products, e.g. not NHS or hospital only, is also given.

The BNF includes a formulary for commonly used 'official' extemporaneous preparations and information on drug interactions, cautionary and advisory labels, etc. for the pharmacist.

Proprietary medicines

ABPI Data Sheet Compendium (updated annually)

This contains copies of the data sheets of the manufactured products of participating companies. Data sheets are prepared in accordance with the Medicines (Data Sheet) Regulations 1972 for most proprietary medicines and include information on the presentation, uses, dosage and administration, contraindications and warnings, pharmaceutical precautions, legal category and package quantities. This is an essential source of information on manufactured medicines.

There is a companion volume for veterinary products.

Monthly Index of Medical Specialities (MIMS)

MIMS is designed as a reference and prescribing guide for doctors in general practice and lists proprietary preparations that can be prescribed or recommended. It is a useful source of up-to-date information on manufactured medicines.

Children's doses

Special care is required in the calculation of doses suitable for young children and specialist information is not always readily available in general texts. The following are recommended information sources for paediatric medicines.

Alder Hey Book of Children's Doses (ABCD)

This lists doses of drugs in common paediatric use.

The Paediatric Vade Mecum

This provides a range of paediatric data including guidance for prescribers.

Regulations and restrictions

Compliance with the following publications is essential for good pharmaceutical practice.

Medicines, Ethics and Practice — A Guide for Pharmacists (updated twice yearly)

A practical guide to the legal classification of medicinal products, particularly for the pharmacist in the community and incorporating the 'Code of Ethics' and the 'Guide to Good Dispensing Practice'.

Medicines and Poisons Guide (1984)

This has been mostly replaced by the above publication. At the time of writing it provides a source of information on veterinary products and non-medicinal poisons.

The Guide to Good Pharmaceutical Manufacturing Practice

This lists the principles of good practice applicable to the compounding and manufacture of medicinal products.

NHS dispensing

The Drug Tariff (HMSO) (updated monthly)

This lists the drugs, appliances and reagents that may be supplied to NHS patients in the community and contains information of fees for the provision of pharmaceutical services.

The Chemist and Druggist Directory

This is a compact source of general information for pharmacists including a tablet and capsule identification guide and lists of names and addresses of suppliers, pharmaceutical organizations, hospital pharmacists and retail and wholesale outlets. There is also a useful summary of the law for pharmaceutical retailers.

PINS (Pharmacy Information and News Service)

This is a facility available from the Royal Pharmaceutical Society and may be accessed by pharmacists with suitable computing equipment.

REFERENCES

ABPI Data Sheet Compendium current edition. Datapharm Publications, London (updated annually)

Alder Hey Book of Children's doses 1982 4th edn. Liverpool Area Health Authority, Liverpool

British National Formulary (current edition) British Medical Association and Royal Pharmaceutical Society of Great Britain, London (updated twice yearly) (use current edition)

British Pharmacopoeia 1980 HMSO, London (and addenda 1982, 1983 and 1986)

British Pharmacopoeia 1988 HMSO, London

Chemist and Druggist Directory current edition. Benn Business Information Services Ltd, Tonbridge, Kent (published annually)

Guide to good pharmaceutical manufacturing practice. Department of Health and Social Security 1983 HMSO, London

Drug Tariff current edition HMSO, London (updated monthly)

European Pharmacopoeia, 2nd edn. First cycle (1980–82), Second cycle (1983–84), Third cycle (1985) Maisonneuve SA, Saint Ruffine, France

Insley J, Wood B (eds) 1986 Paediatric vade mecum, 11th edn. Lloyd-Luke, London

International Pharmacopoeia 1981 vol. 2, Quality specifications, WHO, Geneva

Martindale, see Reynolds J E F

Monthly Index of Medical Specialities (MIMS) Medical Publications Ltd, London

Pearce M E (ed) 1984 Medicines and poisons guide, 4th edn. Pharmaceutical Press, London (with cumulative amendments in the Pharmaceutical Journal)

Pharmaceutical Codex 1979 11th edn (incorporating the British Pharmaceutical Codex) Pharmaceutical Press, London

Reynolds J E F (ed) 1989 Martindale, The Extra Pharmacopoeia, 29th edn. Pharmaceutical Press, London

Royal Pharmaceutical Society of Great Britain current edition

Royal Pharmaceutical Society Code of Ethics (incorporating the Guide to good dispensing practice)

Royal Pharmaceutical Society of Great Britain 1989 Medicines, Ethics and Practice — a guide for pharmacists, no. 1

Royal Pharmaceutical Society of Great Britain, London (updated twice yearly) (use current edition)

United States Pharmacopeia — The National Formulary 1984 (USP XXI–NF XVI)

United States Pharmacopeia Dispensing Information 1986

Wade A (ed) 1980 Pharmaceutical handbook, 19th edn. Pharmaceutical Press, London

Index

Abbreviations
  Latin 455
  Medical 451
ABPI data sheet compendium 464
Absorbent dressings 317
Additives
  Eye drops 258
  Eye ointments 268
  Intravenous 227, 229
  Total parenteral nutrition 252
Adhesive tapes 318
Administration
  Of cytotoxic agents 238
  Of drugs 391
  Total parenteral nutrition 242
Administration sets (i.v. infusions) 227
Adverse drug reactions 413
  Allergic reactions 417
  Classification 415
  Factors affecting 414
  Monitoring 413
  Role of pharmacist 414
Advice to patients 421
Advisory labels 76
Aerosol foams 158
Aerosol inhalations 5, 8
Aerosol sprays 8, 158
Aerosols 157
  Labelling 79
  Patient counselling 157
  see also Pressurized dispensers
Air supply, clean rooms 195
  Pressure gradient 198
Alder Hey Book of Children's Doses 464
Allergic drug reactions 417
Alpha particles 301
Amount of substance, units of 11
Ampholytic surfactants 112
Amphoteric surfactants 112
Ampoules, for parenteral products 218
Anionic surfactants 109
Anticoagulent treatment cards 346
Antioxidants 49, 114
  In ointments 127
  Suppositories 138

Antioxygens 49
Antiseptic 165
  Solutions 92
Apparent volume of distribution 385
Applications 4, 116
  Containers 116
  Labelling 79, 116
  Shelf life 116
Aqueous solutions, sterility testing 291
Aromatic waters 9
Arrhenius equation 47, 230
Aseptic dispensing, operator tests 205
Aseptic production, total parenteral nutrition 250
Aseptic technique 165, 189
  Laminar air flow stations 189
  Operator technique 189
  Personnel 189
  Protective clothing 189
Atmospheric moisture, effect on degradation 49
Autoclave cycle 167
Autoclaves, portable 172
Autoclaving, eye drops 264

Bacterial growth
  Factors affecting 285
  Growth inhibition 287
  Phases 287
Balances 21
Bandages 318
Beta particles 301
Bioburden 165
Biological indicators 168
Blister packs 58
Blood level curves 392
Blood pressure measurement 373
Body temperature measurement 373
Bottles
  Dropper 55
  Medicine 54
British National Formulary 464
British Pharmaceutical Codex 463
British Pharmacopoeia 463
Browne's tubes 168
Buccal route of administration 9
Buffer salts 49

Cachets 4, 147
  Labelling 79
Calculations 13
  Dilutions 13
  Examples 13
  Master formulae 13
  Parts 15
  Percentages 14
  Stock solutions 17
  Triturations 19
Capacity, units of 11
Capsules 4, 152
  Compounding 152
  Formulation 152
  Hard gelatin 152
  Labelling 79, 153
  Shelf life 153
  Soft gelatin 153
Cartons for dispensing 57
Cartridges, for parenteral products 219
Catgut, sterility testing 295
Cationic surfactants 110
Cautionary and Advisory Labels 76
Chelating agents 49
  In gels 128
Chemical degradation 45
  Optical isomerization 46
  Oxidation 45
  Photolysis 46
  Polymerization 46
  Solvolysis 45
  Chemical indicators 168
Chemist and Druggist Directory 464
Child-resistant containers 57, 341
Children's doses 464
Clarification, parenteral products 217
Clean room
  Changing room procedures 201
Design 193
  Environmental control 195
  Premises 193
Operation 193
  Air supply 195
  Cleaning 199
  Contamination 199
  Environmental monitoring 205
  Operator monitoring 205

Clean room (*contd*)
    Settle plates 202
    Swabbing 204
Clearance of drugs from body 390
Closures 53, 54, 56
    For parenteral products 218, 221
    Types 54
    See also Containers
Collodions 4
    Labelling 79
Colostomy 326
Colouring 37
    Agents 37
    Creams 114
    Emulsions 114
    Solutions 89
Committee on Safety of Medicines 379
Communication 339, 342
    Active listening 429
    Advice to patients 431
    Assertiveness 429
    Explaining 430
    Failings 428
    Information leaflets 342
    Persuading 430
    Pharmaceutical information 427
    Report writing 430
    Successful 428
Community pharmacist, role in drug
    therapy 422
Compatibility
    Cytotoxic agents 237
    Infusion additives 229
Competencies 32
Complexing agents 49
Compliance 339
    See also Patient compliance
Compounding
    Calculation 13
    Capsules 152
    Control procedures 30
    Creams 116
    Cytotoxic agents 238
    Dissolution 25
    Documentation 30
    Equipment 29
    Expiry date 30
    Filtration 26
    Formulation 35
      See also Formulation
    Fundamental operations 21
    Gels 129
    Good practice 29
    Granules 145
    Guidelines for students 31
    Information sources 31
    Labelling 30
    Measurement of liquids 23
    Mixing 27
    Ointments 128
    Oral emulsions 115
    Packaging 30
    Parenteral products 217
    Pastes 128

Personal standards 31
Personnel 29
Pessaries 138
Powders 145
Practice 29
Premises 29
Resources 29
Size reduction 28
Size separation 28
Solutions 89
Storage conditions 30
Supervision 30
Suppositories 138
Suspensions 101
Weighing 21
Compression therapy (hosiery)
    321 .
Computer labelling 83
Concentration, units of 11
Conical measures 23
Consumer Protection Act 442
Contact lens preparations 257, 269
    Containers 270
    Information sheets 271
Containers 53
    Antiseptic solutions 92
    Applications 116
    Bottles
      Glass 54
      Plastic 56
    Capsules 153
    Child-resistant 54, 57, 341
    Contact lens preparations 270
    Creams 117
    Disinfectant solutions 92
    Dusting powders 148
    Ear drops 91
    Elixirs 90
    Enemas 91
    External emulsions 116
    External solutions 92
    Eye drops 262
    Eye lotions 269
    Eye ointments 268
    Gargles 90
    Gels 130
    Granules 147
    Ideal properties 53
    Inhalations 103
    Linctuses 92
    Liniments 92, 116
    Lotions 92, 103, 116
    Mixtures 90
    Mouthwashes 90
    Nasal drops 90
    Nasal sprays 90
    Ointments 130
    Oral emulsions 116
    Oral solutions 90
    Oral suspensions 103
    Original pack dispensing 59
    Paints 92
    Parenteral products 218
    Pastes 130

Pessaries 138
Powders 147
Quality assurance aspects 277
Quality assurance considerations
    277
Sealed 54
Semi-solid products 55
Specialist 56
Suppositories 138
Tablets 151
Unit dose 58
Contamination, clean rooms 199
Continuous phase 109
Controlled Drugs 435, 438
    Prescriptions 438
Cosolvency 88
Cough treatment 360
Counselling 339, 346
    See Patient counselling
Cracking of emulsions 115
Creaming of emulsions 115
Creams 5, 109, 116
    Compounding 116
    Containers 117
    Dilution 117
    Examples 117
    Formulation 109
    Labelling 79, 117
    Shelf life 117
    Sterility testing 292, 293
Critical micelle concentration 88
Cytotoxic agents 233
    Administration 238
    Compatibility 237
    Compounding 238
    Disposal 237
    Modes of action 233
    Monitoring exposure 234
    Pharmacist's role in compounding
    238
    Potential hazards 233
      Monitoring exposure 234
    Safe handling 233
    Stability 237

D Values (sterilization) 166
Data sheets 464
Death rates, micro-organisms 166
Decimal reduction time 166
Deflocculated suspensions 100
Degradation
    Chemical 45
      See also Chemical degradation
    Factors influencing 47
      Additives 47
      Moisture (atmospheric) 49
      Solvent 47
      Temperature 47
    Physical 47
      See also Physical degradation
Design of clean rooms 193
Development of a drug 379
Diabetic testing 375

Diagnosis and the pharmacist 357
Diagnostic radiopharmaceuticals 302, 309
Diagnostic tests
  Blood pressure 373
  Body temperature 373
  Diabetic testing 375
  Ovulation testing 375
  Pregnancy testing 374
  Role of the pharmacist 357
  Temperature 373
Diffusible solids 99
Digoxin, pharmacokinetic profile 405
Diluents, for solutions 89
Dilutions, calculations 15
Disease states, effect on
      pharmacokinetics 411
Disinfectant solutions 92, 165
Disinfection 165
Dispensary
  Control procedures 30
  Equipment 29
  Information sources 31
  Personnel 29
  Premises 29
  Requirements 29
Dispensing
  Bottles 55
  Calculations 13
  Cartons 57
  Cytotoxic agents 233
  Definition 61
  Documentation 30
  Expiry date 30
  General procedure 70
  Good practice 29
  Guidelines for students 31
  Labelling 30, 73
    Advisory labels 76
    Cautionary labels 76
    Information 73
    See also Labelling
  Original pack 59
  Packaging 30
  Personal standards 31
  Practice 29
  Resources 29
    See also Compounding
  Storage conditions 30
  Supervision 30
  Tablets 151
  Total parenteral nutrition 253
Dispensing balance 21
Disperse phase 109
Disperse systems, injections 214
Displacement values 139, 142
Disposal, cytotoxic agents 237
Dissolution 25
Distillation 211
Distribution of drugs in the body 385
Divided powders 145
Documentation
  Clean rooms 206
  Compounding 30, 32

Quality assurance 273, 278
Total parenteral nutrition 250
Dosage forms 3
  Formulation see Formulation
  Identification 37
  Labelling 79
    See also individual dosage forms
  Types of 4
  See also individual entries
Dosage regimen design 394
  Effect of pharmacokinetics 396
  In renal failure 398
Dosage regimens 391
Draughts 5
Dressing packs 316
Dressings 315
  See Surgical dressings
Drops
  Ear 5
  Eye 5
    See also Ophthalmic products
  Nasal 6
Drug absorption 396
  Gastrointestinal 419
Drug accumulation 391
Drug administration 391
Drug adverse reactions 413
Drug clearance 390
Drug distribution 385
Drug elimination 387
  Renal excretion 420
Drug information 421, 423
  Centres 427
  Enquiries 421
  Evaluating clinical reports 426
  Responding to enquiries 427
  Sources 424
Drug interactions 418
  Pharmaceutical 418
  Pharmacodynamic 418
  Pharmacokinetic 419
Drug metabolism 397
  Hepatic 419
Drug monitoring 403
Drug pharmacokinetics, profiles 405
  Variable response 380
  See also Pharmacokinetics
Drug plasma concentration 387
Drug Tariff 462
Drug therapy 381, 421
  Pharmacist's role 383
  Selection 382
Dry heat sterilization 176
Dusting powders 5
  Labelling 80
  See Powders

Ear drops 5, 91
  Labelling 80
Elastic hosiery 321
  Role of the pharmacist 322
Elastomers 221
Electrolyte solutions, for injections 215
Electromagnetic radiation 301

Elimination of drugs from the body 387
Elixirs 5
  As a dosage form 89
Emergency supply of medicines 437
Emulgents see Emulsifying agents
Emulsifying agents 109
  Choice of 113
  For suppositories 138
Emulsions 109
  Compounding 115
  Containers
    External 116
    Oral 116
  External 116
  Formulation 109
    HLB method 113
    Preservatives 114
    Stability 114
  Injections 214
  Labelling 80
    External 116
    Oral 116
  Mixing 27
  Oral 7, 116
  As oral dosage forms 115
  Primary 115
  Shelf life
    External 116
    Oral 116
  Types 109
Enemas 5, 91
  Labelling 80
Environmental considerations, sterility
      testing 285
Environmental control, clean rooms
      195
Environmental monitoring, clean
      rooms 202
  Quality assurance aspects 274
Equipment
  For dispensing 29
  Quality control laboratory 28
Ethylene oxide sterilization 169,
      181
Ethylene oxide sterilizers 182
European Pharmacopoeia 463
Expiry date 30
  Labelling 75
External solutions 92
Extra pharmacopoeia (Martindale)
      463
Extracts 9
Eye disorders 369, 370
Eye drop bottle 263
Eye drops 9, 257
  Bioavailability 262
  Containers 262
  Formulation 257
  Labelling 80, 266
  Preparation 264
  Preservatives 258
  Shelf life 262
  Storage 262

Eye lotions 5, 257, 269
  Containers 269
  Formulation 269
  Labelling 80, 269
Eye ointments 5, 257, 267
  Containers 268
  Formulation 267
  Labelling 269
  Preparation 268
  Preservatives 268

F values (sterilization) 167
Filling
  Eye drops 264
  Total parenteral nutrition 252
Filters
  Hepa, radiopharmaceuticals 303
  Media 190
  Membrane 190
  Papers 26
  Sintered glass 26, 191
  Testing 191
Filtration 26
  Air 197
  Eye drops 265
  Eye solutions 265
  Of infusions 228
  Membrane, sterility testing 29
  Parenteral products 217
Filtration sterilization 190
First-pass metabolism 397
Flavouring
  Assessment 40
  Emulsions 114
  Solutions 89
  Stability 40
Flavouring agents 38
  Aromatic oils 39
  Flavoured syrups 39
  Sweetening agents 39
  Synthetic flavours 39
Flocculated suspensions 100
Formaldehyde sterilization 184
Formulation 35
  Capsules 152
  Chemical incompatibility 41
  Colour 37
  Colouring agents 37
  Constraints 36
  Creams 109
  Emulsions 109
  Eye drops 257
  Eye lotions 263
  Eye ointments 267
  Flavouring agents 38
  Gels 127
  Granules 145
  Improvization 43
  Ointments 125
  Parenteral products 209
  Pastes 125
  Patient acceptability 35
  Pessaries 135
  Physical incompatibility 40

Powders 145
Radiopharmaceuticals 305
Routes of administration 35
Solutions 89
Suppositories 135
Suspensions 99
Sweetening agents 39
Total parenteral nutrition 242
FP10 (Prescription form) 63

Gamma radiation 301
Gamma ray sterilization 185
Gargles 5, 90
  Labelling 80
Gaseous sterilization 181
Gases, medicinal 333
Gastrointestinal, drug absorption 419
Gastrointestinal treatment 361
Gels 5, 125
  Compounding 129
  Containers 130
  As a dosage form 129
  Formulation 127
  Labelling 80, 130
  Shelf life 129
General labelling provisions 439
General Sales List medicines 435
Gentamicin, pharmacokinetic profile 406
Giving sets 227
Glass, for parenteral products 218
Glass bottles, eye drops 263
Glass containers 54
Glycerins 9
Glycero-Gelation base 140
GMP See Guide to good pharmaceutical manufacturing practice
Good dispensing practice 29
Good pharmaceutical manufacturing practice 29, 273, 464
Granules 5, 145
  Compounding 145, 146
  Containers 147
  As a dosage form 147
  Formulation 145
  Labelling 80, 147
  Shelf life 147
Grinding 28
Guide to Good Pharmaceutical Manufacturing Practice 273, 464

Half-life
  Drugs 388
  Radioisotopes 301
Hard gelatin capsules 152
Headache 368
Health and Safety at Work, etc Act 442
Heat sterilization 171
  Advantages and disadvantages 179
  Applications 179
Heating with a bactericide 179
  Eye drops 264

Henderson–Hasslebalch equation 230
HEPA filters, radiation 303
Hepatic, drug metabolism 419
High-speed electrons sterilization 185
HLB formulation 113
HLB values 113
Homeopathic preparations 459
Hosiery 321
Hospital pharmacist, role in drug therapy 421
Hot air oven 177
Humectants, in gels 128
Hydrophile–lipophile balance 113

Identification, of dosage forms 37
Ileostomy 325
Imperial system of weights and measures 457
Implants 6
In-process quality controls 279
Incompatibility 40
  Chemical 41
    Complexation 41
    PH effects 41
    Reducing agents 43
    Soaps 41
  Detection 43
  Physical 40
    Immiscibility 40
    Insolubility 41
Incontinence 325
  aids 330
  appliances 325, 327
Indiffusible solids 100
Information leaflets 342
  Contact lens preparations 271
  Multilingual 347
Information sources 463
  Compounding and dispensing 31
Infusion
  Bags 221
  Continuous 230
  Of drugs 391
  Intravenous 227
    Additives 229
    Intermittant 230
Infusions
  Intravenous 7
  Oral 9
Inhalations 5, 103
  Aerosol sprays 8
  Labelling 81
  Pressurized 8
  Route of administration 3
  Therapy, information leaflets 343
Injectable preparations 6
Injections 6
  Disperse systems 214
  Intra-arterial 209
  Intra-articular 209
  Intra-spinal 209
  Intradermal 209
  Intramuscular 209
  Intravenous 209

Non-aqueous vehicles 213
Routes of administration 210
Sterility testing 295
Subcutaneous 209
Inspection, of parenteral preparations 224
Insufflations 6, 153
Labelling 81
Interaction of drugs 418
Intermediate products 8
Intra-arterial injections 209
Intra-articular injections 209
Intra-spinal injections 209
Intradermal injections 209
Intramuscular injections 209
Intravenous
Additives 227, 229
Administration sets 227
Compatibility 229
Giving sets 227
Methods of administration 230
Stability 229
Administration sets 227
Giving sets 227
Infusions 7, 227
Injections 209
Ionising radiations sterilization 185
Irrigation solutions 6
Isotonicity
Adjustment 88
Injections 214

Jellies *See* Gels

Labelling 30
Antiseptic solutions 92
Applications 116
Capsules 153
Computer 83
Creams 117
Diluted products 74
Disinfectant solutions 92
Dosage forms 79
see under individual dosage forms
Dusting powders 148
Ear drops 91
Elixirs 90
Emulsions
External 116
Oral 116
Enemas 91
Expiry date 75
Eye drops 266
Eye lotions 269
Eye ointments 269
Gargles 90
Gels 130
Granules 147
Information to be presented 73
Information leaflets 342
Ingredient details 73
Inhalations 103
Linctuses 90
Liniments 92, 116

Lotions 92, 103, 116
Medicines, legal requirements 439
Mixtures 90
Mouthwashes 91
Nasal drops 91
Nasal sprays 91
Ointments 130
Oral solutions 90
Oral suspensions 103
Paints 92
Parenteral products 226
Pastes 130
Patient compliance 340
Patient details 73
Pessaries 141
Powders 147
Preparation 82
Quality assurance 277
Special instructions 78
Specific dosage forms 79
Suppositories 141
Tablets 152
Total parenteral nutrition 253
Laminar air flow
Cabinets 196, 198
Cytotoxic agents 234
Monitoring 205
Radiation 303
Stations 189
Theory 196
Latin abbreviations 453
Latin terms 453
Legislation 435
Consumer protection act 442
Controlled drugs 438
Health and Safety at Work, etc Act 442
Labelling of medicines 439
Medicines Act 435
Misuse of Drugs Act 437
Prescribed dangerous substances legislation 441
Spirit Regulations 441
Lethality, of sterilization procedures 167
Levigation 28
Limulus amoebocyte lysis (LAL) assay 213
Linctuses 6
As a dosage form 89
Labelling 81
Liniments 6, 92, 116
Containers 116
Labelling 81, 116
Shelf-life 116
Liquids, oral dosage forms 7
Liver disease, effect on pharmacokinetics 412
Lotions 6, 92, 103, 116
Containers 116
Eye 5
Labelling 81, 116
Shelf-life 116
Lozenges 6, 154

Lungs, as a route of administration 3

Manufacture, total parenteral nutrition 250
Manufacturing practice 29
MAOI treatment cards 345
Martindale, The Extra Parmacopoeia 463
Mass, units of 11
Master formulae, calculations 13
Measurement, of liquids 23
Measures, imperial system 459
Mechanical aids to patient compliance 345
Medical abbreviations 449
Medicinal gases
Oxygen 333
Testing 280
Medicine bottle 55
Medicines Act 379, 435
Medicines and Poisons Guide 464
Membrane filters 190
Membrane filtration, sterility testing 291
Metal containers 55
Microbial death 166
Microbiology
Sterilization 165
Total parenteral nutrition preparations 250
MIMS 462
Minimum measurable quantity
Liquids 23
Solids 21
Minor ailments 357
Cough 359
Eye disorders 369, 370
Gastrointestinal 361
Headache 368
Nasal congestion 359
Respiratory tract disorders 358
Skin disorders 363
Sore throat 359
Misuse of Drugs Act 435, 437
Mixing 27
Emulsions 27
Liquids 27
Semi-solids 27
Solids 27
Solutions 27
Suspensions 27
Mixtures 6
As a dosage form 89
Labelling 81
Suspensions, as a dosage form 102
Moist heat sterilization 171
Moisture, effect on degradation 49
Monitoring
Environment, quality assurance aspects 274
Ingredients, quality assurance aspects 274
Mono-amine oxidase inhibitor treatment cards 345

Monthly Index of Medical Specialities 464
Moulds growth, factors affecting 288
Mouthwashes 6, 90
  Labelling 80

Nasal drops 6, 90
  Labelling 81
Nasal sprays 6, 90
Nebulizer therapy 158
Nebulizers 158
NHS dispensing 443
NHS prescriptions 63, 443
Non-heat sterilization 181
Non-ionic surfactants 110
Nose drops 6
  see Nasal drops

Oils, sterility testing 292
Ointments 6, 125
  Bases 125
  Compounding 128
  Containers 130
  As a dosage form 129
  Eye 5
  Labelling 81, 130
  Shelf-life 129
  Sterility testing 292, 293
One-compartment model 385
Ophthalmic products 257
  Contact lens preparations 269
  Eye drops 257
  Eye lotions 269
  Eye ointments 267
  Sterility testing 295
Optical isomerization 46
Oral emulsions 7
Oral liquids 7
Oral powders 7
Oral route of administration 3
Oral solutions, as a dosage form 89
Oral unit dosage forms 151
Original pack dispensing 59
Ostomies 325
Ovulation testing 375
Oxidation 45
Oxygen therapy 333
  Role of pharmacist 334
Oxymels 9

Packaging
  Quality assurance aspects 277
  Total parenteral nutrition 253
Packaging materials 54
  Glass 54
  Metals 56
  Paper and paperboard 57
  Plastics 55
Paints 7, 92
  Labelling 81
Parenteral nutrition 241
Parenteral products 7, 209
  Closures 217, 221
  Compounding 217

Containers 217
  Filling 221
  Filtration 217
  Formulation 209
  Inspection 224
  Labelling 225
  Preparation 217
  Routes of administration 4
  Sealing 221
  Sterilization 217
  Vehicles 213
  see also Injections
Particle sedimentation 47
Particle size, suspensions 99
Particulate radiation 301
Parts, calculations 15
Pastes 7, 125
  Compounding 128
  Containers 130
  As a dosage form 129
  Labelling 81, 130
  Shelf life 129
Pastilles 7, 154
Patient acceptability, of formulations 35
Patient compliance 339
  Mechanical aids 344
  Patient education 348
  And perception 340
  Role of the pharmacist 341
Patient counselling 71, 339, 346
  Aerosols 157
Patient medication profile 422
Patient medication records 351
  Card systems 351
  Computerised systems 354
Patient perceptions 340
Percentages, calculations 14
Personal standards, in dispensing 31
Pessaries 7, 135
  As a dosage form 141
  Compounding 138
  Containers 141
  Examples 142
  Formulation 135
  Labelling 82, 141
  Shelf-life 141
pH adjustment 88
  Injections 216
pH buffers
  Eye drops 261
  Eye ointments 268
Pharmaceutical advice 421
Pharmaceutical Codex 463
Pharmaceutical Handbook 464
Pharmaceutical legislation 435
Pharmaceutical practice 29
Pharmaceutical preparations 85
Pharmacist's role in
  Adverse drug reaction monitoring 414
  Cytotoxic compounding 238
  Diagnosis 357
  Drug therapy 383, 421, 422

Elastic hosiery 322
  Oxygen therapy 334
  Patient advice 421
  Patient compliance 341
  Responding to symptoms 357
  Stoma care 331
  Treating minor ailments 357
Pharmacokinetics 385
  Drug interactions 418
  Drug profiles 405
    Digoxin 405
    Gentamicin 406
    Phenytoin 406
    Theophylline 407
  Effect of
    Age 408
    Diet 410
    Disease states 411
    Gender 410
    Genetic factors 409
    Liver disease 412
    Posture 410
    Renal disease 412
    Social drugs 410
  Influence on dosage regimen design 396
  Non-Linear 400
  Variable 380, 408
Pharmacy information and news service 464
Pharmacy medicines 435
Phase diagram for steam 171
Phase inversion of emulsions 116
Phenytoin, pharmacokinetic profile 406
Photolysis 46
Physical degradation 46
  Particle sedimentation 47
  Polymorphism 46
  Vaporization 47
  Water absorption 47
  Water loss 47
Pills 7
PINS (Pharmacy information and news service) 465
Pipette, use of 24
Plasma protein displacement 419
Plastic
  Containers 55
  Eye drop bottles 263
  For parenteral products 221
Poisons Act 440
Polymerization 46
Polymorphism 46
Potable water 87
Poultices 7
Powders 145
  Compounding 145
  Containers 147
  Divided 145
  As a dosage form 146
  Dusting 5
  Formulation 145
  For injections 7
  Labelling 82, 147, 148

For mixtures 8
Oral 7
Shelf-life 147, 148
Undivided 145
Wrapping 146
Practitioner qualifications 457
Pre-filled syringes, for parenteral
products 220
Pregnancy testing 374
Prescribed Dangerous Substances
legislation 441
Prescription only medicines 435
Prescriptions 61, 436, 443
Bulk 63
Charges 444
Community 63
Disposal 64, 66, 70
Endorsements 445
FP10 63, 64
Hospital 63
Inpatients 66, 69
Outpatients 68, 70
Incomplete 63
Latin terms 453
NHS 63
Private 64
Repeat 62
Requirements 61
Responding to 61
Types of form 63
Preservatives
In emulsions 114
In eye drops 258
In eye ointments 268
In gels 128
In injections 217
In ointments 127
In solutions 89
In suppositories 138
Pressurized dispensers 8, 157
Labelling 79
Shelf-life 158
Storage 158
Pressurized inhalations 8, 157
Labelling 79
Shelf-life 158
Storage 158
Primary emulsions 115
Private prescriptions 64
Product recall 226
Propellants 157, 158
Protective clothing 189
Clean rooms 200
Protein binding 400
Purified water 87
Pyrogens 212
Removal 228
Testing 212
Quality assurance aspects 279

Qualifications of practitioners 457
Qualified person 273
Quality assurance 273
Documentation 273

Environment 274
Environmental monitoring 274
Finished product 277
In-process controls 279
Ingredients 274
Labels 277
Monitoring 274
Packaging 277
Quarantine 279
Release procedures 279
Responsibilities 280
Quality control 273
Laboratory 280
Equipment 281
see also Quality assurance

Radiation 301
Electromagnetic 301
Particulate 301
Sterilization 184
Units of 12
Radionuclides 301
Radiopharmaceuticals 301
Clinical applications 309
Diagnostic 302, 309
Facilities 303
Formulation 305
Indium-111 310
Iodine-123 310
Preparation 303
Production 303
Technetium-99M 305, 309
Therapeutic 301, 311
Radiopharmacy 299
Clinical applications 309
Techniques 301
Records, in dispensing 32
Rectal route of administration 3
Reducing agents 49
Renal disease, effect on
pharmacokinetics 412
Renal excretion of drugs 420
Renal failure, effect on dosage
regimen design 398
Respiratory tract disorders 358
Responding to symptoms 357
Reverse osmosis 211
Role of pharmacist see Pharmacist's
role
Routes of administration 3, 35
Buccal 3
Inhalation 3
Injection 210
Lungs 3
Oral 3, 35
Parenteral 4, 35
Rectal 3, 35
Topical 3, 35
Transdermal 3

Sale of medicinal products 435
Sampling, sterility testing 295
Saturated steam 171
Sealing, parenteral products 223
Sedimentation 47, 99

Semi-solids, mixing 27
Settle plates 202
Shelf life
Antiseptic solutions 92
Applications 116
Capsules 153
Creams 117
Disinfectant solutions 92
Dispensed products 31
Dusting powders 148
Ear drops 91
Elixirs 90
Emulsions
External 116
Oral 116
Enemas 91
Eye drops 262
Gargles 90
Gels 129
Granules 147
Labelling 75
Linctuses 90
Liniments 116, 92
Lotions 116, 92
Mixtures 90
Mouthwashes 90
Nasal drops 90
Nasal sprays 90
Ointments 129
Oral solutions 90
Oral suspensions 103
Paints 92
Pastes 129
Pessaries 141
Powders 147
Pressurized dispensers 158
Suppositories 141
Sintered glass filters 26, 191
Size reduction 28
Size separation 28
Skin disorders 363
Soft gelatin capsules 152
Solids
Mixing 27
Sterility testing 291
Solubility 87
Solubilization 88
Solution tablets 8
Solutions 8, 87
Dissolution 25
As a dosage form 89
External 92
Examples 92
Formulation 87
Irrigations 6
Labelling 82
Mixing 27
Oral 87, 92
Solvent, effect on degradation 47
Solvolysis 45
Sore throat 359
Specific gravity adjustment, injections
216
Spirit regulations 441

Spirits 9
Sprays 8
  Inhalation 8
  Nasal 6
Stability 45
  Cytotoxic agents 237
  Flavours 40
  Infusion additives 229
  Total parenteral nutrition 249
Stabilizers
  Eye drops 261
  In injections 217
  In solutions 89
Standard Labelling Particulars 439
Steam
  Phase diagram 171
  Production 171
  Saturated 171
  Sterilization 172
  Temperature-pressure relationship 171
Sterile manufacturing unit 194
Sterile pharmaceutical preparations 161
  Manufacture 163
Sterility testing 191, 285
  BP test 291
  Creams 292, 293
  EP test 290
  Inactivation of antimicrobials 292
  Injections 295
  Interpretation of results 293
  Methods 290
  Minimum sample size 291
  Ointments 292, 293
  Ophthalmic products 295
  Sampling 295
  Surgical dressings 295
  Sutures 295
  Test methods 290
  Test record 297
  USP test 297
Sterility 165, 290
  Testing 165
Sterilization 165
  Continuous 176
  Criteria 165
  Dry heat 176
  Ethylene oxide 169, 181
  Eye drops 264
  Factors affecting 181
  Filtration 190
  Formaldehyde 181
  Gamma rays 185
  Gaseous 181
  Heat 171
  Heating with a bactericide 179
  High-speed electrons 185
  Ionizing radiations 185
  Moist heat 171
  Monitoring 168
  Non heat 181
  Of clothing 201
  Parenteral products 218

Principles 165
Radiation 184
Steam under pressure 171
Ultraviolet light 184
Validation 168
Sterilizers 172
  Continuous 176
  Ethylene oxide 182
  Hydrostatic 176
  Large scale 173
Stock control 50
Stock solutions, calculations 17
Stokes's law 99
Stoma care 325
  Accessories 328
  Appliances 327
  Prescriptions 329
  Role of pharmacist 331
Storage 045, 049
  Conditions, compounding 30
  Eye drops 262
  Pressurized dispensers 158
  Stock control 50
  Total parenteral nutrition 253
Straining 26
Strip packaging 59
Subcutaneous injections 209
Supply of medicinal products 435
Support stockings 322
Suppositories 8, 135
  Bases 135
  Compounding 138
  Containers 141
  As a dosage form 141
  Examples 142
  Formulation 135
  Labelling 82, 141
  Shelf-life 141
Surfactants 49
  Ampholytic 112
  Amphoteric 112
  Anionic 109
  Cationic 110
  Non-ionic 110
Surgical adhesive tapes 318
Surgical dressings 315
  Absorbent dressings 317
  Bandages 318
  Sterility testing 295
  Surgical adhesive tapes 318
  Wound dressings 315
Suspensions 99
  Compounding 102
  Deflocculated 100
  As a dosage form 102
  Emergency formulations 103
  Examples 104
  External 103
  Flocculated 100
  Formulation 99
  Injections 214
  Mixing 27
  Oral 103
  Particle size 99

Properties 99
Vehicles 99
Sutures, sterility testing 295
Syringes, pre-filled, for parenteral products 219
Syrups 8

Tablets 8, 151
  Containers 151
  Dispensing 151
  Labelling 82, 152
  Solution 8
Technetium-99m 305
  Generation 305
  Use in radiopharmaceuticals 309
Temperature, effect on degradation 47
Theophylline, pharmacokinetic profile 407
Therapeutic aerosols 157
Therapeutic drug monitoring 403
Therapeutic radiopharmaceuticals 301, 311
Therapeutics 379
Thermal death, micro-organisms 171
Thermal destruction value 167
Thickening agents 100
Tinctures 9
Tonicity modifiers, eye drops 260
Topical route of administration 3
Total parenteral nutrition 241
  Administration 242
  Aseptic production 250
  Clinical aspects 241
  Compatibility 249
  Costs 254
  Dispensing 253
  Documentation 250
  Electrolytes 243
  Energy calculations 246
  Equipment 251
  Filling 252
  Fluid requirements 244
  Formulation 242
  Labelling 253
  Lipids 243
  Manufacture 250
  Microbiological considerations 250
  Nitrogen calculations 246
  Nitrogen 242
  Packaging 253
  Regimens 245
  Stability 249
  Storage 253
  Trace elements 244
  Vitamins 244
TPN see Total parenteral nutrition
Transdermal route of administration 3
Trituration, ointments 129
Triturations 19
  Calculations 19
Two-compartment model 385, 386, 390

Ultraviolet light sterilization 184

Unit dosage forms 151
Unit dose, containers 58
United States National Formulary
    465
United States Pharmacopeia 465
Units, amount of substance 11
    Concentration 11, 214
    Length 11
    Mass 11
    Radiation 11
    Volume 11
Urinary incontinence 325
    AIDS 330
Urostomy 326

Vaporization 47
Vehicles
    Eye drops 257
    Formulated products 36

Solution 87
Suspensions 99
Vials, for parenteral products 221
Viscosity modifiers
    Eye drops 260
    Suppositories 138
Vitrellae 8
Volatile substances, measurement
    25
Volume of distribution 385
Volume, units of 11

Water 87
    For injections 87, 210, 211
        Methods of preparation 221
    For preparations 87
    Loss from products 47
    Potable 87
    Purified 87

Waters, aromatic 9
Weighing 21
Weights
    Imperial system 459
    Units of 11
Wetting, of solids 100
Work stations (LAF) *see* Laminar air
    flow cabinets
Wound dressings 315
Wound management 315
Wound management products
    315

Yeasts
    Factors affecting growth 288
    Growth inhibitors 289

Z values (sterilization) 167